Orthopaedic Basic Science:
Foundations of Clinical Practice

Third Edition

Orthopaedic Basic Science: Foundations of Clinical Practice

Third Edition

Edited by

Thomas A. Einhorn, MD
Professor and Chairman
Department of Orthopaedic Surgery
Boston University Medical Center
Boston, Massachusetts

Regis J. O'Keefe, MD, PhD
Professor of Orthopaedics
Director, Center for Musculoskeletal Research
University of Rochester
Rochester, New York

Joseph A. Buckwalter, MD, MS
Professor, Head, and Arthur Steindler Chair
Department of Orthopaedics and Rehabilitation
University of Iowa
Iowa City, Iowa

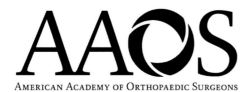

AMERICAN ACADEMY OF ORTHOPAEDIC SURGEONS

The material presented in *Orthopaedic Basic Science, ed 3* has been made available by the American Academy of Orthopaedic Surgeons for educational purposes only. This material is not intended to present the only, or necessarily best, methods or procedures for the medical situations discussed, but rather is intended to represent an approach, view, statement, or opinion of the author(s) or producer(s), which may be helpful to others who face similar situations.

Some drugs or medical devices demonstrated in Academy courses or described in Academy print or electronic publications have not been cleared by the Food and Drug Administration (FDA) or have been cleared for specific uses only. The FDA has stated that it is the responsibility of the physician to determine the FDA clearance status of each drug or device he or she wishes to use in clinical practice.

Furthermore, any statements about commercial products are solely the opinion(s) of the author(s) and do not represent an Academy endorsement or evaluation of these products. These statements may not be used in advertising or for any commercial purpose.

Some of the authors or the departments with which they are affiliated have received something of value from a commercial or other party related directly or indirectly to the subject of their chapter.

Published 2007 by the
American Academy of Orthopaedic Surgeons
6300 North River Road
Rosemont, IL 60018

Copyright 2007
by the American Academy of Orthopaedic Surgeons

ISBN 10: 0892033606
ISBN 13: 9780892033607

Printed in the USA
Library of Congress Cataloging-in-Publication Data

WE 168 O78 2007
Othopaedic basic science : foundations of
clinical practice / edited by Thomas A.
Einhorn, ...
10027487

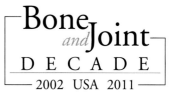

Bone *and* Joint
DECADE
2002 USA 2011

Contributors

Yousef Abu-Amer, PhD
Assistant Professor
Department of Orthopaedic Surgery
Washington University
St. Louis, Missouri

Andrea I. Alford, PhD
Postdoctoral Fellow
Department of Orthopaedic Surgery
University of Michigan
Ann Arbor, Michigan

Kai-Nan An, PhD
Director, Biomechanics Laboratory
Department of Orthopaedic Surgery
Mayo Clinic
Rochester, Minnesota

Robert Tracy Ballock, MD
Associate Professor of Surgery
Head, Section of Pediatric Orthopaedics
Department of Orthopaedic Surgery
The Cleveland Clinic Foundation
Cleveland, Ohio

Mohit Bhandari, MD, MSc, FRCSC
Clinical Fellow
Department of Clinical Epidemiology and
    Biostatistics
Division of Orthopaedic Surgery
McMaster University
Hamilton, Ontario, Canada

Scott D. Boden, MD
Professor of Orthopaedics
Director, The Emory Spine Center
Emory University School of Medicine
Atlanta, Georgia

Barbara D. Boyan, PhD
Price Gilbert Jr. Chair in Tissue Engineering
Wallace H. Coulter Department of Biomedical
    Engineering at Georgia Tech and Emory University
Georgia Institute of Technology
Atlanta, Georgia

Kevin J. Bozic, MD, MBA
Assistant Professor in Residence
Department of Orthopaedic Surgery
University of California, San Francisco
San Francisco, California

Joseph A. Buckwalter, MD, MS
Professor, Head, and Arthur Steindler Chair
Department of Orthopaedics and Rehabilitation
University of Iowa
Iowa City, Iowa

Di Chen, MD, PhD
Assistant Professor
Department of Orthopaedics
University of Rochester
Rochester, New York

John C. Clohisy, MD
Assistant Professor of Orthopaedic Surgery
Department of Orthopaedic Surgery
Barnes-Jewish Hospital at Washington University
    School of Medicine
St. Louis, Missouri

Celine Colnot, PhD
Assistant Researcher
Department of Orthopaedic Surgery
University of California, San Francisco
San Francisco, California

Augustine H. Conduah, MD
Resident in Orthopaedic Surgery
Department of Orthopaedic Surgery
David Geffen School of Medicine at UCLA
Los Angeles, California

Frederick R. Dietz, MD
Professor of Orthopaedic Surgery
Department of Orthopaedic Surgery
University of Iowa
Iowa City, Iowa

M. Hicham Drissi, PhD
Assistant Professor
Department of Orthopaedics
University of Rochester
Rochester, New York

B. Frank Eames, PhD
Department of Orthopaedic Surgery
University of California, San Francisco
San Francisco, California

Thomas A. Einhorn, MD
Professor and Chairman
Department of Orthopaedic Surgery
Boston University Medical Center
Boston, Massachusetts

Cyril B. Frank, MD, FRCSC
McCaig Professor in Joint Injury and Arthritis
  Research
Professor of Surgery
Chief, Division of Orthopaedics
University of Calgary and Calgary Health Region
Calgary, Alberta, Canada

Bruno Fuchs, MD
Mayo Clinic
Rochester, Minnesota

Istvan Gal, MD
Assistant Professor
Department of Orthopedic Surgery
Rush Medical College at Rush-Presbyterian-St. Luke's
  Medical Center
Chicago, Illinois

Jean C. Gan, PhD
Senior Scientist
Department of Research and Development
EBI, L.P.
Parsippany, New Jersey

Steven A. Goldstein, PhD
Henry Ruppenthal Family Professor of Orthopaedic
  Surgery and Bioengineering
Department of Orthopaedic Surgery
University of Michigan
Ann Arbor, Michigan

Alan J. Grodzinsky, ScD
Director, MIT Center for Biomedical Engineering
Professor of Electrical, Mechanical, and Biological
  Engineering
Departments of Electrical Engineering and Computer
  Science, Biological Engineering, and Mechanical
  Engineering
Massachusetts Institute of Technology
Cambridge, Massachusetts

Jonathan M. Gross, MD
Assistant Professor and Assistant Director of the
  Division of Orthopaedic Trauma
Department of Orthopaedic Surgery
University of Rochester
Rochester, New York

Ranjan Gupta, MD
Assistant Professor
Chief, Upper Extremity Surgery
Orthopaedic Surgery
University of California, Irvine
Irvine, California

Kurt D. Hankenson, DVM, PhD
Assistant Professor of Cell Biology
Department of Animal Biology
University of Pennsylvania
Philadelphia, Pennsylvania

David A. Hart, PhD
Professor
Department of Surgery, Medicine, and Microbiology
  and ID
University of Calgary
Calgary, Alberta, Canada

Jill Helms, DDS, PhD
Associate Professor
Department of Plastic and Reconstructive Surgery
Stanford University
Stanford, California

Kenton R. Kaufman, PhD, PE
Director, Biomechanics/Motion Analysis Laboratory
Department of Orthopedic Surgery
Mayo Clinic
Rochester, Minnesota

Sumito Kawamura, MD
Research Fellow
Sports Medicine and Shoulder Service
The Hospital for Special Surgery
New York, New York

Hubert T. Kim, MD, PhD
Assistant Professor
Department of Orthopaedic Surgery
University of California
San Francisco, California

Jack L. Lewis, PhD
Professor of Orthopaedic Surgery and Mechanical
  Engineering
Department of Orthopaedic Surgery
University of Minnesota
Minneapolis, Minnesota

Richard L. Lieber, PhD
Professor of Orthopaedics and Bioengineering
Department of Orthopaedics and Bioengineering
University of California, San Diego
La Jolla, California

Jay R. Lieberman, MD
Director, The New England Musculoskeletal
  Institute
Professor and Chairman
Department of Orthopaedic Surgery
University of Connecticut Health Center
Farmington, Connecticut

Ian Lo, MD, FRCSC
Assistant Professor
Department of Orthopaedic Surgery
University of Calgary
Calgary, Alberta, Canada

Lichun Lu, MD
Associate Professor
Department of Orthopaedics
Mayo Clinic College of Medicine
Rochester, Minnesota

Suzanne A. Maher, PhD
Assistant Scientist
Biomedical Mechanics and Materials
Hospital for Special Surgery
New York, New York

Henry J. Mankin, MD
Edith M. Ashley Professor of Orthopaedics
Harvard Medical School
Orthopaedic Service
Massachusetts General Hospital
Boston, Massachusetts

Barbara R. McCreadie, PhD
Research Assistant Professor
Department of Orthopaedic Surgery
University of Michigan
Ann Arbor, Michigan

Theodore Miclau III, MD
Associate Professor
Department of Orthopaedic Surgery
University of California, San Francisco
San Francisco General Hospital
San Francisco, California

Katalin Mikecz, MD, PhD
Professor
Department of Orthopedic Surgery
Rush Medical College at Rush-Presbyterian-St. Luke's
  Medical Center
Chicago, Illinois

Joshua D. Miller, MD, PhD
Assistant Professor
Department of Orthopaedic Surgery
University of Michigan
Ann Arbor, Michigan

Carol D. Morris, MD
Assistant Professor of Orthopaedic Surgery
Weill Medical College, Cornell University
Attending Surgeon
Department of Orthopaedic Surgery
Memorial Sloan-Kettering Cancer Center
New York, New York

Tahseen Mozaffar, MD
Assistant Professor of Clinical Neurology
Department of Neurology and Pathology
University of California, Irvine
Orange, California

Jeffrey C. Murray, MD
Professor
Department of Pediatrics, Division of Neonatology
University of Iowa, Roy J. and Lucille A. Carver
  College of Medicine
Iowa City, Iowa

Shawn W. O'Driscoll, PhD, MD
Professor of Orthopedic Surgery
Director, Cartilage and Connective Tissue Research
  Laboratory
Department of Orthopedic Surgery
Mayo Clinic
Rochester, Minnesota

Theodore R. Oegema, PhD
Chairman and Professor of Biochemistry
Professor of Orthopaedic Surgery
Department of Biochemistry
Rush Medical College at Rush-Presbyterian-St. Luke's
  Medical Center
Chicago, Illinois

Regis J. O'Keefe, MD, PhD
Professor of Orthopaedics
Director, Center for Musculoskeletal Research
University of Rochester
Rochester, New York

Andrew E. Park, MD
Spine Surgeon
North Texas Spine Care
Baylor Medical Center – Dallas
Department of Orthopaedic Surgery
Dallas, Texas

Christian M. Puttlitz, PhD
Assistant Professor and Director
Orthopaedic Biomechanics Laboratory
Department of Orthopaedic Surgery
University of California, San Francisco
San Francisco, California

Scott A. Rodeo, MD
Associate Professor, Orthopaedic Surgery
Associate Attending Surgeon
Sports Medicine and Shoulder Service
Hospital for Special Surgery
New York, New York

Randy Rosier, MD, PhD
Professor and Chair
Department of Orthopaedics
University of Rochester
Rochester, New York

Daniël B.F. Saris, MD, PhD
Orthopaedic Surgeon
Assistant Professor
Department of Orthopaedics
University Medical Center
Utrecht, The Netherlands

Edward M. Schwarz, PhD
Professor of Orthopaedics and of Microbiology
  and Immunology
University of Rochester Medical Center
Rochester, New York

Sean P. Scully, MD, PhD
Professor
Department of Orthopaedics
Miller School of Medicine
University of Miami
Miami, Florida

Nigel G. Shrive, MA, D. Phil.
Killam Memorial Professor
Department of Civil Engineering
University of Calgary
Calgary, Alberta, Canada

Bobby Tay, MD
Assistant Professor in Residence
Department of Orthopaedics
University of California, San Francisco
San Francisco, California

Timothy M. Wright, PhD
Director
Department of Biomedical Mechanics and Materials
Hospital for Special Surgery
New York, New York

Michael J. Yaszemski, MD, PhD
Professor of Orthopedic Surgery and Biomedical
  Engineering
Department of Orthopedic Surgery
Mayo Clinic
Rochester, Minnesota

Jun Yuan, MD, PhD
Research Fellow
Department of Orthopedics
Mayo Clinic
Rochester, Minnesota

Michael Zuscik, PhD
Assistant Professor of Orthopaedics
Department of Orthopaedics
University of Rochester
Rochester, New York

Peer Reviewers

Roy K. Aaron, MD
Professor
Department of Orthopaedic Surgery
Brown Medical School
Providence, Rhode Island

Gunnar B.J. Andersson, MD, PhD
Professor and Chairman
Department of Orthopedic Surgery
Rush University Medical Center
Chicago, Illinois

Suneel S. Apte, MD, PhD
Staff
Department of Biomedical Engineering
Cleveland Clinic Foundation
Cleveland, Ohio

Susan V. Bukata, MD
Assistant Professor, Department of Orthopaedics,
  Musculoskeletal Oncology
University of Rochester Medical Center
Director, Osteoporosis and Metabolic Bone Disease
  Center
Rochester, New York

Laurence E. Dahners, MD
Professor
Department of Orthopaedics
University of North Carolina School of Medicine
Chapel Hill, North Carolina

Matthew B. Dobbs, MD
Assistant Professor
Department of Orthopaedic Surgery
Washington University School of Medicine
St. Louis, Missouri

Donald C. Fithian, MD
Director, San Diego Sports Medicine Fellowship
Department of Orthopedics
Southern California Permanente Medical Group
San Diego, California

William E. Garrett, Jr, MD, PhD
Professor of Orthopaedic Surgery
Department of Orthopaedic Surgery
Duke University Medical Center
Durham, North Carolina

Stuart B. Goodman, MD, PhD
Ellenburg Professor of Surgery
Professor of Orthopaedic Surgery
Stanford University Medical Center
Stanford, California

Ed Greenfield, PhD
Professor and Director of Research
Department of Orthopaedics
Case Western Reserve University/Case Medical Center
Cleveland, Ohio

John H. Healey, MD
Chief, Orthopaedic Service
Professor of Surgery
Department of Surgery
Memorial Sloan-Kettering Cancer Center
New York, New York

Joshua Jacobs, MD
Crown Family Professor
Department of Orthopaedic Surgery
Rush University Medical Center
Chicago, Illinois

Brian Johnstone, PhD
Adjunct Professor
Director of Research
Department of Orthopaedics and Rehabilitation
Oregon Health and Science University
Portland, Oregon

Nancy E. Lane, MD
Endowed Chair in Geriatrics
Director, UC Davis Center for Healthy Aging
Professor of Medicine and Rheumatology
Department of Internal Medicine
University of California Davis School of Medicine
Sacramento, California

Francis Y. Lee, MD
Columbia University
New York, New York

Patrick Lin, MD
Associate Professor of Surgery
Department of Orthopaedic Oncology
MD Anderson Cancer Center
Houston, Texas

Cahir A. McDevitt, PhD
Professor of Molecular Medicine
Department of Biomedical Engineering
Cleveland Clinic
Cleveland, Ohio

James T. Ninomiya, MD, MS
Associate Professor
Director of Adult Reconstruction
Department of Orthopaedic Surgery
Medical College of Wisconsin
Milwaukee, Wisconsin

Alan Nixon, PhD, DVM
Professor of Orthopedic Surgery
Director, Comparative Orthopaedics Laboratory
Department of Clinical Sciences
Cornell University
Ithaca, New York

Theodore R. Oegema, PhD
Chairman and Professor of Biochemistry
Professor of Orthopaedic Surgery
Department of Biochemistry
Rush Medical College at Rush-Presbyterian-St. Luke's
   Medical Center
Chicago, Illinois

R. Lane Smith, PhD
Professor (Research)
Department of Orthopaedic Surgery
Stanford University School of Medicine
Stanford, California

David Speach, MD
Associate Professor
Department of Orthopaedics and Rehabilitation
University of Rochester School of Medicine and
  Dentistry
Rochester, New York

Marc Swiontkowski, MD
Professor and Chair
Department of Orthopaedic Surgery
University of Minnesota
Minneapolis, Minnesota

Stephen B. Trippel, MD
Professor of Orthopaedic Surgery
Department of Orthopaedic Surgery
Indiana University School of Medicine
Indianapolis, Indiana

Scott W. Wallentine, PT, DPT
Associate Professor of Physical Therapy
Department of Physical Therapy
Missouri State University
Springfield, Missouri

James G. Wright, MD
Surgeon-in-Chief and Chief of Perioperative Services
Department of Surgery
The Hospital for Sick Children
Toronto, Ontario, Canada

Table of Contents

Preface

Advanced technologies for the diagnosis and treatment of musculoskeletal injuries and conditions have changed the way orthopaedic surgeons care for patients. New discoveries about the biology and biomechanics of the musculoskeletal system and the development of more sophisticated tools for probing its many mysteries provide clinicians and scientists with unique opportunities to advance orthopaedic care. This third edition of *Orthopaedic Basic Science: Foundations of Clinical Practice* presents orthopaedic surgeons with the foundations of knowledge required to apply advances in scientific discovery to the decisions they will make in the clinic and operating room. Because of the explosion of knowledge in the fields of musculoskeletal science and medicine, the editors and authors have worked to present this information in a format that is comprehensive yet clinically relevant. To accomplish this, the book is divided into three sections so that the reader can follow a hierarchy of knowledge beginning with an understanding of the basic principles of cell and molecular biology, the genetic basis of orthopaedic disease, the fundamentals of skeletal mechanics, and the science supporting the applications of the biomaterials used in orthopaedic procedures. This is followed by updates on the current knowledge of the physiology of individual musculoskeletal tissues and the way diseases and injuries affect those tissues. In addition, because the multitude of scientific developments now require orthopaedic surgeons to critically evaluate new information in order to determine its potential role in our clinical practices, a chapter has been provided on evidence-based orthopaedics and the issues surrounding research design, analysis, and its critical appraisal.

Perhaps the most exciting new feature of this third edition is its accompaniment by a CD/ROM that presents clinical cases and their scientific basis. This new learning tool is applied to several clinical scenarios that will test the surgeon's scientific understanding of conditions affecting tendons, ligaments, bone, cartilage, and neurologic tissues. It is our intent to continue to add cases in this format so that this electronic accompaniment can be a living, growing part of this comprehensive package to educate orthopaedic surgeons.

The editors and authors wish to express their sincere appreciation to those members of the staff of the American Academy of Orthopaedic Surgeons without whose efforts this text would not have been possible: Marilyn L. Fox, PhD, Director of the Publications Department, Lisa Claxton Moore, Managing Editor, Kathleen Anderson, Associate Senior Editor, Mary Steermann, Manager, Production and Archives, Courtney Astle, Assistant Production Manager, Anne Raci, Production Database Associate, Karen Danca, Production Assistant, and Barbara Reber, Multimedia Producer, worked tirelessly and with incredible commitment to bring this information to you in such a complete, accurate, and attractive format.

Thomas A. Einhorn, MD
Regis J. O'Keefe, MD, PhD
Joseph A. Buckwalter, MD, MS

Basic Principles of Orthopaedic Surgery

Chapter 1

Molecular and Cell Biology in Orthopaedics

Michael J. Zuscik, PhD
M. Hicham Drissi, PhD
Di Chen, PhD
Randy N. Rosier, MD, PhD

Introduction

The insights into DNA and RNA function revealed by modern technology have revolutionized biomedical and biologic science. Understanding the structure and function of genes has led to the identification of the causes of diseases. Recombinant DNA technology has led to novel diagnostic and therapeutic approaches and has paved the way for engineered tissues, genetically altered organisms, and gene therapies. For example, in orthopaedics, the bone morphogenetic proteins (BMPs) are in the vanguard of the application of molecular biology to address clinical problems such as stimulation of fracture healing and regrowth of bone (to create a "living prosthesis"). The discovery, analysis, and production of BMPs for clinical trials would not have occurred without recombinant DNA technology. Thus, for even the general orthopaedist, the future will demand at least a rudimentary understanding of molecular biology.

Several key basic science approaches as well as an overview of orthopaedic biology are presented in this chapter. A general understanding of key methodology will not only frame the discussion of current knowledge, but will enable critical reading of the orthopaedic basic science literature. It is assumed that the reader has a working understanding of basic molecular biology (DNA and RNA structure and function, the processes of transcription and translation).

Molecular and Cell Biology of the Musculoskeletal System

Transcription Factors

Control of Gene Expression

There are numerous points of possible regulation of the level of expression of a given gene, and consequently, of the amount of its protein product. Ultimately, the function and behavior of a cell, its phenotype, will depend on the spectrum of proteins expressed and their relative quantities. Of the estimated 80,000 genes in the human genome, approximately 5,000 are actively expressed in any given cell. Thus, control of gene expression is a critical and powerful determinant of all biologic functions. Some genes are constitutive, or present at constant levels; others are inducible, and expression is turned on by other factors. Genes that are normally expressed but can be turned off by factors are referred to as repressible genes. The major possible levels of regulation include (1) gene activation, or accessibility to interaction with RNA polymerases; (2) interaction of RNA polymerase with the gene (transcription), with both enhancing and suppressing transcriptional factors that can regulate the activity of the polymerase; (3) messenger RNA (mRNA) processing and stability; (4) translation of mRNA to protein; (5) posttranslational processing of protein; and (6) protein degradation.

Genes are organized into transcribed regions, or exons, which contain the coding sequence for the mRNA, and introns, which contain noncoding sequences. Creation of a functional mRNA template requires splicing together the exons during transcription, a phenomenon that occurs in the nucleus. Because of the localization of the transcriptional apparatus and chromosomes within the nuclear envelope, translation does not occur concomitantly in eukaryotes the way it does in bacteria. This allows for posttranscriptional processing of the mRNA, another potential point of regulation of gene transcription in higher organisms. The average sizes of eukaryotic exons are 100 to 200 base pairs, whereas the intronic segments are generally much longer, or an average of 20 kb. Some types of introns contain ribozyme type catalytic activity, and splice themselves out during transcription. Others require extraneous catalytic activity to accomplish the splicing, and use protein-RNA complexes to achieve splicing out of the introns. Exon/intron boundaries are defined by consensus sequences, GT, at the 5' end (GU in the RNA), and AG at the 3' end of the intron, which defines the directionality of the splice site. Splice sites are neither specific to a particular gene nor to a specific cell type. The protein/RNA complexes that mediate splicing consist of large particles containing short nuclear RNA (snRNA) that are referred to as the spliceosomes. This structure cleaves the intron/exon boundary at the 5' end, loops the RNA of the intronic sequence toward the 3' end in a "lariat" formation, cleaves the 3' boundary, and then splices the exons together. This process is complex but occurs rapidly during transcription, with splicing of the 5' introns occurring during transcription of the 3' end of the mRNA. Many genes undergo alternative splicing pathways, where the arrangement of exons varies, enabling production of differing protein products from a single gene. Inclusion or exclusion of specific exons during splicing determines the final form of the transcript and its protein product. Alternative splicing can occur in a tissue- or cell-specific manner during transcription of gene products, and it is increasingly recognized that alternatively spliced forms, or alternative transcripts, exist for a large number of genes. An important example in skeletal tissues is type II collagen. It exists in two forms: as type IIA (full length sequence) that is expressed in embryonic cartilage and is recapitulated during some injury and repair processes such as fracture healing, and as type IIB, the mature form seen in adult cartilage tissues in which exon 2 is spliced out. Parathyroid hormone-related protein (PTHrP), an important regulatory molecule in cartilage, also exists in multiple transcript forms. Overall, increasing numbers of genes exhibiting this phenomenon are being identified. The mechanisms regulating the selection of the alternative splicing pathways have not yet been determined.

The most significant regulation of most class II genes occurs at the level of transcription. The 5' flanking upstream region of the gene contains sequences that allow initiation and control of transcription, and is referred to as the promoter of the gene. The promoter contains binding sites for interaction with RNA polymerase II and several proteins associated with the transcriptional machinery, in addition to sites for interaction with cellular proteins that control transcriptional activity. The promoter region is frequently 100 to 200 base pairs in length, although there is considerable variation in promoter sizes and structures. Unlike DNA synthesis by polymerase activity, RNA transcription does not require a primer. By convention the "sense" strand refers to the strand of DNA that is equivalent to the RNA strand. The DNA strand that serves as the template for RNA synthesis is called the "antisense" or noncoding strand. The transcription initiation site is numbered "+1," and the upstream elements are referred to as negative numbers corresponding to the number of bases 5' to the initiation site. In *Escherichia coli* genes, the promoter region has consensus binding sequences at 10 and 35 nucleotides upstream from the transcription start site (designated positions -10 and -35). The RNA polymerase binds to the consensus binding site at -35, and unwinds the double-stranded DNA as it moves to the -10 binding site, creating a transcription bubble of single-stranded DNA approximately 17 bases in length that will accommodate the transcription complex and allow transcription of the exposed portion of the template DNA. In the promoters of most eukaryotic class II genes there is a consensus sequence known as TATAAA (usually called a TATA box) that is generally located 25 to 30 base pairs upstream from the transcription start site. The TATA box binds the TATA binding protein (TBP) or transcription factor IID (TFIID), which attaches as the initial participant in the assembly of the transcription complex. Associated general transcription factor proteins TFIIA and TFIIB then bind to the promoter, followed by RNA polymerase II, as well as several other factors including TFIIE and TBP associated factors (TAFs). This transcriptional complex then allows initiation of mRNA transcription, and represents the basal transcriptional apparatus.

Other sequences that can function to control transcription in the proximal promoter besides the TATA box include the CCAAT box (5'-GCCAAT-3') and GC box (5'-GGGCGG-3'), which bind the proteins Sp1 and C/EBP. DNA sequences that bind transcriptional regulatory proteins are known as *cis* elements; the proteins that bind to the *cis* elements and influence transcription (which are products of other genes) are called *trans* acting factors. The affinity of binding of a protein to a DNA sequence usually extends over a region of five to seven base pairs, and is strongly influenced by the exact sequence. Consensus sequences are those that bind a given regulatory protein with the highest affinity, although less tight association occurs with increasing mismatch of the consensus sequence from the ideal. Optimal matching of DNA binding sequences to regulatory factors enhances their binding by 10^6 - 10^7 fold. Promoter regions contain activation domains where specific regulatory proteins can bind, and upon doing so interact with the transcription complex in such a way as to enhance the rate of transcription. Similarly, repressor elements bind proteins that either interfere with binding of one of the proteins of the transcriptional complex or the polymerase, or decrease the efficiency of the transcriptional complex in some manner through protein-protein interactions. Regulatory elements such as enhancers can be distant from the proximal promoter region by many kb of DNA, yet influence transcription of the noncontiguous transcribed gene. This is believed to occur through secondary structure of the DNA with loops that bring the enhancer element and its interacting regulatory protein into contact with the transcriptional complex.

The regulatory proteins that interact with *cis* elements in a promoter are loosely termed transcription factors. Several general classes of these proteins exist, all of which contain both DNA binding domains and protein-protein interaction domains through which they influence the transcriptional complex. The first type is the helix-turn-helix form. These are common in prokaryotes, and consist of 20 amino acid segments with two α helices of seven to nine amino acids separated by a β turn. The second type is the zinc finger transcription factor. These proteins contain groups of four cysteine or histidine residues that coordinate a zinc ion. Some regulatory proteins have multiple zinc finger regions, allowing multiple DNA interaction domains and thereby increasing specificity. Steroid receptors such as the vitamin D receptor, thyroid hormone receptor, and retinoid receptors contain a common central domain that binds DNA through two zinc finger regions. Homeodomain transcription factors are related to helix-turn-helix factors, and contain three α helices, one of which is the DNA recognition domain. These proteins are involved in patterning during early development, and are absent in prokaryotes. Another class of factor important in development is the basic helix-loop-helix proteins. These proteins have a basic DNA binding region, and are active as dimers. Myo D, which controls muscle differentiation, is an example of a basic helix-loop-helix factor. The last category of transcription factors is the leucine zipper. These proteins contain α-helical domains containing an exposed series of leucines that interact with similar leucines on a dimerization partner. Leucine zipper transcription factors can be heterodimeric or homodimeric. Activating protein-1 (AP-1) is an important transcription factor in many musculoskeletal tissues and processes, and consists of dimers of the Fos and Jun family members. AP-1 activity is frequently associated with early response gene activation in signaling and control of cell proliferation. Some transcription factors, such as AP-1, can be activated by phosphorylation; the activity of other transcription factors, such as nuclear factor kappa B (NFκB), can be controlled by binding proteins such as inhibitor of NFκB, which prevent translocation of the factor to the nucleus and thereby control access of the transcription factor to DNA binding sites.

Transcription factor expression and function is known to have tissue-specific consequences. For example, deletion of the *Runx2* gene in mouse models results in a perinatal lethal phenotype that fails to develop mineralized bones and fails to express several other osteoblast-specific genes that appear to be under its control. Mutations in *Runx2* have been associated with cleidocranial dysplasia. Deletion of SMAD3, a transcription factor that is involved with signaling downstream of the transforming growth factor-beta (TGF-β) receptor, causes several systemic phenotypes including a defect in articular cartilage that resembles osteoarthritis. An osteoblastic transcriptional coactivator protein, called α NAC (nascent polypeptide-associated complex), has also recently been identified. Furthermore, expression of myo D (mentioned previously) in fibroblasts can transform the cells into myoblasts. Overexpression of *c-fos* in transgenic mice results in development of chondrosarcomas, and *c-fos* overexpression is observed in fibrous dysplasia, although the underlying mutation in this disorder is within a g protein and not *c-fos* itself. Thus, several transcription factors that have specific roles to play in skeletal tissues are the focus of intense scrutiny in the musculoskeletal research arena.

Growth Factors

Local proteins secreted by many cell types that bind to specific receptors and mediate signaling events that modulate cell proliferation and differentiation are called growth factors. Cytokines are similar receptor-activating local protein factors, and in fact, the distinction is somewhat artificial. However, cytokines are historically regarded as secreted factors that were initially characterized in cells of the hematopoietic and immune systems. Essentially all musculoskeletal tissues produce and respond to growth factors, and these proteins are involved in injury, disease, and repair processes as well as in normal growth and development. Growth factors, which are a part of the normal processes that regulate the cell cycle, are also beginning to be used in clinical therapeutic applications. Mutations in growth factors or their signaling pathways can be associated with derangements of cell growth as in certain cancers, or can result in skeletal malformations. Most growth factors are mitogenic, or stimulate cell proliferation. They are secreted by a cell and activate cell surface receptors either on the same cell (autocrine stimulation) or on nearby cells (paracrine stimulation). The activity of some growth factors is regulated extracellularly by specific binding proteins that may either prevent interaction with the receptors, or in some instances be necessary to present the growth factor to the receptor. Growth factors have been named after their apparent functions or tissue of origin.

Transforming Growth Factors

TGF-β is a ubiquitous family of structurally related dimeric growth factors. There are five primary forms of TGF-β and numerous other family members including activins, growth and differentiation factors, and the BMPs. TGF-β 1-4 have been identified in cartilage and bone, and have pleiotropic effects on these tissues. In general, TGFs-β stimulate proliferation of cells of mesenchymal origin except in epithelial cells where these proteins inhibit proliferation. TGFs-β are secreted in a latent propeptide form that requires enzymatic cleavage for activation. Activation can also be achieved by acid pH or heat. A binding protein also is secreted in many TGF-β-producing tissues that sequester the factor(s) and prevent receptor activation. Three receptors have been identified:

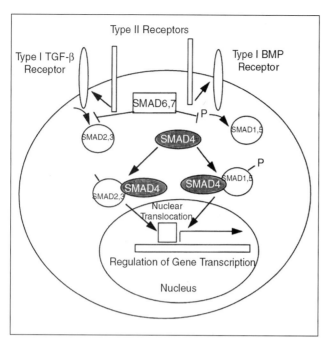

Figure 1 The TGF-β and BMP family members use the SMAD signaling pathways. When the appropriate ligand associates with the type I receptor, the type II receptor binds to and phosphorylates the type I receptor. This in turn results in phosphorylation of the signaling proteins called SMADs. SMAD 2 or 3 can be phosphorylated by the TGF-β type I receptor, and SMAD 1 or 5 by the BMP type I receptor. Upon phosphorylation, the SMADs associate with another protein called SMAD 4, resulting in translocation to the nucleus, where this complex associates with promoter elements and alters gene transcription. *(Reproduced from Rosier RN, Reynolds PR, O'Keefe RJ: Molecular and cell biology in orthopaedics, in Buckwalter JA, Einhorn TA, Simon SR (eds): Orthopaedic Basic Science: Biology and Biomechanics of the Musculoskeletal System, ed 2. Rosemont, IL, American Academy of Orthopaedic Surgeons, 2000, pp 19-76.)*

type I (50 to 60 kd), type II (75 to 80 kd), and type III (200 kd). Biologic effects are believed to be mediated through the type I and II receptors, which function as heterodimeric serine/threonine kinases. All forms of TGF-β bind to these receptors, but generally TGF-β2 has lower affinity than TGF-β1 and TGF-β3 for the type I and II receptors. Type I, II, and III receptors have all been identified in cartilage, and progressive expression of the type II receptor (which may inhibit proliferation) occurs with chondrocyte maturation, and may be responsible for a decreasing mitogenic stimulation as the cells begin to hypertrophy.

Heterodimeric TGF-β receptor complexes initiate signaling via receptor autophosphorylation, and subsequent signaling events partially involving the SMAD family of transcription factors are activated downstream of the receptor (**Figure 1**). It has also been determined that TGF-β receptor activation leads to signaling via mitogen-activated protein kinases/activating transcription factor-2 that may be independent of the SMADs and relevant in cartilage biology. The SMADs are a family of intracellular

proteins that comprise three classes of signaling molecules: receptor-associated SMADs (SMADs 2 and 3 for TGF-β), the cofactor SMAD 4, and the inhibitory SMADs 6 and 7. The receptor-associated SMADs bind to the type I receptor, are phosphorylated following receptor activation, form heteromeric complexes with the cofactor SMAD 4, and translocate to the nucleus where they influence gene transcription. Negative regulation of the TGF-β/BMP signaling pathway occurs in part via a degradation of SMAD proteins facilitated by the SMAD ubiquitination regulatory factors Smurf1 and Smurf2, two members of the HECT (homologous to E6AP carboxyl terminus) family of E3 ubiquitin ligases. In particular, Smurf2 has been shown to target SMAD 2 for degradation thus possessing the ability to at least partially block TGF-β signaling.

The downstream signaling pathways responsible for initiating changes in gene transcription in response to TGF-β receptor activation are not fully understood. In articular chondrocytes, TGF-β stimulates proteoglycan synthesis and may reverse effects of other cytokines such as interleukin-1 (IL-1) that stimulate matrix degradation, but it is not mitogenic in chondrocytes that have not entered the pathway of endochondral ossification. Furthermore, loss of TGF-β signaling in mice (caused by either transgenic overexpression of an inhibitory mutant of the TGF-β receptor in cartilage or a knockout of the *SMAD3* gene) leads to arthritis, confirming that maintenance of the TGF-β signaling axis is necessary in normal articular chondrocytes. In bone, TGFs-β also stimulate osteoblast proliferation as well as matrix synthesis. TGF-β is stored in bone matrix in a latent form. During bone resorption, TGF-β is released from the bone matrix and the acidic pH activates the protein. Therefore, TGF-β has been proposed as one of the molecules that may regulate osteoblast/osteoclast interactions in the local coupling of bone formation and resorption. TGF-β has been used to stimulate cartilage repair, and has shown modest effects in stimulation of fracture healing.

Bone Morphogenetic Proteins
BMPs are a subfamily of the TGF-β superfamily of growth factors. BMPs, which are involved in regulation of growth and development, are dimeric disulfide bonded proteins, but are not secreted as latent polypeptides and consequently do not require proteolysis for activation. Most of the BMPs share the ability to induce differentiation of cartilage and bone through the endochondral calcification pathway when implanted in an ectopic site. BMP-1 is a metalloprotease that functions as a C-propeptidase for types I, II, and III collagen. BMP-2 is an osteoinductive factor, and induces chondrogenic differentiation of mesenchymal cells. BMPs-5, -6, and -7 are closely related, and are also effective osteoinductive agents. BMP-6 and -7 are located in hypertrophic cartilage, and promote cartilage maturation and commitment to the endochondral calcification pathway. Mutations causing overexpression of

BMP-4 in inflammatory cells are responsible for fibrodysplasia ossificans progressiva in which massive spontaneous heterotopic bone formation occurs. BMP expression is also critical to induction of programmed cell death (apoptosis) in the interdigital web spaces to form the digits during embryonic development.

Three BMP receptors have been identified, which are similar to the TGF-β receptors. There are two type I receptors, A and B, and one type II receptor. The receptors dimerize upon binding the ligand, and the receptor autophosphorylates and then phosphorylates members of the SMAD family of signaling proteins (specifically 1, 5, and 8) which heterodimerize with SMAD4 and are transported to the nucleus where they affect gene transcription (Figure 1).

BMPs, in particular BMP-2 and BMP-7 (also known as osteogenic protein-1, [OP-1]), are being used in experimental clinical settings to induce bone regeneration. The typical delivery system for these growth factors is incorporation into a collagen sponge or collagen gel, which is implanted in the prospective site for bone induction. Efficacy in stimulation of critical defect and nonunion models in animals has been established, although data from human trials have been published only for native and not recombinant molecules. Two human clinical trials for nonunions have been published, one using human native BMP with a bone matrix-derived substrate, and a second using a bovine BMP/plaster of Paris delivery system. Both trials demonstrated healing in 16 of 17 patients with this treatment. Delivery of BMPs using gene therapy approaches has successfully been demonstrated in animal models with either direct introduction of the plasmid in a collagen matrix formulated to enhance cellular uptake of the DNA, or introduction of transfected cells. Clinical trials involving spine fusion (in conjunction with titanium cages), osteonecrosis of the hip, and fracture healing are in progress. Trials suggesting efficacy in restoration of alveolar bone loss in periodontal disease have also been reported and further studies are ongoing. Preliminary human results with spinal fusion appear promising.

Parathyroid Hormone-Related Protein and Indian Hedgehog
BMP-6 is regulated in developing cartilage and in growth plate cartilage by other locally produced growth factors including PTHrP and a developmental patterning gene called indian hedgehog (Ihh). PTHrP, unlike PTH, is a locally acting factor rather than a systemic hormone. It was initially identified in malignant tumors that overproduce it, causing hypercalcemia. PTH and PTHrP share a common receptor in most tissues, called the PTH/PTHrP receptor, although a second receptor has been identified that selectively binds PTH. The N-terminal sequence of PTH and PTHrP are similar, and constitute the binding domain for the receptor. The PTH/PTHrP receptor activates multiple signals upon binding ligand through G

proteins that interact with the receptor. These include cyclic adenosine monophosphate (cAMP) stimulation of protein kinase A, and activation of phospholipase C with secondary production of inositol trisphosphate (causing a transient rise in cytosolic calcium levels) and activation of the protein kinase C pathway. The protein kinases phosphorylate intracellular signaling molecules and alter gene transcription. Some of the important transcription factors activated by PTH/PTHrP receptor activation are cAMP response element binding protein (CREB) and AP-1. The effect of PTHrP on chondrocytes is to stimulate proliferation and suppress genes associated with maturation such as alkaline phosphatase, BMP-6, Ihh, and type X collagen. PTH/PTHrP receptor expression is found in growth plate, but not articular or epiphyseal cartilage, and PTHrP produced in the epiphysis is believed to act on receptors in the growth plate chondrocytes in a paracrine fashion, stimulating proliferation and preventing premature hypertrophy, in part by suppression of BMP-6 expression. PTHrP expression is in turn stimulated by Ihh which is expressed in the growth plate chondrocytes. Ihh induces PTHrP expression through a receptor-mediated mechanism via receptors called patched and gli in adjacent perichondrium and possibly the epiphysis, and PTHrP reciprocally inhibits Ihh in a paracrine feedback loop. The balance between these factors controls the rate of chondrocyte proliferation and maturation. The paracrine relationships between the growth plate and articular/epiphyseal cartilage during development is depicted in Figure 2. The critical nature of PTHrP and its receptor, and Ihh have been demonstrated in knockout mouse models. Deletion of the PTHrP expressing gene results in a perinatal lethal dwarfed phenotype, with severe derangements of cartilage maturation typified by decreased proliferation and premature onset of hypertrophy in the growth plates. A similar result occurs with deletion of the PTH/PTHrP receptor. Deletion of Ihh results also in severe disruption of the growth plate, and in addition a failure of mineralized bone formation even in areas of osteoblastic bone formation. The significance of Ihh in developmental regulation of osteoblast function is not yet understood.

Insulin-Like Growth Factors
Insulin-like growth factors (IGFs) are also important in the regulation of many skeletal tissue types. IGF-I, also called somatomedin C, is produced in the liver and also in skeletal tissues in response to activation of cell surface receptors for growth hormone. Locally produced IGF-I in the growth plate has been shown to stimulate proliferation of chondrocytes, and probably contributes significantly to the stimulation of long bone growth by growth hormone. Growth hormone also has been demonstrated to stimulate expression of fibroblast growth factor-2 (FGF-2) in cartilage. IGF-I stimulates proteoglycan synthesis as well as cell proliferation. IGF-II is expressed in bone, and can activate the IGF-II receptor, which is iden-

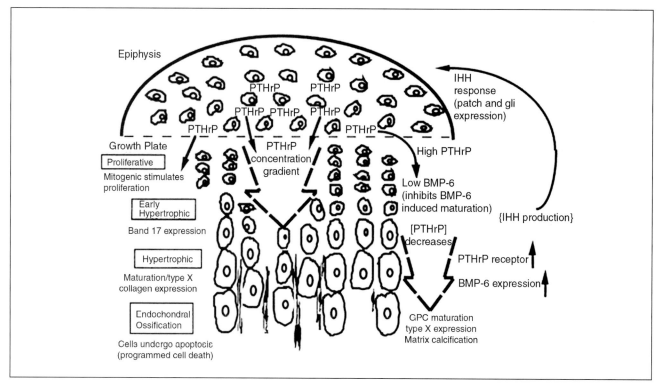

Figure 2   The paracrine regulatory loop of PTHrP and IHH in developing cartilage is illustrated. IHH is produced in the growth plate in response to expression of BMP-6 in the early hypertrophic chondrocytes. IHH in turn signals to cells in the perichondrium and possibly, the epiphysis, through a receptor called patched and its intracellular signaling molecule called gli to stimulate PTHrP expression. PTHrP in the epiphysis then in turn inhibits expression of BMP-6 and IHH in the growth plate cells, suppressing hypertrophy and maturation in a feedback loop. The balance between PTHrP and BMP-6/IHH expression controls the rate of chondrocyte proliferation and maturation. GPC = growth plate chondrocyte. *(Reproduced from Rosier RN, O'Keefe RJ, Reynolds PR, Hicks DG, Puzas JE: Expression and function of TGF-B and PTHrP in the growth plate, in Buckwalter JA, Ehrlich MG, Sandell LJ, Trippel SB (eds): Skeletal Growth and Development. Rosemont, IL, American Academy of Orthopaedic Surgeons, 1998, pp 285-300.)*

tical with the cation-independent mannose-6-phosphate receptor. IGF-II stimulates proliferation and matrix synthesis by osteoblasts. Cells that secrete IGFs also secrete binding proteins that control the activity of IGFs. Six IGF binding proteins have been identified, and most of the binding proteins inhibit IGF function, although IGF binding protein 5 actually enhances the effect of IGFs on bone cells.

Fibroblast Growth Factors

FGFs are a family of 11 growth factors, of which the most abundant are FGF-1 and FGF-2. FGFs are found in cartilage matrix and in bone, and stimulate proliferation of both cell types. Four different FGF receptors have been identified. FGF inhibits proliferation in vivo in the growth plate or in organ cultures, although FGF is stimulatory in monolayer cultures of chondrocytes. Mutations of the FGF receptors have been implicated in several human chondrodysplasias, including identification of an activating mutation of FGF receptor 3 as the cause of achondroplasia. FGFs are also angiogenic, stimulating growth of vasculature. The angiogenic properties of FGF-2 have been used experimentally in patients to revascularize in-

farcted areas of myocardium by implantation of the growth factor at the time of coronary bypass surgery. FGFs are tightly bound by many extracellular matrix molecules, including heparin-like carbohydrates and proteoglycans. The FGF receptors function as tyrosine kinases, triggering intracellular signaling pathways usually via direct phosphorylation of kinase targets. Although they have no effect on fracture repair, FGFs can have a synergistic impact on the stimulation of chondrocyte proliferation when combined with IGF-I and TGF-β and they have been used to stimulate tendon, ligament, and cartilage repair.

Vascular Endothelial Growth Factor

Vascular endothelial growth factor (VEGF) is another angiogenic growth factor expressed by endothelial cells. This growth factor stimulates endothelial cell proliferation in vitro, and in vivo it markedly stimulates formation of new vasculature. VEGF has been identified in the lower hypertrophic zone of the growth plate, where it likely plays a role in stimulating vascular ingrowth into the calcified cartilage, triggering its conversion to bone. VEGF has also been localized to the tissue within the distraction gap during distraction osteogenesis lengthening of long bones. In fact, with each microdistraction caused by lengthening the fixation device there is a wave of VEGF expression. The histology of the distraction gap tissue, which demonstrates a highly vascularized fibrous interzone that develops abundant osteoblastic activity and bone formation along the vessels that develop, supports the central role of VEGF in driving the vascularization necessary to support osteoblastic bone formation. VEGF does not appear to be highly expressed in normal bone, but is involved in angiogenesis in bone repair and in malignant tumors. VEGF has been used in experimental clinical trials of gene therapy for vascular ischemic disease and myocardial infarction. In one clinical trial, injection of naked plasmid DNA encoding VEGF intra-arterially resulted in dramatic clinical improvement in lower limb ischemia; promising results in myocardial revascularization have been reported in animal models.

Wnt Proteins
The Wnt family consists of several small, cysteine-rich, secreted glycoproteins involved in regulation of a variety of cellular activities and plays critical roles during early development, for instance controlling mesoderm induction, patterning, cell fate determination and morphogenesis. However, a role for these proteins beyond development has not been demonstrated. At the surface of cells, Wnts interact with two kinds of protein: Frizzled receptor and low-density lipoprotein receptor-related protein 5 or 6. There are many genes encoding Frizzled proteins (10 in the human genome), and different Frizzled proteins probably have different affinities for various types of Wnt proteins. Wnt proteins can form a complex with the cysteine-rich domain of Frizzled proteins and with low-density lipoprotein receptor-related protein 5 of 6, leading to the formation of a dual-receptor complex. The intracellular parts of the receptors pass on this information, turning on the pathways that feed through β-catenin inside the cell.

Wnt proteins trigger signaling pathways inside cells that proceed through several protein complexes. One protein in these pathways is β-catenin. The canonical Wnt signaling pathway affects cellular functions by regulating β-catenin expression and its subcellular localization. In the absence of Wnts, β-catenin levels are kept at a steady-state. Any β-catenin molecules that are not bridging cadherins to the actin cytoskeleton or participating in other activities are conjugated with and degraded by the 26S proteasome. A multiprotein complex containing kinases (glycogen synthase kinase [GSK] 3β and casein kinase [CK] 1) and scaffolding proteins (axin, axin2, adenomatous polyposis coli [APC] and disheveled [Dsh]) mediate the degradation of excess β-catenin by phosphorylating specific N-terminal residues and creating docking sites for F-box protein/E3 ligase complexes. Therefore, inhibition of β-catenin phosphorylation prevents its degradation and increases its cytoplasmic level and nuclear translocation. Signaling from Wnt releases β-catenin from its binding proteins, allowing it to move to the nucleus, where it interacts with cytoplasmic transcription factor/lymphoid enhancer factor, to activate expression of target genes.

In addition to the recent realization that chondrocytes are influenced by Wnt/β-catenin signaling, osteoblasts are a major target of this pathway. Leucine-responsive regulatory protein 5 (Lrp5) is expressed by osteoblasts of the endosteal and trabecular bone surfaces but not osteoclasts, and regulates osteoblastic proliferation, survival, and activity. Human mesenchymal stem cells express various members of the Wnt, Frizzled-related proteins and Lrp5 coreceptor Frizzled families as well as Lrp5 and DKK1 during osteogenesis. Wnt-Lrp5 stimulates expression of alkaline phosphatase, a marker of osteoblastic differentiation, in pluripotent mesenchymal cell lines, C3H10T1/2, C2C12, and ST2 cells and the osteoblast cell line MC3T3-E1 cells. Effects of BMP-2 on osteoblast differentiation and extracellular matrix mineralization are enhanced by Wnts. In addition, BMP-2 stimulates Lrp5 and Lrp6 expression in ST2 bone marrow stromal cells. In the same cells, Wnt1, Wnt2, Wnt3a, and Wnt7b but not Wnt4 and Wnt5a induce expression of alkaline phosphatase. Overexpression of Lrp5 did not enhance Wnt3a-induced alkaline phosphatase activity, whereas a gain-of-function mutation in this gene does induce the high bone mass phenotype in humans. This suggests that other Wnts, or even other ligands, may be involved in signaling through Lrp5, or that Wnt-induced alkaline phosphatase stimulation may reflect only one aspect of their activity.

Cytokines
Cytokines are a diverse group of soluble peptide signaling molecules; more than 100 such molecules have been identified. Although cytokines are widely known for their role in inflammation, they also have a multitude of other effects, including tissue homeostasis and repair. Cytokines are produced by a variety of cells, but are sometimes referred to as lymphokines or monokines to denote a relative specificity of production by either activated lymphocytes or monocytes. The term chemokine is sometimes used to designate cytokines with chemoattractant activity for fibroblasts or leukocytes. Cytokines are typically produced locally and act in a paracrine or autocrine manner. However, cytokines also can have systemic effects ranging from an infection-mediated febrile response to the cachexia of malignancy. Elevated systemic cytokine levels have been associated with hypercalcemia of malignancy secondary to increased osteoclastic bone resorption.

Cytokines act on specific cell membrane receptors and have pleiotropic effects on a variety of target cells. One of the most important effects of these molecules is their role in immunomodulation. Activation of monocytes/macrophages by phagocytosis or stimulation with bacterial lipopolysaccharide results in the synthesis of several important proinflammatory cytokines, including IL-1, IL-6, and tumor necrosis factor-alpha (TNF-α). These molecules increase vascular permeability, attract additional mononuclear cells to the site of inflammation, lead to the proliferation and differentiation of lymphocytes, and stimulate additional proinflammatory cytokine release. Thus, the action of these molecules is to enhance and amplify the inflammatory response. Although important for the control of infection, if unchecked, the inflammatory response results in tissue catabolism.

Regulation of the inflammatory response is probably provided in part by one or more anti-inflammatory cytokines, such as IL-4 or IL-10. IL-4 is made predominantly by lymphocytes, whereas IL-10 is produced by both monocytes and lymphocytes. Both peptides act via specific cell membrane receptors and decrease the expression and secretion of the proinflammatory cytokines in activated mononuclear cells. IL-10 also decreases monocyte expression of HLA-DR. Because it is involved in antigen presentation to CD4+ lymphocytes, HLA-DR is essential for the immunologic activity of macrophages. Thus, IL-10 also indirectly downregulates the cell-mediated immune response. There is evidence to suggest that downregulation of IL-10 may play an important role in the pathogenesis and progression of some human inflammatory diseases, a concept supported by the limited lifespan of transgenic mice lacking the expression of IL-10. These animals die prematurely because of the development of chronic inflammatory disease. Similarly, experimental studies show the ability of exogenously administered IL-4 to control inflammatory arthritis in animal models. Thus, normal tissue homeostasis may depend on a balance between proinflammatory and anti-inflammatory cytokines.

Cytokines play a major role in both the health and disease of the musculoskeletal system. Inflammatory arthritis is associated with high levels of cytokine release, including the proinflammatory cytokines. These cytokines lead to tissue catabolism through both direct and indirect mechanisms. The proinflammatory cytokines stimulate matrix metalloproteinase (MMP) activity in synovial lining cells and incite the development of a proliferative, erosive pannus that invades and destroys the cartilage surface. However, the proinflammatory cytokines have a wide range of direct effects on chondrocyte metabolism. Cytokine-stimulated articular chondrocytes secrete MMPs, which leads to cartilage degradation via aggrecanases, which induce the breakdown of proteoglycans. Proinflammatory cytokine-stimulated articular chondrocytes also have diminished collagen and proteoglycan synthesis and secretion, furthering the catabolic effect of these agents.

Several recently conducted human trials have demonstrated that strategies aimed at blocking the proinflammatory cytokines can improve the clinical course of inflammatory arthritis. Administration of IL-1 receptor antagonist, a naturally occurring soluble IL-1 blocking protein that binds and sequesters IL-1, resulted in improvements in clinical parameters and in radiographic evidence of joint damage over a 6-month period of investigation. Human gene therapy trials using vectors expressing IL-1 receptor antagonist are currently underway with promising early results. Recently, the US Food and Drug Administration has approved the use of a recombinantly produced soluble fusion protein containing TNF-α type I receptor binding sequences for use in the treatment of rheumatoid arthritis. Injection of the fusion protein, which sequesters TNF-α, has resulted in marked and continuous improvement in most patients with arthritis unresponsive to traditional therapies.

The proinflammatory cytokines IL-1, IL-6, and TNF-α are also important regulators of bone resorption. These cytokines stimulate osteoclast recruitment from undifferentiated cells in the granulocyte/macrophage lineage and induce mature osteoclast function. Thus, these cytokines have been implicated in the increase in bone resorption observed in several pathologic inflammatory conditions, including infection, periprosthetic osteolysis and loosening, and inflammatory arthritis. Recently, tumor-associated bone loss has been shown to be mediated by osteoclasts in response to cytokine production by tumor cells. Proinflammatory cytokine synthesis has been demonstrated in benign tumors such as pigmented villonodular synovitis, primary bone tumors such as Ewing's sarcoma, and in most metastatic tumors involving bone. Animal studies have suggested that the increase in bone resorption that occurs during estrogen deficiency is related to increased levels of IL-6 secretion in marrow stromal cells, an effect that is blocked by the exogenous administration of estrogens. These proteins may have a role in the treatment of postmenopausal osteoporosis. Osteoclasts also synthesize IL-1, IL-6, and TNF-α, and may stimulate further bone resorption through an autocrine mechanism in conditions such as giant cell tumor of bone, where there are excess numbers of osteoclasts.

In addition to their responsiveness to cytokines, cells of the musculoskeletal system also secrete cytokines. Osteoblasts synthesize and secrete IL-6 in response to PTH as well as after stimulation with prostaglandins. Because PTH does not have a direct effect on osteoclasts, the well-established bone resorptive effects of PTH are probably mediated in part through the synthesis of IL-6 by osteoblasts. In addition to its effects on osteoblasts, IL-6 has been shown to stimulate both the differentiation and proliferation of osteoblasts and is a putative stimulator of bone formation. IL-6 demonstrates the pleiotropic effects characteristic of the cytokines.

TGF-β is another multifunctional cytokine that acts as an autocrine and paracrine factor in musculoskeletal tissues. TGF-β is synthesized by both articular and growth plate chondrocytes and bone cells. In articular cartilage, TGF-β increases matrix synthesis, and activation of its

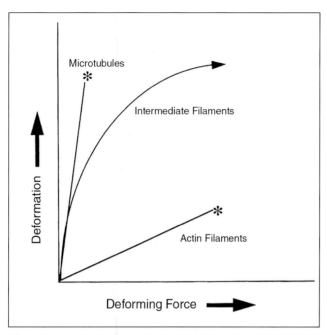

Figure 3   Mechanical properties of different cytoskeletal elements subjected to shear force. Microtubules readily deform with minimal force, whereas actin filaments are much more rigid, tolerating greater force with less deformation. The intermediate filaments such as vimentin are easily deformed, but withstand large forces without rupture. *(Adapted with permission from Janmey P, Euteneur V, Troub P, Schliwa M: Viscoelastic properties of vimentin compared with other filamentous biopolymer networks.* J Cell Biol *1991;113:155-160.)*

signaling pathways may protect against the development of arthritis. Animals with defects in TGF-β signaling develop severe degenerative arthritis. TGF-β stimulates the proliferation of growth plate chondrocytes, although its role in endochondral bone formation remains uncertain. However, TGF-β probably has an important role in wound healing and probably in the early events of fracture healing. In fracture healing, TGF-β is present in high concentrations in early fracture callus.

Cell-Matrix Interactions

The matrix is a key factor in influencing gene expression in skeletal tissues, and in allowing the cells to receive signals from the environment. This is particularly important in the musculoskeletal system because of the load-bearing functions of the tissues, which require responsiveness and adaptability to mechanical forces. Matrix proteins interact with cell surface receptors in a manner similar to growth factors, and transduction of this array of stimuli occurs with the integration of intracellular signaling pathways. This process in turn causes activation of genes that control the cell cycle and the expression of proteins that define differentiated functions of target cells.

Some interactions of cells with surrounding matrix are mediated through the cytoskeleton. Cytoskeletal proteins are essential for numerous cellular functions, includ-

ing mitosis, cell motility, intracellular movement, and organization of organelles. The cytoskeleton is composed of three major types of filaments made by reversible polymerization of specific proteins: actin filaments (actin polymer), microtubules (tubulin polymer), and intermediate filaments (polymers of vimentin or lamin). Cell surface movements are controlled by interactions of the actin molecules with myosins in the cytoplasm, enabling contractility and cell movement. Actin fiber formation is regulated by the Rho family of G proteins. Actin filaments are flexible, whereas microtubules are more rigid structures. Microtubules polymerize and depolymerize continuously in the cell, and mediate organelle transport and subcellular organization. Microtubules are critically involved in organizing the events of cell division, and radiate outward through the cell from origin sites within the centrosome, a structure adjacent to the nucleus. Proteins called kinesins and dyneins are cytoplasmic adenosine triphosphate-dependent motors that move in opposite directions along microtubules, carrying bound proteins or vesicles. The cytoplasmic intermediate filaments are believed to function within the cell to resist deformation to external mechanical stress, and have greater strength than actin and tubulin (**Figure 3**). Numerous cytoplasmic proteins associate with the cytoskeletal proteins and control their structure, contractility, and stability.

One common mechanism linking cells to matrix is the integrin family of cell surface receptors that interact with specific matrix proteins. Integrins consist of transmembrane heterodimeric signaling molecules that reside on the cell surface and interact with matrix proteins containing a specific sequence of amino acids (arginine-glycine-aspartate, or RGD). Many extracellular matrix proteins, including collagens, contain RGD sequences that enable interaction with integrin receptors. The receptor dimers consist of α and β subunits that associate in specific combinations in different cell types. All mesenchymal cells express specific subsets of integrin receptors on the cell surface. Over 20 heterodimers have been identified between 9 types of β subunits and 14 types of α subunits. In addition to the numerous isoforms of the two integrin subunits, some isoforms have several alternatively spliced forms of the protein, further increasing the diversity of this receptor family. The different heterodimers possess differing and sometimes overlapping specificity for particular matrix RGD-containing proteins. Integrin receptors have relatively lower affinities for their ligands than do growth factor and hormone receptors, and are 10 to 100 times more abundant on cell surfaces. The β subunit contains a binding domain that interacts with the cytoskeletal proteins talin and α-actinin, and upon ligand binding causes formation of linkages to the actin cytoskeleton. These areas of focal receptor/cytoskeletal contact can activate kinases such as the focal adhesion kinase or the tyrosine kinase product of the *src* gene. This in turn leads to a signal cascade that can result in changes in gene expression. Because cells are attached to their matrix by the integrins, perturbations of the mechanical environment couple to effects on the cytoskeleton and associated kinases, providing one mechanism whereby cells can respond with changes in gene expression to changes in mechanical loading.

Another class of adhesion molecules known as the hyaluronan receptor family recognize carbohydrates related to hyaluronate. This is also known as the CD44 receptor group, and consists of several isoforms. CD44 has been implicated in the attachment of tumor cells to matrix in target tissues during metastasis. Like other cell surface receptors, CD44 can activate intracellular processes. Some types of cell surface receptors, such as cadherins and receptors with some homology to immunoglobulins, cell-cell adhesion molecules mediate cell-cell contact events rather than cell-matrix interactions. Activation of cadherins results in binding of these receptors to cytoplasmic proteins called catenins, which interact with the actin cytoskeleton analogous to the manner in which talin and α-actinin link integrin activation to actin. Cadherins and cell-cell adhesion molecules are homophilic receptors (bind to a like receptor on a different cell to mediate signaling events). Alterations in cadherin expression can change chondrocyte differentiation pathways in embryogenesis, indicating dependence of gene expression on cell-cell interactions as well as cell-matrix interactions.

Most cells possess stretch-activated ion channels in the plasma membrane, which provide another means of cellular response to mechanical stimuli. These channels control influx of K^+ or Ca^{2+}, two cations that the cell actively maintains at low intracellular levels through the actions of plasma membrane-based energy-dependent pumps. When the matrix adjacent to an attached cell is mechanically deformed, transient elevations of cations can occur through the action of the stretch-activated channels. These cations can influence other signaling pathways within the cell, thus enabling mechanical input to influence the cell's transcriptional machinery. Stretch-activated channels have been demonstrated in fibroblasts, osteoblasts, and chondrocytes. A family of matrix-cell binding proteins called annexins has characteristics of both a matrix receptor and an ion channel. Annexins are ubiquitous extracellular proteins that associate with the plasma membrane under certain conditions. Annexins II, V, and VI bind to collagen and to the plasma membrane, providing another mechanism for cell-matrix attachment. In addition, some annexins function as calcium channels in the plasma membrane. In chondrocytes, annexins V and VI may function as calcium channels that are activated by binding of type II and type X collagen. The phospholipid composition of the plasma membrane influences annexin association with the membrane, with acidic phospholipids enhancing membrane binding. Annexin V binding is enhanced by changes in the phospholipids of the plasma membrane, which occur as part of the cascade of events in apoptosis;

binding of this annexin has been used as a marker for apoptosis. Annexins provide another connection between the matrix and intracellular signaling pathways.

Bone remodeling provides an excellent prototypical example of matrix control of cell behavior and communication, and integration of multiple signal inputs by cell-matrix interactions. Osteoblasts secrete the matrix of bone, incorporating growth factors that can be released and activated upon matrix resorption. Osteoblasts provide the initial signals for bone resorption by osteoclasts, responding to stimuli such as PTH with production of collagenase, which appears to clear an area for osteoclast attachment, as well as producing cytokines that stimulate osteoclast formation and activation. The osteoclast begins resorbing bone, organizing its functional apparatus in response to integrin signals upon contact with the bone matrix. The osteoclast releases and activates growth factors from the bone matrix as it is resorbed; the growth factors in turn stimulate nearby osteoblast progenitors to differentiate. In addition, the osteoclast deposits signals on the resorption surface before moving on or undergoing apoptosis. These signals attract osteoblasts and stimulate matrix deposition at the previously resorbed surface, replacing the bone matrix. This functional cooperation of osteoblasts and osteoclasts, coupled by the matrix, is under modulation of systemic hormonal controls such as PTH and vitamin D, which regulate systemic calcium metabolism. However, the remodeling process is also under local control through mechanical signal transduction through the bone matrix to the osteoblasts and/or osteoclasts, allowing the bone to remodel according to local mechanical stress. Finally, pathologic processes such as inflammation or tumors can produce local cytokines that alter the balance between formation and resorption, leading to pathologic loss of bone matrix.

Expression of Cellular Phenotype

The genotype of an organism or a cell refers to the genes present in its genome. However, in any somatic cell, only a fraction of the genes are expressed and that expression profile is usually regulated by specific interactions with the matrix and various factors (**Figure 4**). The phenotype of a cell is defined by the array of genes that are expressed, and their relative levels of expression. When the phenotype of a cell is characterized, the focus tends to be on the genes expressed that are unique or relatively unique to that cell type, because there are thousands of genes that all cells express in common. Differentiation of cells refers to acquisition of a specific profile of gene expression that sets the cell apart from other types of cells, and determines its structure and its function. In general, cell proliferation and differentiation tend to be inversely regulated. Proliferation of normal cells is prevented by cell-cell contacts, a phenomenon known as contact inhibition. When cells are plated at low densities in culture, there is no contact inhi-

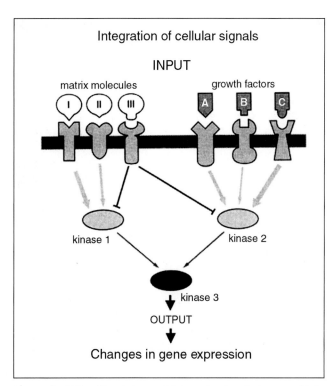

Figure 4   Cells ultimately must integrate signals from multiple pathways and stimuli into net changes in gene expression. Matrix/cell interactions cause kinase signals through integrins and other receptors, as does stimulation of multiple cell surface receptors by various growth factors or hormones. These signals have varying positive and negative influences on tissue-specific gene expression controlling proliferation and differentiated function, which integrate through kinase signaling pathways into a net resultant effect on the cell's behavior. *(Reproduced with permission from Alberts B, Bray D, Lewis J, Raff M, Roberts K, Watson JD:* Molecular Biology of the Cell, *ed 3. New York, NY, Garland Publishing, 1994, p 781.)*

bition and they tend to enter the cell cycle and proliferate. During active proliferation, the expression of tissue-specific proteins by the cells diminishes. When confluency is attained, contact inhibition triggers mechanisms that inhibit the cell cycle, and cells tend to differentiate, expressing specific characteristics of the tissue from which they were derived. This paradigm has been well established in several skeletally relevant tissues, including osteoblasts in culture. For example, when initially plated in culture, osteoblasts proliferate and exhibit minimal expression of proteins associated with normal osteoblasts in vivo. In the presence of appropriate differentiation-stimulating agents, the cells progressively express proteins characteristic of differentiation at confluency such as alkaline phosphatase, osteocalcin, and osteopontin, and ultimately produce a mineralized osteoid matrix (**Figure 5**). A more detailed description of the behavior of these cells can be found below.

The cells of most skeletal tissues, including muscle, tendon, ligament, connective tissue, bone, and cartilage, are derived from multipotent cells called mesenchymal stem cells. Mesenchymal stem cells give rise to the devel-

opment of all the skeletal elements during development, and remain present in low numbers in sites such as periosteum and bone marrow throughout life. It is these cells that can differentiate into bone, cartilage, and fibrous tissue following a fracture and generate a reparative callus. Mesenchymal stem cells can be isolated from bone marrow, and under the correct culture conditions can be induced to differentiate into lipoblasts, myoblasts, fibroblasts, osteoblasts, or chondrocytes. Most likely they can also be induced to form tenocytes or fibrochondrocytes, although this has not yet been demonstrated specifically. The number of mesenchymal stem cells declines with age, as does their responsiveness to growth factors; hence, the ability to regenerate various mesenchymal tissues declines as a function of aging. Use of mesenchymal stem cells for regenerating bone and repairing osteochondral defects is well underway and feasibility has been demonstrated in several animal models. Several markers that are putatively specific for mesenchymal stem cells have been reported, such as STRO1, but further work needs to be done to fully characterize these markers.

Osteoblast Phenotype

There are several phenotypic parameters that characterize the osteoblast. Osteoblasts produce and secrete both structural proteins such as collagen, and regulatory proteins such as growth factors. Study of osteoblasts has been facilitated by development of methods of isolating them from intact bone tissue, usually by collagenase digestions of calvarial or long bone specimens from rats or mice, or from trabecular bone specimens in humans. The cells can be grown in culture, and also several transformed osteoblastic cell lines have been developed from mouse, human, and rat bone cells derived from tumors or immortalized by viral transformations. Commonly used cell lines include ROS 17.28 (rat), UMR106 (rat), SAOS2 (human), MG63 (human), and MC3T3 (murine). The abundant extracellular matrix produced by osteoblasts is called osteoid, and when mineralized with crystalline hydroxyapatite becomes bone. The major matrix protein synthesized by osteoblastic cells, which comprises more than 90% of the organic matrix of bone, is type I collagen. Type I collagen is synthesized and secreted as a triple helix with two $\alpha 1$ and one $\alpha 2$ chains (genes designated *COLIA1* and *COLIA2*). The N-terminal and carboxyterminal propeptides are cleaved extracellularly, and the collagen molecules spontaneously self assemble into collagen microfibrils and fibrils, with a quarter-staggered arrangement of the individual molecules. The C-propeptide is cleaved by proteolytic activity of BMP-1, which lacks osteoinductive capacity but has some homology to the other members. The C-propeptide and N-propeptide fragments can be detected in serum, and are indicative of bone formation rates. Bone matrix also contains small amounts of type III and type V collagens. The collagen fibrils are laid down parallel to the surface of

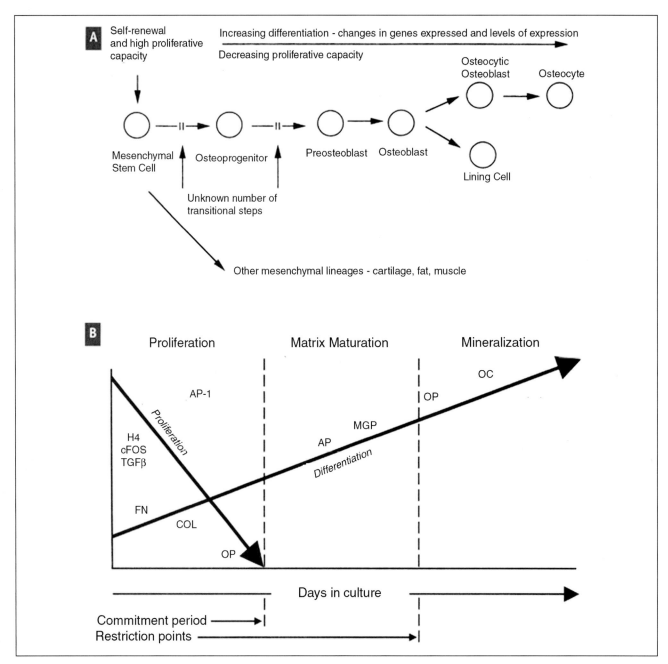

Figure 5 **A,** The pathways of bone cell progenitor differentiation from mesenchymal stem cell to osteoblast and osteocyte *(Reproduced with permission from Aubin JE, Kahn A: The osteoblast lineage: Embryologic origins and differentiation sequence, in Favus MJ (ed): Primer on the Metabolic Bone Disease and Disorders of Mineral Metabolism, ed 3. Philadelphia, PA, Lippincott-Raven, 1996, p 36.)* **B,** Reciprocal relationship between genes associated with proliferation and differentiation in an osteoblast culture model. During early culture, genes associated with proliferation such as histone H4, c-fos, TGF-β and AP-1 activity are downregulated, while matrix genes such as fibronectin (FN) and type I collagen (COL) begin to increase. This continues through matrix maturation, when proliferation ceases and onset of expression of alkaline phosphatase (AP) and matrix glutamic acid containing protein (MGP) begins. During the final phases of differentiation the matrix mineralizes, and osteopontin (OP) and osteocalcin (OC) are expressed. *(Reproduced with permission from Lian JB, Stein GS: Development of the osteoblast phenotype: Molecular mechanisms mediating osteoblast growth and differentiation. Iowa Orthop J 1995;15:118-140.)*

the osteoblast, and spontaneously nucleate hydroxyapatite crystals, which initially form preferentially in the "hole zones" between the quarter-staggered collagen molecules. With a periodicity related to the bone formation rate, the orientation of the fibrils changes 90° to the preceding layer, resulting in a plywood-like layered structure that maximizes the tensile strength of the material. The mechanism that controls this ordered orientation of the matrix is unknown. Normal bone formation in this layered arrangement is referred to as lamellar bone, and is an important feature that distinguishes normal bone from bone formed by tumors or in injury and repair processes.

The carboxyglutamic acid-containing glycoprotein osteocalcin, along with two other glycoproteins (osteopontin and osteonectin), are the next most abundant extracellular matrix protein constituents produced by osteoblasts. Osteonectin may function to enhance binding of hydroxyapatite crystals to the collagen matrix as mineralization proceeds. Osteocalcin is believed to play a role in recruitment of osteoclasts to bone surfaces for bone resorption; the function of osteopontin is unclear. Bone matrix also contains a sialoprotein and small amounts of several other glycoproteins and phosphoproteins of uncertain function. The extracellular matrix structural proteins are one set of phenotypic parameters that define the osteoblast. During osteoblast differentiation, there are several shifts in protein synthesis: from a mixture of type III and type I collagen to predominantly type I collagen; from low to high levels of alkaline phosphatase; from versican to fibronectin expression, and from expression of an attachment protein called thrombospondin to expression of the bone glycoproteins osteonectin, osteocalcin, osteopontin, and sialoprotein.

Bone matrix also contains several regulatory proteins deposited by osteoblasts. These include growth factors such as TGF-β, IGF-I and IGF-II, FGFs, platelet-derived growth factor (PDGF), and BMPs. Although present quantitatively in minute amounts, these proteins are extremely important in regulation of bone remodeling and in conferring osteoinductive capacity on bone, which enables bone grafting and transplantation.

Osteoblasts also express many genes as part of their phenotype that are not incorporated into the bone matrix. For instance, bone-specific alkaline phosphatase is an enzyme probably involved in mineralization of osteoid. Osteoblasts express the PTH/PTHrP receptor, and exhibit intracellular signaling responses to PTH or PTHrP. Osteoblasts also express the vitamin D receptor and consequently vitamin D responsiveness. Some transcription factors such as Runx2 and a transcriptional coactivator called αNAC have been identified. Glucocorticoids have complex effects on bone, stimulating differentiation of preosteoblasts in culture through a BMP-6 mediated pathway, while inhibiting bone cell proliferation and decreasing bone formation, resorption, and net mass when given systemically in vivo.

Osteocytes are fully differentiated osteoblasts that become encased in the secreted matrix. Because they are completely embedded in bone, culture and study of osteocytes has been difficult, and less is known about their phenotype and function than for osteoblasts. Osteocytes have numerous long cell processes that extend throughout the bone matrix and are in contact with the cell processes of other osteocytes. The channels in the matrix through which these numerous connecting cell processes extend are called canaliculi. It has been demonstrated that osteocytes express cell-cell channels (gap junctions) called connexins, through which small molecules such as second messengers can pass. This implies that the network of osteocytes is in communication with one another. It is also known that bone exhibits piezoelectric properties under mechanical loading because of its anisotropic nature; that is, it develops surface electrical charges that are asymmetrically distributed when mechanically loaded. One putative function of osteocyte-osteocyte communication within the larger organization of bone as a tissue may be in sensing and modulating signals that control osteoblastic and osteoclastic activity, enabling the observed ability of bone to increase its mass in areas that are loaded and decrease mass in response to unloading. Osteocytes also express osteocalcin and fibronectin, although the role of these proteins in osteocyte function is unknown.

Chondrocyte Phenotype

Chondrocytes are derived from similar undifferentiated mesenchymal precursor cells to those that give rise to osteoblasts. As chondrocytes differentiate, they also express a pattern of specific genes that define their function. Chondrocytes are characterized, like osteoblasts, by production of an abundant extracellular matrix. Chondrocytes undergo differentiation along two major distinct pathways: one in which the cells undergo maturation, hypertrophy, and matrix calcification (the endochondral calcification pathway), and one in which the cells are relatively quiescent, carrying out load bearing and structural functions (**Figure 6**). Induction of chondrocyte differentiation from mesenchymal stem cell precursors occurs during embryogenesis, and also in injury and repair such as in fracture callus. The nonendochondral calcification pathway can be activated in quiescent chondrocytes as demonstrated by the onset of maturation and calcification in the deep layers of the articular cartilage during cartilage degeneration. Growth plate chondrocytes generate bone growth through proliferation and hypertrophy during maturation along the endochondral calcification pathway. Chondrocytes can be isolated from cartilage by digestion of the tissue with collagenase or combinations of collagenase, hyaluronidase, and trypsin, and the cells can be grown and studied in culture. Chondrocytes in monolayer culture tend to dedifferentiate, and lose expression of type II collagen and other phenotypic markers such as proteoglycan synthesis. Instead they take on a more fibroblastic phenotype and express type I collagen. When cultured in a suspension culture or in a three-dimensional gel made of collagen, agar, or alginate, the cells will maintain a chondrocytic phenotype, emphasizing the importance of cell-matrix interactions in controlling gene expression.

The predominant matrix protein in cartilage is type II collagen, which is composed of a single type chain forming a triple helix. Like type I collagen, it is secreted as triple helical proprotein that is cleaved extracellularly (gene designated as *COLIIA1*). The C-propeptide of type II col-

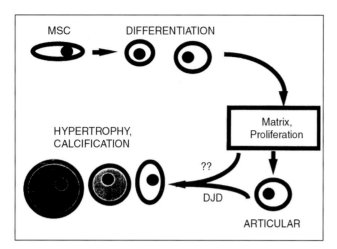

Figure 6 Under proper circumstances, mesenchymal stem cells (MSC) undergo differentiation to prechondroblast and chondroblast, associated with expression of chondrocyte specific genes such as type II and type IX collagen, and aggrecan. The cartilaginous matrix thus produced defines the phoenotype. Chondrocytes can then differentiate along two pathways: the first is toward articular chondrocyte phenotype, in which the cells are not actively dividing although they are metabolically active in maintenance and turnover of the matrix; the second pathway is endochondral maturation, which results in hypertrophy, expression of type X collagen, and mineralization as a precursor to bone formation. The pathway of maturation may be activated during osteoarthritis, as evidenced by chondrocyte cloning (proliferation), hypertrophy, and type X collagen expression. DJD = degenerative joint disease. (*Reproduced from Rosier RN, Reynolds PR, O'Keefe RJ: Molecular and cell biology in orthopaedics, in Buckwalter JA, Einhorn TA, Simon SR (eds): Orthopaedic Basic Science: Biology and Biomechanics of the Musculoskeletal System, ed 2. Rosemont, IL, American Academy of Orthopaedic Surgeons, 2000, pp 19-76.*)

lagen may also be cleaved by BMP-1, which is constitutively expressed in cartilage. Type II collagen exists in two alternatively spliced forms, as previously mentioned. The embryonic form, type IIA, differs from the more mature IIB form by inclusion of exon 2. The other major organic component of the matrix is proteoglycan, which includes several proteins containing covalently bound glycosaminoglycan side chains. The major proteoglycan is aggrecan, which consists of a protein core and chondroitin sulfate and keratan sulfate side chains. The proteoglycans confer many of the unique mechanical properties on cartilage, including its ability to absorb repetitive compressive mechanical loads without damage. Aggrecan molecules form noncovalently bound aggregates with hyaluronic acid and a link glycoprotein. In addition, cartilage contains small proteoglycans such as decorin and biglycan. There are a series of minor collagens also associated with the chondrocyte phenotype. These include type VI, IX, X, and XI collagens. Type VI collagen is a pericellular matrix protein, and type IX is a collagen molecule with a proteoglycan moiety. Type IX collagen molecules coat the outer surface of type II collagen fibrils and interact with the

matrix proteoglycan via their own proteoglycan moieties. This is believed to interconnect the collagen and proteoglycan matrix. Type XI collagen is localized within the type II fibrils, and may regulate fibril diameter.

Several chondrocyte phenotypic markers are specific to the differentiation pathway of the chondrocyte. For instance, type X collagen is only expressed by hypertrophic chondrocytes, and is a highly specific marker for this phenotype. In addition these cells express high levels of alkaline phosphatase, in contrast to minimal expression in chondrocytes not committed to maturation. Chondrocytes committed to the endochondral calcification pathway also express several growth factors, including BMP-6 and BMP-7, which promote maturation. Differential expression of these genes in articular and growth plate chondrocytes demonstrates the critical role that regulatory gene products can play as determinants of phenotypes.

Osteoclast Phenotype

The osteoclast is the cell responsible for carrying out bone resorption. These are extremely specialized cells, with an array of proteins used for accomplishing the complex task of resorbing calcified matrix. Osteoclasts are derived from monocytic precursors, and share some of the characteristics of monocytes and macrophages. Osteoclasts are multinucleated, and arise through syncytial fusion of several precursor cells under the influence of specific growth factors in the bone marrow. Functional osteoclasts have been isolated from animal and human models using several techniques. Rinsing the marrow cavity of long bones of egg-laying chicks on low calcium diets was one of the earliest methods of obtaining sufficient numbers of osteoclasts for study. Later, cells with osteoclast-like characteristics were isolated from human giant cell tumors. Functional osteoclasts can also be generated from the marrow of long bones of neonatal rats or mice, and are cultured on wafers of cortical bone in the presence of vitamin D and PTH. This procedure readily enables the study of osteoclasts in vitro.

Osteoclasts attach to bone surfaces through a specific cell attachment receptor called an integrin. The osteoclast integrin receptor is also known as $\alpha v \beta 3$, or the vitronectin receptor. Several bone matrix proteins, including collagen, fibronectin, and osteopontin, contain the attachment RGD sequences. After attachment to a bone surface, the integrins activate focal adhesion kinases that induce intracellular signals, including activation of c-src, a regulatory kinase that contributes to the induction of polarization of the osteoclast. An extensive series of microscopic invaginations of the plasma membrane surface against the bone matrix surface forms, called the ruffled border, which serves to markedly increase the surface area of membrane next to the bone. A plasma membrane proton pump moves to the ruffled border and pumps protons from the cytosol into the space between the osteo-

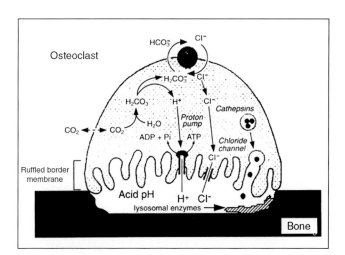

Figure 7 The osteoclast is an extraordinarily complex and functionally specific cell type. The cell attaches to bone through the vitronectin receptor, resulting in a series of intracellular activation steps that cause formation of the microvillous ruffled border and increase dramatically the amount of cell surface adjacent to the bone. The cell polarizes, with migration of the proton pump to the ruffled border and consequent acidification of the space between the cell and the bone, causing dissolution of mineral. Carbonic anhydrase II expression generates protons for this activity. Lysosomal enzymes, including cathepsins, are secreted by exocytosis into the region and degrade collagen and other proteins. Some of these lysosomal proteins are retained on the bone surface after the osteoclast undergoes apoptosis, possibly defining sites for subsequent osteoblastic bone formation. (*Reproduced from Rosier RN, Reynolds PR, O'Keefe RJ: Molecular and cell biology in orthopaedics, in Buckwalter JA, Einhorn TA, Simon SR (eds): Orthopaedic Basic Science: Biology and Biomechanics of the Musculoskeletal System, ed 2. Rosemont, IL, American Academy of Orthopaedic Surgeons, 2000, pp 19-76.*)

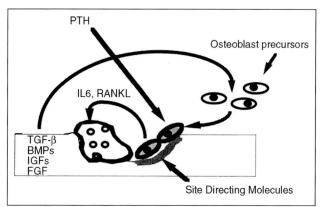

Figure 8 Osteoblasts and osteoclasts communicate in a process known as coupling of bone formation and resorption. Upon resorption of bone by osteoclasts, bone matrix growth factors such as TGF-β and BMPs are released and activated. These anabolic factors may stimulate osteoblastic precursors to differentiate into osteoblasts and begin bone formation. The carbohydrates of the glycosylated lysosomal enzymes deposited on the resorption surface by the osteoclasts may induce osteoblast attachment and matrix synthesis through cell surface receptors such as the mannose-6-phosphate/IGFII receptor, thus site-directing the replacement of the resorbed bone. The overall process is controlled by systemic hormones such as PTH, which activates receptors of osteoclast stimulating molecules such as IL-6, and the recently identified TNF-like molecule called osteoprotegerin ligand or RANKL. These effector molecules in turn stimulate osteoclast differentiation and function. (*Reproduced from Rosier RN, Reynolds PR, O'Keefe RJ: Molecular and cell biology in orthopaedics, in Buckwalter JA, Einhorn TA, Simon SR (eds): Orthopaedic Basic Science: Biology and Biomechanics of the Musculoskeletal System, ed 2. Rosemont, IL, American Academy of Orthopaedic Surgeons, 2000, pp 19-76.*)

clast and the bone (**Figure 7**). This acidifies the bone surface, resulting in a dissolution of the hydroxyapatite mineral phase of the bone.

Lysosomes move to the ruffled border and discharge their contents of lysosomal enzymes into the resorption region. This includes acid-activated hydrolases such as cathepsins, which degrade the collagen in the matrix. Osteoclasts also express a matrix metalloproteinase (gelatinase B, or MMP-9), although its function is unknown. An isoform of carbonic anhydrase (CAII) is expressed and generates intracellular protons for the acidification process. Osteoclasts also express a specific phosphatase called tartrate-resistant acid phosphatase, but its function is unknown. Tartrate-resistant acid phosphatase and other glycosylated lysosomal enzymes are deposited on the resorption surface and remain there after the osteoclast has moved away. It is possible that these residues are important in attracting osteoblasts to the resorption sites (**Figure 8**). Many of these enzymes contain glycosylations that can bind to receptors such as the IFGII/mannose-6-phosphate receptor. This receptor is expressed in osteoblasts, and when stimulated causes anabolic effects and matrix synthesis. Theoretically,

the residue of glycosylated enzymes on the resorption surface may function to target osteoblasts to this location and initiate bone formation, thus representing part of the site-directing coupling mechanism between bone formation and resorption. Osteoclasts contain a calcium receptor that may be involved in the induction of movement of the pseudopodia of the motile osteoclasts, which creep along the bone surface as they excavate the matrix. When the pseudopodia lift up from the bone surface and move to reattach, the accumulated high concentration of inorganic ions such as calcium and phosphate resulting from the resorption of bone matrix are discharged into the extracellular space. Some of the matrix and mineral may be removed by endocytosis and transport across the osteoclast, but this is controversial. Osteoclasts have a finite lifetime, and are active in bone resorption for an estimated 10 to 14 days, after which they undergo apoptosis.

Several key hormones and local factors control osteoclast function. Systemically, PTH stimulates bone resorption. However, only osteoblasts and not osteoclasts express the PTH receptor. Therefore the stimulation of resorption is by PTH is mediated through signals from the osteoblast. One of these signals may be IL-6, a stimulator of osteoclast formation and resorption. TNF-α is an extremely potent stimulator of osteoclast progenitor proliferation, fusion, and activation of osteoclastic bone resorption, as is IL-1. TNF, IL-1, and IL-6 are produced in many inflammatory processes, and are known as proinflammatory cytokines. These factors are critical to many important clinical disorders, and have been implicated in pathologic bone resorption in metastatic and primary bone tumors, infection, prosthetic loosening, nonunion of fractures, osteoporosis, and periarticular bone loss in inflammatory arthropathies.

Fibroblastic Phenotype

The hallmarks of the fibroblastic phenotype are synthesis of types I and III collagen, and a spindle cell shape with cell processes. There are relatively few specific markers for the fibroblastic phenotype, and it appears in some ways to be a default differentiation pathway for mesenchymal cells. Fibroblastic cells express fibronectin, and can differentiate along some specialized pathways in generation of cells of tendon and ligament. Ligaments and tendons contain primarily type I collagen, as well as type XII, which coats the type I fibrils and is analogous to type IX collagen in cartilage in that it contains a proteoglycan-like moiety that is believed to interact with the proteoglycans within the matrix. Tendon and ligament contain only small proteoglycans, biglycan and decorin, rather than aggrecan. During compression, tendon can develop a more fibrocartilaginous phenotype with expression of aggrecan. This occurs where tendons are under chronic compressive force, such as in the posterior tibial tendon. Other important components of tendon and ligament are tenascin and elastin. Recently two new BMPs (BMP-12 and BMP-13), which are homologous to previously identified murine growth and differentiation factors (gdf7 and gdf6, respectively), have been identified through molecular cloning techniques. When implanted ectopically these molecules induce the formation of an organized fibrous tissue resembling tendon or ligament. This tissue also expresses tenascin, small proteoglycans, and elastin, which may play a role in regulating tendon and ligament morphogenesis. Embryologic studies have identified expression of these molecules during formation of the joint capsule, tendinous attachments to bone, and ligament sites. In addition, a recent study has shown stimulation of patellar tendon healing in an animal model by implantation of BMP-12. Growth factors such as bFGF, PDGF, and TGF-ß have also been demonstrated in animal models to enhance the healing of ligaments and tendons.

Tendon and ligament fibroblastic-like cells also respond to mechanical stress, and this controls reorganization of the matrix during healing, both to decrease the excessive amount of type III collagen that is expressed early in healing in favor of increased expression of type I, and to allow realignment of the fibrils with the direction of mechanical force that increases the strength of the struc-ture. The realignment is believed to occur through matrix remodeling, but little is known about this process. The strength and rate of remodeling of healing tendons or ligaments is enhanced by application of mechanical tensile force, as long as it is not excessive (which will lead to laxity). In addition, crosslinking of collagen increases with progressive healing, as does the fibril diameter; both factors enhance the mechanical structure of the healing tissue.

Neoplasia

The numerous regulatory genes involved in control of cell proliferation offer numerous points of potential disruption because of mutations, which can result in loss of growth control, or neoplasia. Genes whose function becomes disrupted leading to malignant transformation of the cell are known as oncogenes. A large number of genes have been identified in which mutations are associated with specific types of cancer. Oncogenes are classified as either proto-oncogenes or antioncogenes. Proto-oncogenes are mutations in genes that stimulate cell proliferation, and are dominant mutations, because mutation in a single allele of the gene can lead to loss of growth control. Proto-oncogenes, the normal counterparts of mutated genes in cancers, were initially identified from viruses that induced malignant transformations in cells or caused tumors in animals. Some viruses can incorporate an oncogene through recombinant events, and overexpression of this gene in association with viral infection of a cell can cause uncontrolled cell proliferation, or neoplastic transformation. These oncogenes were later identified as normal growth regulators in cells, hence the term proto-oncogene. Some proto-oncogenes associated with human cancers include *erbB1* (squamous cell carcinoma), *c-myc* (Burkitt's lymphoma), *brca1* and *brca2* (breast cancer), *L-myc* (lung carcinoma), *bcl-2* (follicular lymphoma), *ras* (lung carcinoma), *c-fos* (osteosarcoma, chondrosarcoma), and *c-src* (colon cancer).

Antioncogenes are also known as tumor suppressor genes, such as the *RB* and *p53* genes previously mentioned. These genes normally function to prevent cell proliferation, and when mutated in a way that interferes with their suppressive ability, excessive cell division results. Antioncogenes are also known as recessive oncogenes because the absence of their function leads to malignancy. Some tumor suppressor gene mutations and associated cancers include *RB* (retinoblastoma, breast cancer, lung carcinoma, osteosarcoma), *APC* (colonic carcinoma in familial polyposis), *p53* (diverse mutations associated with 50% of cancers; colon carcinoma, osteosarcoma, breast, and others), *NF* (neurofibromatosis), and *WT* (Wilms' tumor). Mutations can also occur in either somatic cells or in germline cells, as a result of errors during replication, or environmental mutagens such as toxic chemicals (carcinogens) or radiation. Germline mutations are heritable, whereas somatic mutations obviously are not. Li-Fraumeni syndrome is a germline mutation in *p53* that causes a strong hereditary predisposition to several cancers, including colonic carcinoma and osteosarcoma. Approximately 50% of osteosarcomas have mutations in *p53*, mostly somatic. p53 is bound by another protein called MDM2, which prevents its tumor suppressor activity. Overexpression of MDM2 reduces p53 activity, and has been identified in 37% of soft-tissue sarcomas, 10% of osteosarcomas, and 13% of Ewing's sarcomas, where the overexpression appears to result from amplification of the gene. A new group of genes associated with tumor formation are the *EXT* genes, named for their association with hereditary multiple exostoses. Three *EXT* genes have been cloned (*EXT1, 2,* and *3*) with three different chromosomal locations; mutations in these genes are associated with multiple exostoses as well as with chondrosarcomas. The function of the *EXT* genes is not yet known, but they are hypothesized to be tumor-suppressor genes, and are related to a group of *Drosophila* genes with a regulatory role in development.

Because of the redundancy of growth regulatory proteins, frequently more than one gene must be altered for a cell to become malignant, particularly in the case of anti-oncogenes. The need for multiple "hits" to express a fully malignant phenotype is well accepted. In some instances, such as with the *RB* gene, a combination of a germline mutation that confers a susceptibility does not lead to a malignancy until a second somatic mutation occurs affecting the other *RB* allele. Rare instances exist where a malignant tumor spontaneously regresses or disappears, this is theorized to result from a further somatic mutation that interferes with cell proliferation or induces apoptosis. An example is the change of a neuroblastoma to a benign ganglioneuroma.

Another class of genetic abnormalities that can cause neoplasia are chromosomal translocations. These are somatic cell defects that occur during mitosis with recombinations of nonhomologous portions of chromosomes. Ewing's sarcoma is one of the best examples of a malignancy resulting from a chromosomal translocation. In 95% of Ewing's sarcomas (as well as in the closely related peripheral neuroectodermal tumor) there is a translocation between chromosome 11 and 22, designated t(11;22), (q24;q12). The translocation results in joining two genes together, creating a fusion protein. The fused genes are the *EWS* gene and a member of the ETS transcription factor family called *Fli-1*. Presumably resulting dysregulation of the *Fli-1* gene contributes to the malignant cell phenotype. Alveolar rhabdomyosarcoma has a t(2;13,(q35;q14) translocation that creates a fusion protein product of the *PAX3* and *ALV* genes, which encode developmental transcription factors. Synovial sarcomas also have a chromosomal translocation in 95% of patients, a t(X;18) translocation, which creates a fusion of the *SSX* and *SYT* genes. Myxoid chondrosarcoma has a t(9;22) in 50% of patients, and myxoid liposarcomas a t(12;16) translocation in 75%

of patients. Liposarcomas, clear cell sarcomas, and several other tumors also have various chromosomal abnormalities that likely are involved in their oncogenesis.

Another important gene family that is a strong determinant of responsiveness to chemotherapy in musculoskeletal malignancies is the family of multidrug resistance genes, the best characterized being *MDR1*. Chemotherapeutic agents interfere with various aspects of cell proliferation, including DNA synthesis and protein synthesis. Many cells possess mechanisms to detoxify the cell of foreign chemicals by actively pumping them out of the cell. MDR1 (also known as p-glycoprotein) is one such mechanism, which is a transmembrane adenosine triphosphatase that pumps a wide range of weakly charged organic compounds from the cytoplasm to the extracellular fluid. Multidrug resistance-related protein is a related gene. Chemotherapeutic agents such as doxorubicin are efficiently extruded from cells expressing MDR1. A significant percentage of osteosarcomas express MDR1, and several studies have demonstrated an inverse correlation between the responsiveness of the tumor, judged by the amount of necrosis following neoadjuvant chemotherapy, and gene expression. In some cancers, including lymphomas and sarcomas, attempts have been made to use pharmacologic agents to block MDR1 function to increase the efficacy of chemotherapy. However, drug toxicity to normal tissues is also enhanced, and results of this approach have been limited. Chondrosarcomas have recently been shown to constitutively express MDR1, with a tendency for increased levels of expression in higher grade tumors. This may explain the notorious lack of sensitivity of chondrosarcomas to chemotherapy.

Metastasis

The hallmark of malignancy, in addition to the loss of growth control, is the ability cancer cells acquire to migrate to other organs, or metastasize (**Figure 9**). Metastasis is an extremely complex process requiring a series of coordinated cellular events and unique behaviors: (1) cell motility; (2) invasion of normal tissue matrices; (3) transgression of endothelial basement membranes, or intravasation; (4) attachment to endothelium at a remote site; (5) transgression of the endothelial basement membrane in the organ of implantation, or extravasation; (6) invasion of the local host organ; (7) establishing a colony and proliferating in a new environment; (8) inducing local angiogenesis to support tumor growth; (9) possibly repeating the cycle of metastasis from the new site. In addition to all of the required steps, there is a site selectivity that may depend on many host factors. For instance, sarcomas almost always metastasize to the lungs as the most common initial site. Clinical patterns of metastatic disease are common and are specific to different tumor types. Certain carcinomas such as breast, prostate, and lung cancer have a strong predilection for bone as a metastatic site, and specific locations show an order of preference: axial skeleton, proximal ap-

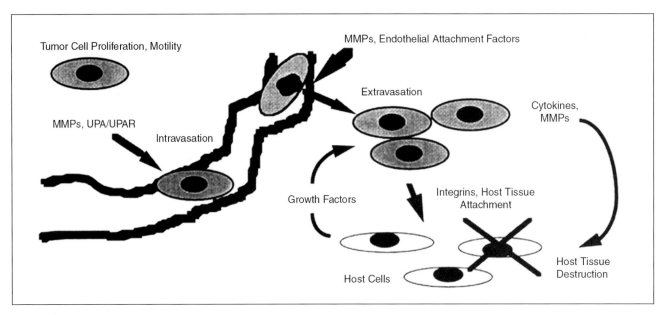

Figure 9 The process of metastasis involves a complex series of events. Tumor cells proliferate at the primary site and exhibit motility, allowing them to invade tissues and vascular or lymphatic channels. MMP-9 and the urokinase-like plasminogen activator/urokinase-like plasminogen activator receptor (UPA/UPAR) expression are essential to vascular invasion, possibly concentrating proteolytic activity at the invading leading edge of the cell along the vessel basement membrane. After intravasation, the cells attach to endothelium at a remote organ site via attachment factors, and extravasate using MMP proteolytic activity again. The cells may attach to the host tissue through integrins, CD44, or other cell/matrix receptors, and then proliferate at the host site, elaborating MMPs which contribute to host tissue matrix destruction, and cytokines that can induce these and other degradative enzymes in the tumor and host cells. The host tissues in turn may produce growth factors that further stimulate the tumor cell growth. (*Reproduced from Rosier RN, Reynolds PR, O'Keefe RJ: Molecular and cell biology in orthopaedics, in Buckwalter JA, Einhorn TA, Simon SR (eds): Orthopaedic Basic Science: Biology and Biomechanics of the Musculskeletal System, ed 2. Rosemont, IL, American Academy of Orthopaedic Surgeons, 2000, pp 19-76.*)

pendicular skeleton, distal appendicular skeleton. Metastasis is still presumed to operate on the seed and soil concept. Both the tumor and the host tissue express factors that facilitate the metastatic localization. Local growth factors and cytokines may play a key role in this site selection. In an interesting experiment, an osteosarcoma model was developed in which metastasis of cells to the lungs occurred after intravascular inoculation. When pieces of lung were removed from the animals before inoculation and placed subcutaneously as ectopic explants, tumor metastasis occurred not only to the lungs, but also to the lung explants. If the lung tissue was digested and the cells implanted subcutaneously as pellets, metastasis occurred again both to the lung and the ectopic lung cells. This clearly demonstrates that host site selectivity is related to interactions between the tumor cell and local tissue and cell-specific factors.

Metastasis also requires several cellular properties, which include (1) expression of degradative enzymes such as MMPs; (2) extracellular matrix receptors such as integrins or CD44; (3) cytoskeletal elements which facilitate motility; (4) expression of angiogenic molecules such as FGFs or VEGFs; (5) systems to activate MMPs, including other proteases and urokinase-like plasminogen activator; and, for metastasis to bone, (6) cytokines to stimulate osteoclastic bone resorption.

Immunobiology

The immune system provides defense against foreign pathogens and is dependent on an exquisitely regulated interaction between several different cell types. At the apex of the immune response is the antigen-presenting cell. Antigen-presenting cells phagocytose and present exogenous antigens to CD4 T lymphocyte cells. Following phagocytosis, antigens are processed in the cell within the lysosomal compartment. The processing includes in part proteolysis, and 10 to 18 amino acid fragments are noncovalently complexed with the type II major histocompatibility complex (MHC) molecule, HLA-DR, and transported to the plasma membrane. In contrast with type I MHC molecules, which are expressed on all cells, type II MHC molecules are expressed only on phagocytic antigen processing cells. T lymphocytes possessing the CD4 receptor (T-helper cells) are able to interact with MHC type II expressing cells.

The immune response, depicted in **Figure 10**, is dependent on the activation of CD4 cells. CD4 cells determine whether the antigen is "self," in which case there is no activation, or "non-self," which results in initiation of the immune response. A CD3 receptor complex is responsible for this determination and is also referred to as the T cell antigen receptor (TCR). The TCR contains disulfide linked

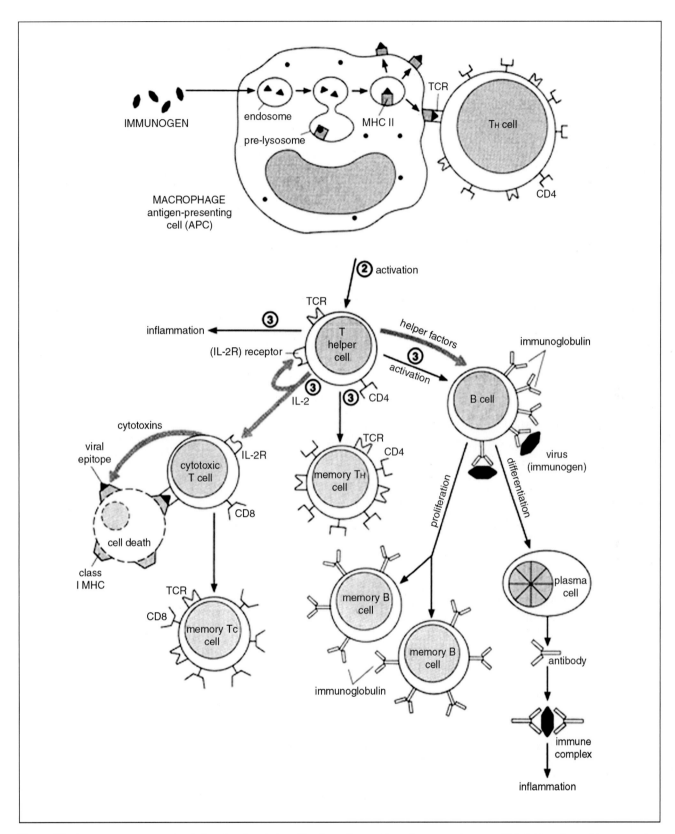

Figure 10   Immune response stimulation involves internalization of an antigen by macrophages, which is then bound to a receptor, MHC II, and expressed on the cell surface. The CD4-expressing helper T cells are activated by receptor interaction with the antigen (2) if it is recognized as foreign. The activated CD4 cell elaborates factors which stimulate B cells to express antibody, and also inflammatory cytokines. B cells can differentiate into antibody-producing plasma cells, or remain as memory cells. Similarly, the sensitized T cells can expand by proliferation and mediate cytotoxicity, or be retained as memory cells. *(Reproduced with permission from Stites DP, Terr AI, Parslow TG: Medical Immunology, ed 8. Norwalk, CT, Appleton & Lange, 1994, pp 43-44.)*

α and β chains derived from genes that undergo combinatorial joining of variable regions. In this process, which is also used to generate the diversity of immunoglobulins, variable regions are randomly mixed to create an unlimited number binding sites with different specificity. As with B cells, which produce immunoglobulins, each CD4 cell produces a single CD3 receptor complex. The diversity of the immune system is derived from the large number of CD4 cells, each with unique binding specificity.

Upon recognizing an antigen, the CD3 receptor complex initiates a signal transduction pathway which results in the synthesis and secretion of IL-2. IL-2 leads to clonal expansion of the CD4 cells and results in stimulation of CD8 lymphocytes (cytotoxic T cells). Stimulated CD8 cells also undergo clonal expansion and develop cytotoxic activity. Although B lymphocytes have the capacity to respond to exogenous antigens directly and undergo clonal expansion with antigen binding, this process is markedly enhanced by IL-2 and results in both clonal proliferation and differentiation into immunoglobulin producing plasma cells. Activation of CD4 lymphocytes is the critical event in immune activation. Depletion of CD4 cells occurs in the setting of human immunodeficiency virus infection and is associated with increased rates of opportunistic infection.

Cytotoxic T cells, through expression of the CD8 receptor, recognizes type I MHC molecule rather than the type II MHC molecules. Type I MHC molecules are less complex and have less antigen binding specificity than type II MHC molecules. Class I MHC molecules are composed of an α chain encoded by genes at the A, B, and C loci of the HLA complex on chromosome 6. The α chains are polymorphic (with variable sequences) and are noncovalently associated with a small protein called β2-microglobulin. β2 microglobulin is probably associated with the transport of small endogenously produced peptide fragments (8 to 10 amino acids) to the cell surface where they become associated with the polymorphic regions of the α chain of the type I MHC molecule. This complex can subsequently interact with the CD3 antigen receptor complex (TCR) on cytotoxic T-cells. When activated CD8 cells recognize foreign antigens, the cytotoxic response is initiated. Thus, a cell infected with a viral particle would present viral antigens to CD8 cells through type I MHC molecules and the cytotoxic response would be initiated. MHC I molecules present endogenous antigens, whereas MHC II molecules present exogenous antigens.

Inflammatory processes can occur in the absence of immunologic activation. An example of this is the inflammatory reaction that occurs in association with aseptic implant loosening. Although phagocytosis of particulate material by macrophages results in the secretion of proinflammatory cytokines such as TNF-α, IL-1, and IL-6 with subsequent tissue fibrosis, inflammation, and bone resorption, there is no evidence demonstrating immune activation during this process. In contrast, autoimmune disorders such as rheumatoid arthritis are associated with loss of self-tolerance and immune activation in response to the host's own proteins. The cause of autoimmune disease is unknown, but is multifactorial and probably includes a complex interplay of elements such as genetic susceptibility, infectious agents, and environmental factors.

Rejection of allograft tissues is understandable considering the cellular immune response mediated by type I MHC molecules. Allogeneic tissues present "non-self" antigens to CD8 lymphocytes. CD8 cells activation is enhanced by CD4 activation by antigen presenting cells that scavenge shed MHC I and MHC II molecules from the allogeneic tissue. Thus, live, vascularized allograft organs typically require the delivery of immunomodulatory agents to prevent rejection. In contrast, the implantation of allogeneic tissue with minimal cellular content (freeze-dried allograft bone) is not associated with inflammation or rejection. The importance of the immune response to fresh or fresh-frozen allografts, which are poorly revascularized and potentially have living cells only in avascular articular cartilage, is not clear. However, it is likely that the success of allograft implants is caused in part to subtle differences in the immune response to the implanted bone.

Selected Bibliography

Alberts B, Bray D, Lewis J, Raff M, Roberts K, Watson JD: *Molecular Biology of the Cell*, ed 4. New York, NY, Garland Publishing, 2002.

Ashkenazi A, Dixit VM: Death receptors: Signaling and modulation. *Science* 1998;281:1305-1308.

Bejsovec A: Wnt signaling: An embarrassment of receptors. *Curr Biol* 2000;10:R919-R922.

Bilezikian JP, Raisz LG, Rodan GA (eds): *Principles of Bone Biology*. San Diego, CA, Academic Press, 1996.

Boland GM, Perkins G, Hall DJ, Tuan RS: Wnt 3a promotes proliferation and suppresses osteogenic differentiation of adult human mesenchymal stem cells. *J Cell Biochem* 2004;93:1210-1230.

Buckwalter JA, Ehrlich MG, Sandell LJ, Trippel SB (eds): *Skeletal Growth and Development: Clinical Issues and Basic Science Advances*. Rosemont, IL, American Academy of Orthopaedic Surgeons, 1998.

Ebisawa T, Fukuchi M, Murakami G, et al: Smurf1 interacts with transforming growth factor-β type I receptor through Smad7 and induces receptor degradation. *J Biol Chem* 2001;276:12477-12480.

Etheridge SL, Spencer GJ, Heath DJ, Genever PG: Expression profiling and functional analysis of wnt signaling mechanisms in mesenchymal stem cells. *Stem Cells* 2004;22:849-860.

Evan G, Littlewood T: A matter of life and death. *Science* 1998;281:1317-1322.

Favus MJ, Christakos S (eds): *Primer on the Metabolic Bone Diseases and Disorders of Mineral Metabolism*, ed 3. Philadelphia, PA, Lippincott-Raven, 1996.

Gong Y, Slee RB, Fukai N, et al: LDL receptor-related protein 5 (LRP5) affects bone accrual and eye development. *Cell* 2001;107:513-523.

Hoffmann A, Gross G: BMP signaling pathways in cartilage and bone formation. *Crit Rev Eukaryot Gene Expr* 2001;11:23-45.

Huelsken J, Birchmeier W: New aspects of Wnt signaling pathways in higher vertebrates. *Curr Opin Genet Dev* 2001;11:547-553.

Hunter T: Oncoprotein networks. *Cell* 1997;88:333-346.

Ionescu AM, Schwarz EM, Vinson C, et al: PTHrP modulates chondrocyte differentiation through AP-1 and CREB signaling. *J Biol Chem* 2001;276:11639-11647.

Ionescu AM, Schwarz EM, Zuscik MJ, et al: ATF-2 cooperates with Smad3 to mediate TGF-beta effects on chondrocyte maturation. *Exp Cell Res* 2003;288:198-207.

Jacobson MD, Weil M, Raff MC: Programmed cell death in animal development. *Cell* 1997;88:347-354.

Levine AJ: The cellular gatekeeper for growth and division. *Cell* 1997;88:323-331.

Li TF, O'Keefe RJ, Chen D: TGF-beta signaling in chondrocytes. *Front Biosci* 2005;10:681-688.

Lukashev ME, Werb Z: ECM signaling: Orchestrating cell behaviour and misbehaviour. *Trends Cell Biol* 1998;8:437-441.

Rawadi G, Vayssiere B, Dunn F, Baron R, Roman-Roman S: BMP-2 controls alkaline phosphatase expression and osteoblast mineralization by a Wnt autocrine loop. *J Bone Miner Res* 2003;18:1842-1853.

Schenk PW, Snaar-Jagalska BE: Signal perception and transduction: The role of protein kinases. *Biochim Biophys Acta* 1999;1449:1-24.

Schipani E, Provot S: PTHrP, PTH, and the PTH/PTHrP receptor in endochondral bone development. *Birth Defects Res C Embryo Today* 2003;69:352-362.

Schubert S, Kurreck J: Oligonucleotide-based antiviral strategies. *Handb Exp Pharmacol* 2006;173:261-287.

Serra R, Johnson M, Filvaroff EH, et al: Expression of truncated, kinase-defective TGF-beta type II receptor in mouse skeletal muscle promotes terminal chondrocyte differentiation and osteoarthritis. *J Cell Biol* 1997;139:541-552.

Stites DP, Terr AI, Parslow TG (eds): *Medical Immunology*, ed 8. Norwalk, CT, Appleton & Lange, 1994.

Thomson AW (ed): *The Cytokine Handbook*, ed 3. San Diego, CA, Academic Press, 1998.

Thornberry NA, Lazebnik Y: Caspases: Enemies within. *Science* 1998;281:1312-1316.

Westendorf JJ, Kahler RA, Schroeder TM: Wnt signaling in osteoblasts and bone diseases. *Gene* 2004;341:19-39.

Yang X, Chen L, Xu X, Li C, Huang C, Deng CX: TGF-beta/Smad3 signals repress chondrocyte hypertrophic differentiation and are required for maintaining articular cartilage. *J Cell Biol* 2001;153:35-46.

Yates KE, Shortkroff S, Reish RG: Wnt influence on chondrocyte differentiation and cartilage function. *DNA Cell Biol* 2005;24:446-457.

Yoshida CA, Komori T: Role of Runx proteins in chondrogenesis. *Crit Rev Eukaryot Gene Expr* 2005;15:243-254.

Zhang Y, Chang C, Gehlin DJ, Hemmati-Brivanlou A, Derynck R: Regulation of Smad degradation and activity by Smurf2, an E3 ubiquitin ligase. *Proc Natl Acad Sci USA* 2001;98:974-979.

Zhou S, Eid K, Glowacki J: Cooperation between TGF-beta and Wnt pathways during chondrocyte and adipocyte differentiation of human marrow stromal cells. *J Bone Miner Res* 2004;19:463-470.

Chapter 2

Genetic Basis of Disorders With Orthopaedic Manifestations

Frederick R. Dietz, MD
Jeffrey C. Murray, MD

Introduction

New technology in molecular biology and quantitative analysis has led to an explosion in the knowledge and understanding of inherited diseases. Over 99.9% of the human DNA sequence is publicly available. Gene therapy is being investigated for the treatment of a host of diseases ranging from cystic fibrosis to cancer. Presymptomatic diagnosis is possible for people at risk for some diseases with delayed onset, such as Huntington's disease, Alzheimer's disease, and familial breast cancer.

The availability of the human DNA sequence and computer-based resources for manipulating that sequence enable quick identification of a gene once it is localized by genetic mapping. A current estimate of the number of human genes identified is 25,000, and the sequences of other useful organisms such as the mouse also are being rapidly completed. With the completion of the first reference sequence for humans, emphasis has shifted to finding the normal DNA sequence variations between individuals that will allow characterization of the specific variations that play a role in disease severity or progression. It is estimated that as many as 30 million DNA sequence differences can be found between any two individuals and more than 2 million of these are now in public databases. Referred to as single nucleotide polymorphisms, these individual changes in sequence can underlie something as well known as the ABO blood group differences or as complex as a variant that could increase the risk for chondrosarcoma or osteoporosis. It is the work of the next generation of physicians to move from medicine and surgery for people as a group to medicine and surgery for a specific person based on underlying genetic makeup. For example, the individual genetic makeup contributes to how an individual might respond to a course of medication or a surgical intervention based on genetic differences in drug metabolism or wound healing. Over the next decade, a shift to personalized medicine will dramatically alter treatment plans and patient evaluations. This shift will be particularly true for those disorders that have a complex etiology such as clubfoot, scoliosis, arthritis, osteoporosis, and other disorders where the interaction of genetic and environmental factors (that may number in the dozens) makes studies of causes challenging. Progress has been made in the study of these more common disorders that will eventually lead to early diagnosis and more effective treatment.

For a patient to have the best care, it is important that the orthopaedic surgeon is aware of the genetic cause of the disease being treated. In addition, a familiarity with new knowledge is necessary for appropriate referrals for genetic counseling. Specific diagnoses based on genotype as well as phenotype will refine the prognosis for many disorders. Patients form a resource from which new knowledge is gained, and awareness of investigations in progress will allow physician collaboration with researchers. A single patient with a rare gene translocation or deletion can provide the key for identifying a disease-causing gene, as occurred in the search for the gene causing Duchenne muscular dystrophy. The orthopaedic surgeon's knowledge of primarily orthopaedic disorders can aid in the search for their causes. Accuracy in diagnosis in the patients studied is vital in the common approaches used for isolating disease-causing genes. Also, knowledge of the pathology of orthopaedic disorders can help in selecting appropriate candidate genes for investigation.

Information and searching services relevant to genetics is accessible on the Internet. This information ranges from clinically oriented services to specific information about the molecular biology of particular organisms such as yeast or the fruit fly. A few of these resources are listed in **Table 1**. This chapter will summarize current genetic in-

Table 1   Internet Resources Relevant to Genetics

Database	Function	Address
Online Mendelian Inheritance in Man (OMIM)	Provides profiles of specific disorders with clinical and gene mapping data Provides an extensive list of references Searchable using key words	http://www3.ncbi.nlm.nih.gov/omim/
The Human Genome Database (GDB)	A general collection of information about gene mapping, genetic polymorphisms, genetic and physical maps, and DNA sequences Connected to other related databases via links	http://gdbwww.gdb.org
Gene Tests	A public access database of laboratories doing research and/or clinical testing for specific disorders Provides contacts to arrange for genetic testing Provides information on groups involved in research on rare disorders	http://www.genetests.org

Table 2   Listing of Genes Identified as Causing Musculoskeletal Abnormalities With Their Associated Disorders and Gene Product Function

Gene	Disease	Gene Function
ARSE	Chondrodysplasia punctata X-linked	Unknown
ANKH	Premature osteoarthrosis with chondrocalcinosis	Transport molecule
Cathepsin K	Pycnodysostosis	
CBFA1	Cleidocranial dysplasia	Transcription molecule
C7orf2	Acheiropodia Preaxial polydactyly (some)?	Signaling molecule
COL1A1, COL1A2	Osteogenesis imperfecta I-IV	Structural molecule
COL2A1	Achondrogenesis II	Structural molecule
	Hypochondrogenesis	Structural molecule
	Kniest dysplasia	Structural molecule
	Precocious osteoarthrosis (one type)	Structural molecule
	Spondyloepiphyseal dysplasia congenital	Structural molecule
	Spondyloepimetaphyseal dysplasia	Structural molecule
	Stickler's syndrome 1	Structural molecule
COL9A2	Multiple epiphyseal dysplasias (EDM2) some cases	Structural molecule
COL10A1	Schmid metaphyseal chondrodysplasia,	Structural molecule
COL11A1	Stickler syndrome II (without eye findings)	Structural molecule
COL11A2	Stickler syndrome II	Structural molecule
	Otospondylomegaepiphyseal dysplasia (OSMED)	Structural molecule
COMP	Multiple epiphyseal dysplasia	Structural molecule
	(EDM2) some cases	Structural molecule
	Multiple epiphyseal dysplasia (EDM1)	Structural molecule
	Pseudoachondroplasia	Structural molecule
DHAPAT	Chondrodysplasia punctata type 2	Enzyme for structural synthesis
DTDST	Diastrophic dysplasia	Transport molecule
	Achondrogenesis 1B	Transport molecule
	Atelosteogenesis II	Transport molecule
	Meekeren-Ehlers-Danlos Syndrome (autosomal recessive)	Transport molecule
EBP	Chondrodysplasia punctata, x-linked type 2	Signaling pathway molecule
EVC	Ellis-Van Creveld syndrome	Unknown
FBLN1	Complex synpolydactyly (one form)	Structural molecule

Table 2 Listing of Genes Identified as Causing Musculoskeletal Abnormalities With Their Associated Disorders and Gene Product Function (cont)

Gene	Disease	Gene Function
FBLN1	Complex synpolydactyly (one form)	Structural molecule
FGFR3	Achondroplasia	Cell signaling molecule
	Hypochondroplasia	Cell signaling molecule
	Thanatophoric dysplasias I and II	Cell signaling molecule
FGFR2	Apert syndrome	Cell signaling molecule
	Jackson-Weiss syndrome	Cell signaling molecule
	Crouzon syndrome	Cell signaling molecule
	Pfeiffer syndrome (most)	Cell signaling molecule
	Antley-Bixler syndrome	Cell signaling molecule
FGFR1	Pfeiffer syndrome (some)	Cell signaling molecule
FLJ90130	Dyggve-Melchior-Clausen dysplasia	Unknown, probably cell signaling
GLI3	Greig cephalopolysyndactyly	Transcription factor
	Pallister-Hall syndrome	Transcription factor
	Postaxial polydactyly type A	Transcription factor
	Postaxial polydactyly A/B	Transcription factor
GJA1	Oculodentodigital dysplasia	Structural protein
	Preaxial polydactyly IV	Transcription factor
	Acrocallosal syndrome	Transcription factor
HOXA13	Hand-foot-genital syndrome	Transcription factor
HOXD13	Synpolydactyly	Transcription factor
	Brachydactyly D and E (some cases)	Transcription factor
IHH	Brachydactyly A1	Transcription factor
LMX1B	Nail-patella syndrome	Transcription factor
MATN3	Meekeren-Ehlers-Danlos syndrome (one type of autosomal dominant)	Structural molecule
	Hand osteoarthrosis (small percentage)	
MSX2	Boston-type craniosynostosis	Transcription factor
OFD1	Oral-facial-digital type I syndrome	Unknown
P63	Split hand-split foot (some of nonsyndromic cases)	Cell signaling protein
	Ectrodactyly-ectodermal dysplasia clefting syndrome	Cell signaling protein
	Ankyloblepharon-ectodermal dysplasia clefting syndrome	Cell signaling protein
	ADULT syndrome	Cell signaling protein
PEX7	Chondrodysplasia punctata type 1	Transcription factor
PTH-PTHrP	Jansen metaphyseal chondrodysplasia	Cell signaling protein
RMRP	McKusick metaphyseal chondrodysplasia	Enzyme for RNA processing
ROR2	Brachydactyly type B	Cell signaling protein
	Robinow syndrome	Cell signaling protein
SALL1	Townes-Brocks syndrome	Transcription factor
SEDL	X-linked spondyloepiphyseal dysplasia	Transport molecule
SK2	Spondyloepimetaphyseal dysplasia	Transcription factor
SHOX	Leri-Weill dyschondrosteosis	Transcription factor
	Idiopathic short stature (some cases)	Transcription factor
	Langer mesomelic dysplasia	Transcription factor
	Turner syndrome (part of the cause)	Transcription factor
SOST	Bone dysplasia sclerosteosis	??
SOX9	Campomelic dysplasia	Transcription factor
TBX3	Ulnar-mammary syndrome	Transcription factor
TBX5	Holt-Oram syndrome	Transcription factor
TGFB1	Camurati-Engelmann disease	Signaling molecule
TWIST	Saethre-Chotzen syndrome	Signaling molecule
WISP3	Spondyloepimetaphyseal dysplasia with progressive osteoarthropathy	??

formation about disorders with orthopaedic manifestations, which will include a discussion of disorders with specific skeletal manifestations, allelic disorders, metabolic bone diseases, connective tissue and neuromuscular disorders, and other conditions of interest to the orthopaedic surgeon.

Skeletal Dysplasias and Disorders With Specific Skeletal Manifestations

A nearly complete listing (as of the time of manuscript preparation) of disorders with musculoskeletal manifestations whose genetic cause is known is presented in Table 2. Only the more common and/or orthopaedically relevant disorders will be discussed in more detail in this chapter.

Fibroblast Growth Factor Receptor 3 Disorders

Four fibroblast growth factor receptors (FGFRs) have been identified. They participate in complex signaling pathways involving the various fibroblast growth factors (FGFs) (their ligands) and heparan sulfate proteoglycans. These pathways are critical in developmental biology. The FGFRs regulate cell replication, growth, differentiation, and migration. Their function in homeostasis in the mature organism is not well defined. Only two disorders have been identified for a mutation in an FGF (probably because most FGF mutations are not compatible with embryonic development), but many have been defined for three of the four identified FGFRs.

The four FGFRs differ in their distribution in body tissues and the strength of their affinity for different FGFs. The FGFRs are similar in that all have three extracellular immunoglobulin-like domains, a single transmembrane domain, and two intracellular tyrosine kinase domains. Binding of the ligand results in phosphorylation of the tyrosine kinase domain, which initiates signal transduction within the cell.

All FGFR disorders are inherited as autosomal dominant traits and all involve gain of function—that is, the receptors are active without ligand binding or are overactive when ligand binding occurs. Specific mutations result in differences in genotype that result in phenotypes of varying characteristics and severity.

Achondroplasia

Achondroplasia, the most common form of dwarfism, is an autosomal dominant disorder. Most affected individuals represent new mutations. People with achondroplasia often have varus deformity of the legs and are at risk for atlantoaxial instability and spinal stenosis. Achondroplasia is caused by a point mutation in the gene coding for FGFR3 This mutation is almost always at the same nucleotide (nucleotide number 1138) and causes a single

amino acid change (arginine to glycine) in the transmembrane portion of this cell surface receptor. This receptor is expressed in all prebone cartilage as well as diffusely in the central nervous system. The remarkable homogeneity of the phenotype in achondroplasia results from the remarkable homogeneity of the mutation in this disorder. No other autosomal dominant disorder whose gene defect is known has such a homogeneous mutation. This is the most mutable single nucleotide known in the entire human genome. DNA testing for the common mutations is clinically available.

The function of FGFR3 has been studied in mice by disrupting the normal gene. FGFR3-deficient mice have elongated vertebral columns and long bone because of accelerated and prolonged growth compared with normal mice. Malfunction of FGFR3 causes inhibition of chondrocyte proliferation in the proliferative zone of the physis. Thus, FGFR3 seems to regulate bone growth by limiting endochondral ossification. A possible explanation for the dwarfing phenotype in humans with an abnormal gene for FGFR3 is that the human mutation results in a receptor that is active even without the binding of a FGF ligand to the receptor. The receptor function in limiting endochondral ossification is overactive (a gain of function mutation).

Hypochondroplasia

Hypochondroplasia is similar to achondroplasia, but affected individuals experience milder dwarfing and their skulls and facies are normal. Associated conditions, such as spinal stenosis and severe genu varum, are less common in patients with hypochondroplasia. Sixty percent of patients studied have a mutation of the *FGFR3* gene. The mutation in hypochondroplasia affects the first tyrosine kinase domain, which is intracellular, instead of the transmembrane domain of FGFR3 found in achondroplasia. A gain of function mutation occurs with increased tyrosine phosphorylation. Gain of function mutations result when the gene mutation causes unregulated production of the gene product. Forty percent of individuals with the hypochondroplasia phenotype do not have the typical mutation. In some individuals with hypochondroplasia, a *FGFR3* mutation has been excluded, implicating genetic heterogeneity for the hypochondroplasia phenotype.

Thanatophoric Dysplasia Types I and II

Thanatophoric dysplasia types I and II, the most common neonatal lethal skeletal dysplasias, are also caused by mutations of the *FGFR3* gene. This association was suggested by a phenotypic similarity between thanatophoric dysplasia and homozygous achondroplasia. Most reported mutations in thanatophoric dysplasia type I occur in the extra cellular portion of the FGFR3 receptor between the second and third immunoglobulin loops or between the third immunoglobulin loop and the transmembrane por-

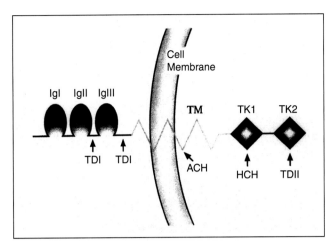

Figure 1 IgI, IgII, and IgIII are extracellular immunoglobulin-like domains. TM is the transmembrane domain. TK1 and TK2 are the tryosine kinase domains. The common sites for mutations causing achondroplasia (ACH), hypochondroplasia (HCH), and thanatophoric dysplasias I and II are labeled with arrows

tion of the protein. Thanatophoric dysplasia type II is caused by mutations in the second intracellular tyrosine kinase domain (Figure 1).

Craniosynostosis

Although most syndromes with craniosynostosis are caused by a mutation in FGFR1 or FGFR2, nonsyndromic craniosynostosis is caused by a mutation of FGFR3. This syndrome has been defined in 61 individuals from 20 unrelated families, all of whom have a single amino acid substitution. All affected individuals have coronal synostosis. Variable features include abnormalities of the hands and feet, including syndactyly, brachydactyly, thimble-like middle phalanges, cone epiphyses, and carpal and tarsal fusions. A small number of individuals have developmental delay and/or sensorineural hearing loss. Affected individuals have normal stature, a factor that differentiates this disorder from other known FGFR3 disorders. The mutation occurs between the second and third immunoglobulin-like domains of the FGFR3 protein, which is analogous to the location of mutations in FGFR 1 and 2, which cause Pfeiffer and Apert syndromes, respectively.

Other rare disorders caused by FGFR3 mutations include Crouzon syndrome with acanthosis nigricans, platyspondylic lethal dysplasia—San Diego type, and severe achondroplasia with developmental delay and acanthosis nigricans.

FGFR2 Disorders

Several disorders with premature fusion of the cranial suture and variable anomalies of the hands and feet are caused by mutation of the gene for FGFR2; for example, autosomal dominant disorders such as Apert, Jackson-

Weiss, Crouzon, and most Pfeiffer syndromes. Of these disorders, Apert syndrome has the most extensive syndactyly of the fingers and toes. Specific mutations within the *FGFR2* gene have been correlated with different phenotypes, both between diseases and for different phenotypes within diseases, such as the severity of syndactyly and cleft palate in Apert syndrome. New mutations in 57 families with Apert syndrome were all found to be of paternal origin, which explains the paternal age effect for new mutations causing Apert syndrome. Antley-Bixler syndrome is a severe form of craniosynostosis and is characterized by radiohumeral synostosis and femoral bowing. Many patients have severe respiratory distress that results in early death. FGFR2 mutations have been identified in some of these patients. Some also have a defect in steroid biosynthesis, suggesting a possible digenic cause of this syndrome.

Pfeiffer syndrome is sometimes caused by a mutation in FGFR1. Boston-type craniosynostosis has been shown to be caused by mutations in the *MSX2* gene—a DNA transcription factor called a homeobox gene.

Cartilage Oligomeric Matrix Protein Disorders

Cartilage oligomeric matrix protein (COMP), an extracellular protein with seven calcium-binding regions, is present in high levels in developing bone and tendon.

COMP is normally involved in cartilage cell proliferation and migration through calcium-dependent proteoglycan binding. COMP is made of five identical protein chains that are assembled into a bouquet-like structure. Therefore, a single mutation results in only 3% of COMP molecules having five normal subunits. This causes the "dominant negative" effect of a mutation in one allele on COMP function.

Pseudoachondroplasia

Pseudoachondroplasia is one of the more common skeletal dysplasias and is characterized by disproportionate short-limbed dwarfism and ligamentous laxity. Pseudoachondroplasia is not clinically apparent at birth, although platyspondyly is evident on radiographs. Growth retardation becomes apparent between 1 and 3 years of age. The disproportionate limb shortness increases with growth. The hands and feet are short and broad. The facies are normal, but patients with pseudoachondroplasia tend to have similar features.

Electron microscopy shows dilated rough endoplasmic reticulum containing material that shows a laminar structure in epiphyseal and physeal chondrocytes. Immunostaining suggests that this material includes proteoglycan link protein and aggrecan. A single patient has been studied showing retention in the rough endoplasmic reticulum of COMP, fibromodulin, decorin, and collagen types IX, XI, and XII. The cause of this disorder is a mutation in the calmodulin-like calcium binding region of the gene coding for COMP. The mutations causing pseudoachondroplasia are deletions or alterations causing important changes in protein structure as a result of improper folding of the molecule. This protein is present at high levels in the territorial matrix of cartilage. The mechanism by which this defective gene causes pseudoachondroplasia is probably through an increase in cell death of physeal chondrocytes as well as by defective collagen assembly in the extraterritorial matrix of cartilage and tendon. Although most instances of pseudoachondroplasia are new mutations, it is a dominant disorder because of the pentameric structure of COMP.

Multiple Epiphyseal Dysplasia Type I

Multiple epiphyseal dysplasia denotes a group of disorders with dysplasia of the epiphyses of the tubular bones and normal or near-normal vertebrae. Dwarfing is mild and presentation varies from childhood (a waddling gait and difficulties with running or stair climbing) to adulthood (premature osteoarthrosis). Pain, limp, or decreased range of motion in the weight-bearing joints prompt evaluation.

Several disorders with different causes are subsumed under the multiple epiphyseal dysplasia label. The cause of one type that shows dilated rough endoplasmic reticulum with lamellar inclusions (similar to those seen in pseudoachondroplasia) is known. It is a mutation in the gene coding for COMP. The mutations occur in the calmodulin-like domain as in pseudoachondroplasia, but appear to cause a more subtle structural alteration in the protein. Different types of mutations in the *COMP* gene result in the differing phenotypes of these two disorders. Also, analysis of different mutations consists of clarifying the phenotypic variation within both the pseudoachondroplasia and multiple epiphyseal dysplasia disorders.

Autosomal dominant multiple epiphyseal dysplasia phenotype is also caused by a mutation in the gene coding for the alpha 1, 2, and 3 polypeptide chains of collagen type IX. Collagen IX is located on the surface of collagen II fibrils. Because defects in collagen IX cause early, noninflammatory articular cartilage degeneration in both humans and mice, it is hypothesized that collagen IX is essential in the long-term integrity of articular cartilage. Another autosomal dominant form of multiple epiphyseal dysplasia is caused by mutation of the *MATN3* gene, which encodes matrilin-3, a oligomeric protein expressed in cartilage extracellular matrix. Families with autosomal recessive inheritance who have the multiple epiphyseal dysplasia phenotype have been identified with mutations in the diastrophic dysplasia sulfate transporter gene.

Precocious Osteoarthrosis

A four-generation family with precocious osteoarthrosis without short stature or brachydactyly has been identified with a mutation in the *COMP* gene. Serum levels of COMP are being investigated as a marker for susceptibility to osteoarthrosis. Serum COMP levels have been found to be significantly higher in patients with symptoms of hip osteoarthrosis (before radiographic findings of osteoarthritis) than in control patients. The difference between skeletal dysplasias and milder forms of osteochondral dysfunction that were previously considered variations of normal is becoming less clear. Identification of a continuous spectrum of disorders based on mutations of varying severity is currently underway.

Type II Collagen Disorders

Type II collagen is the major structural component of cartilage. It is composed of water, proteoglycans, and types IX and XI collagen (which bind to the surface of type II collagen) as well as other matrix components. Different mutations of type II collagen cause different chondrodysplasias of varying severity. Single codon mutations causing a substitution for glycine in the triple helix cause one half of the reported mutations in human disorders. Glycine, the smallest amino acid, is normally present as every third amino acid in the restricted space at the center of the type II collagen triple helix. Substitution by bulkier amino acids disrupts the integrity of the collagen fibril. The perinatally lethal type II collagen disorders usually have such a substitution for glycine. Other mutations are caused by duplications, deletions, insertions, or premature stop codons, which often cause a quantitative defect in type II collagen rather than a severe structural defect.

The type II collagen disorders (also called type II collagenopathies or the spondyloepiphyseal dysplasia family of osteochondrodysplasias) are named descriptively based on phenotypic or radiographic features. Some are commonly referred to by eponym. A better understanding of the cause of these disorders will lead to improved classification in the near future. Families of chondrodysplasias are being defined because all the members possess the same known or presumed abnormal gene. The type II collagen family denotes a group of allelic chondrodysplasias that are caused by different mutations in the gene coding for type II collagen. The most severe disorders in this family are the perinatally lethal achondrogenesis type II disorders and hypochondrogenesis. Spondyloepiphyseal dysplasia congenital, Kniest type spondyloepiphyseal dysplasia, Stickler syndrome, and precocious osteoarthropathy are progressively milder disorders.

Spondyloepiphyseal Dysplasia Congenita

Spondyloepiphyseal dysplasia congenita is a clinically heterogeneous disorder that is evident at birth and is characterized by disproportionate short trunk dwarfing. The facies show mild midface flattening. The neck is short and the chest is barrel-shaped. There is usually a thoracolumbar kyphosis with excessive lordosis in children of walking age. Rhizomelic shortening of the limbs is present with fairly normal hands and feet. The vertebral bodies are ovoid in the newborn and become markedly flattened with irregular end plates during childhood. The iliac bones are short and square. The tubular bones are short with mild metaphyseal irregularity. The epiphyses show delayed ossification and are usually fragmented in appearance. These changes are most pronounced in the capital femoral epiphyses. The features of spondyloepiphyseal dysplasia become more apparent with growth. Biochemical investigations of individuals with spondyloepiphyseal dysplasia congenita have shown abnormal α1(II) chains that form triple helical fibrils but make structurally abnormal type II collagen, resulting in a moderately severe phenotype.

X-Linked Spondyloepiphyseal Dysplasia

Patients with x-linked spondyloepiphyseal dysplasia tarda have disproportionately short stature at age 5 to 10 years, with severe degenerative changes of the spine and hips during middle age. The condition is caused by mutations in a gene encoding the protein sedlin. This gene is expressed in many tissues, including fetal cartilage, and may have a role in vesicular transport from the endoplasmic reticulum to the Golgi apparatus. The reason that phenotypic expression is limited to cartilage tissue is unknown.

Spondyloepiphyseal Dysplasia With Progressive Osteoarthropathy

Spondyloepiphyseal dysplasia with progressive osteoarthropathy (also called progressive pseudorheumatoid dysplasia) mimics polyarticular juvenile rheumatoid arthritis and is caused by *WISP3*, a gene encoding a cystine-rich protein involved in cell growth and differentiation. Its function in cartilage growth and/or homeostasis is unknown.

Kniest Type Spondyloepiphyseal Dysplasia

Kniest type spondyloepiphyseal dysplasia or metatrophic dwarfism type II is characterized by short stature, a disproportionately short trunk, kyphoscoliosis, enlarged and stiff joints, cleft palate, hearing loss, and a flat nasal bridge. Multiple mutations that cause the Kniest phenotype have been identified. Disrupted triple helix formation, abnormal fibril formation, and significant errors in α1(II) chain formation have been found.

Stickler Syndrome

Stickler syndrome (hereditary arthro-ophthalmopathy) is an autosomal dominant disorder that is characterized by myopia, vitreoretinal degeneration, retinal detachment, and premature osteoarthritis. Approximately two thirds of families with this phenotype have a mutation of the type II collagen gene. Mutations causing this form of Stickler syndrome typically result in a premature stop codon causing a truncated type II collagen chain. This results in a quantitative decrease in type II collagen, rather than an increase in abnormal type II collagen molecules seen in other more severe type II collagenopathies.

Stickler syndrome without eye involvement is caused by a gene coding for type XI collagen. This collagen is a minor fibrillar collagen important in determining type II collagen fiber diameter and orientation. Given the biologically intimate association between types II and XI collagen, it is not surprising that certain mutations in either gene result in a similar phenotype. Refined classification based on the gene mutation will enhance diagnostic and prognostic accuracy in individuals with Stickler syndrome.

Osteoarthrosis

That osteoarthrosis is hereditary has been long recognized. That some people will never develop osteoarthrosis, barring trauma or infection, is also clear. The age of onset of nontraumatic osteoarthrosis varies greatly. Osteoarthrosis has been considered a multifactorial disorder; a combination of genetic predisposition and unknown environmental factors is believed to be the cause. In a prospective epidemiologic study of patients undergoing total joint replacement of the hip or knee, the heritability of primary osteoarthritis was assessed by comparing siblings of the probands with the probands' spouses. The siblings were at significantly higher risk of osteoarthritis than were spouses with a heritability estimate of 27% in this population. Stronger evidence comes from a study of 500 female twins age 45 to 70 years. Radiographically proven osteoarthritis was twice as common in the 130 monozygotic twins compared with the 120 dizygotic twins. The genetic contribution to the likelihood of developing osteoarthrosis was estimated to be 35% to 65% in this study.

One reason that disorders with nonmendelian inheritance patterns may be categorized as multifactorial is the mixing of several different disorders, with different causes and inheritance patterns. It is important to be as specific about the phenotype that causes inclusion in a group as possible. Although all end-stage arthritic joints look alike, perhaps individuals who develop arthrosis in the second to fifth decades have a different etiology than those who develop arthritic joints in their 70s or 80s. This concept appears to be true in osteoarthrosis.

Familial, generalized precocious osteoarthrosis has been associated with a mutation in the gene coding for collagen II in several large families. Furthermore, a small percentage of primary osteoarthrosis results from a rare allele coding for type II collagen that causes reduced gene expression. Some occurrence of premature osteoarthrosis accompanied by chondrocalcinosis is caused by a mutation in the *ANKH* gene. This gene is the human homolog to a mouse gene that causes a severe form of joint calcification and arthritis. Distal interphalangeal joint osteoarthritis has been linked to a region on chromosome 2q and psoriatic arthritis has been linked to chromosome 16q (with evidence of paternal transmission only, suggesting an imprinting effect). Although specific genetic causes have been identified for only a small proportion of patients with osteoarthrosis, discovery of involved genes will provide diagnostic, prognostic, and therapeutic insights. Much of what is now considered primary osteoarthrosis may have a detectable genetic cause or predisposition.

Diastrophic Dysplasia Sulfate Transporter Disorders

The diastrophic dysplasia sulfate transporter gene (*DTDST*) mediates sulfate entry into chondrocytes. *DTDST* has 12 membrane-spanning domains and, although it is expressed in many tissues, it appears to have two distinct forms in cartilage cells. Cartilage requires properly sulfated glycosaminoglycan side chains for normal proteoglycan function, which is impaired by *DTDST* mutations. *DTDST* mutations also appear to blunt the normal cellular response to FGFs, which may help account for the often severe phenotypes.

Diastrophic Dysplasia

Diastrophic dysplasia is a well-characterized skeletal dysplasia; characteristics include short limbs, short stature, kyphoscoliosis, generalized joint dysplasia with limitation of finger flexion, hitchhiker thumbs, and foot deformities ranging from the more common valgus of the hindfoot and adductus of the forefoot to clubfeet. The joint abnormalities associated with this disorder result in painful osteoarthrosis at an early age. These patients, who are of normal intelligence, are severely handicapped by their joint abnormalities. Although there is increased mortality in infancy, life span after that time is not markedly decreased. Diastrophic dysplasia is caused by a mutation in a gene coding for a sulfate transporter protein located on chromosome 5. The sulfate transporter function of the gene product was suggested by protein sequence analysis that showed an amino acid sequence similar to that of known sulfate transporter proteins, and was supported by greatly diminished sulfate uptake in skin fibroblasts from a patient with diastrophic dysplasia.

In normal cartilage, proper sulfation and a sufficient negative charge are necessary for proteoglycans to function properly. There is evidence that the sulfation of proteoglycans is sensitive to both extracellular and intracellular sulfate concentrations. A defect in the sulfate transporter protein could easily explain the defective cartilage in this disorder. The gene responsible for the synthesis of this protein is expressed in virtually all cell types. That its effects are most pronounced in cartilage-producing cells may simply be because of the greater requirement for sulfate for proteoglycan synthesis in cartilage than in other tissues. Specifically, a defect in sulfate transport across the cell membrane results in inadequate intracellular sulfate and undersulfation of proteoglycans.

Atelosteogenesis Type II/Achondrogenesis Type 1B

Mutations of the diastrophic dysplasia sulfate transporter also have been found to cause the neonatally lethal achondrogenesis type IB and atelosteogenesis type II disorders. The most severe cases of diastrophic dysplasia overlap phenotypically and by mutation analysis with atelosteogenesis type II. The severity of these three autosomal recessive chondrodysplasias correlates well with the severity of dysfunction of DTDST protein that is predicted by mutation analysis.

Multiple Epiphyseal Dysplasia (Autosomal Recessive Type)

The relatively mild phenotype seen in multiple epiphyseal dysplasia (autosomal recessive) results from a different gene mutation than found in the other disorders.

SHOX Gene Disorders

The short stature homeobox-containing gene (*SHOX*) encodes several isoforms of a transcription factor (containing a homeodomain) and is important in limb development. *SHOX* maps to the pseudoautosomal region of the X and Y chromosomes. Idiopathic short stature, Leri-Weill dyschondrosteosis (bilateral Madelung's deformity and mesomelic short stature), and Turner's syndrome (XO) all have one nonfunctional copy of the *SHOX* gene; this is usually because of microdeletions (except in Turner's syndrome where the entire copy from the Y chromosome is missing), although point mutations have been described. Langer mesomelic dysplasia is a severe mesomelic dwarfing condition with marked hypoplasia of the ulna, fibula, and mandible, with a normal trunk. This condition results from a homozygous mutation of the *SHOX* gene, causing complete *SHOX* deficiency. This homozygous mutation explains the autosomal recessive inheritance of Langer mesomelic dysplasia as opposed to the autosomal dominant inheritance of Leri-Weill dyschondrosteosis.

p63 Disorders

p63 is a member of a family of proteins involved in regulating cell proliferation, apoptosis, and differentiation by sensing multiple inputs to cells. p63 is expressed in the basal layer of several epithelial tissues, including the epidermis and urogenital tract. It has been shown to have a critical role in the formation and differentiation of the apical ectodermal ridge, which is required for normal limb outgrowth and patterning. These are autosomal dominant mutations that act through gain of function, loss of function, or change in function effect. The five syndromes described are caused by specific mutation of p63, giving a strong though not perfect genotype-phenotype correlation.

Specific Syndromes

Approximately 10% of nonsyndromic split hand-split foot malformation (also called ectrodactyly or lobster claw deformity) is caused by p63 mutation. Two additional loci have been identified for this genetically heterogeneous disorder but the specific genes have not been identified. Almost all instances of ectrodactyly-ectodermal dysplasia-clefting syndrome (EEC syndrome) are caused by a mutation resulting in a small number of amino acid substitutions in the DNA binding region of p63. Ankyloblepharon-ectodermal dysplasia-clefting syndrome is characterized by ectodemal dysplasia that is more severe than in EEC, cleft lip with or without cleft palate, and generally minimal or absent limb deformity. Limb-mammary syndrome is characterized by ectrodactyly and hypoplastic or absent mammary glands and nipples. ADULT (acro-dermato-ungual-lacrimal-tooth) syndrome has many overlapping features with EEC and is characterized by ectrodactyly, syndactyly, nail dysplasia, hypoplastic mammary glands, underdeveloped teeth, and intense freckling. These allelic deformities support the search for single gene causes of disorders with clinically similar features.

HOX Gene Disorders

HOX genes are the human homolog of the basic body segment patterning genes in fruit flies. The *HOX* genes are DNA binding transcription factors and are critical in the development and patterning of the axial skeleton, limbs, central nervous system, urogenital tract, genitalia, and gut. The 39 human *HOX* genes are labeled *HOXA*, *HOXB*, *HOXC*, and *HOXD* for the anterior to posterior positioning of different clusters of genes in the developing limb. They are further identified with numbers, such as *HOXA 3* and *HOXB 5*, to describe similar genes within the larger clusters. The *HOX* clusters are expressed in an overlapping and nested fashion with complex feedback loops in the developing limb and are necessary for proper tissue differentiation and patterning. Three human disorders resulting from *HOX* gene mutations have been identified. It is surprising that mutations in such fundamental genes for development result in relatively mild phenotypes. It seems likely that redundancy of functions might exist in these very important genes and, also, that many mutations are not compatible with embryonic development.

Synpolydactyly is an autosomal dominant disorder characterized by syndactyly between the middle and ring fingers and between the fourth and fifth toes with variable presence of hypoplastic digit duplications in the webs. Almost all instances of this condition result from a polyala-

nine tract expansion in *HOXD 13*. These expansions are stable in size within families (as opposed to trinucleotide repeats) and act by disrupting normal protein-protein interactions. Deletions causing frame shifts have been identified in a few families who have atypical foot deformities for this condition. Hand-foot-genital syndrome is characterized by short thumbs and great toes, urinary tract malformation and hypospadias in males/müllerian duct fusion defects in females. This autosomal dominant disorder is commonly caused by a *HOXA 13* nonsense mutation, although polyalanine repeat expansions have been reported. In one study, a single child born with mutations of both *HOXA 13* and *HOXD 13* demonstrated more severe digital anomalies than patients with only one mutation, suggesting that these genes act synergistically. Guttmacher syndrome has features similar to hand-foot-genital syndrome but differs in the occurrence of postaxial polydactyly of the hands and uniphalangeal second toes. This may be a distinct entity and would then be a third *HOX* gene disorder in humans.

Another cause of one form of complex synpolydactyly is a mutation in the fibulin-1 gene (*FBLN1*). *FBLN1* encodes a protein that is expressed in the extracellular matrix in the developing digits. Normal digital development is partially dependent on the influence of the extracellular matrix in determining cell fates.

GLI 3 Disorders

GLI 3 is a DNA-binding transcription factor expressed in the interdigital mesenchyme and joint-forming regions of the digits as well as being part of the sonic hedgehog-patched-GLI pathway. This pathway is an evolutionarily conserved pathway that has been adapted to many functions that are critical in development. It functions in embryonic development of the notochord, neural tube, brain, limb (including the critical zone of polarizing activity, which specifies AP axis in the limb bud), and gut.

There are 119 human disorders with origins primarily or exclusively related to polydactyly, and 39 causative genes have been identified. Six polydactyly disorders are caused by mutations in the *GLI 3* gene: postaxial polydactyly A/B, postaxial polydactyly A, preaxial polydactyly IV, Greig cephalopolysyndactyly syndrome (postaxial polysyndactyly of hands, preaxial polysyndactyly of feet, and dysmorphic facies), Pallister-Hall syndrome (congenital hypothalamic hypopituitarism, imperforate anus, polydactyly, and various visceral anomalies), and acrocallosal syndrome (postaxial polydactyly, hallux duplication, macrocephaly, absence of the corpus callosum). Sonic hedgehog uses cholesterol as a carrier molecule, and Smith-Lemli-Opitz syndrome, which has defective cholesterol synthesis, is characterized by polydactyly and brachydactyly.

The brachydactylies (BDA) consist of a group of autosomal dominant inherited disorders of the hands that have been categorized clinically by the pattern of digital involvement into five major types, A through E. A causative gene has been found for some patients with four of the phenotypes (types A, B, D, and E). BDA type A is characterized by shortening of the middle phalanges. BDA type A1 (there are two other A subtypes) has distal or terminal symphalangism and is caused by a mutation in the indian hedgehog gene (*IHH*). Indian hedgehog is a member of the hedgehog proteins, morphogens that regulate the patterning of many embryonic structures including the limbs. Indian hedgehog is expressed in developing cartilage.

BDA type B is characterized by shortening of the distal phalanges, nail dysplasia, hypoplastic middle phalanges, and variable proximal and distal symphalangism. Mutations of *ROR2* (an orphan receptor tyrosine kinase) cause this disorder. ROR2 is a transmembrane tyrosine kinase receptor that is necessary for normal chondrocyte differentiation. Knockout mice lacking this gene have severely foreshortened and deformed skeletons and abnormal growth plates. The autosomal recessive Robinow's syndrome (generalized limb shortening, segmental defects of the spine, brachydactyly and typical, abnormal facies) is also cause by an *ROR2* mutation. This mutation in Robinow's syndrome results in complete absence ROR2 activity.

BDA type D is characterized by a broad, short terminal thumb phalanx and BDA type E is characterized by shortening confined to the metacarpals. Families with both these phenotypes have been found; the condition is caused by specific mutations in the *HOXD 13* gene, which was previously discussed.

Brachydactyly is also a consistent feature, along with short stature and obesity that is characteristic of Albright hereditary osteodystrophy. More than half of affected patients have heterotopic ossification and some have end organ resistance to parathyroid hormone, resulting in pseudohypoparathyroidism; other patients with normal endocrine function are said to have pseudopseudohypoparathyroidism. Albright hereditary osteodystrophy is caused by a mutation in the gene *GNAS1*.

Miscellaneous syndromes with bone and joint abnormalities are outlined in **Table 3**.

Metabolic Bone Diseases
Osteoporosis
Osteoporosis affects many individuals and remains a public health concern. Femoral neck fracture caused by senile osteoporosis continues to result in a high rate of mortality. Peak bone mass is a major determinant of the occurrence of osteoporosis. Multiple nongenetic factors, including exercise, drug use, alcohol intake, nutrition (including calcium intake), and smoking, are important in determining peak bone mass. Twin studies suggest that 80% of the variation among individuals' bone density is genetic.

In Tamai and associates' study of Caucasians of Anglo-Irish background living in Australia, it was shown that the genetic contribution to peak bone mass can be explained by differing alleles for the gene coding for the receptor for 1,25 dihydroxyvitamin D. Other studies have not found an association between vitamin D receptor genotype and osteoporosis, or have found a minor effect that is overwhelmed by other variables such as obesity. This same study found a correlation between bone mineral density and vitamin D receptor genotype in nonobese postmenopausal women, but not in obese postmenopausal women. Twin studies comparing bone mineral density and vitamin D receptor genotype found that dizygotic twins sharing the same vitamin D receptor genotype are similar to monozygotic twins and different from dizygotic twins not sharing the same vitamin D receptor genotype, with respect to bone mineral density. Susceptibility to osteoporosis in some families is associated with specific polymorphisms in estrogen receptor 1, calcitonin receptor, and type I collagen alpha 1 chain. Linkage studies have suggested several other susceptibility loci for which no specific gene has been identified.

Although a genetic influence seems likely, there are methodologic issues that make all associations reported to date tentative. It must be established that the alleles associated with low bone mass are the proximate cause and not merely a chance association with some other process that actually results in low bone mass. If different alleles coding for this vitamin D receptor (or different alleles in other genes affecting bone turnover such as TGF-α1) result in clinically important differences in peak bone mass, specific allele identification could be used clinically to identify a population at particular risk early in life. This population could be targeted for aggressive prophylactic treatment and education before bone mass falls below the critical level necessary to avoid osteoporotic fractures.

Hypophosphatemic Rickets
The most common cause of vitamin D-resistant rickets is X-linked hypophosphatemic rickets. This disorder causes short stature, lower extremity deformities, and bone pain. A decrease in proximal tubular resorption of phosphate causing hypophosphatemia causes the disorder. Recent evidence indicates that an intrinsic renal defect is not responsible for this disorder but rather a humeral factor is produced that actively induces phosphate wasting. This has been shown by performing transplant experiments in an analogous disorder in mice. Normal kidneys transplanted into mice with X-linked hypophosphatemia waste phosphate; kidneys from phosphate-wasting mice function normally in normal mice. Furthermore, the gene in humans that codes for the sodium phosphate transport protein is on chromosome 5; X-linked hypophosphatemic rickets has been linked to an area of the X chromosome (the X P 22.1 region).

A gene called *PEX* (phosphate regulating gene with homologies to endopeptidases, on the X chromosome) was identified by linkage studies and confirmed by mutation analysis to cause hypophosphatemic rickets. Not all families studied have shown mutations in this gene. The gene has not been completely characterized; therefore, mutations in some families may have been missed. PEX is similar to a class of endopeptidases that function to activate or inactivate hormones. The tissue of origin of PEX and its possible target hormone have not been identified.

The rare autosomal dominant form of hypophosphatemic rickets is caused by mutations in the *FGF23* gene. The only other reported human disease from a FGF is autosomal dominant cerebral ataxia caused by a *FGF14* mutation.

Connective Tissue Disorders

Type I Fibrillinopathies

Marfan syndrome is an autosomal dominant disorder affecting 1 in 10,000 to 20,000 people. The expression of the disorder is variable within and among different families. Several named variants with phenotype similarity include severe neonatal Marfan syndrome, dominantly inherited ectopia lentis, isolated skeletal features of Marfan syndrome, and Shprintzen-Goldberg syndrome. Typical Marfan syndrome is characterized by dolichostenomelia (long, thin limbs), pectus excavatum or carinatum, scoliosis, high and narrow palate, ectopia lentis, myopia, dilatation of the ascending aorta, aortic dissection, and dural ectasia. Because of the wide distribution of affected tissues, a connective tissue defect was suspected for decades.

In 1991 the defective gene causing Marfan syndrome, located on chromosome 15, was found to encode for fibrillin (FBN1). Fibrillin is a large glycoprotein that is a structural component of elastin-containing microfibrils and is present in many tissues. The gene defect usually results in decreased amounts of fibrillin and, presumably, a structurally weakened elastin. The gene mutations occur throughout this large gene and are usually unique to the affected individual. Clear genotype/phenotype correlations are not apparent except for a clustering of mutations causing the severe, neonatal forms in a specific region of the gene. The entire gene has been sequenced and gene-based diagnosis is now possible through research laboratories.

A second, distinct, fibrillin protein is coded for by a gene on chromosome 5 (*FBN2*). An autosomal dominant disorder, congenital contractural arachnodactyly, has the same skeletal features as Marfan syndrome; but joints are contracted instead of loose. This disorder is caused by a mutation in the fibrillin gene on chromosome 5.

Osteogenesis Imperfecta

With rare exceptions, osteogenesis imperfecta is an autosomal dominant disorder caused by a mutation in either of the two chains that form type I collagen. Two copies of the α1 chain (coded for on chromosome 17) and one copy of the α2 chain (coded for on chromosome 7) form a triple helix approximately 1,000 amino acids long with repeated triplets of glycine-X-Y. Three triple helices wind around each other to form a superhelix. Type I collagen is the predominant structural protein in bone and connective tissue. Clinically, osteogenesis imperfecta is classified as type I, mild; type II, perinatally lethal; type III, progressively deforming; and type IV, moderately severe (between types I and III in severity).

Most type I disease (mild) is caused by mutations that result in type I collagen that is not incorporated into the collagen fibril. The phenotype results from a diminished quantity of collagen I being formed. The mutated messenger RNA is rapidly degraded and does not, therefore, result in the formation of structurally abnormal collagen. Most mutations (about 85%) are point mutations that cause a substitution for the repeated glycine amino acid. Severe phenotypes result from the incorporation of structurally abnormal chains into the collagen fibril, resulting in ubiquitous, abnormal collagen I. Similar to the situation with achondroplasia and Apert syndrome, many severe forms of osteogenesis imperfecta (types II and III) result from new, dominantly acting mutations often arising in the paternal germ line. In rare cases, clinically unaffected parents may be germ line mosaics for a predisposing mutation so that the risk of a subsequent affected child is greater (1% to 5%) than the new mutation rate alone.

Two approaches to gene therapy are being actively explored in cell culture and/or animal models. Bone marrow transplantation holds some promise for increasing the amount of normal type I collagen. Antisense therapy seeks to form complementary molecules that will bind with the mutated RNA, thus stopping expression of the abnormal chain. This would result in a diminished amount of type I collagen and would seek to transform severe phenotypes into the type I, mild phenotype.

Ehlers-Danlos Syndromes

Ehlers-Danlos syndromes (EDS) are a heterogeneous group of disorders characterized by laxity and weakness of the dermis, ligaments, and blood vessels. Nine clinical and genetic subtypes have been described and all, whose etiology is known, are caused by mutations in fibrillar collagen genes or genes for enzymes that modify the fibrillar collagens.

EDS I is an autosomal dominant condition characterized by lax joints, hyperextensible skin, and wide, atrophic scars. EDS II is a milder form with the same clinical characteristics. Both disorders result from mutation of the gene coding for collagen V. Collagen V is coexpressed with collagen I in many tissues and is important for proper formation of collagen I fibrils.

Table 3 Miscellaneous Syndromes With Bone and Joint Abnormalities

Syndrome	Clinical Characteristics	Inheritance	Gene	Gene Characteristic
Acheiropodia	Bilateral congenital amputations of the upper and lower extremities with aplasia of the hands and feet	Autosomal recessive	C7orf2	C7orf2 is the human ortholog of the mouse gene Lmbr1, which is expressed in the developing limb Mutations in mice cause preaxial polydactyly-like mutant A decrease in expression of these genes may allow ectopic anterior expression of sonic hedgehog (a key-axis determining gene) C7orf2 mutation may cause preaxial polydactyly in humans as well as the much more severe acheiropodia.
Bone dysplasia sclerosteosis	A sclerosing bone dysplasia with over-growth throughout life causing gigantism Syndactyly is inconsistent feature	Autosomal recessive	SOST	SOST encodes a novel protein with characteristics of a class of "cystine-knot" factors Expressed in long bones and cartilage Is apparently a new, important regulator of bone growth
Camptomelic dysplasia	Short and bowed long bones Genetic males show sex reversal. Usually lethal in infancy because of tracheomalacia and respiratory failure	Autosomal dominant	SOX9 (SYR-related box gene)	SOX9 encodes a transcription factor that has strong similarity to SYR, which is located on the Y chromosome and determines male gender. SOX9 regulates transcription of the anti-müllerian hormone gene (accounting for the sex reversal) Regulates type II collagen formation in the precartilage mesenchymal anlage of bones.
Camurati-Engelmann disease	Progressive gene dysplasia with sclerosis and hyperostosis of long bone diaphyses	Autosomal dominant	TGF-β (transforming growth factor-β 1)	Widely expressed, circulating proteins with a wide range of functions Important influence on bone modelling and remodeling Clarification of the effect of TGFβ-1 on bone in vivo will supply significant information on its natural and possible therapeutic effects
Chondrodysplasia punctata: Rhizomelic chondrodysplasia punctata type 1	Nasal hypoplasia and severe rhizomelic shortening of limbs Cataracts and ichthyosis are usually present in infancy	Autosomal recessive	PEX7 (peroxisomal assembly gene 7)	PEX genes encode proteins that are necessary for importing proteins into peroxisomes Peroxisome malfunction results in accumulation of very long chain fatty acids and phytanic acid PEX7 encodes a peroxisomal targeting signal receptor necessary for importation of several proteins
Chondrodysplasia punctata: Rhizomelic chondrodysplasia punctata type 2	Nasal hypoplasia and severe rhizomelic shortening of limbs. Cataracts and ichtyosis usually present in less than 30% of patients Respiratory failure often causes death in infancy.	Autosomal recessive	DHAPAT (encodes acyl-CoA: dihydroxyacetone-phosphate acyltransferase	DHAPAT encodes a protein necessary for plasmalogen synthesis
Chondrodysplasia punctata: X-linked type	Nasal hypoplasia with mild limb shortening and hypoplastic digits	X-linked recessive	ARSE (encodes arylsulfatase E)	Unknown
Chondrodysplasia punctata: X-linked type 2	Lethal in males Dwarfing with asymmetric limb shortening, scoliosis, and ichthyosis	X-linked dominant	EBP (encodes a sterol isomerase emopamil binding protein)	The encoded sterol isomerase aids in conversion of lanostero to cholesterol Mutation results in accumulation of precursors and may act through the cholesterol-dependent sonic hedgehog signaling pathway
Cleidocramial dysplasia	A generalized skeletal dysplasia Most prominent features include hypoplasia or aplasia of the clavicles, persistently open skull sutures, midface hypoplasia, wide symphysis pubis, mild to moderate short stature, short middle phalanx of the little finger, dental anomalies, and often vertebral malformation	Autosomal dominant	CBFA1	CBFA1 has homology to the 'runt' family of genes in mice, which are bone-specific nuclear-matrix-binding transcription factors Shown to cause cleidocranial dysplasia by mutation analysis Encodes a protein that is the α subunit of an osteoblast-specific transcription factor, RUNX2

Disorder	Inheritance	Gene	Clinical features	Function
Dyggve-Melchior-Clausen dysplasia	Autosomal recessive	FLJ90130	Marked disproportionate short stature with a barrel chest and limitation of joint motion; Mental retardation; Developmental delay	Unproven function; Its structure shows similarity to proteins that are present in many species with the characteristics of a transmembrane protein; May be important in proteoglycan metabolism; Smith-McCort dysplasia is caused by different mutations of this gene
Ellis-Van Creveld syndrome (Chondroectodermal dysplasia)	Autosomal recessive	EVC (" mutated in" Ellis-van Creveld)	Short stature with disproportionate short limbs and often postaxial polydactyly; Sparse and thin hair; Dysplastic nails	Encodes a protein that is expressed in early development in bone, kidney, heart, and lung; Role in normal development and its mechanism of action in causing this disorder are unknown
Jansen metaphyseal chondrodysplasia	Autosomal dominant	PTH-PTHrP (encodes the parathyroid hormone-parathyroid hormone-related peptide receptor)	Rare disorder characterized at birth by severe limb shortening with a prominent forehead and micrognathia; Tubular bones are short and the metaphyses are markedly flared with irregular ossification; asymptomatic hypercalcemia	PTH-PTHrP receptor normally mediates the activity of parathyroid hormone-related peptide (PTHrP), which causes hypercalcemia of malignancy syndrome and is an autocrine/paracrine regulator of chondrocyte proliferation and differentiation; The mutation is a gain of function mutation of the PTH-PTHrP receptor; gain of function of the receptor causes severe delay in chondrocyte differentiation and delay in ossification
McKusick metaphyseal chondrodysplasia (cartilage-hair hypoplasia)	Autosomal recessive	RMRP (RNA component of mitochondrial RNA processing endoribonuclease)	Disproportionate short limbed dwarfing with sparse and fine body hair; Joint laxity, impaired cellular immunity, anemia, Hirschsprung's disease, and malignancies	Encodes a protein that is involved in cleavage or mitochondrial RNA and processing of RNA to become ribosomal RNA in the nucleus; Particular proteins that result in the McKusick phenotype have not been identified
Nail-patella syndrome	Autosomal dominant	LMX1b	Dysplastic nails, hypoplastic patellae; Iliac horns (exostoses), dysplastic elbows; Occasionally nephropathy or glaucoma	LMX1b is a member of a family of regulatory proteins containing zinc finger motifs and a homeodomain; Involved in dorsal-ventral patterning during development; Inadequate quantities of LMX1b at critical developmental stages may result in inadequate ventral specification, resulting in the NPS phenotype
Oculodentodigital dysplasia	Autosomal dominant	GJA1 (or connexin 43)	Syndactyly of the long, ring, and little fingers and second, third, and fourth toes; Camptodactyly and clinodactyly; microcephaly and a constellation of typical orofacial abnormalities	Encodes a transmembrane protein that forms gap junction channels for passage of ions and small molecules; Expressed in the developing brain, neural tube, prevertebrae, and limb at various stages of development (pleiotropic effects)
Oral-facial-digital type 1 syndrome	X-linked dominant	OFD1 (oral-facial-digital 1)	Facial malformations, cleft palate and tongue; Syndactyly, brachydactly, clinodactyly, and polydactyly; Lethal in males	Shares no homology to known proteins involved in mammalian development, although apparently important for normal development of several organ systems; Expression is highest in craniofacial structures and the nervous system with lower levels of expression in the integument, lung, thymus, and kidney; unknown effect on hands and feet
Schmid metaphyseal chondrodysplasia	Autosomal dominant	Type X collagen.	Short stature, bowed legs, coxa vara and a waddling gait; The metaphyses of the long bones are flared and the physes are wide and irregular	Exists as a homotrimer in the pericellular matrix of hypertrophic chondrocytes; The mutations in this disease occur in the C-terminal, noncollagenous domain of the protein and may limit the ability of the collagen to form trimers; Appears to play a role in organizing matrix components of cartilage; Absence results in alteration of the supporting properties of the physis as well as mild decrease in trabecular bone formation and mild disorganization of mineralization

EDS IV is a clinically heterogeneous subtype but is characterized by the tendency for rupture of large and medium-sized arteries. Fatal ruptures often occur in the second or third decade of life. The etiology of EDS IV is a mutation in the gene coding for a chain of type III collagen that interrupts the helical structure of this fibular collagen. Type III collagen constitutes 50% of the collagen in blood vessel walls (most of the remaining collagen is type I) and 15% of the collagen in skin.

EDS VII A and B are caused by mutations in the structural gene coding for type I collagen, whereas EDS VI and VIIC have mutations in genes coding for enzymes involved in collagen I synthesis.

Neuromuscular Disorders
Duchenne and Becker's Muscular Dystrophy
The dystrophinopathies, Duchenne and Becker's muscular dystrophy, have traditionally been considered two different diseases. When the gene, dystrophin, was cloned in 1987, it became clear that these diseases represent different phenotypes resulting from different mutations in a single gene.

The most severe form of the disease, Duchenne muscular dystrophy, presents in early childhood with proximal muscle weakness and calf hypertrophy. Affected boys experience a slight delay in attaining motor milestones. Toe walking may be an early manifestation of the disease. The course is one of steadily worsening weakness.

The milder dystrophinopathies are varied in clinical phenotype. Affected males who present in childhood with proximal weakness, calf hypertrophy, and very high creatine kinase values, but follow a more indolent course than the Duchenne muscular dystrophy patients, are given the diagnosis of Becker's muscular dystrophy. Dystrophinopathies may be indistinguishable from limb girdle dystrophy. Seven of 41 (17%) patients with the clinical diagnosis of limb girdle dystrophy had dystrophin mutations in one study. Carrier females may be symptomatic on the basis of skewed X-inactivation. They usually present with limb girdle weakness and elevated creatine kinase levels. Cardiomyopathy can be clinically significant, and rarely is the primary manifestation of dystrophinopathy.

Dystrophin is an intracellular protein that is associated with two transmembrane complexes—the dystroglycan complex and the sarcoglycan complex. Loss of dystrophin leads to loss of all components of these complexes. The dystrophin gene is the largest human gene yet identified, making it a very large target for new mutations. One third of patients with dystrophinopathy have new mutations. Most patients can be identified by DNA testing. In these patients a muscle biopsy is not necessary to make the diagnosis, although it may be performed to allow more accurate predictions about the clinical course.

(Duchenne muscular dystrophy has absent dystrophin in muscle, the milder phenotypes have decreased or abnormal dystrophin.)

Because there is no effective treatment for the dystrophinopathies, there is great interest in the possibility of introducing a functional dystrophin gene into the muscle fibers, and thus curing the disease (gene therapy). There are many issues to be addressed before this is a viable treatment option; among these are identifying an appropriate vector for the new gene, overcoming host immune response to the vector or the expressed new protein, targeting muscle, and regulating the expression of the gene. These issues are the focus of active research. Most of the hurdles to be overcome before gene therapy is clinically useful in treating muscular dystrophy are not specific to one missing protein, such as dystrophin. If the problems are solved for one muscular dystrophy, it is likely that the protocol will be adapted relatively quickly for other muscular dystrophies with similar pathogenesis.

Autosomal Recessive Limb Girdle Dystrophies
The autosomal recessive limb girdle dystrophies are progressive muscular dystrophies that predominantly affect the pelvic and shoulder girdle musculature. The severity ranges from severe forms manifesting weakness in the first decade of life with rapid progression (called Duchenne-like muscular dystrophy) to mild forms with late onset and slow progression.

Eight genetic loci have been identified in families with this phenotype. Four loci code for proteins that are part of the sarcoglycan complex (the alpha, beta, gamma, and delta-sarcoglycans). The sarcoglycan complex and the dystroglycan complex are part of the dystrophin-glycoprotein complex that spans the muscle membrane from the cytoskeleton to the basal lamina. One hypothesis is that the dystrophin-glycoprotein complex functions to stabilize the sarcolemma, thereby protecting the muscle fiber from damage caused by repeated contractions. Another form is caused by a mutation in the gene coding for calpain-3, a muscle-specific proteolytic enzyme. The sixth form with an identified gene is caused by a mutation in dysferlin. Two other forms have been linked to regions on chromosomes 9 and 17.

Hereditary Spastic Paraplegia
The hereditary spastic paraplegias (familial spastic paraparesis, Strumpell-Lorrain syndrome) are characterized by progressive spasticity of the legs. Symptoms usually manifest during the second to fourth decades, and gait slowly and steadily worsens. These disorders have been classified by mode of inheritance and whether the lower extremity spasticity is the only finding (uncomplicated) or whether other neurologic conditions, such as optic neuropathy, dementia, ataxia, mental retardation, or deafness are present

(complicated). Inheritance may be autosomal dominant, autosomal recessive, or X-linked.

Autosomal dominant forms have been linked to 11 different loci, and four causative genes have been identified—*atlastin* (involved with vesicle behavior that is important for neurotropic factor activity), *spastin* (involved in microtubular dynamics), *KIF5A* (a component of the microtubule transport system), and *HSP60* (encodes a mitochondrial chaperone protein). Autosomal recessive forms have been linked to six loci, and two causative genes have been identified—*paraplegin* (encodes a mitochondrial metalloprotease necessary for axonal transport) and *spartin* (may be involved in endosome protein pathways). Three loci have been located for the X-linked form and two genes identified—*L1-CAM* (encodes a transmembrane glycoprotein that mediates both cell adhesion and neurite growth) and *PLP1*(encodes a major protein component of myelin). It appears that disruption of normal intracellular-trafficking dynamics may be the common link in the various gene defects causing this disorder. The clinical phenotype is similar among families with mutations at the same loci. Other loci will be found for this extremely heterogeneous group of disorders.

Charcot-Marie-Tooth Disease (Hereditary Motor Sensory Neuropathies)

This is a heterogeneous group of inherited peripheral neuropathies. Charcot-Marie-Tooth disease is the most common of these disorders. Charcot-Marie-Tooth 1A (CMT-1A) is an autosomal dominant disorder and is characterized by progressive distal muscle wasting and weakness, areflexia, and foot deformities—most commonly cavovarus feet. Nerve conduction velocities show severe slowing and nerve pathology reveals simultaneous demyelination and remyelination. This disorder has variable expression but usually begins in childhood. Patients with foot deformities usually present to the orthopaedic surgeon in late childhood or early adolescence.

At the molecular level, 70% to 80% of affected individuals have a duplication of the gene coding for peripheral myelin protein 22 (PMP22). This protein appears to modulate cell proliferation. Rare patients with point mutations in this gene have also had the CMT-IA phenotype, providing strong evidence for the primary role of PMP22 in disease causation. CMT-1B, causing 5% of CMT-1 phenotype, is caused by a mutation in the *MPZ* gene, which encodes the protein myelin protein 0. This gene encodes a protein that makes up nearly 50% of all protein in peripheral myelin. Some families with the CMT-1 phenotype have a gene cause that has not been located and are designated CMT-1C. Additional families with the CMT-1 phenotype are caused by a mutation in the early growth response gene (*EGR2*), a transcription factor involved in early myelination, and are designated CMT-1D. This gene is also involved in some cases of Dejerine-Sottas disease.

CMT type 2 is an autosomal dominant, axonal polyneuropathy with age of onset in the second or third decade of life, characterized by near-normal motor nerve conduction velocity. Nomenclature is in flux as new variants are found. Of five presently described subtypes, four have been linked to chromosomal regions. The gene cause has been identified in three. The gene encoding kinesin (*KIF1B*), part of a family of mitochondrial motor transport proteins, causes CMT-2A. CMT-2D is caused by mutations in the glycyl transcription RNA synthetase gene. This is the first transcription RNA synthetase enzyme known to cause a human disease. The neurofilament-light gene (*NF-L*), which encodes neurofilament proteins involved in axonal structure, causes CMT-2E. A few families with the CMT-2 phenotype have been found with point mutations in the *MPZ* gene. An autosomal recessive form of CMT-2 is caused by mutations in the *LMNA* gene, which encodes lamin A/C nuclear-envelope proteins—a component of the nuclear envelope.

X-linked CMT comprises approximately 14% of CMT cases. Two forms (CMT-X1 and CMT-X2) have been localized and the gene cause has been identified for CMT-X1 (connexin 32). This gene encodes a major protein in myelin at the nodes of Ranvier and the Schmidt-Lanterman incisures.

Dejerine-Sottas disease is a severe form of hypertrophic demyelinating neuropathy with early childhood onset. Motor nerve conduction velocities are very slow and sensory nerve conduction velocities are absent. Mutations in both the *PMP22* and *MPZ* genes have been identified in most instances. A few instances have been found with mutations in the *periaxin* gene (periaxin is a constituent of the dystroglycan-dystrophin-related protein-2 complex linking the Schwann cell cytoskeleton to the extracellular matrix) and connexin 32. Not all mutations are linked to these genes. Dejerine-Sottas disease was believed in the past to be an autosomal recessive disorder. It is now believed to be autosomal dominant with most cases being new mutations.

Congenital hypomyelination begins in infancy with hypotonia, areflexia, distal muscle weakness, and slow nerve conduction velocities. The clinical course is extremely variable, from early death to improvement in clinical signs. Affected families have been found with mutations in genes coding for myelin protein 0 and early growth response gene 2.

Hereditary neuropathy with a liability for pressure palsies, another autosomal dominant neuropathy, has recurrent, episodic peripheral nerve palsies as a result of mechanical compression. A chromosome 17 deletion reciprocal to the hereditary motor sensory neuropathy IA duplication in the *PMP-22* gene is the cause.

Several autosomal recessive forms of CMT have been identified and eight have been linked to specific chromosomal locations. Six genes, which cause forms of this rare disorder, have been identified. Several of these genes are

Disorder	Gene	Function
Table 4 Charcot-Marie-Tooth Disease and Related Disorders		
	Charcot-Marie-Tooth Type 1 (CMT-1)	
CMT-1A	Peripheral myelin protein 22 (*PMP22*)	Regulated cell proliferation?
CMT-1B	Myelin protein 0 (P0), myelin structure (50%)	
CMT-1C	Unknown	Unknown
CMT-1D	Early growth response gene (*EGR2*)	Transcription factor for early myelination
	Charcot-Marie-Tooth Type 2 (CMT-2)	
CMT-2A	Kinesin (*KIF1B*)	Mitochondrial transport protein
CMT-2B	Unknown but linked (3q13-922)	Unknown
CMT-2C	Unknown	Unknown
CMT-2D	Glycyl tRNA synthetase gene	tRNA synthesis
CMT-2E	Neurofilament-light gene (*NF-L*)	Axonal filament protein
CMT-2 autosomal recessive	Lamin A/C nuclear-envelope protein (LMNA)	Nuclear envelope protein
	Charcot-Marie-Tooth X-Linked (CMT-X)	
CMT-X1	*Connexin 32*	Myelin structure
CMT-X2	Unknown but linked (Xq24-q26)	Unknown
	Dejerine-Sottas Syndrome (DSS)	
DSS-A	*PMP-22*	Regulated cell proliferation?
DSS-B	*P0*	Myelin structure
DSS (other)	*periaxin (PRX)*	Dystroglycan-dystrophin related protein complex-2
	Connexin 32	Myelin structure
Congenital hypomyelination	*P0*	Myelin structure
	EGR2	Transcription factor for early myelination
Hereditary neuropathy with liability to pressure palsies (HNPP)	*PMP-22*	Regulated cell proliferation?
	Recessive Forms of Charcot-Marie-Tooth Disease	
CMT-4A	Ganglioside-induced differentiation-associated protein 1 (*GDAP1a*)	Unknown
CMT-4B	Myotubularin-related protein-2 (*MTMR2*)	Myotubularin phosphatase (gene transcription regulator?)
	Myotubularin-related protein-13 (MTMR13)	Myotubularin pseudophosphatase of unknown function
	SET binding factor (*SBF2*)	Myotubularin pseudophosphatase of unknown function
CMT-4C	Unknown but linked (5q23-q33)	Unknown
CMT-4F	Periaxin (*PRX*)	Dystroglycan-dystrophin-related protein complex-2
CMT-4L	N-myc downstream-regulated gene 1 (*NDRG1*)	Schwann cell signaling?

myotubularin-related proteins that contain phosphatases or pseudophosphatases. The pseudophosphatses were believed to be inactive copies until they were found to be the cause of these rare disorders (Table 4).

Spinal Muscular Atrophy

Spinal muscular atrophy has been classified into three clinical forms: (1) Werdnig-Hoffmann disease is charac-terized by generalized muscle weakness and hypotonia at birth, and early death. (2) The intermediate type of spinal muscular atrophy afflicts patients who initially achieve normal motor milestones, but never gain the ability to walk. (3) Kugelberg-Welander is the mildest type; patients have muscle weakness, which becomes evident after age 2 years. All three types of spinal muscular atrophy are char-acterized by anterior horn cell degeneration and result in limb and trunk paralysis with muscle atrophy. Major orthopaedic conditions include scoliosis and hip instability. It has long been recognized that there is a continuum from the most severe early forms through the milder later onset disease. This clinical impression has been borne out by the mapping of all forms of spinal muscular atrophy to one small region of chromosome 5. Several genes have been identified in this region, including the survival motor neuron gene (*SMN*), the neuronal apoptosis inhibitory protein, and the *p44* gene. This is a very complex and unstable segment of the genome. Two copies of the *SMN* gene with very minor differences are present in this region; one centromeric and one telomeric to each other. More than 90% of spinal muscular atrophy patients have deletions (or conversion of the telomeric *SMN* to the centromeric *SMN* type) in a specific portion (exons 7 and 8) of the telomeric *SMN* gene. Spinal muscular atrophy types II and III appear to have a conversion of the telomeric *SMN* to the centromeric *SMN* gene and have more copies of the centromeric *SMN* gene than exist in type I disease. The telomeric *SMN* gene encodes the fully functional protein, whereas the centromeric *SMN* gene encodes a transcript lacking exon 7.

The neuronal apoptosis inhibitory protein may provide an additional explanation for the variations in genotype/phenotype correlation. The neuronal apoptosis inhibitory protein gene functions to inhibit motor neuron programmed cell death. Programmed cell death is a normal occurrence in the development of the nervous system. Failure to inhibit cell death at the appropriate time could be part of the explanation for the anterior horn cell loss seen in spinal muscular atrophy. In a group of patients with the most severe type of spinal muscular atrophy, a high percentage of deletions in this gene was found. However, deletion of this gene may simply be coincidentally associated with more disease because of a more severe interruption in the *SMN* gene function.

Trinucleotide Repeat Disorders

Repeated sequences of nucleotides occur throughout the human genome and are the basis for inherited polymorphisms that have allowed the dramatic increase in identification of disease-causing genes in the last decade. Expansion of certain trinucleotide repeats causes 11 known neurologic disorders: Friedreich's ataxia, myotonic dystrophy, fragile X syndrome, X-linked spinal and bulbar muscular atrophy, Huntington's disease, spinocerebellar ataxia type 1, spinocerebellar ataxia type 2, spinocerebellar ataxia type 6, spinocerebellar ataxia type 7, spinocerebellar ataxia type 3 (Machado-Joseph disease), and dentatorubral-pallidoluysian atrophy. The repeated sequences are unstable and change size in successive generations, usually becoming longer. Myotonic dystrophy and fragile X syndrome contain repeat sequences that are not within the protein coding region and, probably, cause disease by altering gene expression rather than by altering the protein product. Expansion of trinucleotide repeats (CAG repeats) in the coding region cause Huntington's disease, spinal and bulbar muscular atrophy, spinocerebellar ataxia type 1 and 6, dentatorubral-pallidoluysian atrophy, and Machado-Joseph disease. The CAG repeat results in polyglutamine amino acid sequences and evidence suggests these polyglutamine regions are specifically neurotoxic by themselves. The trinucleotide repeat expansion provides a molecular basis for "anticipation," a phenomenon recognized by astute clinical geneticists, but discounted by colleagues in part because it failed to conform to classic mendelian genetics. "Anticipation" is the worsening of the clinical phenotype (earlier onset, more severe disease) in succeeding generations. It is now clear that the trinucleotide repeats tend to lengthen in succeeding generations and the severity of the disease correlates, although not perfectly, with the length of the repeat segment.

Not all trinucleotide repeat disorders cause neurologic diseases. In fact, grouping of trinucleotide repeat disorders is somewhat artificial in that the gene involved and the nature of the trinucleotide repeat are often more important in determining the disease characteristics than the fact that a trinucleotide repeat is the type of mutation. For example, synpolydactyly is an inherited disorder that affects the hands and/or feet with various combinations of syndactyly and polydactyly. It is caused by a trinucleotide repeat resulting in an expansion of a polyalanine stretch in the amino terminal region of *HOXD 13*. Increasing size of the polyalanine repeat regions may correlate with increasing numbers of involved limbs, from monomelic through tetramelic involvement.

Myotonic Dystrophy

Myotonic dystrophy is an autosomal dominant, multisystem disease with marked clinical variability with an incidence of 1 per 8,000 patients. The most severely affected patients are babies with congenital myotonic dystrophy. These children have severe hypotonia and weakness. They often require ventilatory support and nasogastric feedings. Clubfeet and dislocated hips are common. These children are almost always born to myotonic mothers rather than affected fathers. If they survive the neonatal period, these children show improvement in strength, but have persistent motor disability. In addition, they are uniformly mentally retarded. At the other extreme, the only manifestation of myotonic dystrophy in the most mildly affected individuals may be cataracts.

After the neonatal period, the disease presents with mild muscle weakness, and myotonia exacerbated by cold. Wasting of the temporalis muscles contributes to the typical phenotype of long narrow faces with bitemporal narrowing. Cardiac conduction defects are common, and may necessitate a pacemaker. Diabetes mellitus, male pattern baldness, infertility, and mental retardation are also manifestations of myotonic dystrophy.

The abnormal gene, *myotonin*, is a protein kinase. The substrate for the kinase and the pathophysiology of the disease remain unknown. Recent data suggest that the adjacent *DMAHP* gene may play a complementary or even primary role in the pathogenesis of myotonic dystrophy. The protein location has been shown by immunoelectron microscopy to be membrane-bound in the terminal cisternae of the sarcoplasmic reticulum, mainly in the I-band. The mutation is an expansion of a trinucleotide repeat in the 3' untranslated region of the gene. The normal gene has 5 to 30 copies of this CTG repeat. This is expanded in myotonic dystrophy patients, reaching thousands of copies. The congenitally affected infants have the largest expansions, on average, and the mildest phenotypes are associated with the smallest expansions into the disease-associated range.

Friedreich's Ataxia

Friedreich's ataxia is the most common early onset hereditary ataxia and occurs in approximately 2 to 4 per 100,000 patients in ethnically European populations. It is an autosomal recessive disorder characterized by progressive ataxia beginning before age 25 years. Muscle weakness, cardiomyopathy, and diabetes mellitus are frequent accompanying conditions. Scoliosis and pes cavus are common orthopaedic manifestations that often require treatment. The cause of Friedreich's ataxia is a mutation of the gene *FRADA*, which codes for the protein named frataxin. Friedreich's ataxia is caused by a GAA repeat expansion in introns 1 of the gene *FRADA*. The mutation appears to cause an accumulation of iron in mitochondria leading to excess free radical production and subsequent cell damage/death. Earlier age of onset and more frequent occurrence of associated conditions such as diabetes and cardiomyopathy are associated with larger repeat expansions.

Hereditary Multiple Exostosis

This autosomal dominant disorder is viewed as a single clinical phenotype, but has localized to three different chromosomal locations: chromosome 8q24.1 (*EXT 1*), chromosome 11p11-p13 (*EXT2*), and chromosome 19p (EXT3). The *EXT 1* and *EXT 2* genes have been cloned and are hypothesized to be a new family of tumor suppressor genes. The main evidence for this is that mutations of both alleles of the *EXT* genes have been identified in chondrosarcomas arising from both sporadic and hereditary exostoses. The *EXT 1* gene has been shown to be expressed in many tissues, but the only known effect is on growing bones.

A current hypothesis is that exostosis formation fits the "two-hit" model of tumorigenesis. Both alleles must be mutated for an exostosis to form; therefore, hereditary exostoses occur at a younger age and in more sites than sporadic exostoses. That is, individuals who inherit an abnormal allele need a cartilage cell to undergo a mutation of only the second allele to form an exostosis, whereas sporadic exostoses require new mutations of both alleles in a cell. Presumably, malignant degeneration occurs when an additional mutation happens to another tumor-suppressor gene or proto-oncogene.

Neurofibromatosis

Neurofibromatosis (NF) is the most common single gene disorder. It is autosomal dominant, with a nearly complete penetrance. Half of reported cases are new mutations.

There are two forms of neurofibromatosis. NF-1 has an incidence of 1 in 3,500 live births. The clinical features of NF-1 include café-au-lait spots, neurofibromas, dysostosis, congenital pseudarthrosis of the tibia, and scoliosis. The responsible gene codes for a protein named neurofibromin. Neurofibromin is believed to be a tumor-suppresser gene that normally functions to control cell growth and differentiation. Neurofibromin negatively regulates the gene *RAS*. Increased *RAS* activity results in cell proliferation. Neurofibromas occur if the unaffected allele coding for neurofibromin (that is, the allele not carrying the mutation causing NF-1) undergoes a somatic mutation. This "two-hit" hypothesis of neurofibroma causation is supported by mutation analysis of neurofibromas from a large number of individuals in different families. Approximately 250 different mutations of neurofibromin have been identified in persons with NF-1. No phenotype-genotype correlations have been found except for complete deletion of the gene, which results in a severe phenotype of mental retardation and development of many neurofibromas at a young age.

NF-2, with a gene location on chromosome 22, is far less common, with a prevalence of 1 in 50,000 births. NF-2 is associated with a high prevalence of acoustic neuromas and rarely has orthopaedic complications. The mutant gene codes for merlin or schwannomin, which is a protein that links the cytoskeleton to the plasma membrane. This gene is a tumor suppressor gene and inhibits cell proliferation, adhesion and migration. The severity of the disorder correlates with the severity of truncation of the protein.

McCune-Albright Syndrome/ Monostotic Fibrous Dysplasia

McCune-Albright syndrome occurs sporadically and is characterized by polyostotic fibrous dysplasia, sexual precocity, hyperplastic endocrine disorders, and café-au-lait spots. A mutation of the gene for the alpha subunit of stimulatory guanine-nucleotide-binding protein (Gs), a protein that stimulates cyclic adenosine monophosphate formation, has been found in patients affected with this disorder. The mutation seems to result in an inappropriate stimulation of adenyl cyclase. There is strong evidence that the mutation of this gene is a somatic rather than a germline mutation—meaning that the mutation occurred after fertilization in some subsequent cell division. The variation in the distribution of the abnormality in individuals can be explained by the tissues that have the mutated gene as opposed to the normal gene. In all patients studied so far, the abnormal gene was found in fibrous dysplasia material.

Abnormal tissues in this disease have been found by in situ hybridization to have increased expression of the c-*fos* proto-oncogene. Transgenic mice that overexpress the c-*fos* proto-oncogene have bone marrow fibrosis, increased formation of woven bone, and disordered bone remodeling. The abnormal stimulatory guanine-nucleotide-binding protein may create the abnormal cells by increasing the level of cyclic adenosine monophosphate in affected tissues and, thereby, increasing the expression of the c-*fos* proto-oncogene, which is responsive to increased levels of cyclic adenosine monophosphate.

Mutations in this gene have also been found in patients with monostotic fibrous dysplasia. It seems likely that different mutations within this gene might result in lesser or greater involvement of bones and other tissues. Both monostotic and polyostotic fibrous dysplasia lesions show an increase in cell proliferation with a diminished synthesis of osteocalcin suggesting a reduction in cell differentiation as the cause of the lesions.

Paget's Disease

Paget's disease is an extremely common disorder of bone remodeling with an incidence of approximately 3.3% in individuals older than 40 years. Paget's disease has long been known to have a strong familiarity, with more than 40% of affected people having a first-degree relative with the disease. Because paramyxovirus-like nuclear inclusion has been found in osteoclasts, a viral etiology has been suggested as the cause. In a single large family in which Paget's disease had an autosomal dominant segregation pattern, Paget's disease was found to be strongly linked to a region on chromosome 18. Leach and associates surmise that a gene mutation might either confer a susceptibility to viral infection or be involved directly in osteoclast function. The authors searched this region of the genome because of the histologic similarity of Paget's disease to an extremely rare disorder—familial expansile osteolysis—that had previously been linked to the same region of chromosome 18. At least four susceptible loci for Paget's disease have been identified. A mutation in the gene encoding sequestosome 1 (*SQSTM1*) has been found to be a common cause of familial and sporadic Paget's disease in a French-Canadian population. *SQSTM1* appears to function in a complex signaling pathway that controls osteoclast activity, differentiation, or survival.

The Orthopaedic Surgeon and the Geneticist at the Start of the 21st Century

Genetic research will alter the understanding and treatment of many disorders in the future. Prenatal and presymptomatic diagnosis are available for an increasing number of diseases. Gene therapy or gene product replacement may one day be available with the potential for ameliorating or eliminating the effects of abnormal genes. The study of gene expression is already changing how tumors are diagnosed and treated. The orthopaedist must stay abreast of this knowledge to participate in advances in diagnosis and treatment, and to appropriately counsel patients. Molecular genetics and biology will find inherited susceptibilities to diseases that are not mendelian in inheritance. Identifying a subpopulation of patients within a single disease phenotype based on differing genetic backgrounds may allow improved treatment for individual patients. The orthopaedic community must stay informed of and involved with the revolution in understanding the genetic and molecular bases of diseases.

It is probably prudent for the orthopaedic surgeon who takes care of patients with heritable disorders to work closely with a medical geneticist annually or biannually. The new information is accumulating too rapidly for most practicing orthopaedic surgeons to stay abreast of new developments. Patients expect orthopaedic surgeons to be at least as informed as they are. Educational lecture series in teaching institutions should include medical geneticists to relate new information concerning orthopaedic disorders. National educational meetings should include guest speakers with expertise in genetics to allow a broad dispersion of this new knowledge in the orthopaedic community. The Internet offers many tools of use to the orthopaedist and is commonly used by patients who may show great apparent familiarity with a rare disease.

A large family with an inherited disorder of unknown etiology should prompt a call or referral to a medical geneticist, who will be able to discover if active research into that disorder is occurring. If so, participation by the family in ongoing research may result in identification of the disease-causing gene.

A geneticist should be consulted before a diagnostic biopsy is performed if any question exists about the availability of gene-based diagnosis. Most instances of Duchenne muscular dystrophy and Charcot-Marie-Tooth disease, for example, can be diagnosed by blood analysis, rather than muscle or nerve biopsy.

If the orthopaedic surgeon is unfamiliar with the empirical risk of recurrence of a disorder, a medical geneticist should be consulted. Idiopathic clubfoot is an example of a disorder for which treating orthopaedic surgeons commonly underestimate the recurrence risk.

Patients with multisystem congenital anomalies should be referred to a geneticist to attempt to identify a unifying diagnosis.

Families with diseases with mendelian inheritance should be offered referral for genetic counseling. The practicing orthopaedist does not have the time or teaching aids to adequately explain genetics to most families.

Selected Bibliography

Skeletal Dysplasias and Disorders With Specific Skeletal Manifestations

Alman BA: A classification for genetic disorders of interest to orthopaedists. *Clin Orthop Relat Res* 2002; 401:17-26.

Anderson IJ, Goldberg RB, Marion RW, et al: Spondyloepiphyseal dysplasia congenital: Genetic linkage to type II collagen (COL2A1). *Am J Hum Genet* 1990;46: 896-901.

Bellus GA, McIntosh I, Smith EA, et al: A recurrent mutation in the tyrosine kinase domain of fibroblast growth factor receptor 3 causes hypochondroplasia. *Nat Genet* 1995;10:357-362.

Briggs MD, Chapman KL: Pseudoachondroplasia and multiple epiphyseal dysplasia: Mutation review, molecular interactions, and genotype to phenotype correlations. *Hum Mutat* 2002;19:465-478.

Briggs MD, Hoffman SM, King LM, et al: Pseudoachondroplasia and multiple epiphyseal dysplasia due to mutations in the cartilage oligomeric matrix protein gene. *Nat Genet* 1995;10:330-336.

Chapman KL, Mortier GR, Chapman K, et al: Mutations in the region encoding the von Willebrand factor A domain of matrilin-3 area associated with multiple epiphyseal dysplasia. *Nat Genet* 2001;28:393-396.

Cohn DH, Briggs MD, King LM, et al: Mutations in the cartilage oligomeric matrix protein (COMP) gene in pseudoachondroplasia and multiple epiphyseal dysplasia. *Ann N Y Acad Sci* 1996;785:188-194.

Dragomir AD, Kraus VB, Renner JB, et al: Serum cartilage oligomeric matrix protein and clinical signs and symptoms of potential pre-radiographic hip and knee pathology. *Osteoarthritis Cartilage* 2002;10:687-691.

Gedeon AK, Colley A, Jamieson R, et al: Identification of the gene (SSEDL) causing X-linked spondyloepiphyseal dysplasia tarda. *Nat Genet* 1999;22:400-404.

Gofflot F, Hars C, Illien F: Molecular mechanism underlying limb anomalies associated with cholesterol deficiency during gestation: Implications of Hedgehog signaling. *Hum Mol Genet* 2003;12:1187-1198.

Hastbacka J, Superti-Furga A, Wilcox WR, et al: Atelosteogenesis type II is caused by mutations in the diastrophic dysplasia sulfate-transporter gene (DTDST): Evidence for a phenotypic series involving three chondrodysplasias. *Am J Hum Genet* 1996;58: 255-262.

Kawaji H, Nishimura G, Watanabe S, et al: Autosomal dominant precocious osteoarthropathy due to a mutation of the cartilage oligomeric matrix protein (COMP) gene: Further expansion of the phenotypic variations of COMP defects. *Skeletal Radiol* 2002; 31(12):730-737.

Knowlton RG, Patzenstein PL, Moskowitz RW, et al: Genetic linkage of a polymorphism in the type 11 procollagen gene (COL2A1) to primary osteoarthrosis associated with mild chondrodysplasia. *N Engl J Med* 1990;322:526-530.

Mabuchi A, Manabe N, Haga N, et al: Novel types of COMP mutations and genotype-phenotype association in pseudoachondroplasia and multiple epiphyseal dysplasia. *Hum Genet* 2003;112:84-90.

Muenke M, Gripp KW, McDonald-McGinn DM: A unique point mutation in the fibroblast growth factor receptor 3 gene (FGFR3) defines a new craniosynostosis syndrome. *Am J Hum Genet* 1997;60:555-564.

Muragaki Y, Mariman EC, van Beersum SE, et al: A mutation in COL9A2 causes multiple epiphyseal dysplasia (EDM2). *Ann N Y Acad Sci* 1996;785:303-306.

Park WJ, Theda C, Maestri NE, et al: Analysis of phenotypic features and FGFR2 mutations in Apert Syndrome. *Am J Hum Genet* 1995;57:321-328.

Pendleton A, Johnson MD, Hughes A: Mutations in ANKH cause chondrocalcinosis. *Am J Hum Genet* 2002;71:933-940.

Stefansson S, Jonsson H, Ingvarsson T, et al: Genome-wide scan for hand osteoarthritis: A novel mutation in matrilin-3. *Am J Hum Genet* 2003;72:1448-1459.

Tiller GE, Polumbo PA, Weis MA, et al: Dominant mutations in the type II collagen gene, COL2A1, produce spondyloepimetaphyseal dysplasia, Strudwick type. *Nat Genet* 1995;11:87-89.

p63 Disorders

Biesecker LG: Polydactyly: How many disorders and how many genes? *Am J Med Genet* 2002;112:279-283.

Debeer P, Schoenmakers EF, Twal WO: The fibulin-1 gene (FMLN1) is disrupted in at (12;22) associated with a complex type of synpolydactyly. *J Med Genet* 2002;39:98-104.

Goodman FR: Limb malformations and the human HOX genes. *Am J Med Genet* 2002;112:256-265.

Goodman FR, Majewski F, Collins AL, Scambler PJ: A 117-kb microdeletion removing HOXD9-HOXD13 and EVX2 causes synpolydactyly. *Am J Hum Genet* 2002;70:547-555.

Ianakiev P, Kilpatrick MW, Toudjarska I, et al: Split-Hand/split-foot malformation is caused by mutations in the p63 gene in 3q27. *Am J Hum Genet* 2000;67:59-66.

Johnson D, Kan S, Oldridge M, et al: Missense mutations in the homeodomain of HOXD13 are associated with brachydactyly types D and E. *Am J Hum Genet* 2003;72:984-997.

Kang S: GLI3 frameshift mutations cause autosomal dominant Pallister-Hall syndrome. *Nat Genet* 1997;15:266-268.

Kirkpatrick TJ, Mastrobattista JM, McCready ME, et al: Identification of a mutation in the Indian Hedgehog (IHH) gene causing brachydactyly type A1 and evidence for a third locus. *J Med Genet* 2003;40:42-44.

Polinkovsky A: Mutations in CDMP1 cause autosomal dominant brachydactyly type C. *Nat Genet* 1997;17:18-19.

Schwabe GC, Tinschert S, Buschow C, et al: Distinct mutations in the receptor tyrosine kinase gene ROR2 cause brachydactyly type B. *Am J Hum Genet* 2000;67:822-831.

Utsch B, Becker K, Brock D, et al: A novel stable poly-alanine [poly(A)] expansion in the HOXA13 gene associated with hand-foot-genital syndrome: Proper function of poly(A)-harbouring transcription factors depends on a critical repeat length? *Hum Genet* 2002;110:488-494.

van Bokhoven H, Hamel BC, Banshad M: p63 Gene mutations in EEC syndrome, limb-mammary syndrome, and isolated split hand-split foot malformation suggest a genotype-phenotype correlation. *Am J Hum Genet* 2001;69:481-492.

Warren ST: Polyalanine expansion in synpolydactyly might result from unequal crossing over of HOXD13. *Science* 1997;275:408-409.

Wild A: Point mutations in human GLI3 cause Greig syndrome. *Hum Mol Genet* 1997;6:1979-1984.

HOX Gene Disorders

Goodman FA: Limb malformations and the human Hox genes. *Am J Med Genet* 2002;112:256-265.

GLI 3 Disorders

Dharmavaram RM, Elberson MA, Peng M, et al: Identification of a mutation in type X collagen in a family with Schmidt metaphyseal chondrodysplasia. *Hum Mol Genet* 1994;3:507-509.

Hintz RL: SHOX mutations. *Rev Endocr Metab Disord* 2002;3:363-367.

Ianakiev P, van Baren MJ, Daly MJ, et al: Acheiropodia is caused by a genomic deletion in C7 orf2, the human orthologue of the Lmbr1 gene. *Am J Hum Genet* 2001;68:38-45.

McIntosh I, Abbot MH, Warman ML, Olsen BR, Francomano CA: Additional mutations of type X collagen confirm COL10A1 as the Schmidt metaphyseal chondrodysplasia locus. *Hum Mol Genet* 1994;3:303-307.

McIntosh I, Dreyer D, Clough M, et al: Mutations analysis of LMX1B gene in nail-patella syndrome patients. *Am J Hum Genet* 1998;63:1651-1658.

Motley A, Brites P, Gerez L, et al: Mutational spectrum in the PEX7 gene and functional analysis of mutant alleles in 78 patients with rhizomelic chondrodysplasia puncata type 1. *Am J Hum Genet* 2002;70:612-624.

Powell C, Michaelis RC: Townes-Brocks syndrome. *J Med Genet* 1999;36:89-93.

Reichenberger E, Tiziani V, Watanabe S, et al: Autosomal dominant craniometaphyseal dysplasia is caused by mutations in the transmembrane protein ANK. *Am J Hum Genet* 2001;68:1321-1326.

Metabolic Bone Diseases

Eisman JA, Morrison NA, Kelly PJ, et al: Genetics of osteoporosis and vitamin D receptor alleles. *Calcif Tissue Int* 1995;56(suppl 1):S48-S49.

Holm IA, Huang X, Kunkel LM: Mutational analysis of the PEX gene in patients with x-linked hypophosphatemic rickets. *Am J Hum Genet* 1997;60:790-797.

Langdahl BL, Knudsen JY, Jensen HK, et al: A sequence variation: 713-8delC in the transforming growth factor-beta 1 gene has higher prevalence in osteoporotic women than in normal women and is associated with very low bone mass in osteoporotic women and increased bone turnover in both osteoporotic and normal women. *Bone* 1997;20:289-294.

Lania A, Mantovani G, Spada A: G protein mutations in endocrine diseases. *Eur J Endocrinol* 2001;145:543-559.

Tamai M, Yokouchi M, Komiya S, et al: Correlation between vitamin D receptor genotypes and bone mineral density in Japanese patients with osteoporosis. *Calcif Tissue Int* 1997;60:229-232.

Connective Tissue Disorders
De Paepe A, Nuytinck L, Hausser I, et al: Mutations in the COL5A1 gene as causal in the Ehlers-Danlos syndrome I and II. *Am J Hum Genet* 1997;60:547-554.

Dietz HC, Cutting GR, Pyeritz RE, et al: Marfan syndrome caused by a recurrent de novo missense mutation in the fibrillin gene. *Nature* 1991;352:337-339.

Giunta C, Superti-Furga A, Spranger S, Cole WG, Steinmann B: Ehlers-Danlos syndrome type VII: Clinical features and molecular defects. *J Bone Joint Surg Am* 1999;81:225-238.

Hewett D, Lynch J, Child A, Firth H, Sykes B: Differential allelic expression of a fibrillin gene (FBN1) in patients with Marfan syndrome. *Am J Hum Genet* 1994;55:447-452.

Mackay K, Raghunath M, Superti-Furga A, Steinmann B, Dalgleish R: Ehlers-Danlos syndrome type IV caused by Gly400Glu, Gly595Cys and Gly1003Asp substitutions in collagen III: Clinical features, biochemical screening, and molecular confirmation. *Clin Genet* 1996;49:286-295.

Nuytinck L, Freund M, Lagae L: Classical Ehlers-Danlos syndrome caused by a mutation in type 1 collagen. *Am J Hum Genet* 2000;66:1398-1402.

Robinson PN, Godfrey M: The molecular genetics of Marfan syndrome and related microfibrillopathies. *J Med Genet* 2000;37:9-25.

Tsipouras P, Del Mastro R, Sarfarazi M, et al: Genetic linkage of the Marfan syndrome, ectopia lentis, and congenital contractural arachnodactyly to the fibrillin genes on chromosomes 15 and 5. *N Engl J Med* 1992;326:905-909.

Wenstrup RJ, Florer JB, Willing MC: COL5a1 haploinsufficiency is a common molecular mechanism underlying the classical form of EDS. *Am J Hum Genet* 2000;66:1766-1776.

Neuromuscular Disorders
Antonellis A, Ellsworth RE, Sambuughin N: Glycyl tRNA synthetase mutations in Charcot-Marie-Tooth disease type 2D and distal spinal muscular atrophy type V. *Am J Hum Genet* 2003;72:1293-1299.

Azzedine H, Bolino A, Taieb T, et al: Mutations in MTMR13, a new pseudophosphatase homologue of MTMR2 and Sbf1, in two families with an autosomal recessive demyelinating form of Charcot-Marie-Tooth disease associated with early-onset glaucoma. *Am J Hum Genet* 2003;72:1141-1153.

Berger P, Bonneick S, Willi S: Loss of phosphatase activity in myotubularin-related protein 2 is associated with Charcot-Marie-Tooth disease type 4B1. *Hum Mol Genet* 2002;11:1569-1579.

Bijlsma EK, Aalfs CM, Sluijter S, et al: Familial cryptic translocation between chromosomes 2qter and 8quter: Further delineation of the Albright hereditary osteodystrophy-like phenotype. *J Med Genet* 1999;36:604-609.

Bovee JV, Cleton-Jansen AM, Wuyts W, et al: EXT-mutation analysis and loss of heterozygosity in sporadic and hereditary osteochondromas and secondary chondrosarcomas. *Am J Hum Genet* 1999;65:689-698.

Candeliere GA, Glorieux FH: Prud'Homme J, St-Arnaud R: Increased expression of the c-fos proto-oncogene in bone from patients with fibrous dysplasia. *N Engl J Med* 1995;332:1546-1551.

Crosby AH, Proukakis C: Is the transportation highway the right road for hereditary spastic paraplegia? *Am J Hum Genet* 2002;71:1009-1016.

Delatycki M, Williamson R, Forrest SM: Friedreich ataxia: An overview. *J Med Genet* 2000;37:1-8.

Fabrizi GM, Simonati A, Taioli F: PMP22 related congenital hypomyelination neuropathy. *J Neurol Neurosurg Psychiatry* 2001;70:123-126.

Gennarelli M: Novelli, Bassi FA, et al: Prediction of myotonic dystrophy clinical severity based on the number of intragenic [CTG]n trinucleotide repeats. *Am J Med Genet* 1996;65:342-347.

Hallam PJ, Harding AE, Berciano J, Barker DF, Malcolm S: Duplication of part of chromosome 17 is commonly associated with hereditary motor and sensory neuropathy type I (Charcot-Marie-Tooth disease type 1). *Ann Neurol* 1992;31:570-572.

Hecht JT, Hogue D, Wang Y, et al: Hereditary multiple exostoses (EXT): Mutational studies of familial EXT1 cases and EXT-associated malignancies. *Am J Hum Genet* 1997;60:80-86.

Laurin N, Brown J, Lemainque A, et al: Paget disease of bone: Mapping of two loci at 5q35-qter and 5q31. *Am J Hum Genet* 2001;69:528-543.

Laurin N, Brown JP, Morissette J, Raymond V: Recurrent mutation of the gene encoding sequestosome 1 (SQSTM1/p62) in Paget disease of bone. *Am J Hum Genet* 2002;70:1582-1588.

Leach RJ, Singer FR, Roodman GD: The genetics of Paget's disease of the bone. *J Clin Endocrinol Metab* 2001;86:24-28.

Lumbroso S, Paris F, Sultan C: McCune-Albright syndrome: Molecular genetics. *J Pediatr Endocrinol Metab* 2002;15(suppl 3):875-882.

Marie PJ, dePollak C, Chanson P, Lomri A: Increased proliferation of osteoblastic cells expressing the activating Gs alpha mutation in monostotic and polyostotic fibrous dysplasia. *Am J Pathol* 1997;150:1059-1069.

Nelis E, Erdem S, Van Den Bergh PY, et al: Mutations in GDAP1: Autosomal recessive CMT with demyelination and axonopathy. *Neurology* 2002;59:1865-1872.

Plante-Bordeneuve V, Said G: Dejerine-Sottas disease and hereditary demyelinating polyneuropathy of infancy. *Muscle Nerve* 2002;26:608-621.

Ruttledge MH, Andermann AA, Phelan CM, et al: Type of mutation in the neurofibromatosis type 2 gene (NF2) frequently determines severity of disease. *Am J Hum Genet* 1996;59:331-342.

Senderek J, Bergmann C, Weber S: Mutation of the SBF2 gene, encoding a novel member of the myotubularin family, in Charcot-Marie-Tooth neuropathy type 4B2/11p15. *Hum Mol Genet* 2003;12:349-356.

Serra E, Puig S, Otero D, et al: Confirmation of a double-hit model for the NF1 gene in benign neurofibromas. *Am J Hum Genet* 1997;61:512-519.

Shahbazian MD, Zoghbi HY: Rett syndrome and MeCP2: Linking epigenetics and neuronal function. *Am J Hum Genet* 2002;71:1259-1272.

van Swieten JC, Brusse E, de Graaf BM: A mutation in the fibroblast growth factor 14 gene is associated with autosomal dominant cerebral ataxia. *Am J Hum Genet* 2003;72:191-199.

Zhao C, Takita J, Tanaka Y: Charcot-Marie-Tooth disease type 2A caused by mutation in a microtubule motor KIF1Bß. *Cell* 2001;105:587-597.

Chapter 3

Biomechanics

Lichun Lu, PhD
Kenton R. Kaufman, PhD, PE
Michael J. Yaszemski, MD, PhD

Introduction

Biomechanics is the science of applying the principles and methods of engineering mechanics to biologic tissues and to the analysis of medical problems. The behavior of the human musculoskeletal system, although complex and dynamic, can be described by, and obeys, Newton's laws of mechanics. Orthopaedic biomechanics focuses on the effects, motions, and deformations that result from forces and moments acting on various tissues such as bone, cartilage, growth plate, ligament, tendon, meniscus, synovial fluid, and intervertebral disks.

The study of biomechanics has been important in the understanding of the normal structure and function of the musculoskeletal system, in the examination of specific pathologic conditions, in the development and design of devices used in orthopaedic surgery, in the evaluation of surgical procedures for the restoration of normal mechanics, and in improving postoperative rehabilitation treatments. For instance, human joints are subjected to a wide range of forces during activities of daily living. Most human joints can undergo millions of loading cycles per year, even under forces that can be several times body weight during strenuous activities. However, abnormal joint forces are believed to play a central role in cartilage degeneration that leads to osteoarthritis. In addition, many issues in total joint arthroplasty, such as the wear and deformation of the articulating surface, the stress distribution in the implant, the mechanical behavior of the bone-implant interface, and the load-bearing characteristics of the remaining bone, are intimately related to the joint loads. Therefore, a thorough understanding of joint forces is important.

In this chapter, selected fundamental principles of mechanics are reviewed and examples provided of how these principles are used in orthopaedic biomechanics. The chapter begins with a presentation of basic definitions of forces and moments and their analysis. The concepts of static equilibrium of a rigid body are then developed and representative calculations demonstrated. The procedures for analyzing the strength of materials are discussed.

Definitions and Basic Concepts

The study of mechanics can be described as the study of the conditions of rest or motion of bodies under the action of forces. Mechanics can be subdivided into the study of solids and fluids. Solid body mechanics can be further subdivided into rigid body mechanics and deformable body mechanics.

Rigid Bodies

If a body, when subjected to externally applied forces or heat, maintains the relative positions of any two particles within it, then that body is defined as being rigid. Actually, all structures deform under load, but if the deformations are small compared with the body size, they can be ignored for static equilibrium and motion (dynamics) calculations. The assumption of rigidity is therefore only relative, depending on the circumstances and applications. Rigid body mechanics includes the study of statics and dynamics. Dynamics includes both the study of motion without consideration of the forces that cause that motion (kinematics), and the study of the relationship between forces and the motion that results from their application (kinetics).

Deformable Bodies

If a body subjected to external forces or heat demonstrates relative displacements between its component particles, then it is defined as deformable. Deformable body mechanics is the study of the internal force density (stress) and the associated deformation (strain) of a body subjected to various external loading conditions or changing ambient temperature.

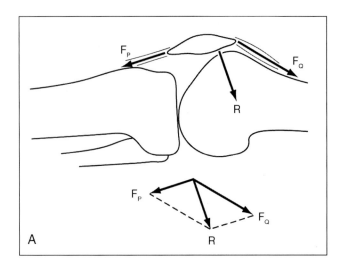

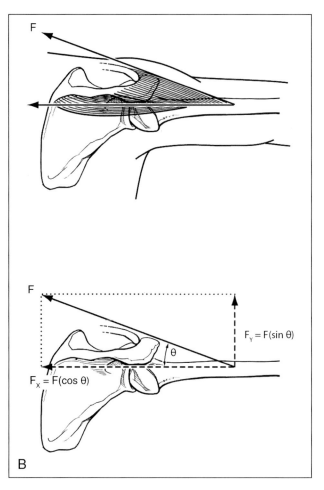

Figure 1   **A,** The addition of the force of the quadriceps F_Q and the force of the patellar tendon F_p, according to the parallelogram law, produces the resultant force R, which tends to compress the patella against the femur. *(Reproduced from Mow VC, Flatow EL, Ateshian GA: Biomechanics, in Buckwalter JA, Einhorn TA, Simon SR (eds): Orthopaedic Basic Science: Biology and Biomechanics of the Musculoskeletal System, ed 2. Rosemont, IL, American Academy of Orthopaedic Surgeons, 2000, pp 134-180.)* **B,** The deltoid force F, can be resolved into a stabilizing component F_x, and a rotatory component F_y, by using the trigonometric relationships for the right triangle. The angle of force application is θ. *(Adapted with permission from An KW, Chao EYS, Kaufman KR: Analysis of muscle and joint loads, in Mow VC, Hayes WC (eds): Basic Orthopaedic Biomechanics, ed 2. Philadelphia, PA, Lippincott Williams & Wilkins, 1997.)*

Fluids

A fluid is a continuum that is unable to withstand a static shear stress. Fluid mechanics, also called fluid dynamics, is the branch of mechanics that studies the properties of liquids and gases, such as viscosity and flow conditions, as a function of space and time.

Vectors and Forces

There are several types of physical quantities. Two of these are scalars and vectors. Scalars are quantities that are completely specified by a single number, which describes their magnitude. Examples include mass (kg), volume (m^3), density (kg/m^3), time (sec), and speed (m/s). Vectors are composed of four components: magnitude, direction, sense, and position (also called point of application). Examples of vectors are force, stress, strain, velocity, torque, and displacement. Vectors are denoted by several different symbols. These symbols include either a boldface letter or a letter with an arrow (→), or bar (—) over it.

Force represents an interaction between two bodies. Forces can be contact forces (bodies touching each other) or field forces (bodies separated by a distance, such as gravitational, electric, or magnetic forces). The International System of Units (SI) unit for force is newton (N),

with 1 N defined as the force that causes a 1-kg mass to accelerate at 1 m/s^2.

Mechanics experiments show that any set of coplanar forces may be replaced by a single force having the same effect. This single force, obtained by combining the given forces according to the parallelogram law of vector addition, is called the resultant force. Vectors are added by joining the head of one vector to the tail of the next vector while retaining the magnitude and direction of each vector (**Figure 1,** *A*). The resultant vector is represented by the distance between the last head and the first tail.

The original vector may be broken down or resolved into several component forces, usually along specified mutually perpendicular coordinate axes. The original vector **F** is the sum of its components along these axes (**Figure 1,** *B*).

$$\mathbf{F} = \mathbf{F}_x + \mathbf{F}_y$$

The magnitudes of $\mathbf{F}_x$ and $\mathbf{F}_y$ are denoted by F_x and F_y or $|\mathbf{F}_x|$ and $|\mathbf{F}_y|$, respectively. According to the trigonometric relationships of combining and resolving forces, the magnitude and direction of the resultant force may be calculated by:

$$F^2 = F_x{}^2 + F_y{}^2$$
$$\tan \theta = F_y / F_x$$

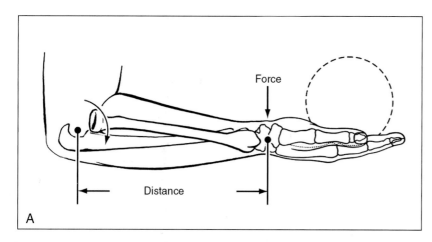

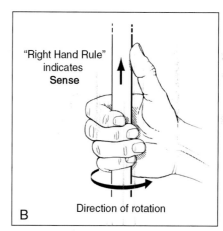

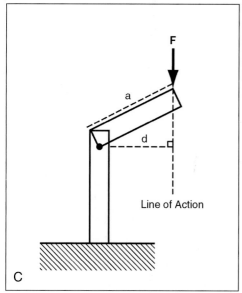

Figure 2   A, The magnitude of a moment is the product of a force and the perpendicular distance from an axis of rotation. **B,** The direction of a moment is given by the right-hand rule. **C,** The action arm, a, is the direct distance along the structure, whereas the moment arm, d, is the perpendicular distance from the line of action of the force to the axis of rotation.

The values of F_x and F_y also can be obtained if **F** is known by using the sine and cosine functions:

$$F_x = F\cos\theta$$
$$F_y = F\sin\theta$$

In orthopaedic biomechanics, it is often useful to describe forces as tensile, compressive, or shear. Tensile and compressive forces are perpendicular (normal) to the surface under consideration, whereas shear forces are parallel (tangential) to the surface under consideration. The surfaces to be considered for force analysis are chosen such that the desired information can be obtained in the most expeditious mathematical method possible. These surfaces are the external boundaries of the free body chosen for analysis, whether the system consists of a rigid body, a deformable body, or a fluid.

Moments

A moment represents the turning, twisting, or rotational effect of a force. Skeletal motions are the result of the moments applied by muscles that cross the joints on which they act. A moment is defined as the product of a force and the perpendicular distance between the line of action of the force and the axis of rotation of the motion that the force produces (**Figure 2, A**). The SI unit for a moment is the newton-meter (Nm). A moment is a vector. Its magnitude is the force-perpendicular distance product mentioned above. The direction of a moment is defined by the "right-hand rule" (**Figure 2, B**), where the positive moment direction is identified by the thumb of the right hand when the fingers of the right hand are curled in the direction of rotation caused by the force. The direction of a moment is along the axis of rotation (or potential rotation) and thus perpendicular to the plane in which the twisting force is applied. Moment arm, the distance used to calculate the moment, is the distance from the action line to the actual or potential pivot point of the system, regardless of the state of motion. The moment arm is chosen so that it is perpendicular to the action line of the force that is responsible for the motion or potential motion. The moment arm (d) may or may not be the same as the action

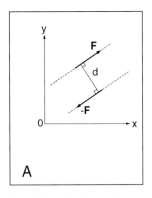

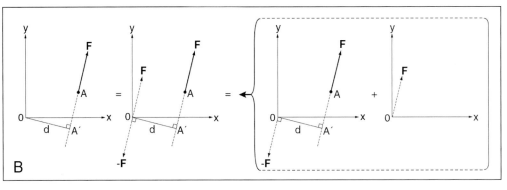

Figure 3   **A,** A couple is created by two equal, noncollinear, parallel but oppositely directed forces **F** and **–F**. The magnitude of the couple is Fd, where d is the perpendicular distance between the two forces. **B,** A single force applied at point A, acting along A-A', whose perpendicular distance to point O is d, is equivalent to a force acting at O and a couple of magnitude Fd.

arm (a), which is the shortest distance along the structure from the point of force application to the pivot point (**Figure 2,** *C*).

When a pair of forces **F** and **–F** that have equal magnitude, parallel lines of action, and opposite senses act on a body, the moment created is called a couple (**Figure 3,** *A*). The resultant force of a couple is zero. The magnitude of the couple is Fd, where d is the perpendicular distance between the two forces. As illustrated in **Figure 3,** *B*, any system of forces on a rigid body may be replaced by an equivalent system that consists of a single force acting at a chosen point and a couple. The force **F** at point A is shown in the xy plane with an origin of O. The line of action of **F** is closest to O at point A'. The distance d is thus the moment arm relative to point O. A pair of imaginary forces **F** and **–F** can be added to the point O because they cancel each other. The pair of forces composed of the original force **F** at A and **–F** at O is a couple, which is a free pure moment acting in the xy plane. Thus, the original force **F** at A is equal to a couple and a force **F** at O. The concept of couple is very useful in understanding the effects of muscle action around a joint.

Newton's Laws

Newton's three laws of mechanics form the basis for understanding force equilibrium. The first law states that if the resultant force acting on a body is zero, the body is either at rest, or remains in motion at a constant speed and direction (that is, it has constant velocity). The second law states that if the resultant force acting on a body is not zero, the body will have an acceleration proportional to the magnitude and in the direction of the resultant force. The force is equal to the mass multiplied by acceleration **F = ma**. The third law states that the forces of action and reaction between bodies in contact have equal magnitude and same line of action but opposite sense.

Static Equilibrium

A rigid body is an idealized model of a real object because it assumes that there is no deformation of the body no matter how large the forces and moments acting on it. Gait analysis uses rigid body models to describe the kinetics and kinematics of human locomotion. In the musculoskeletal system, bones are assumed to be rigid rods, and joints to be frictionless hinges. The important elements of rigid body mechanics are: (1) the magnitude, direction, line of action, and point of application of forces acting on the body; (2) the total mass of, and its distribution within, the body; and (3) the size and geometric form of the body.

When the sum of all forces and moments acting on the body is zero, there will be no linear accelerations because of unbalanced forces or angular (rotational) accelerations because of unbalanced moments. Under these conditions, the system is considered to be in equilibrium, either at rest or at constant velocity. Because ΣF and ΣM must be zero regardless of the location on a rigid body where one chooses to calculate them, the choice can be made in a manner that optimizes the ability to perform the calculations for the equilibrium condition.

Statics is the study of forces acting on an object at rest. When performing a force analysis of a rigid body, the body or part of a body at equilibrium may be isolated from the environment, and the environment is replaced by forces acting on the system. This is called a free-body diagram. Because both forces and moments are vectors, they must sum to zero in each of the three perpendicular directions (reference system). Thus, there are a total of six equations of equilibrium, and a maximum of six unknowns may be solved, in a three-dimensional system.

Mechanics problems in which the number of unknown forces and moments is equal to the number of available equations are called statically determinate problems. In statically indeterminate problems, however, the number of unknowns exceeds the number of equations,

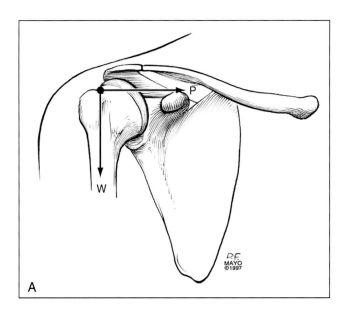

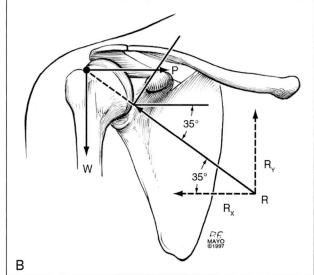

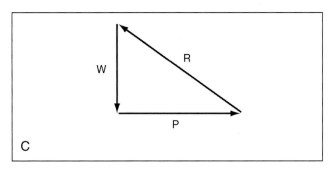

Figure 4   **A,** Static forces on the glenohumeral joint during standing. **B,** Free-body diagram. **C,** Graphic solution. *(Adapted with permission from An KW, Chao EYS, Kaufman KR: Analysis of muscle and joint loads, in Mow VC, Hayes WC (eds):* Basic Orthopaedic Biomechanics, *ed 2. Philadelphia, PA, Lippincott Williams & Wilkins, 1997.)*

and no unique solution can be found. In virtually all problems in orthopaedic biomechanics that determine muscle and joint forces, the situations are statically indeterminate because of the large number of muscles spanning the joint. In these situations, assumptions are often made to simplify the models to estimate the important muscle and joint forces. For instance, a muscle force is often assumed to exist only in tension, whereas the joint reaction-force is considered to be always compressive. The line of action of the muscle force is defined by assuming that it always acts along the center of the cross-sectional area of the muscle mass, and a joint may be modeled as a simple hinge, thus eliminating two of three possible axes of rotation and ignoring translations.

Many joint force problems are further simplified into a two-dimensional analysis. For the body to be in equilibrium, there are two sets of conditions that must be satisfied: translational equilibrium and rotational equilibrium.

In translational equilibrium, there must be no unbalanced forces acting in either the x or y direction. This situation is equivalent to requiring that both the x and y components of the resultant force acting on the object are zero. The condition for translational equilibrium can be written $\Sigma\mathbf{F} = 0$. This vector equation is equivalent to:

$$\Sigma F_x = 0$$
$$\text{and } \Sigma F_y = 0$$

In this notation, a component is positive if it points in the direction of the positive axis and negative if it points in the other direction.

Example 1. In the example shown in **Figure 4,** *A,* if the weight (W) of the upper limb is 50 N and the slope of the glenoid fossa at the point of joint contact is 35° from the horizontal, calculate the force, P, in the supraspinatus muscle that is necessary to prevent subluxation of the humeral head. In addition, calculate the glenohumeral joint reaction force, R.

Solution: A free-body diagram (**Figure 4,** *B*) is drawn first, with the y-axis parallel to the direction of the force of gravity. Because the magnitude, the direction, and line of action of the force due to gravity, W, and the direction and line of action of the muscle force are known, vector analysis can be used to determine the magnitude of the muscle force and the direction and magnitude of the joint reaction force. The direction of the joint reaction force is assumed to be perpendicular to the joint surface because healthy articular cartilage surfaces transmit nearly no frictional forces parallel to the joint surface. The reaction

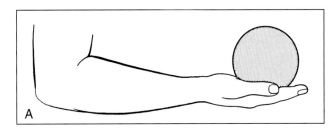

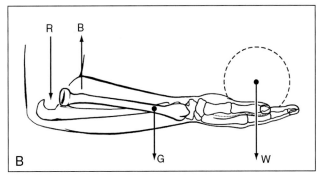

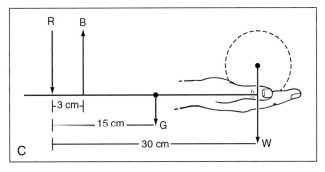

Figure 5   A parallel force system acting on the forearm. *(Adapted with permission from An KW, Chao EYS, Kaufman KR: Analysis of muscle and joint loads, in Mow VC, Hayes WC (eds): Basic Orthopaedic Biomechanics, ed 2. Philadelphia, PA, Lippincott Williams & Wilkins, 1997.)*

force can be resolved into two components, the horizontal component $R_x = R\cos35°$, and the vertical component $R_y = R\sin35°$. The equilibrium equations become:

$$\Sigma F_x = P - R_x = P - R\cos35° = 0$$
$$\text{and } \Sigma F_y = R_y - W = R\sin35° - W = 0$$

which give

$$R = W / \sin35° = 50 / 0.574 = 87.1 \text{ N}$$
$$\text{and } P = R_x = R\cos35° = (87.1)(0.819) = 71.3 \text{ N}$$

The graphic solution is illustrated in **Figure 4**, *C*.

In rotational equilibrium, there must be no unbalanced moments that would tend to cause rotation. The sum of moments (ΣM) about a point must be zero, that is, the sum of the clockwise moments (ΣM_{cw}) must be equal to the sum of the counterclockwise moments (ΣM_{ccw}). Thus, the condition for rotational equilibrium is:

$$\Sigma M = 0$$
$$\text{or } \Sigma M_{CW} = \Sigma M_{CCW}$$

Example 2. Consider the flexed arm that is holding a ball, as shown in **Figure 5**. The biceps muscle provides force B to counterbalance the moment exerted by the forces of gravity on the forearm (G) and the ball (W). With the biceps muscle supporting the forearm at 90° of elbow flexion, the lever arm is the perpendicular distance from the tendon to the axis of the elbow joint.

Solution: Suppose the forearm weighs 15 N, its center of mass is 15 cm from the elbow joint, the ball weighs 20 N and is placed in the hand at 30 cm from the elbow center, and the biceps muscle has a lever arm of 3 cm. The elbow joint is the axis of rotation (or potential rotation). Note that the reaction force produces no moment about the elbow because its distance from the axis is zero. Thus the moments produced by each force are added to obtain rotational equilibrium:

$$\Sigma M = \Sigma M_{CW} - \Sigma M_{CCW} = 0$$
$$(B \times 3 \text{ cm}) - [(G \times 15 \text{ cm}) + (W \times 30 \text{ cm})] = 0$$
$$\text{Thus, } 3B = 15G + 30W = (15 \text{ cm} \times 15 \text{ N}) +$$
$$(30 \text{ cm} \times 20 \text{ N}) = 825 \text{ N·cm}$$
$$B = 275 \text{ N}$$

In this example it could instead be assumed that the potential axis of rotation is at the point of application of force B, and the equation could be solved for the elbow joint reaction force R. This illustrates that in using the rotational equilibrium condition, it makes no difference which axis is used for the purpose of summing moments. Note also that, by convention, counterclockwise moments are positive, and clockwise moments are negative.

In many situations, the forces acting on a body are neither parallel nor concurrent. This is described as a general force system. Both translational and rotational equilibrium need to be maintained in such a system, which can be described by the following equations, referred to as the planar equilibrium conditions:

$$\Sigma F_x = 0$$
$$\Sigma F_y = 0$$
$$\Sigma M = 0$$

To summarize, when an object is known to be at rest, the steps in the solution of the equilibrium problem are:
(1) Select the free body appropriate to the solution of the problem.
(2) Draw the free-body diagram to show all forces acting (both magnitude and direction).
(3) Choose coordinate axes and the axis to be used for summing moments.
(4) Resolve each force into orthogonal components and apply the pertinent equations of equilibrium ($\Sigma F = 0$; $\Sigma M = 0$).
(5) Solve the equations of equilibrium to obtain unknown values.

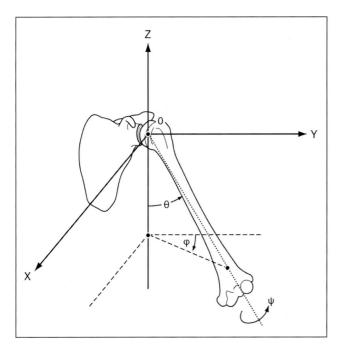

Figure 6   Illustration of the six degrees of freedom of a rigid body: the position of the humeral head is specified by the three coordinates in the xyz orthogonal system, and the position of the humerus relative to the xyz coordinate axes is defined by the three angular orientations θ, φ, and ψ.

Dynamics

When there are unbalanced forces or moments acting on a rigid body, it is under a nonequilibrium, or dynamic condition, resulting in motion. The study of dynamics of a rigid body includes kinematics and kinetics. Kinematics is used to describe motion without regard to the forces and moments producing the motion. It is the study of the relationships between positions, velocities, and accelerations of a rigid body. Kinetics is the study of the forces that cause motion of a rigid body.

The position of an object is defined relative to a reference frame. In a rigid body, there is no internal deformation and the mutual distances between all particles remain constant. Degrees of freedom is a term that describes the number of independent coordinates necessary to describe the motion of a rigid body in space. In three dimensions, six coordinates are required to locate and orient the rigid body. Therefore, a rigid body in space without any constraint has six degrees of freedom. The six coordinates may be defined as: (1) the three coordinates of a point in the x, y, z reference frame, and (2) the three orientation angles of the body relative to the reference frame. In such a system, a rigid body may translate in any of three mutually perpendicular directions, and may rotate about any of those same three axes. As an example, shown in **Figure 6**, the center of the humeral head is placed at the origin O defined by the three coordinates (0,0,0) in the x, y, z reference frame. The position of the humerus relative to the

three orthogonal axes x, y, and z is defined by the three angles θ, φ, and ψ. The humerus may translate in an antero-posterior (x) direction, toward or away from the glenoid (joint compression or distraction; y-direction), or in a superior-inferior (z) direction. Possible rotations of the humerus are abduction/adduction, θ, in the scapular plane, flexion/extension, φ, perpendicular to the scapular plane, or axial rotation, ψ, around the longitudinal axis of the humerus.

The change of position of a point in space is represented by a vector called displacement. The displacement vector is independent of the path of motion, and can be either linear or angular. Velocity is defined as the change of position with respect to time. Because velocity is a vector, the change in velocity could mean a change of direction or speed (magnitude) or both. Translation is the movement of a body such that all points in the body move along parallel paths and have the same velocity and acceleration at any given instant. Rotatory, or angular, motion is the movement of a body around an axis, called the axis of rotation. During rotatory motion, all parts of the body travel in the same direction through the same angle of rotation. With rotation, all parts of the body, except those that lie on the axis of rotation, move in parallel planes along concentric circles centered on the same fixed axis. The angle of rotation is measured on a plane perpendicular to the axis. In general, the motion of any rigid body can be described as a combination of translation and rotation. At any given instant, the general motion is equivalent to the sum of translation along and rotation about an instantaneous axis.

Hip Abductor Forces

The free-body method of solution will be illustrated by calculating the abductor and joint reaction forces at the hip. **Figure 7,** *A* illustrates a free-body diagram of the hip of a person standing on the right leg. The body and the left leg weigh 5/6 W, where W is the total weight of the person. When in equilibrium, the known clockwise moment (M_{cw}, negative by convention) created by the gravitational force 5/6 W, which tends to rotate the upper body about the center of the femoral head O, must be balanced by the unknown counterclockwise moment (M_{ccw}, positive by convention) created by the abductor muscles on the pelvis, F_{AB}. Because the point of application and direction of the abductor force F_{AB} are assumed to be known from the anatomic data, the magnitude of F_{AB} can be calculated. The moment arm for the force F_{AB} is 5 cm (distance "a" in the figure) and that for 5/6 W is 15 cm (distance "b" in the figure). Thus, magnitudes of the corresponding moments are $M_{ccw} = \{(F_{AB}) \times (a)\}$ and $M_{cw} = \{- (5/6 \, W) \times (b) \}$. Because the sum of these two moments must equal zero at equilibrium, the magnitude of the abductor muscle force F_{AB} is determined to be 2.5W:

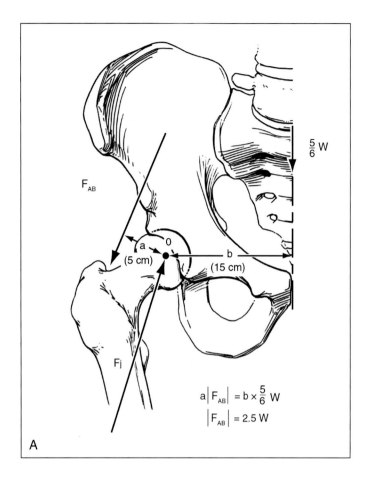

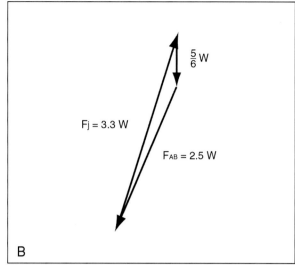

$$a \left| F_{AB} \right| = b \times \frac{5}{6} W$$
$$\left| F_{AB} \right| = 2.5 \ W$$

A

Figure 7   A, A free-body diagram of the hip of a person standing on the right leg. The body and the left leg weights 5/6 W, where W is the total weight of the person. The magnitude of the abductor muscle force F_{AB} (its direction is known), may be determined by setting the sum of the moments about point O equal to zero. **B,** A force triangle may be constructed to determine the joint-reaction force F_j. *(Reproduced from Mow VC, Flatow EL, Ateshian GA: Biomechanics, in Buckwalter JA, Einhorn TA, Simon SR (eds): Orthopaedic Basic Science: Biology and Biomechanics of the Musculoskeletal System, ed 2. Rosemont, IL, American Academy of Orthopaedic Surgeons, 2000, pp 134-180.)*

$$\Sigma \ M_{ccw} + \Sigma \ M_{cw} = 0$$

$$\{(F_{AB}) \ x \ (a)\} + \{- \ (5/6 \ W) \ x \ (b)\ \} = 0$$

$$F_{AB} = (5/6 \ W) \ x \ (b) \ / \ (a) = (5)(15) \ W \ / \ (6)(5) = 2.5 \ W$$

The hip joint reaction force acting on the right acetabulum, F_j, does not create a moment about the joint center, similar to the reaction force at the hinge in a seesaw. To calculate F_j, the force equilibrium condition is applied, which stipulates that the sum of all forces acting on the pelvis must equal zero. **Figure 7,** *B* illustrates the force triangle based on the parallelogram law of vector addition. With the two known forces, 5/6 W and 2.5 W, drawn to scale, the third unknown force F_j can also be drawn to scale, with the length of the third side of the triangle being the magnitude of the force F_j and the direction of the arrow being the direction of F_j. In this example, the magnitude of F_j is calculated to be 3.3 W. Both the muscle force and the joint-reaction force are considerably greater than the weight of the body and leg they are supporting because of the lever action of muscle forces around the hip joint. The joint reaction force is the compressive force between the opposing cartilage surfaces of the femoral head and the acetabulum. This is the force that the cartilage must bear in carrying out its function as the joint-bearing surface.

This example also illustrates that the force calculation can be done either graphically, as in the determination of the joint reaction force, or analytically, as in the calculation of the hip abductor muscle force.

Shoulder Forces

The free-body diagram in **Figure 8** shows three forces acting on an extended arm: the weight W that is held in the hand, the deltoid muscle force Fd, and the joint-reaction force F_j between the humeral head and the glenoid fossa. For the purposes of this example, the weight of the arm has been neglected in the determination of the deltoid muscle force and the glenohumeral joint force resulting from the weight held in the hand. This free-body diagram is obtained by using the following four modeling assumptions for the unknown forces: (1) a two-dimensional plane model is chosen; (2) the location of the deltoid force is at the centroid of the muscle (d = 5 cm from the center of the humeral head); (3) the deltoid force is tensile; and (4) the glenohumeral joint force is compressive. The held weight W is 100 N in the direction of gravity, and is located 60 cm from the center of the humeral head O.

When the arm is in equilibrium, the three forces and their moments must sum to zero. Because the clockwise moment of the deltoid muscle force about the point O $[-(F_d) \times 5]$ must equal the counterclockwise moment of

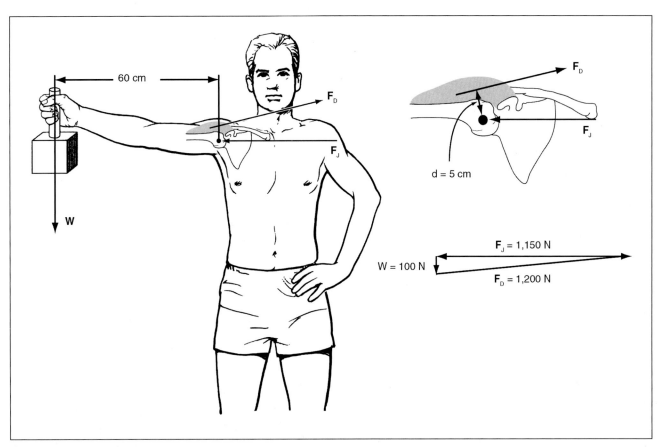

Figure 8   A person holds a weight W at a distance of 60 cm from the center of rotation of the humeral head. After determining the magnitude of the deltoid muscle force F_d (its direction is known) by summing the moments about point O, F_j may be found from the force triangle. *(Adapted from Mow VC, Flatow EL, Ateshian GA: Biomechanics, in Buckwalter JA, Einhorn TA, Simon SR (eds): Orthopaedic Basic Science: Biology and Biomechanics of the Musculoskeletal System, ed 2. Rosemont, IL, American Academy of Orthopaedic Surgeons, 2000, pp 134-180.)*

the weight $[+ (W) \times 60]$, then $F_d = 1,200$ N, which is about 1.5 times the average body weight of an adult. The joint-reaction force F_j can be found by using the force triangle concept described earlier. By drawing the two known sides of the triangle proportional to the length of the forces, F_j is found to be 1,150 N in the direction shown.

Spine Forces

The free-body diagram in **Figure 9** is used to show how the musculoskeletal lever system can magnify the compressive force acting on the spine during an ordinary daily activity such as holding a weight W_1 with an outstretched hand. The moment equilibrium condition about the center of a vertebral body O can be used to calculate the compressive force F_n in the spine. The clockwise moment is produced by both the held weight W_1 $[-(W_1) \times b]$ and the upper body weight $[-(W) \times c]$, while the counterclockwise moment is generated by the extensor muscle force F_e $[+(F_e) \times a]$. Assume $W = 500$ N, $W_1 = 100$ N, $a = 5$ cm, $b = 50$ cm, and $c = 8$ cm, then $F_e = (1,000 + 800)$ N. Note that the 100-N weight held at 50 cm produces a 1,000-N force in F_e while the

500-N upper body weight produces only 800 N in F_e. The transverse force acting on the vertebral body (and disk) is F_t. This would be the force that tends to produce a spondylolisthesis, for example.

For the upper body to be at equilibrium, the sum of the vertical components of all forces must equal to zero: $F_n\cos\theta - F_e\cos\theta - W - W_1 + F_t\sin\theta = 0$. In addition, the horizontal components of all forces must add to zero: $F_n\sin\theta - F_e\sin\theta - F_t\cos\theta = 0$. If $\theta = 60°$, then the two equations can be solved to give $F_t = (W+W_1) \sin60° = 520$ N and $F_n = F_e + (W+W_1) \cos60° = 2,100$ N. Hence, the compressive force acting perpendicular to the face of the vertebral body F_n is many times the weight supported, which derives mostly from the extensor muscle force (1,800 N), and the major component of that force (1,000 N) is a result of holding a relatively small weight (100 N) at a 50 cm distance from the spine. The normal compressive force F_n acting on the vertebral body can be reduced dramatically if the distance b is reduced by holding the weight closer to the body. This example illustrates that large forces may be generated in the spine from simple activities, causing fracture in some patients, especially those with osteoporosis.

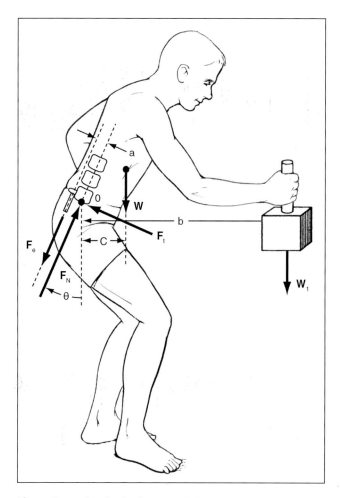

Figure 9   A free-body diagram of the spine. The normal compressive force F_n acting on the spine is 2,100 N even during an ordinary daily activity such as holding a 100-N weight by an outstretched hand at a 50-cm distance. *(Adapted from Mow VC, Flatow EL, Ateshian GA: Biomechanics, in Buckwalter JA, Einhorn TA, Simon SR (eds): Orthopaedic Basic Science: Biology and Biomechanics of the Musculoskeletal System, ed 2. Rosemont, IL, American Academy of Orthopaedic Surgeons, 2000, pp 134-180.)*

Mechanical Properties of Materials

The study of mechanics of deformable bodies is also known as the mechanics of materials or strength of materials. This topic includes the study of externally applied forces, internal constraint forces, deformation associated with the forces, material properties, and physical laws to relate the forces and deformations based on the material properties of the specimen.

Normal Stress and Strain

Consider the example given in **Figure 10**. An axial force F produces a uniform stretching of a prismatic bar of cross-sectional area A, resulting in an elongation of δ. A prismatic bar is a bar that has a constant cross section along its entire length. To investigate the stress and strain, the part of the bar to the left of an imaginary cut section (cross sec-

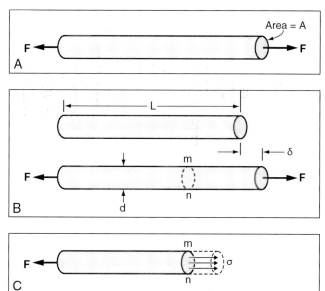

Figure 10   Prismatic bar with an initial length of L and cross-sectional area of A under tensile forces F.

tion mn) is isolated as a free body. To balance the tensile load F at the left end, the forces at the other end represent the action of the removed part of the bar upon the free body. The force per unit area is defined as the stress σ. Assuming a uniform distribution of force over the cross-sectional area A, the stress is written $\sigma = F/A$.

When the force acts perpendicular to the surface, the resulting stress is called normal stress. It is further classified as tensile stress if the bar is stretched by the force, and as compressive stress if the bar is compressed by the force. In SI units, the stress is expressed as N/m^2 or pascals (Pa). In order for the equation $\sigma = F/A$ to be valid, the stress must be uniformly distributed over the cross section of the bar. This is realized if the axial force F acts through the centroid of the cross-sectional area. The centroid is the geometric center of an area and is a single point that represents the entire cross section such that a force applied at the centroid would tend to translate, but not rotate, the entire cross section. It is equivalent in concept to the center of gravity of a three-dimensional object that is under the influence of a gravitational force. If the force on a prismatic bar acts at a point other than the centroid, then bending occurs.

In the example given, the uniform stress condition exists throughout the length of the bar except near the ends. If the load F is applied over a small area, high localized stresses will result in stress concentrations. Moving away from the ends of the bar, the stress distribution gradually approaches the uniform distribution. It is usually assumed that the formula $\sigma = F/A$ is valid for distances larger than d from the ends, where d is the largest transverse dimension of the bar.

The axially loaded bar undergoes a change in length,

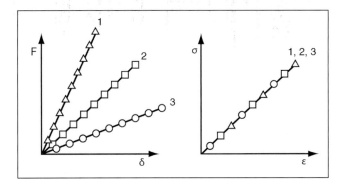

Figure 11　Load-deformation (F-δ) and the corresponding stress-strain (σ-ε) curves of three different structures made from the same material.

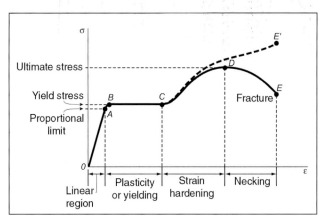

Figure 12　Stress-strain diagram for a typical structural steel in tension (not to scale).

becoming longer in tension and shorter in compression. The change in length is denoted by δ, which is the cumulative result of the stretching of all elements of the material throughout the length L of the bar. Assuming that the material is homogeneous, the strain, or the elongation per unit length, can be expressed as: $\varepsilon = \delta/L$. The strain that is associated with normal stress is called normal strain. It can be further classified as either tensile strain or compressive strain as a result of the corresponding tensile or compressive forces applied.

Forces can be applied to any structure, which results in stresses and strains within the structure. The analysis method presented here requires that the deformation of the bar is uniform, which in turn requires that the bar is prismatic, loads act through the centroid, and the material is homogeneous. The resulting state of stress and strain is called uniaxial stress and strain. The stress and strain obtained by calculations using the initial geometry of the specimen are called nominal stress and strain. However, after the loads are applied, the surface area A becomes smaller under the action of tensile forces and larger under the action of compressive forces, and the corresponding length L is respectively either larger or smaller. If these actual areas and lengths are used in the calculations, the true stress and strain are obtained.

Structural Versus Material Properties

The relationship between the load, F, and the elongation, δ, can be considered a structural property because it depends on both the material and the geometry of the specimen. The relationship between stress σ and strain ε, on the other hand, provides a characterization of a material property of the specimen, independent of its size and shape.

As illustrated in **Figure 11**, the slope of the load-deformation (F-δ) curve for a linear elastic material is k (rigidity) and the slope of the stress-strain (σ-ε) curve is E (modulus of elasticity). Using the definitions of σ and ε,

the equation $\sigma = E\varepsilon$ can be rewritten as:

$$F/A = E\,(\delta/L) \text{ or } F = k\,\delta$$

Where k = AE/L is the structural stiffness of the specimen (in N/m), depending on both its geometry (A and L), and an intrinsic property (Young's modulus) of the material from which it is made. The three structures made of the same material shown here have different F-δ curves but each of them has an identical σ-ε curve.

Stress-Strain Diagrams

The structural and/or material properties of a device are typically determined by mechanical testing. For tests done at different sites and at different times to be comparable, the dimensions of test specimens and the methods of applying loads have been standardized for many commonly encountered materials and structures. The American Society for Testing and Materials (ASTM) is a volunteer standards organization that produces such standardized test conditions. During a static test, the load is applied very slowly and the rate of loading need not be measured. However, during a dynamic test, the rate of loading may be high and because it can affect the material properties, it must be specified and recorded.

As an example, the stress-stain diagram of structural steel under tension is presented in **Figure 12**. The point A is called the proportional limit, and because the curve from origin O to A is linear, the slope of this straight line is the modulus of elasticity. As the stress increases, the slope of the stress-strain curve becomes smaller, until it reaches point B, the yield point. The corresponding stress is the yield stress. This is the transition point between elastic and plastic deformation. From this point on, the stress does not increase or increases only slightly, while considerable elongation occurs up to point C. This phenomenon is called yielding and the material has demonstrated plastic behavior from point B to point C. Beyond point C, the

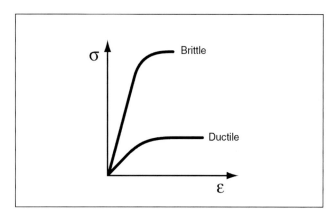

Figure 13 Stress-strain curves of brittle versus ductile materials.

material starts to strain harden, during which period the atomic and crystalline structures of the material change, resulting in increased resistance to further deformation. This is shown as a positive slope from point C to D, reaching a maximal stress called ultimate stress at point D. If the material is further stretched, the stress is decreased and fracture or failure of the material eventually occurs at point E.

Because of lateral contraction, the cross-sectional area of the specimen decreases during stretching. The reduction in area is usually negligible to about point C, beyond which it starts to affect the calculated stress. In the vicinity of the ultimate stress, the reduction in area is clearly visible, creating a phenomenon called necking of the material. When the actual cross-sectional area is used to calculate the stress, the true stress-strain curve that follows the dashed line is obtained. From this curve, it is clear that the material withstands an increase in stress up to failure point E'. Practically, the conventional stress-strain curve OABCDE provides satisfactory information for most design purposes.

Based on the characteristics of the stress-strain curve, a material can be classified as either ductile or brittle (Figure 13). Ductile materials undergo large strains during plastic deformation before failure, and include mild steel, aluminum, copper, magnesium, lead, nickel, brass, bronze, nylon, Teflon, and many others. The ductility of a material in tension can be characterized by its elongation and the percent reduction in area at the fracture section. The percent elongation is defined by:

$$\text{Percent elongation} = \frac{L_f - L_o}{L_o} \times 100\%$$

where L_o is the original gage length during tension testing and L_f is the distance between gage marks at fracture. The gage length is the distance between the attachment points of the extensometer to the specimen during testing. Because the elongation is usually concentrated in the region of necking and is not uniform over the length of the specimen, the percent elongation depends on the gage length.

The amount of necking is measured by the percent reduction in area defined by:

$$\text{Percent reduction in area} = \frac{A_o - A_f}{A_o} \times 100\%$$

where A_o is the original cross-sectional area and A_f is the final area at the fracture surface. The reduction is about 50% for ductile steels.

When a material exhibits no obvious yield point, yet undergoes large strains after the proportional limit, an offset method is often used to determine an arbitrary yield stress. A line is drawn on the stress-strain curve parallel to the initial linear portion of curve, but offset by some standard amount of strain, such as 0.002 or 0.2%. The intersection of this line with the curve is defined as the yield point, and the corresponding stress is the yield stress. Because this stress is not an inherent physical property of the material, it is referred to as the offset yield stress.

A brittle material exhibits very little plastic deformation before fracture, and fails in tension at relatively low strain. Brittle materials include concrete, stone, cast iron, glass, ceramic materials, and many common metallic alloys. Some of these materials, such as glass fibers, demonstrate large strengths and can resist high stresses.

The stress-strain curve under compression may differ from the tension curve. For ductile materials, the proportional limits in compression are very close to those in tension, and therefore the initial regions of their compression curves are similar to the tension curves. However, when yielding begins, instead of necking as would occur under tensile loading, the material bulges outward on the sides, and flattens out as the load increases, thus offering increased resistance to further shortening. The stress-strain curve therefore has a positive slope in its plastic deformation region. For brittle materials, the compression stress-strain diagram has a shape similar to that of the tensile diagram. However, brittle materials usually reach much higher ultimate stresses in compression than in tension. Unlike ductile materials, brittle materials in compression actually fracture or break at the ultimate stress.

Elasticity and Plasticity

As described previously, when the specimen is statically loaded in tension or compression, the corresponding stress-strain diagrams can be obtained. The behavior of the material during unloading when the load is slowly removed is also an important characteristic of the material. As an example, in Figure 14, a tensile load is applied to a specimen and the stress-strain curve goes from point O to A. When the load is removed, the material follows exactly the same curve back to the origin O, meaning it returns to its original dimensions after unloading. Such a material is considered elastic, and this behavior is called elasticity. The curve OA needs not to be linear in order for the material to be elastic.

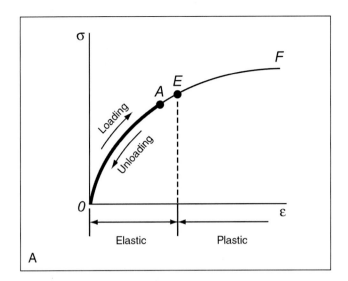

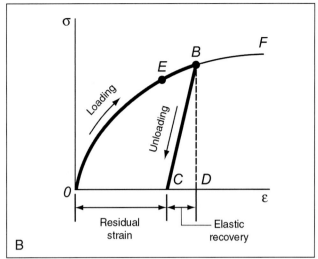

Figure 14   Stress-strain diagrams illustrating **A,** elastic behavior and **B,** partially elastic behavior.

If the material is loaded to a much higher point B on the diagram (**Figure 14,** *B)*, the material follows line BC during unloading. The unloading line is typically parallel to the initial portion of the loading curve (that is, parallel to a line that is tangential to that portion of the curve near O). The strain OC that remains in the material is called the residual strain or permanent strain. The strain CD is that part of the strain that resolves after unloading and is called the elastic recovery. A material that behaves in this manner returns partially to its original shape and is said to be partially elastic. The upper limit of the elastic region is known as the elastic limit of the material, and is very close to the proportional limit. The behavior of a material that undergoes inelastic strains beyond the elastic limit is called plasticity. When large deformations occur in a ductile material loaded into the plastic region, the material is said to undergo plastic flow.

Toughness

The amount of energy per volume a material can absorb before failure defines the intrinsic toughness of the material (**Figure 15**). It is calculated as the area under the stress-strain curve up to the failure point. Materials such as ceramics and cast iron are brittle and are easily fractured. Although they are stiff, these materials are not tough because they cannot absorb much energy. Ductile steel and cortical bone are intrinsically stiff and tough because they fail only after significant stretching. Plastics and rubber are intrinsically soft and tough because they stretch a great amount before failure. Collagenous tissues are soft and not particularly tough.

Fatigue

When materials are subjected to a large number of loading cycles, they will fail at a stress lower than their ultimate stress, which is the stress at failure from a single

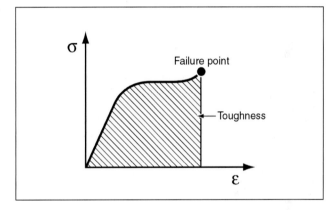

Figure 15   Toughness is the area under the stress-strain curve up to the failure point.

loading cycle. The number of loading cycles required to cause failure is determined by performing a cyclic stress-strain experiment. A stress-cycle (σ-n) curve is generated by plotting the number of loading cycles (n) required to cause failure against the maximum stress level attained during those n loading cycles (**Figure 16**). As the number of cycles increases, the stress at failure decreases. When a stress is reached such that the material will not fail no many how many cycles are repeated, that stress is called the endurance limit σ_E.

Linear Elasticity

Many materials have an initial region on the stress-strain diagram in which they behave both elastically and linearly. The material behavior in this region is called linearly elastic. Many materials are designed to function at these levels to avoid permanent deformation or plastic flow. The linear relationship between stress and strain for a bar in simple tension or compression is expressed as: $\sigma = E\varepsilon$

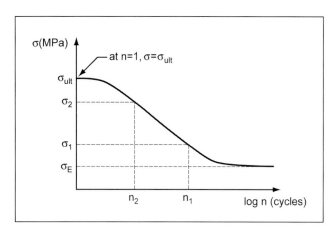

Figure 16   The number of loading cycles, n, required to cause failure of the specimen, plotted against the maximum stress level σ attained during the cyclic test. Cyclic fatigue failure will occur at n_1 cycles of stress σ_1, or n_2 cycles of stress σ_2.

where E is the modulus of elasticity, also called Young's modulus. This equation, which describes the bar's material properties in the linearly elastic region, is an analog of Hooke's law for a spring. Hooke's law describes the linear relationship between the applied load and the resulting deformation.

The modulus of elasticity is specific for a particular material. It is the slope of the stress-strain curve in the linear elastic region, and has the same units as stress, because strain is a dimensionless quantity. As the Young's modulus of a material increases, so does the stiffness of a structure made from it. The moduli of some common materials, arranged from lower to higher values are: ligaments, cartilage, cancellous bone, ultra-high molecular weight polyethylene, polymethylmethacrylate bone cement, cortical bone, titanium, stainless steel, cobalt-chromium-molybdenum alloy, zirconium, and aluminum.

Poisson's Ratio

When a prismatic bar is loaded in tension, the axial elongation is accompanied by a lateral contraction. In the linearly elastic region, the lateral strain is proportional to the axial strain. For the lateral strain to be the same throughout the bar, the material needs to be homogeneous. This means that the composition needs to be identical at all points throughout the specimen. In addition, the specimen's elastic properties need to be identical in all directions perpendicular to its longitudinal axis. The ratio of the lateral strain to the axial strain is known as Poisson's ratio, denoted by the Greek letter ν:

$$\nu = -\frac{\text{lateral strain}}{\text{axial strain}}$$

For many metals and other materials, the Poisson's ratio is in the range of 0.25-0.35. Concrete has values of 0.1-0.2, whereas rubber is between 0.45-0.5, approaching the theoretical upper limit of Poisson's ratio of 0.5.

Directional Properties

Materials having the same properties in all directions are called isotropic. Their intrinsic material properties do not depend on the direction of loading. Typically, the internal structure of such materials is randomly dispersed and its characteristic repeating geometric units (for example, grains in a metal) are small. The elastic properties of isotropic materials can be fully characterized by only two material constants: Young's modulus (E) and Poisson's ratio (ν).

A material is called anisotropic if its intrinsic properties differ in various directions. The internal structure of such materials is typically composed of large units that are arranged in an orderly fashion. Almost all materials in the musculoskeletal system are anisotropic. As a special case of anisotropy, when material properties are identical in a particular direction throughout the material, and the properties in all directions perpendicular to that direction are identical to each other, but different from the properties in the first direction, the material is classified as orthotropic. For example, articular cartilage and meniscus are considered orthotropic and their elastic modulus in the direction parallel to the predominant collagen fiber direction is different from that in all directions perpendicular to the collagen fiber direction.

Creep and Stress Relaxation

A material may fail because of the phenomenon called creep. Creep occurs as a material deforms when it is loaded at a constant load for a long time. The greater the load, the faster the material will deform. Stress relaxation is similar to creep, in that it is a time-dependent phenomenon. It occurs when a material is strained (deformed) to a given dimension and then maintained at that strain. In this situation, the stress within the material gradually decreases with time.

The difference between creep and stress relaxation is that creep occurs with a constant load applied and strain increases (**Figure 17, A**), whereas stress relaxation has a constant strain and stress decreases (**Figure 17, B**).

Viscoelasticity

Linear elasticity has previously been discussed as an idealized model for analyzing the stress-strain behavior of some real materials. Such a structure is often designated by a spring (**Figure 18, A**) with the relationship between load F, deformation x, and stiffness k expressed as: F = kx. This behavior does not depend on time or the rate of loading.

Soft collagenous tissues such as articular cartilage, intervertebral disk, ligament, and tendon, however, exhibit viscoelastic behavior that does depend on time and rate of loading. This behavior can be modeled by a linear viscous dashpot (**Figure 18, B**) the following relationship: F = ηs where F is the applied force, η is the viscosity, and s is the rate of deformation.

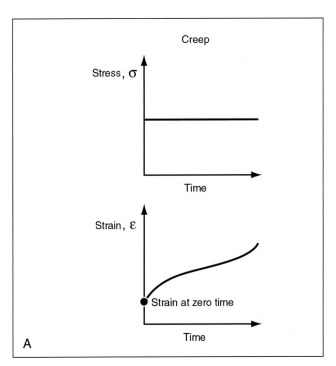

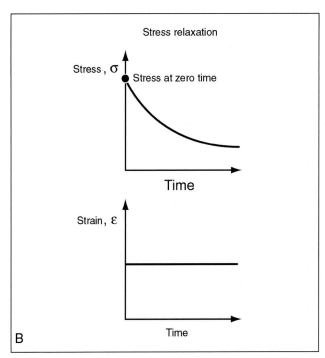

Figure 17   Stress (σ) and strain (ε) as a function of time during **A,** creep and **B,** stress relaxation.

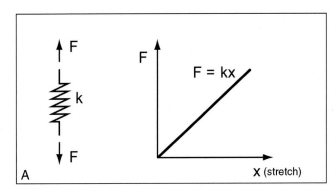

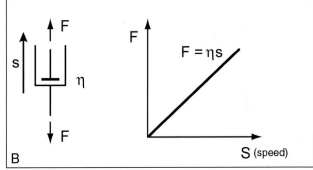

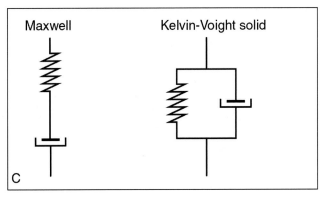

Figure 18   **A,** A linear elastic spring element and its linear load-deformation (stretch) response. **B,** A linear viscous dashpot element and its linear load-rate of deformation (speed) response. **C,** A Maxwell viscoelastic fluid modeled with a spring and dashpot linked in series and a Kelvin-Voigt viscoelastic solid modeled with a spring and dashpot linked in parallel.

Actual viscoelastic materials are often modeled by combining elastic springs and viscous dashpots (**Figure 18,** *C*). For example, a Maxwell viscoelastic fluid is modeled with the spring and dashpot linked in series, and a Kelvin-Voigt solid with the spring and dashpot linked in parallel.

Summary

Loading issues are almost always considered in the care of patients who have musculoskeletal conditions. These issues may include physiologic loads that occur during the activities of daily living, or traumatic loads that the body experiences during accidents, strenuous athletic activities, or injuries. The load-deformation relationships that occur between the human body and these physiologic or traumatic forces all obey Newton's laws of mechanics. The postinjury assessment of the direction of force application that occurred at the moment of injury may help predict likely bony and ligamentous injury patterns. The Allen-Ferguson classification of cervical spine fractures is an example of such a system. The intraoperative assessment of corrective force application to the spine or extremities helps to predict whether the desired fracture reduction or spine deformity correction will occur, or whether an additional injury is more likely to happen. Postoperative instructions for brace or cast wear, weight-bearing restrictions, and the gradual resumption of work, home, and recreational activities are all based on an assessment of the musculoskeletal system's ability to safely bear the loads that each of these activities will impose on it. Therefore, an understanding of methods of newtonian mechanics analysis that are applicable to the musculoskeletal system will contribute to the effective care of both surgical and nonsurgical orthopaedic patients.

Selected Bibliography

Beer FP, Johnston ER Jr: *Vector Mechanics for Engineers: Statics,* ed 6. New York, NY, McGraw-Hill, 1996.

Beer FP, Johnston ER Jr, Clausen WE: *Vector Mechanics for Engineers: Dynamics,* ed 7. New York, NY, McGraw-Hill, 2004.

Gere JM, Timoshenko SP: *Mechanics of Materials*, ed 3. Boston, MA, PWS-KENT, 1991.

Lardner TJ, Archer RR: *Mechanics of Solids*. New York, NY, McGraw-Hill, 1994.

Mow VC, Hayes WC (eds): *Basic Orthopaedic Biomechanics,* ed 2. Philadelphia, PA, Lippincott-Raven Publishers, 1997.

Panjabi MM, White AA III: *Biomechanics in the Musculoskeletal System*. Philadelphia, PA, Churchill Livingstone, 2001.

Schmid-Schönbein GW, Woo S-LY, Zweifach BW (eds): *Frontiers in Biomechanics*. New York, NY, Springer-Verlag, 1986.

Chapter 4

Biomaterials

Timothy M. Wright, PhD
Suzanne A. Maher, PhD

Requirements for Orthopaedic Biomaterials

The term biomaterials refers to all synthetic and natural materials that are used in clinical practice to replace, stabilize, or augment damaged tissue. In orthopaedic surgery, biomaterials are used to fabricate devices for internal fixation of fractures, osteotomies and arthrodeses, wound closure, tissue substitution, and total joint arthroplasty. To ensure their safety and functionality under such varied and demanding conditions, orthopaedic biomaterials must be biocompatible (able to function in vivo without eliciting detrimental local or systemic responses in the body), resistant to corrosion and degradation (able to withstand the harsh in vivo environment without being adversely affected), and have adequate mechanical and wear properties. These criteria are especially important when replacing or reinforcing load-bearing skeletal structures such as long bones and joints. In addition, biomaterials must reflect high standards of quality at a reasonable cost. Knowing the link between structure and composition of commonly used metallic, polymeric, and ceramic orthopaedic biomaterials and their ability to meet necessary performance criteria is essential to understanding their efficacy in clinical practice.

Biocompatibility

Because they are foreign to the in vivo environment, orthopaedic biomaterials initiate a cascade of events when implanted that can be harmful or toxic to living tissue. Biocompatibility, therefore, is defined on the basis of the level of adverse reactions that occur at implantation. For example, biomaterials that elicit little or no host response (such as cobalt-chromium metallic alloys) can be thought of as inert. Interactive biomaterials, on the other hand, are designed to elicit specific beneficial responses such as tissue ingrowth (for example, porous tantalum). Biomaterials incorporating or attracting cells that are then resorbed or remodeled (such as biodegradable polymeric scaffolds

for functional tissue engineering) are best described as viable. Finally, replant biomaterials consist of native tissue that has been cultured in vitro from cells obtained from a specific patient (for example, chondroplasty for the treatment of focal cartilage defects). Materials that elicit more severe biologic reactions than those covered by these definitions should be considered not biocompatible.

An acceptable degree of biocompatibility has been established for most traditional orthopaedic biomaterials. Nonetheless, biocompatibility issues remain, particularly for multicomponent devices such as bone-plate combinations or devices with articulations such as in joint arthroplasties. These devices are prone to releasing particulate debris known to accumulate both locally and systemically. Although the biomaterials (such as ultra-high molecular weight polyethylene [UHMWPE]) are biocompatible in bulk form, in particulate form they can elicit detrimental tissue reactions such as osteolysis that lead to tissue destruction and treatment failure.

Corrosion and Degradation Resistance

The in vivo environment of the human body can be highly corrosive. Corrosion creates two problems: it often leaves behind damaged regions on the surface of orthopaedic implants that act as stress risers, markedly decreasing implant strength, and it releases to the surrounding environment corrosion products that can adversely affect biocompatibility, causing pain, swelling, and destruction of nearby tissue. Orthopaedic implants can be susceptible to several corrosion modes, depending on their geometry and manufacturing history, the in vivo conditions under which they perform, and the presence of surface defects.

Galvanic corrosion occurs as a result of the electrochemical potential created between two metals in physical contact and immersed in a conductive medium such as serum or interstitial fluid. Galvanic corrosion typically is seen in fracture fixation plates at the interface between the plate and the screws that secure it to the bone. Even

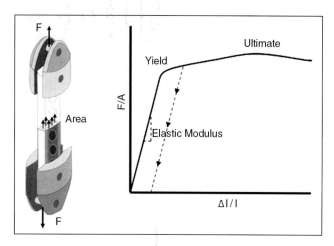

Figure 1   A tensile test on a stainless steel plate can be used to measure the steel's mechanical properties by plotting the stress (the applied tensile load divided by the plate's cross-sectional area) versus the strain (the normalized elongation that the plate experiences as a result of the applied load). After an initial elastic portion, in which strains are recoverable, the steel yields and begins to undergo larger plastic strains with less increase in stress. If the load is removed, elastic strain is recovered (dotted line) and permanent deformation remains. With high enough loads, the steel eventually reaches the ultimate stress it can withstand before failure. *(Adapted with permission from Burstein AH, Wright TM (eds):* Fundamentals of Orthopaedic Biomechanics. *Baltimore, MD, Williams & Wilkins, 1994.)*

when the plate and screws are manufactured from the same metallic alloy, differences in manufacturing methods between the two components can translate to localized variations in microstructure and chemical composition, eliciting a galvanic response during contact. Galvanic corrosion also can be caused by impurities within an implant (also called intergranular corrosion). Although rare, intergranular corrosion has been found in retrieved hip prostheses where cracks propagated between several pits, leading to catastrophic fracture. Galvanic corrosion is best avoided by ensuring raw material purity, by minimizing additional impurities that can enter the material during manufacture, and by ensuring that consistent heat treatment procedures are used on different components of multicomponent devices.

Fretting corrosion occurs at contact sites between materials that are subject to relative micromotion when under load. The introduction of modularity into joint arthroplasty devices has increased the incidence of fretting corrosion by introducing tapered junctions, for example, between the femoral head and the neck of the stem replacements. Fretting corrosion also can be a problem in stainless steel screw-plate systems through a combination of mechanical damage caused by screw tightening and subsequent micromotion while implanted, both of which cause mechanical destruction of the protective oxide layer. This mode of corrosion can be avoided by not overtightening screws, maintaining taper connections free from de-

bris, and optimizing taper design to reduce relative micromotion.

Crevice corrosion occurs because of differences in oxygen tension within and outside of a crevice with an associated concentration of electrolytes and changes in pH. Crevices and thus the potential for crevice corrosion are common in orthopaedic implants, most notably between the countersunk region of holes in devices such as plates and cementless acetabular components and the head of a screw used to secure the device to adjacent bone. For example, crevice and fretting corrosion were observed on nearly 90% of stainless steel bone plates at retrieval. Crevice corrosion can be avoided by minimizing surface defects that might be created during manufacture and during intraoperative handling.

Degradation of orthopaedic biomaterials such as polymers is also a form of corrosion resulting from exposure to harsh environments. In some instances, degradation is programmed into the material, such as biodegradable polymers intended to lose strength or to deliver drugs in a timed manner. In certain instances, however, degradation can be detrimental to the performance of an implant. Perhaps the most widely recognized complication associated with degradation in orthopaedic implants has been oxidative degradation of UHMWPE components for total joint arthroplasties. Exposure to radiation in an ambient environment causes scission of the polymer chains and the creation of free radicals that in turn react with oxygen. The result is a decrease in molecular weight and an increase in crystallinity and density. These changes, in turn, cause a decrease in the polyethylene's toughness and resistance to crack propagation and an increase in elastic modulus. Therefore, degraded polyethylene implants are less resistant to fatigue-type wear mechanisms such as pitting and delamination and yet experience high contact stresses because of their increased stiffness. Degradation has been avoided by alterations in packaging and sterilization techniques and by thermal treatments intended to quench the material of free radicals.

Mechanical Properties

Designing a device for an orthopaedic application requires the ability to predict its mechanical performance through consideration of its geometry and the material from which it is manufactured. Predicting a device's mechanical performance depends on several factors: the forces to which it is subjected (see chapter 3), the mechanical burdens that those forces place internally on the material, and the material's capability to withstand those burdens over the device's lifetime.

Stress and Strain

Consider a metallic bone plate manufactured from stainless steel and gripped at the ends (**Figure 1**). A tensile load is applied through the grips, causing the bone plate to elongate. The external load is resisted by an internal load acting perpendicular to the cross section of the plate and evenly distributed over the plate's cross-sectional area. The resulting tensile stress within the bone plate has a magnitude equal to the applied load divided by the cross-sectional area (F/A). The elongation is described as tensile strain by dividing the amount of elongation occurring between the gripped regions by the original length of that region when no load was applied (ΔL/L).

If the load is removed during the initial straight line portion of the resulting stress-strain curve (**Figure 1**), both stress and strain will return to zero (that is, the stress-strain curve retraces itself back to the origin). Such fully reversible stress-strain behavior implies no change in the plate's shape and, therefore, no damage to the metal; the stainless steel is behaving elastically. The ratio of stress to strain is called the modulus of elasticity (E) and is a material property of the stainless steel and not of the bone plate. For example, repeating the loading experiment on a stainless steel plate with twice the cross-sectional area would require twice the load to achieve the same elongation, but the modulus would not change because the stress (F/A) to achieve that elongation would be the same. The elastic modulus is, therefore, a measure of the material's ability to maintain shape under the application of external loads. A material with a higher elastic modulus is said to be stiffer and more resistant to deformation for any particular shape and loading than a material with a lower elastic modulus.

Yield and Ultimate Stress

If tensile load is applied to the bone plate again and allowed to continually increase, the stress-strain curve eventually becomes nonlinear. Removal of the load reveals permanent elongation (or plastic deformation) of the stainless steel plate (**Figure 1**). The stress at which plastic deformation begins is called the yield stress (or also the yield strength). As the load continues to increase, plastic damage accumulates in the stainless steel, and the bone plate eventually ruptures. The maximum stress reached after yield but before rupture is called the ultimate stress (or ultimate strength).

The yield strength is an important failure criterion. For example, the maximum load that can be imposed on a hip nail plate before it permanently deforms (its yield strength) defines whether the device can keep fracture fragments in a fixed relative position to facilitate healing. The material and plate geometry specifications must be such that the stresses to which the nail plate is subjected are lower than its yield strength.

Materials that can exhibit a clearly defined yield point followed by permanent strain before failure are defined as ductile materials, whereas those that undergo little or no permanent deformation before fracture are defined as brittle. Ductility can be beneficial, for example, in allowing energy to be absorbed without catastrophic failure such as might occur in a structure made from a brittle material (such as a ceramic femoral head for a total hip replacement). Moderate ductility also is useful in certain bone plates, allowing them to be contoured in the operating room.

Fatigue

Failure based on yield strength is pertinent to trauma or other situations involving a single application of a very large load. Most orthopaedic implants, however, are subjected to repetitive, cyclic loads. Such repeated loading and unloading can cause failure, even though each individually applied load creates stresses in the implant that are below its ultimate strength. Fatigue failure is the most common mode of mechanical failure experienced by orthopaedic devices. Bone plates, femoral components from total hip replacements, tibial trays from total knee replacements, intramedullary nails, and other devices fabricated from metallic alloys have all undergone fatigue failure in clinical use. Even articular surfaces of polyethylene tibial knee components fail by fatigue-related wear mechanisms because of the cyclic nature of the applied contact loads.

Under fatigue conditions, the number of stress cycles that the material can withstand is inversely proportional to the magnitude of the applied stress; that is, the number of stress cycles the material can withstand increases as the stress intensity is reduced. Typically, the stress at which the material can withstand 10 million stress cycles without failure is called the endurance limit (or the fatigue strength). Given that patients apply millions of stress cycles each year to their musculoskeletal systems, orthopaedic implants such as total joint arthroplasties that are intended to be permanent must possess an adequate combination of size, shape, and material choice to ensure that induced stresses are below the endurance limit.

Fatigue consists of three steps: the initiation of a crack in the material, the propagation of the crack through the material, and final catastrophic failure when the crack reaches a length for which the remaining material cannot withstand applied stress. Any factor that encourages crack initiation markedly reduces the fatigue life of the material. For example, scratching or nicking the surface of a metallic orthopaedic device creates damage that under cyclic loading could quickly become a crack, thus greatly decreasing the device's useful lifetime. Conversely, any factor that acts to arrest or slow crack propagation will increase fatigue life. A crack growing through a fiber-reinforced matrix will stop growing when it reaches the boundary of a strong fiber within the matrix. The crack will remain stagnant until enough damage accumulates to move the crack through the fiber.

Isotropic and Anisotropic Behavior

Materials that have the same mechanical properties in all directions are called isotropic. Metallic and ceramic materials used in orthopaedics are generally isotropic. Musculoskeletal tissues (bone, cartilage, muscle, ligament, and tendon) and composites (fiberglass and carbon fiber–reinforced resins) have directionally dependent properties and are called anisotropic. Cortical bone tissue from the appendicular skeleton, for example, exhibits very different stress-strain and fatigue behavior when loaded in a longitudinal as opposed to a transverse direction. When loaded transversely, the tissue is much weaker in terms of yield and ultimate strength, is much less ductile, and has a much lower elastic modulus. The anisotropic behavior reflects the bone's structure, being a composite at both the ultrastructural level, where both collagen fibrils and hydroxyapatite crystals generally align in a longitudinal direction, and at a microstructural scale, where osteons generally also are aligned longitudinally.

Man-made composite materials are often anisotropic. For example, strong fibers can be aligned in preferred directions and then impregnated with a weaker matrix. The resulting material displays mechanical properties that depend on the fiber and matrix material properties, the relative amounts of fiber and matrix, the bonding between the fiber and matrix, and the geometry and orientation of the fibers. Composite materials have been developed for artificial ligaments, biodegradable fracture fixation devices, tissue engineering scaffolds, and even total joint components. The anisotropic behavior of materials underscores the importance of testing devices in more than just one loading direction for adequate evaluation of their potential clinical performance.

Combined Stress States

Although simple loading regimens are useful for measuring mechanical properties (**Figure 1**), most orthopaedic devices usually experience combinations of axial, bending, and torsion loads (see chapter 3) that result in complex stress distributions in the materials from which they are made. Even under simple tension, combined stresses exist on planes other than the one perpendicular to the applied load. In the more realistic loading situations encountered in the musculoskeletal system, calculating the types, magnitudes, and distributions of stresses within the material can be difficult, given the complex shapes of implants and skeletal structures. Computer techniques, such as finite element analysis, often are used to determine the stresses and to predict failure by comparing the predicted stresses to failure criteria for the material.

Viscoelasticity

If the tensile test of the stainless steel bone plate is performed at many different rates of loading, the resulting stress-strain behavior will be the same (**Figure 1**). This statement is true for other metallic alloys and ceramics. However, for many other materials, such as polymers, the loading rate profoundly affects the material's mechanical properties. A material with properties that are rate-dependent is said to be viscoelastic.

Consider a viscoelastic material that is subjected to a suddenly applied strain. Stress will instantaneously occur within the material, but the stress required to maintain the strain reduces with time; the material experiences stress relaxation. If the material is subjected instead to a suddenly applied load, stress and strain again will occur instantaneously in the material. However, even though the stress remains constant with time, the strain in the viscoelastic material continues to increase with time, a phenomenon called creep.

Another characteristic of viscoelastic materials is hysteresis. For example, consider a tensile test similar to that performed on the stainless steel bone plate (**Figure 1**) but performed on a plate fabricated from a viscoelastic material. When the specimen is loaded, the area under the stress-strain curve represents the strain energy stored in the material. When unloaded, the curve follows a different, less steep path. The closed loop formed between the loading and unloading plots reflects energy lost in the material as a result of inefficiency in the process of storing and releasing energy (for example, by internal friction within the microstructure). Polymers, for example, are often viscoelastic, with energy dissipated through friction between the polymer chains as the material is deformed. When cyclically loaded and unloaded, such viscoelastic materials actually generate heat as a result of the friction. Metallic materials, on the other hand, have crystalline, ordered material structures with few mechanisms for internal friction and typically do not exhibit a hysteresis loop as part of their stress-strain behavior.

Wear Resistance

Metallic, polymeric, and ceramic particulate by-products of orthopaedic implant wear are nondegradable. The subsequent reaction, especially to very small particles, can initiate a cascade of biologic events, leading eventually to tissue destruction and treatment failure (for a more detailed review of the host response to foreign objects, see chapter 20).

The exact relationship between material properties and wear resistance is poorly understood; hence, wear resistance often is established empirically through screening tests such as joint simulators and more simplified wear tests (such as pin-on-disk tests). The ability for such tests to provide meaningful results depends on the ability to recreate the loading, kinematics, and environmental conditions. Test validation currently lies solely in the ability to create wear rates equal to those found on average in patients (based on estimates from serial radiographs) and particulate debris matching the size and shape of that recovered from periprosthetic tissues at revision surgeries.

In general, materials with high hardness, such as ceramics, have demonstrated better wear resistance than those with metallic or polymeric surfaces. Ceramics may have better wear resistance because they can be polished to a smoother surface finish and because they have better wettability, creating the possibility of protective lubricating films to exist between the articular surfaces. Materials that are softer and, therefore, more prone to scratching, such as titanium alloys, have proven more susceptible to wear. UHMWPE wear has been associated with osteolysis on the basis of the volume of small submicron particles generated from polyethylene articular surfaces. Therefore, considerable efforts have been undertaken to improve the wear resistance of UHMWPE.

Quality Control and Cost

Quality control of orthopaedic biomaterials is essential to the performance of the end product. The importance of quality control is reflected in the level of federal regulation and the large number of voluntary standards devoted to ensuring that raw materials, manufacturing processes, and treatments such as cleaning, sterilization, and packaging conform to acceptable specifications. All stages in the manufacture of medical devices that are marketed or manufactured in the United States are regulated by the Food and Drug Administration (FDA) to ensure that they are safe and effective for their intended use. To acquire and maintain FDA approval, manufacturing facilities must conform to the Good Manufacturing Practices regulations. The regulations require, for example, that specifications and controls be established for devices; that devices be designed and manufactured under a controlled quality system; that finished devices meet these specifications; that devices be correctly installed, checked, and serviced; that quality data be analyzed to identify and correct problems; and that customer complaints about quality be processed and reported to the FDA. The FDA routinely monitors device problem data and inspects the operations and records of device developers and manufacturers to determine that they have complied with the Good Manufacturing Practices regulations.

Despite the best efforts of manufacturers and the scrutiny of the FDA, manufacturing problems that adversely affect the performance of orthopaedic implants occasionally arise. Recent examples include contamination of hip and knee replacement components that led to premature failure and the need for revision surgery, and problems with zirconia femoral heads for hip replacement that increased the likelihood for fracture. The FDA has estimated that between 1995 and 2004, 13 orthopaedic device products have been recalled for manufacturing or design flaws. One of the largest recalls occurred in December 2000 when Sulzer Orthopaedics (Alton, England) issued a recall for 40,000 acetabular shells of the InterOP design, followed shortly thereafter by a recall for tibial baseplates. The recall was in response to an unusually high early loosening rate believed to be related to a residue of lubricant oil used during one of the manufacturing steps.

In general, conventional orthopaedic biomaterials can be fabricated and used to manufacture products with a high degree of quality control and at a reasonable cost. Nearly all of these materials, however, were adopted for use in implants. In most instances, developing new materials that would match biocompatibility, corrosion, and mechanical property requirements better than existing materials is prohibitive given reasonable profits in comparison to development costs based on the size of the orthopaedic marketplace.

Metallic Materials

Alloys are metals composed of mixtures or solutions of metallic and nonmetallic elements added to impart workability, strength, ductility, elastic modulus, corrosion resistance, and biocompatibility required for specific load-bearing applications. Metallic alloys have a range of features that make them attractive for use as structural load-bearing implants; consequently, they are widely used in orthopaedic surgery. Metal alloys can be fabricated using a variety of techniques that lend flexibility in terms of both mechanical properties and shape.

Metallic Bonding

Consider a molten metal that is being cooled to form a solid material. As the temperature drops, many small crystals nucleate, each growing by the addition of atoms. Within each crystal the atoms are regularly spaced with respect to one another and pack together in specific configurations, depending on the thermodynamic conditions and the mix of atoms of different elements present in the molten solution (**Figure 2**). The atoms bond together, sharing their outer electrons; this mobility of electrons between atoms gives rise to the excellent heat and electrical conductivity of metals. The more tightly packed the atoms become, the more the strength of the metallic bond increases. These strong metallic bonds account for the high strengths and melting points of metals.

Microstructure

As the molten metal continues to cool, more atoms join the nucleation sites (**Figure 3**, *A* and *B*), and the individual crystals grow in size (**Figure 3**, *C*). The outer arms of the crystal begin to make contact with those of its neighbors, so that when solidification is complete, the resulting solid is an array of irregularly shaped individual crystals called grains (**Figure 3**, *D*). Often, impurities that cannot fit into the crystalline configuration remain in solution, eventually ending up in the grain boundaries. The microstructure can be revealed by polishing a flat surface of the metal, etching the surface with a mild corrosive agent to reveal the grain boundaries, and viewing the surface under a microscope (**Figure 4**).

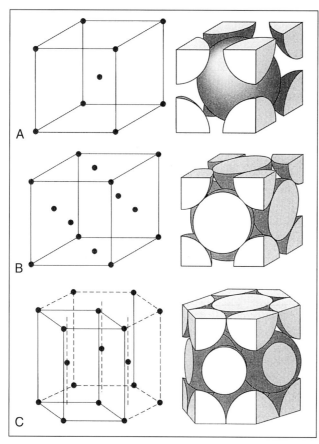

Figure 2 Common unit cell structures for crystalline arrangements of atoms can be body-centered cubic **(A)**, face-centered cubic **(B)**, or hexagonal close-packed **(C)**. *(Adapted with permission from Rolls KM, Courtney TH, Wulff J: Introduction to Materials Science and Engineering. New York, NY, John Wiley and Sons, 1976.)*

The rate at which a molten metal cools affects the size of the crystals that form. A slow drop in temperature promotes the formation of relatively few dispersed nuclei around which crystals will form, resulting in large crystals. Rapid cooling allows for the formation of a large number of nucleation sites so that a large number of small grains or crystals will form.

Mechanical properties also are optimized by uniformity in grain size and by avoidance of voids or impurities and depend on the atomic configuration (**Figure 2**), the geometry and size of the grains (**Figure 3**), and the constituents of the grain boundaries. For example, plastic deformation in metals occurs by sliding rows of atoms past each other and is facilitated by atomic defects called dislocations. The dislocations move through the grain, eventually reaching the boundary. Because the neighboring grain has a different orientation of atomic planes, the dislocation is temporarily halted. The smaller the grain size, the more rapidly dislocation progress is stopped. Therefore, smaller grain sizes impart greater strength to the alloy.

Grain size and, hence, mechanical properties can be controlled during manufacturing. Thus, the steps used to produce an orthopaedic implant can be manipulated to produce the desired properties.

Processing of Metallic Alloys

Metallurgic implants typically are fabricated by casting, forging, or extrusion, followed by postprocessing thermal treatments such as mechanical working and annealing. Casting is a process during which molten metal is poured into a mold (**Figure 5,** *A*) that allows heat to be rapidly transferred away from the molten metal, facilitating rapid

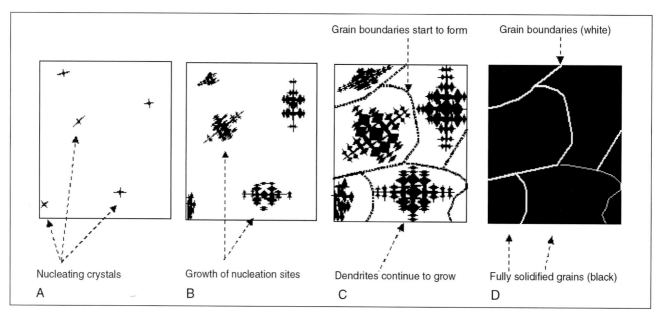

Figure 3 The solidification of molten metal. *(Adapted with permission from Higgins RA: The crystalline structure of metals, in Engineering Metallurgy, 1. Applied Physical Metallurgy, ed 5. United Kingdom, Edward Arnold of Hodder and Stoughton Ltd, 1983.)*

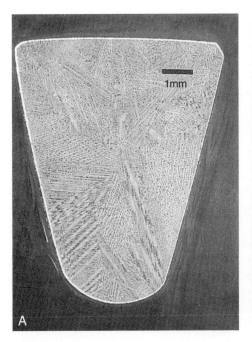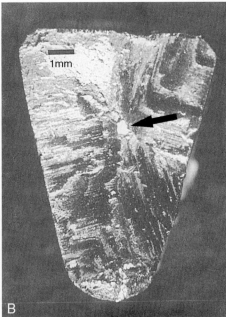

Figure 4 Etched cross section of the femoral component of a total hip replacement fabricated from cast cobalt alloy showing dendritic structure and very large grain size **(A)**. The fracture surface of the same component, which failed in vivo, including a large inclusion *(arrow)* that probably contributed to the failure **(B)**. *(Reproduced with permission from Ratner BD, Hoffman AS, Schoen FJ, Lemons JE (eds):* Biomaterials Science: An Introduction to Materials in Medicine. *San Diego, CA, Academic Press, 1996.)*

cooling and allowing for abundant nucleating sites and a corresponding fine grain structure. Quality control can be an issue during the casting process. If solidification proceeds too slowly, grains have too much time to grow, and alloying elements intended to strengthen the material by being evenly distributed throughout the grains can segregate to the boundaries; both factors markedly diminish the metal's strength and even can decrease corrosion resistance. If solidification proceeds too quickly, gases that are released during the solidification process can become entrapped in the microstructure, generating voids that can act as stress risers, decreasing the fatigue strength.

Forging is a process by which one half of a die is attached to a hammer, the other half is attached to an anvil, and the metal to be formed is heated and placed in the working space between the two (**Figure 5,** *B*). As the hammer falls it forces the metal to fit the shape of the die. Conventional forging processes often require two or three individual forging operations to reach the final desired shape. Extrusion is a process by which the metal is heated and forced through a die to obtain a long piece of uniform cross section (**Figure 5,** *C*). This process is well suited for fabricating cylindrical objects such as wire, pins, and circular cross sections from which rods and screws subsequently can be machined.

Quality control during the fabrication process itself can be difficult. Defects in cast materials, nonuniform crystalline structures in forged materials, and large residual stresses in extrusions are common. Postprocessing thermal treatments (cold and hot working, annealing, and hot isostatic pressing) are used to reduce these problems. Stainless steel, for example, often is strengthened by squeezing the material between rollers to reduce the cross-sectional size of the material or drawing the mate-

rial through a series of dies to achieve the same result. Both methods are performed at temperatures well below the melting point of the steel (hence, the term cold work). When stainless steel is worked in this manner, the microstructure of the material is altered and the grain size is reduced. As a result of this strain hardening, the steel's surface hardness and strength are increased (**Figure 6**). Hot working, on the other hand, involves plastic deformation of a metal at a high enough temperature and strain rate that recrystallization takes place simultaneously with deformation. The result is a more regular, smaller grain size and the removal of any residual stresses within the material. Such treatments (either hot or cold working) of cast alloys frequently are used to close voids between crystals, redistribute alloying elements, and improve mechanical properties.

During annealing, a component is heated to a temperature below its melting point, maintained at that temperature for a fixed time, then cooled at a predetermined rate. Final grain size can be selected by carefully choosing the annealing temperature, the time at that temperature, and the cooling rate. Furthermore, annealing can encourage diffusion of alloying elements throughout the microstructure, resulting in a more homogenous distribution of the alloys.

Hot isostatic pressing is a heat treatment procedure during which heat (to a temperature just below the melting point of the alloy) and pressure (of at least 1,000 atmospheres) are applied in an oxygen-free environment to consolidate a part. Hot isostatic pressing frequently is applied after casting to consolidate voids. The process produces plastic flow of the alloy, thereby collapsing voids and cavities in the material that otherwise would have acted as potential sites for fatigue crack initiation during use.

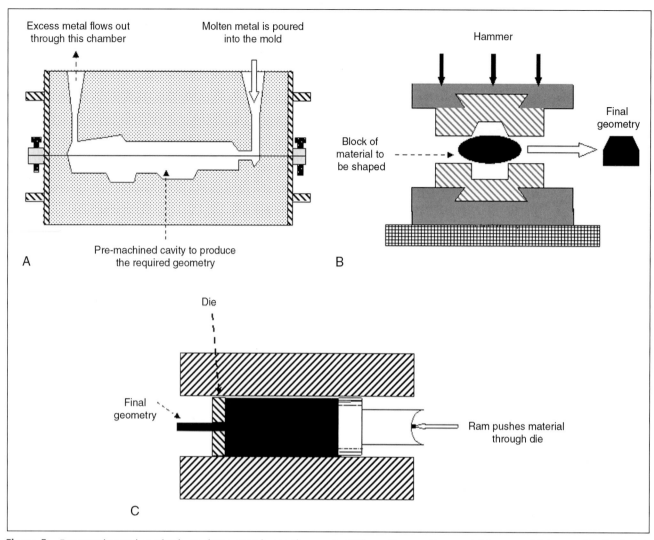

Excess metal flows out through this chamber

Molten metal is poured into the mold

A

Pre-machined cavity to produce the required geometry

Hammer

Block of material to be shaped

Final geometry

B

Die

Final geometry

Ram pushes material through die

C

Figure 5   Frequently used methods to shape metals are shown. **A,** With casting, molten metal is poured into a split die that is pinned together. After solidification the pins are removed, the mold opened, and the solidified metallic piece removed. **B,** With forging, solid metal is placed between molds mounted to a hammer and anvil. The hammer is forced onto the metal solid, forcing it to conform to the shape of the split mold. **C,** With extrusion, metal is rammed through a die, conferring a cross-sectional geometry on the final shape that matches the geometry of the cutout in the die. *(Adapted with permission from Higgins RA: The crystalline structure of metals, in* Engineering Metallurgy 1: Applied Physical Metallurgy, *ed 5. United Kingdom, Edward Arnold of Hodder and Stoughton, 1983, pp 124-131.)*

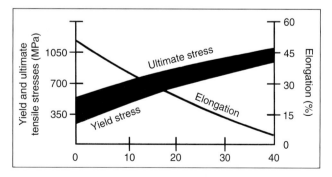

Figure 6   Metallic materials such as 316L stainless steel can be cold worked to improve the yield and ultimate stress, although the ductility is decreased. Stainless steel in orthopaedic implants is often cold worked about 30%. *(Reproduced with permission from Burstein AH, Wright TM:* Fundamentals of Orthopaedic Biomechanics, *Baltimore, MD, Williams and Wilkins, 1994.)*

Metals Used in Orthopaedic Devices

Nearly all metallic materials used in orthopaedic devices are alloys, either steel (an iron-based alloy), titanium-based, or cobalt-based (**Figure 7**). The alloying elements used, the generic names of the alloys, and their most typical orthopaedic applications are summarized in **Table 1**. Their mechanical properties are summarized in **Table 2**.

Stainless Steels

Stainless steels are used predominantly in temporary implant devices, such as fracture plates, screws, and hip nails, although stainless steel also is used in some Charnley-style femoral components for hip replacement. Like any steel, stainless steel is predominantly an iron-carbon alloy. Other alloying elements for stainless steel in-

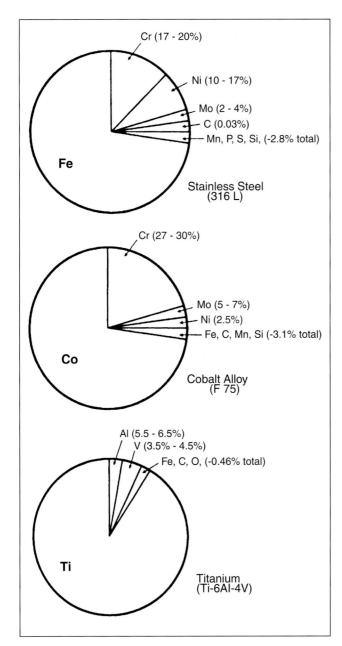

Figure 7 The composition of the three common orthopaedic metallic alloys. *(Reproduced from Litsky AS, Spector M: Biomaterials, in Simon SR (ed): Orthopaedic Basic Science. Rosemont, IL, American Academy of Orthopaedic Surgeons, 1994, pp 447-486.)*

harder than the surrounding material, and a uniform distribution of carbides provides strength to the steel. Additions of other alloying elements such as molybdenum stabilize the carbides. If carbon concentrations are too high, carbides segregate at the grain boundaries, significantly weakening the steel by making it prone to corrosion-related fracture. To ensure superior corrosive characteristics for medical grade stainless steel, carbide contents are kept low (0.03% to 0.08%).

Chromium provides the stainless quality to stainless steel. It forms a strongly adherent oxide (Cr_2O_3) on the surfaces, which provides corrosion resistance by forming a passive layer between the environment and the bulk steel. Chromium also stabilizes the body-centered cubic phase of stainless steel (**Figure 2**), which is more malleable than the face-centered cubic phase. This facilitates the shaping of stainless steel into its required final geometry.

Nickel is added to counteract the tendency of chromium to cause grain growth. The tendency of nickel to favor graphitization of the carbides (which reduces strength and hardness) is, in turn, counteracted by the strong carbide-forming tendency of chromium. The addition of both materials increases strength and corrosion resistance. New nickel-free stainless steel screws recently have been developed, primarily to combat the issue of nickel sensitivity.

Because molybdenum helps form carbides that can harden the steel and make it difficult to form, molybdenum contents are kept to a minimum (2.5% to 3.5%). Molybdenum enhances corrosion resistance and improves impact strength. The addition of small amounts of vanadium helps to resist grain growth. Like molybdenum, vanadium has a strong tendency to form into carbides and nitrides that are finely dispersed in the microstructure.

Stainless steel is susceptible to galvanic and crevice corrosion, although corrosion resistance can be improved by increasing chromium, molybdenum, and nitrogen concentrations. To ensure the creation of the oxide layer, stainless steel devices are passivated by immersion in a strong nitric acid bath; a cobalt, chromium, and nickel oxide layer is formed on the surface of an implant.

Stainless steel can be cast, forged, or extruded; however, the cooling of steel to ambient temperature should be controlled to ensure that slow cooling does not cause carbide precipitation. The predominant postprocessing treatment applied to stainless steels is cold working. Stainless steel strain hardens very rapidly and, therefore, cannot be cold worked without intermediate treatments.

Cobalt Alloys

The three basic elements of cobalt alloys are cobalt, chromium, and molybdenum (**Table 1**). Chromium is added for increased hardness and corrosion resistance, particularly resistance to crevice corrosion. As with stainless steel, the chromium forms a strongly adherent oxide film that provides a passive layer shielding the bulk material from

clude molybdenum, chromium, and small amounts of manganese and silicon (**Figure 7**). The properties of medical grade stainless steel are such that it provides a balance between high strength, good ductility, and good fatigue performance (**Table 2**). The ductility of this alloy is important in applications such as bone screws where a definite yield point allows the surgeon to feel the onset of plastic deformation, thus avoiding screw failure through the application of too much torque.

Carbon is added to allow the formation of metallic carbides within the microstructure. Carbides are much

Table 1   Metallic Alloys and Their Typical Orthopaedic Applications

Generic Name	Base Element	Principal Alloying Elements	Typical Applications
Steels	Fe (Iron)	Carbon, chrome, nickel, manganese, molybdenum, vanadium, phosphorous, selenium, silicon	Fracture hardware, braces, surgical instruments, guide wires, nails
Super alloys or cobalt-based alloys	Co (Cobalt)	Chrome, nickel, manganese, tungsten, molybdenum, niobium, iron, carbon	Joint arthroplasty components, nails, screws, fracture plates
Titanium-based alloys	Ti (Titanium)	Aluminum, vanadium, iron, niobium, zinc	Fracture hardware, joint arthroplasty components, screws, wires, nails, plates, screws for fixation and stabilization of fractures/artificial joints

Table 2   Typical Mechanical Properties of Implant Materials

Material	Condition	Elastic Modulus	Yield Strength (MPa)	Ultimate Strength (MPa)	Endurance Limit (MPa)
Stainless steels	Annealed	190	331	586	241-276
	30% cold worked	190	792	930	310-448
	Cold forged	190	1213	1351	820
Cobalt alloys	As cast/annealed	210	448-517	655-889	207-310
	HIP*	253	841	1277	725-950
	Hot forged	210	896-1200	1399-1586	600-896
	44% cold worked	210	1606	1896	586
	Cold forged/aged	232	1500	1795	689-793
Titanium alloys	30% cold worked	110	485	760	300
	Forged annealed	116	896	965	620

* HIP = hot isostatic pressing
(Adapted with permission from Ratner BD, Hoffman AS, Schoen FJ, Lemons JE (eds): Biomaterials Science: An Introduction to Materials in Medicine. San Diego, CA, Academic Press, 1996.)

the environment. Long-term clinical use has proved that these alloys also have exceptional biocompatibility in bulk form. Molybdenum is added to produce fine grain structures with high strength after casting or forging.

Standard cobalt alloy contains significant amounts of carbon and, hence, great quantities of hard carbides, which make forging the alloy difficult. Cobalt alloy is also particularly susceptible to strain hardening, which makes machining of the alloy difficult. The predominant fabrication technique for this alloy, therefore, is casting with emphasis on achieving a small grain size and evenly distributed carbides. Unacceptably large grain sizes can lead to insufficient fatigue strength and clinical failures (Figure 4). Hot isostatic processing is particularly suitable for improving the mechanical properties of cast cobalt alloy components.

Significant amounts of nickel can be added to cobalt alloys to form an alloy suitable for forging. Nickel stabilizes the high temperature, face-centered cubic form of the alloy, decreasing the resistance to deformation and facilitating the forging process. Forged cobalt alloys strain harden during forging, which promotes recrystallization; thus they must be reheated frequently to lower the power required for subsequent forging.

Postprocessing thermal treatments of forged cobalt alloys include cold working and annealing. Cold working provides additional energy for the transformation of some of the face-centered cubic phase into a hexagonal phase that emerges as fine platelets throughout the microstructure. A very fine grain size (the face-centered cubic grains are less than 0.1 μm in any dimension) in combination with dispersed platelets impede plastic deformation, strengthening the material. Tungsten is added to improve machinability and fabrication via cold working. In addition, the material can be treated thermally to form a uniform distribution of very fine cobalt-molybdenum (Co_3Mo) precipitates that act to further strengthen the material. The resulting alloy is among the strongest of the orthopaedic implant biomaterials (Table 2). The superior fatigue and ultimate tensile strength of the forged alloy make it suitable for high load applications that require long service life. As with other alloys, however, increased strength is accompanied by decreased ductility.

Titanium Alloys
Pure titanium has somewhat unique tissue and bone adhesion characteristics that can be attributed to an adherent passive layer of titanium oxide (TiO_2) that provides

corrosion resistance significantly exceeding that of stainless steel and the cobalt alloys. Uniform corrosion, even in saline solutions, is extremely limited, and resistance to pitting, intergranular, and crevice corrosion is excellent. Unalloyed titanium typically is used for fracture fixation devices where large loads are not expected (maxillofacial, phalanges, and the wrist). However, pure titanium is less ductile than stainless steel, and an increased incidence of titanium screw breakage during implantation and removal has been attributed to the lower ductility. The tactile warning given when titanium screws are overtightened is less than that for stainless steel screws.

The major limitation of unalloyed titanium is its low tensile strength. For higher strength, titanium alloys must be used. The most commonly used alloy in orthopaedic applications is titanium-aluminum-vanadium alloy. Developed by the aerospace industry, it has a high strength-to-weight ratio. The primary alloying elements, aluminum and vanadium, are limited to 5.5% to 6.5% and 3.5% to 4.5%, respectively, so the alloy often is called Ti-6Al-4V or simply Ti-6-4. Titanium has the ability to self-passivate, forming its own oxide that has a high degree of resistance to corrosion and chemical attack. Oxygen, however, readily dissolves in titanium and causes it to become brittle; therefore, oxygen concentration is kept very low to maximize strength and ductility. The microstructure of Ti-6Al-4V is a fine-grained two-phase structure, consisting of a hexagonal close-packed phase stabilized by aluminum and a body-centered cubic phase stabilized by vanadium. The manipulation of these crystallographic variations through adding alloys and thermal-mechanical processing treatments can provide a wide range of properties.

Forging is a common method of producing wrought titanium alloy components. Titanium alloys can be strain hardened by cold working, increasing tensile and yield strength and slightly decreasing ductility. Titanium alloys are particularly suitable for casting and, unlike castings of other metals, they may have tensile fracture toughness, strength, and creep-rupture strength equal or nearly equal to their wrought counterparts. Although fatigue strength may be lower for cast titanium alloys, it can be enhanced by heat treatments such as high isostatic pressing.

Titanium alloy has an elastic modulus roughly half that of stainless steel and cobalt alloy (Table 2). Thus, the structural stiffness of a device, which is proportional to the elastic modulus of the material from which it is made (see chapter 3), can be reduced without changing its shape. For example, the axial, bending, and torsional stiffness of a bone plate fabricated from titanium alloy will be half that of a bone plate of the same size and shape made from stainless steel or cobalt alloy. Thus, the severity of stress shielding when the plate is rigidly attached to the bone (so that the bone and the plate share load) will be less for the titanium alloy plate. This consideration has led to the use of titanium alloy in fracture and spinal fixation devices, including plates, nails, and screws.

Ti-6Al-4V alloy is notch sensitive; sharp corners, holes, notches, and other stress concentrations lower the fatigue life of the device considerably. Applying a porous coating to a joint arthroplasty component to allow for fixation by bone ingrowth could have the same detrimental effect. Clinical observations have demonstrated significant scratching and wear of total hip femoral heads made from titanium alloy, particularly where evidence exists of third-body wear caused by debris becoming entrapped between the articular surfaces. Despite the long-term clinical evidence of the excellent biocompatibility of titanium alloy, concern persists that the release of cytotoxic elements such as vanadium as part of the wear process could cause local and systemic problems (see chapter 20). In response to this concern, other titanium alloys in which the vanadium is replaced by more inert elements such as niobium have been introduced into the orthopaedic marketplace.

Tantalum

Tantalum, like titanium, is a highly biocompatible, corrosion resistant, osteoconductive material. Recently, porous forms of tantalum deposited on pyrolytic carbon backbones have been promoted as superior structures for bone ingrowth. Possible orthopaedic applications include coatings for joint arthroplasty components (acetabular cups and tibial trays) and spinal cages. Experimental work in animal models and randomized trials in humans suggest that this may be a useful material for achieving fixation to bone.

Polymers

Polymers are large molecules made from combinations of smaller molecules. These small molecules are called "mer" units from the Greek word "meros," which means part. For the purposes of this discussion, polymers will be made up only of organic monomers, molecules based predominantly on carbon, hydrogen, oxygen, and nitrogen. Table 3 provides a list of polymers commonly used in orthopaedic applications.

Definitions and Properties

The properties of a polymer are dictated by its chemical structure (the monomers used to make the polymer), the molecular weight (the number of monomers in the polymer), the physical structure (the way in which monomers are attached to each other), isomerism (the different orientations of atoms in some polymers), and crystallinity (the packing of polymer chains into ordered atomic arrays).

Polyethylene is the simplest polymer, consisting entirely of ethylene monomer units. The number of ethylene units in a polymer chain determines its molecular weight. For instance, each ethylene monomer has a molecular weight of 28. A polymer made up of 1,000 ethylene units

Table 3   Polymers in Medicine and Orthopaedics

Name	Use
Polyethylene	Joint arthroplasties
Polypropylene	Ligament augmentation
Polytetrafluoroethylene	Early joint arthroplasties
Polyvinyl chloride (PVC)	Surgical tubing, clips
Polymethylmethacrylate	Bone cement
Methacrylic acid	Bone cement copolymer
Polyglycolic acid	Resorbable polymer
Polylactic acid	Resorbable polymer
Polyethylene oxide (polyacetal)	Early joint arthroplasties, plastic trial inserts, surgical clips
Polystyrene	Tissue culture plates, bone cement copolymer

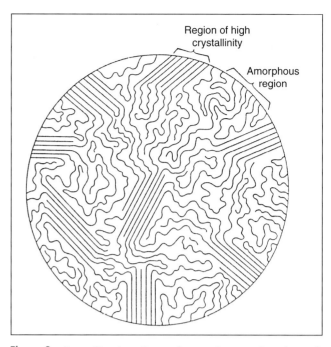

Figure 8   Crystalline lamellae and amorphous regions in semi-crystalline polymer. *(Reproduced from Wright TM, Li S: Biomaterials, in Buckwalter JA, Einhorn TA, Simon SR (eds): Orthopaedic Basic Science, ed 2. Rosemont, IL, American Academy of Orthopaedic Surgeons, 2000, pp 181-215.)*

has a molecular weight of 28,000. However, during polymerization of ethylene, not all chains will end up with the same number of units; therefore, not all chains will have the same molecular weight, resulting in a distribution of molecular weights. Both the breadth of the distribution and the magnitudes of the molecular weights can markedly influence the stiffness, strength, toughness, and wear properties of a polymer such as polyethylene.

Copolymers are polymers that contain more than one type of monomer. For instance, polymethylmethacrylate, commonly called bone cement or PMMA, can contain copolymers of methyl methacrylate and polystyrene or methyl methacrylate and methacrylic acid. In copolymers, the distribution of the different monomers can substantially affect polymer properties, depending on whether they are randomly distributed (AABABBBABAAABB...) or alternate sequentially (ABABAB...) or in blocks (AAABBBAAABBBAAA...). Furthermore, the manner by which each monomer is linked to the overall polymer structure also can provide different structural arrangements. In linear polymers, the monomers are linked end to end. In branched polymers, side chains (branches) of monomers are attached to the main chain, and the length of each branch, the number of branches, and the distribution of branches will affect the polymer's properties. In cross-linked polymers, the chains are covalently bonded to each other at various locations along their lengths. Other structural possibilities can occur within polymers. For example, three possibilities exist for the CH_3 group in each monomer segment of polypropylene: all segments can be on the same side of the backbone (isotactic), on alternating sides (syndiotactic), or randomly placed (atactic). Isomerism can be especially important in determining the biologic activity and physical properties of polymers.

Temperature also can greatly affect a polymer's properties. At temperatures below the glass transition temperature (Tg), a polymer is glassy in nature and is generally stiff, strong, and brittle. Above the Tg, the polymer is leathery and is tougher and less rigid. The Tg for UHMWPE is approximately −40°C; thus, for orthopaedic applications, UHMWPE behaves in a leathery fashion. In contrast, the Tg for PMMA bone cement is greater than 60°C; thus in orthopaedic applications it behaves in a glassy fashion.

Segments of polymer chains can align themselves in a structured, crystalline order, much like the atomic planes in metallic alloys. Virtually all polymers are semicrystalline in that only some areas of the structure are ordered; in other parts of the polymer the chains are randomly oriented in an amorphous manner (**Figure 8**). The degree of crystallinity can greatly influence the polymer's properties, depending on the size, orientation, and distribution of crystalline areas.

Polymers Used in Joint Arthroplasty
PMMA Bone Cement
PMMA bone cement has been the polymer of choice as a grouting agent to secure implant components to bone since its introduction by Charnley in the 1970s. The PMMA used in orthopaedics is provided in two parts: a liquid in a sealed glass ampule and a powder in a bag. The liquid is predominantly methylmethacrylate monomer but also contains hydroquinone and N,N-dimethyl-*p*-toluidine. Hydroquinone inhibits polymerization, ensuring that the liquid does not polymerize prematurely because of heat or light; N,N-dimethyl-*p*-toluidine acts to

accelerate polymerization and offset the effect of the hydroquinone once the liquid and powder are mixed, and the reaction has begun. That process begins once the liquid monomer comes into contact with an initiator, dibenzoyl peroxide, which is mixed into the powder. In addition to the initiator, the powder is composed mainly of already polymerized PMMA or a blend of PMMA with a copolymer of either PMMA and polystyrene or PMMA and methacrylic acid, depending on the grade and manufacturer of the cement. The copolymers increase toughness. A radiopaque material, either barium sulfate ($BaSO_4$) or zirconia (ZrO_2), is also dispersed throughout the powder to allow the cement to be visualized on radiographs. The average molecular weight of a typical bone cement mixture after curing is 242,000, although the range of molecular weights in the final mixed and set form is large.

Once the polymerization process begins, the original carbon-to-carbon double bonds in methylmethacrylate are broken, and new carbon-to-carbon single bonds are formed in the polymer chain. The heat given off during this process is approximately 130 cal/g of methylmethacrylate monomer. The actual temperature rise, however, is dictated by the amount and thickness of the cement bulk and the heat transfer to surrounding structures. Bone cement temperatures during in vivo polymerization are as low as 40°C, below the 56°C that causes protein denaturation and the 47°C reported to cause bone necrosis. The long-term clinical success of cemented joint arthroplasty implants and bone filling applications such as vertebroplasty strongly indicates that thermal necrosis is not an important factor affecting overall performance.

Antibiotics can be added to bone cement to provide prophylaxis or treatment of infection. The elution of antibiotic from the cement is dictated by the preparation technique, chemistry, and surface area of the cement. For instance, among commercial cements, elution of gentamicin from Simplex cement (Stryker Orthopaedics, Mahway, NJ) or CMW cement (DePuy Orthopaedics, Warsaw, IN) is significantly less than that from Palacos (Zimmer, Warsaw, IN). Bone cement properties can be detrimentally altered by the addition of antibiotics during the mixing process, an important clinical concern when antibiotics are mixed into the cement at surgery. The FDA has recently approved commercially prepared antibiotic cements for commercial distribution in the United States, markedly reducing this potential problem.

The performance of cement as a grout for fixation of joint arthroplasty components has been enhanced by improved protocols in cement handling, bone preparation, and cement delivery. For example, vacuum mixer or low viscosity formulations of cement that are then delivered into the bone under pressure using a cement gun significantly reduce the porosity of the cement compared with hand-mixed cement. Reducing the porosity results in more cement in the mantle and increases its structural strength, even though the material properties of the cement itself remain unaltered. Although difficult to prove clinically, porosity reduction should reduce the chances of cement mantle fracture and subsequent implant loosening. Typical mechanical properties of bone cement include a compressive ultimate strength of 85 to 110 MPa, a tensile strength of 25 to 45 MPa, a fatigue strength of 10 to 15 MPa, and an elastic modulus of 1 to 4 GPa.

Ultra-High Molecular Weight Polyethylene

The first hips using UHMWPE as a bearing surface were implanted in the 1960s. The UHMWPE family remains the material of choice as the bearing surface in total joint arthroplasties. The distinctions between types of polyethylene are a result of molecular weight differences and the extent and type of branching. UHMWPE, as the name implies, has a very high molecular weight (typically exceeding one million), imparting significantly higher impact strength and toughness and better abrasive wear characteristics than high-density polyethylene (with a molecular weight in the range of 500,000).

Three methods are used to fabricate UHMWPE orthopaedic components. In ram extrusion, UHMWPE resin is extruded through a circular die under heat and pressure to form a cylindrical bar that, in turn, is machined into the final shape. In compression molding, the resin is molded (again under heat and pressure) into a large sheet, which is cut into smaller pieces to use in machining final components. Finally, in net shape or direct compression molding, the resin is directly molded into the finished part. In the direct molding process, additional machining usually is necessary to create detailed features such as locking mechanisms or backside profile of acetabular and tibial inserts; the articular surfaces are not machined.

The dominant method for sterilizing UHMWPE components has been by exposure to gamma radiation. Although it has been known for some time that oxidation of UHMWPE occurred after gamma sterilization, the oxidation did not become a major concern until the connection between polyethylene wear debris and osteolysis was suggested in the 1980s. Postirradiation oxidation increases the elastic modulus, decreases the ductility, and decreases the fracture toughness of UHMWPE. The extent of oxidation is determined by the radiation dose, the environment in which the component is irradiated, and subsequent shelf aging.

Postirradiation oxidation is initiated by the gamma radiation used during sterilization. The gamma rays can break both the carbon-hydrogen and carbon-carbon bonds, resulting in the formation of free radicals (atoms with an unpaired electron) that then can react to recombine, to cause chain scission, or to form cross-links. Recombination simply reforms the bonds that were broken and provides no net change in chemistry. In chain scission, a fragment is removed from the original polymer chain. Chain scission is driven by the presence of oxygen,

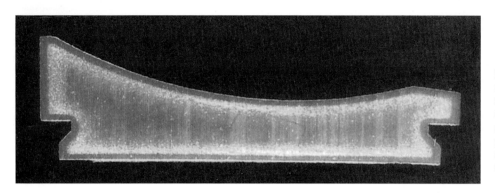

Figure 9 Subsurface white bands in cross-sectional view of postirradiation aged tibial insert. *(Reproduced from Wright TM, Li S: Biomaterials, in Buckwalter JA, Einhorn TA, Simon SR (eds): Orthopaedic Basic Science, ed 2. Rosemont, IL, American Academy of Orthopaedic Surgeons, 2000, pp 181-215.)*

which reacts readily with free radicals, resulting in a lower molecular weight (shorter chains) and increased density (because the smaller chains pack together more tightly). In cross-linking, radicals from different polymer chains react to form chemical bonds (cross-links) between the chains. A cross-linked polymer can be more abrasion-resistant than its non–cross-linked precursor. However, extremely high levels of cross-links may result in the material becoming brittle.

The maximum effects of postirradiation oxidation occur below the surface of irradiated UHMWPE components. In this region the density is quite high, as much as 0.007 to 0.02 g/mL higher than in the bulk, and the material properties are quite poor—so poor, in fact, that on sectioning, the brittle, oxidized material in the subsurface region fractures form a white band (**Figure 9**). Unfortunately, the subsurface oxidation coincides with the region where contact stresses can be quite high in devices such as tibial knee joint components that typically have nonconforming articular surfaces. The result is a propensity for wear surface damage in the form of pitting and delamination that can alter implant function and contribute to osteolysis.

Postirradiation degradation can be avoided by altering the sterilization method. For example, some manufacturers have converted to nonirradiation sterilization methods such as exposing UHMWPE devices to ethylene oxide or gas plasma. These nonirradiation methods sterilize the surface without forming the free radicals that lead to oxidative degradation. Nonirradiation methods do not, however, provide any cross-linking, which is known to reduce abrasive and adhesive wear. Many other manufacturers have continued to use gamma irradiation, but conduct the sterilization in an oxygen-free environment to minimize free-radical degradation and maximize cross-linking. Recent clinical studies of patients with total hip replacements have demonstrated a significant reduction in wear with radiation sterilization in comparison with ethylene oxide and gas plasma.

Postirradiation aging continues after sterilization because of the presence of free radicals. For conventional sterilization in air, exposure to an oxygen-containing environment results in continued degradation of the material properties as the free radicals react with oxygen. The degradation in properties has been correlated with clinical failures secondary to excessive polyethylene wear in patients with total knee replacements, results that have been supported by observations on retrieved total joint components and in vitro wear simulator and mechanical studies. These radicals, however, can be quenched by thermal treatments of the irradiated polyethylene, so that subsequent shelf aging no longer will occur.

The benefits of cross-linking in improving the adhesive and abrasive wear resistance of UHMWPE total joint components has been known since the mid 1970s, although cross-linking has gained widespread clinical acceptance only over the past few years. The first clinical use of highly cross-linked UHMWPE occurred in 1971 with the implantation of polyethylene acetabular components that had been irradiated with 100 Mrad of gamma irradiation, based on the results of reciprocating ball-on-flat laboratory wear tests that demonstrated a large decrease in wear when polyethylene was cross-linked by exposure to radiation greater than 50 Mrad. More recently, hip simulator tests have confirmed a marked decrease in wear rate with radiation doses as low as 5 to 10 Mrad (**Figure 10**). Based on these results, several companies have introduced versions of elevated cross-linked UHMWPE that differ in the resins used, the manner in which the resin is formed into the device, and the irradiation and posttreatment conditions.

Although cross-linking reduces wear rate, it adversely affects fracture and fatigue properties, so that in the final manufacturing process, a balance exists between low wear and reduction of other important properties. Concern has been raised that because of the reduced toughness and resistance to fatigue crack propagation, elevated cross-linked polyethylene components may be susceptible to gross fracture and other forms of fatigue-related wear, including pitting and delamination. These situations could occur whenever high stresses would be expected, such as in thin polyethylene inserts, in inserts with stress concentrations associated with locking mechanisms, or during impingement between the femoral neck and the acetabular rim in hip replacements.

Resistance to fatigue-related wear is especially impor-

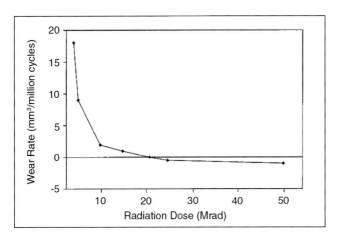

Figure 10 Wear rates of acetabular cups tested in a hip simulator are lower the higher the doses of radiation to which the UHMWPE is exposed before the start of the test. *(Adapted with permission from McKellop H, Shen FW, Lu B, Campbell P, Salovey R: Development of an extremely wear-resistant ultra high molecular weight polyethylene for total hip replacements. J Orthop Res 1999;17:157-167.)*

tant in knee replacements and other nonconforming joint arthroplasties, in which the need for reduced conformity to impart appropriate function and joint kinematics leads to high surface and subsurface stresses and moving contact areas. Although the reduced toughness and fatigue properties might portend an even worse performance for elevated cross-linked UHMWPE in these conditions, it has not been verified with in vitro wear tests. This worsened performance may be a result of the post–cross-linking thermal treatments developed to quench free radicals. These treatments involve heating the polyethylene to temperatures near or exceeding its melting point; the stabilization process is accompanied by a decrease in elastic modulus. The lower elastic modulus related to larger contact areas and smaller contact stresses may account for the resistance of elevated cross-linked polyethylene to fatigue wear, despite the accompanying decrease in other mechanical properties.

In joint arthroplasty the clinical benefits of elevated cross-linked UHMWPE in joint arthroplasty remain to be proven. Use of the material is in the early stages, with few reports of in vivo wear rate measurements based on serial radiographs. Only long-term clinical studies can demonstrate that elevated cross-linked UHMWPE can provide an overall patient benefit.

Biodegradable Polymers
Biodegradable polymers can be synthesized to degrade chemically and physically in a controlled manner over time. Such polymers are used in orthopaedic applications to replace more permanent biomaterials by providing immediate primary support, such as in sutures, screws, anchors, and pins, that is then slowly lost as the polymer resorbs and the tissue heals. Resorption allows the tissue to

assume its normal mechanical role because the load-sharing capabilities of the polymer decrease as it resorbs. Resorption also eliminates the need for a second surgical procedure to remove the device. Resorbable polymers also can be used for drug delivery, releasing the drug as the polymer degrades. Biodegradable scaffolds for tissue engineering are currently being researched and developed. This last application is a daunting one. The scaffold must provide a suitable biologic environment for the cells that are to be delivered to the defect. It must also provide a suitable mechanical environment so that the cells are encouraged to manufacture extracellular matrix with the appropriate biomechanical properties, while at the same time degrading at an adequate rate for tissue to replace the scaffold without adversely affecting the cells or the tissue.

Bioresorbable polymers include variations of polylactic acid, polyglycolic acid, polydioxanone, and polycaprolactone. The properties of these resorbable polymers can span large ranges. For example, elastic modulus values can range from 0.1 to 30 MPa and ultimate strength values from 3 to 290 MPa, depending on polymer type, the addition of copolymers, molecular weight, fabrication technique, and the addition of reinforcing materials such as fibers. Property changes are accompanied by marked differences in degradation rates and biologic activity.

Lactic acid, for example, can be made from either D (poly-D-lactic acid, PDLA) or L (poly-L-lactic acid) monomers of lactic acid or as a combination made from both monomers. Poly-L-lactic acid has long been considered a desirable choice as the basis for a bioresorbable polymer because the degradation product is lactic acid, a natural constituent. However, the form of the lactic acid (D or L) and the high concentration of lactic acid released to the region surrounding the device may nonetheless present biocompatibility problems. Molecular weight increases in poly-D or L lactic acid can vary biodegradation rates considerably; for example, with a molecular weight of 5,200, the polymer loses 50% of its mass in about 8 weeks, whereas with a molecular weight of 89,000, the same polymer takes 45 weeks to lose 21% of its mass. Unfortunately, mechanical properties often decrease faster than the mass loss, a factor that has limited the use of these materials to applications where load demands are low.

Another class of biodegradable materials receiving attention in orthopaedics is hydrogels. Hydrogels are a soft, porous-permeable group of polymers that are nontoxic, nonirritant, nonmutagenic, nonallergenic, and biocompatible. They readily absorb water (and thus have high water contents). They have low coefficients of friction and time-dependent mechanical properties that can be varied through altering the material's composition and structure. Hydrogels have been considered for use in a wide range of biomedical and pharmaceutical applications; orthopaedic applications include tissue engineering of cartilage and bone and for drug delivery.

Polymers Used in Orthotics and Prosthetics

Polymers play an important role in orthotics; two major groups, thermoplastics and thermosets, are used for orthotic design. Low-temperature thermoplastics, those classified as requiring temperatures no higher than 80°C to become workable, may be molded directly to the body. These materials are popular for upper extremity applications in which the rapid provision of an assistive or protective orthosis is desirable. Minimal equipment is required: a source of hot water, scissors, and a heat gun. However, low-temperature thermoplastics typically are ineffective when high loads are anticipated because they are not very strong. High-temperature thermoplastics require higher temperatures to become workable and usually are molded under vacuum to the prescribed shape of a plaster model prepared by the orthotist. Polyethylene and polypropylene are the most widely used high-temperature thermoplastics.

Low-, medium-, and high-density polyethylenes are used, depending on the required mechanical properties. Low-density polyethylene is a good option for non–weight-bearing applications, such as a supportive wrist and hand orthosis. High-density polyethylene is commonly used in spinal orthotic treatments where greater strength and elastic modulus are required. Polypropylene's unique flexing capability and excellent fatigue resistance are particularly useful for lower extremity orthotics. However, the plastic most often used for orthotic design is a copolymer of polyethylene and polypropylene. This copolymer is mostly polypropylene with 5% to 25% polyethylene and has much better fatigue resistance than either constituent polymer.

The range of material properties possible by combining different copolymers and the ability to alter structural properties by changing the shape and thickness of the device provide a wide range of structural stiffness and strength for orthotic designs. The design of foot orthoses is an area in which the choice of materials is of paramount importance. Weight, for example, is important because of its effect on the moment of inertia of the lower extremity and, thus, on the amount of muscle power required to move the lower extremity. Shock absorption and comfort are required to relieve pain. If the function of the orthosis is support, leather or felt with or without a sturdier underliner may be more appropriate than polymers; if the function is to reduce shear force, a viscoelastic polymer may be best. Commonly, foot orthoses are required to cushion or absorb shock; closed-cell polyethylene foams and nitrogen-filled rubbers have proved successful. As is the case in most areas of prosthetic and orthotic design, clinical devices typically are manufactured from more than one material because the functional requirements demand varying characteristics from each component; for example, the patient with diabetes who has

significant tissue loss and adherent scar tissue will require both shock absorption and shear reduction.

The current selection of materials allows amputees to be fit with lightweight functional prostheses constructed from thermoplastics, improved acrylic resins, titanium, graphite, and carbon fiber composites. Exoskeletal prostheses provide strength via the hard laminated surface of the prosthesis; endoskeletal prostheses provide strength through a central pylon commonly constructed of aluminum alloy or a graphite composite to give the patient a strong, lightweight prosthesis. Cost and durability are advantages of the exoskeletal design; however, endoskeletal prostheses allow for interchange of modular components, incorporation of soft cosmetic coverings, and convenience in making alignment changes.

Typically, only the socket of the prosthesis is custom fabricated; the other components are manufactured in an array of sizes and varying levels of sophistication. Components and their materials are selected by the prosthetist to match the biomechanical and functional needs of each patient. Prosthetic sockets can be manufactured from either thermoplastic materials or fiber-reinforced thermosetting plastics. The use of thermoplastics for this important part of the prosthesis has gained wider acceptance as both patient and prosthetist have come to appreciate the advantages, including reduced manufacturing time.

Ceramic Materials

Ceramic materials are solid, inorganic compounds consisting of metallic and nonmetallic elements held together by ionic or covalent bonding. Ceramics include compounds such as silica (SiO_2) and alumina (Al_2O_3). When processed appropriately to high purity, they possess excellent biocompatibility (a function of their insolubility and chemical inertness) and exceptional wear resistance (with hard, smooth, hydrophilic surfaces). Ceramic materials are very stiff and brittle, but are very strong under compressive loads. In orthopaedics, ceramics have gained favor as biomaterials for two quite different applications. The first involves their use in total joint arthroplasty components as fully dense ceramics, such as alumina and zirconia, with inertness and wear resistance superior to those of metallic alloys. The second involves the use of ceramics, such as calcium phosphate and bioglass (SiO_2-Na_2O-CaO-P_2O_5), as bone graft substitutes and as osteoconductive coatings for metallic implants, providing surfaces to which bone will bond. The success and the limitations of ceramics in these applications can be understood by considering their bonding, structure, and properties.

Ionic and Covalent Bonding

Ceramics are typically three-dimensional arrays of positively charged metal ions and negatively charged nonmetal ions, often oxygen. Positively charged ions form from elements that easily release outer electrons, and negatively charged ions form from elements that readily accept electrons in their outer atomic shells. Positively charged ions surround themselves with as many negatively charged ions as possible, and vice versa, resulting in a closely packed arrangement of strongly bonded nuclei for which the total charge is zero. This localization of the sharing of electrons between nuclei makes most ceramics excellent electrical and thermal insulators.

Other ceramic materials are held together by covalent bonds. Covalent bonds are formed through the mutual sharing of electrons between adjacent atoms so that the shared electrons complete the outer valence shell of each atom. Both ionically and covalently bonded materials are good insulators. The potential high strength of covalent bonds can be understood by considering diamond, a material composed only of covalently bonded carbon atoms.

Ceramic Microstructures

Most ceramic materials have polygranular microstructures similar to those of metallic alloys. The properties of ceramics are dictated to a large extent by the characteristics of the microstructure, including grain size, porosity, and the types and distribution of phases within each grain. As with metallic alloys, ceramic microstructures can be altered significantly by thermal processing techniques.

A common technique for fabricating ceramic materials is to mix fine particulates of the material with water and an organic binder and press them into a mold of the desired shape. The resulting part is dried by heating to evaporate the water and burn away the binder. The part is then fired or sintered at a much higher temperature. This process results in densification as the particles come into close contact driven by mechanisms such as diffusion, evaporation, and condensation that reduce the total surface energy in the part. As with the casting of metallic alloys, the resulting microstructure (and therefore properties) of the ceramic part will depend on the control of key variables in the processing. For example, strength is inversely proportional to both grain size and porosity. Grain size can be controlled by the starting size of the particles used to form the part; the smaller the particles, the smaller the grain size. However, grain size will increase during processing, whereas porosity will be reduced, so sintering times are critical.

Ceramics Used in Joint Arthroplasty

Ceramic-on-polyethylene bearings have been commercially available for some time as alternatives to conventional metal-on-polyethylene. Ceramic-ceramic bearings have only recently received regulatory approval for commercial distribution in the United States. Both types of bearings were introduced to address the problem of polyethylene wear because they have few other mechanical advantages for joint arthroplasty. Ceramics have high hardness and high elastic modulus, allowing them to be polished to a

very smooth finish and to resist roughening while in use as a bearing surface. They have good wettability, suggesting the possibility of forming lubricating layers between ceramic couplings to reduce adhesive forms of wear.

Alumina

Aluminum oxide (Al_2O_3) has excellent abrasion resistance and when highly polished creates a very low coefficient of friction surface against both UHMWPE and itself. Long-term experience with alumina-on-polyethylene bearings for hip replacement shows reduced wear rates over those typically seen with metal-on-polyethylene bearings, as well as an associated decrease in osteolysis, suggesting that these types of bearings are indeed beneficial in improving clinical performance. The use of alumina-on-polyethylene bearings in knee replacements has been limited, and only midterm results are available. Results are excellent but the absence of direct comparisons with conventional metal-on-polyethylene bearing surfaces of the same design and the lack of long-term results make it difficult to assess the clinical benefits.

Early clinical experience showed fracture of alumina femoral heads to be a significant complication, with an incidence of more than 5% in some reported series. Improvements and standardization in alumina processing, including refinement of the grain size, hot isostatic pressing of the material after sintering to further increase the density, and improved manufacturing taper connections have led to a dramatic improvement in performance. Grain sizes, for example, typically exceeded 4 µm in the 1970s with densities of about 4 g/mm^3; grain sizes are now maintained at about 0.5 µm with densities of about 6 g/mm^3. The resulting refinement creates a 45% increase in strength. Even though alumina is considered highly biocompatible, periprosthetic osteolysis secondary to alumina debris reinforces the concern that small particles ingested by cells can elicit an adverse biologic reaction regardless of their chemical nature.

Ceramic-on-ceramic bearings have been used extensively in total hip arthroplasty in Europe. In general, alumina-on-alumina joints have shown very low wear rates clinically. However, the results are design dependent, and even these bearings can show excessive wear if incorporated into an inferior design. Recent reports also show excellent wear resistance in young patients, with no measurable wear and no evidence of osteolysis in more than 10 years of follow-up. Furthermore, head fractures have not been observed in this high-demand patient population, lending further credence to the improved mechanical properties of alumina ceramic materials.

Zirconia

The use of zirconia as a bearing surface against polyethylene has not proved as successful clinically as the use of alumina. A direct comparison between alumina-, zirconia-, and metal-on-conventional polyethylene bearings in pa-

tients with total hip replacements revealed the highest wear rate in the zirconia group, consistent with an increased monoclinic content on the surface of retrieved zirconia heads from the same series. The propensity for zirconia to transform from a tetragonal crystalline form, which is stable at elevated temperatures, to the less tough monoclinic form is a disadvantage of this material and has led to US FDA warnings against autoclave resterilization of zirconia heads. The decrease in toughness makes the material more susceptible to roughening and increased wear. Problems with manufacturing processes that led to a high incidence of fracture prompted a recent voluntary recall of nine batches of zirconia heads, further undermining confidence in this material. Nonetheless, zirconia has found clinical use as an alternative bearing material to metallic alloys for articulating against UHMWPE. Zirconia does not, however, wear well against itself or against other ceramics such as alumina.

Recently, a ceramic composite of zirconia oxide at the surface of zirconium alloy components has been introduced into both femoral components for total knee replacement and femoral heads for total hip replacement. The oxide is formed by thermally driving oxygen diffusion into a metallic zirconium alloy surface with the goal of providing a hardened ceramic articular surface with the strength and ductility of a metal alloy base. As with other ceramic surfaces, laboratory wear tests show a clear advantage of the oxide surface in comparison with conventional metallic alloy (such as cobalt alloy). Clinical experience is short, however, so the advantages in terms of wear and osteolysis remain to be demonstrated. Recent problems with early clinical failures of porous versions of this technology intended for biologic fixation led to a voluntary recall of these products by the manufacturer.

Ceramics as Bone Substitutes

The second application of ceramic materials is in the area of bone substitutes. Certain ceramic and glass materials have been found to be osteoconductive in nature, such that osteoblasts form bone when the mineral phase is in direct contact with the ceramic surface. The chemical or physical bond that forms between the ceramic and the bone is not well understood, but results in sufficient interfacial strength that applications such as ceramic coatings on implants have been used in an attempt to improve implant fixation to bone.

Most applications of bioceramics are aimed at the eventual resorption or removal of the bioceramic through substitution with remodeled bone. The mineral phase of bone is hydroxyapatite, which is a calcium phosphate ($Ca_{10}[PO_4]_6[OH]_2$). The stability of calcium phosphate ceramics depends on the temperature and the environment and can be affected by substitution (for example, of a carbonate for a phosphate). Hydroxyapatite coatings for fixation of load-bearing implants have been in clinical use for more than a decade. However, the true composition of these coatings can be quite variable because of differences in manufacturing processes and changes with time in vivo. Studies of coatings on retrieved implants show that although the coatings are often osteoconductive, bonding with bone is not uniform, and the coatings themselves may not, in fact, be true hydroxyapatite, but a mixture of phases, including calcium oxide, tricalcium phosphate, and amorphous calcium phosphate. Coatings have been shown to dissolve and fracture from the implant substrate and can be removed by an osteoclastic remodeling process.

Hydroxyapatite cements (either alone or in combination with PMMA bone cement) have also been developed. Injectable cements that cure isothermally to an apatite similar to that in bone and have strength comparable to cancellous bone have been tested in animal models and have been used clinically, especially in maxillofacial applications. The cement appears to maintain its strength as it is remodeled, making it a candidate for bone graft material. Hydroxyapatite cement has been shown to be as effective as autograft for treating bone defects.

Bioactive glasses are based typically on combinations of SiO_2, CaO, Na_2O, and P_2O_5. These materials partially solubilize in vivo, forming a surface hydrogel that is rich in calcium and phosphate ions. Crystallization leads to the formation of apatite and thus a bond with the bone. The brittleness and inherent stability of these materials restrict their use to nonstructural applications such as coatings and fillers.

Summary

Biomaterials used for orthopaedic applications have unique functional and safety requirements. Ideally materials should be biocompatible, resistant to corrosion and degradation, and have adequate mechanical properties for their specific application. The ability of a material to meet these requirements necessitates an understanding of its chemical nature, microstructure, and how that microstructure is affected by the mode of manufacture. Furthermore, when fashioned into a device, mechanical strength and stiffness are dictated by consideration of the material from which the device is manufactured, the loads to which it is subjected, and its shape. The microstructure, composition, and mechanical properties of metallic, polymeric, and ceramic biomaterials traditionally used in the orthopaedic sciences have been reviewed in this chapter along with a brief review of the effect of geometry and mode of loading on mechanical performance.

Selected Bibliography
Requirements for Orthopaedic Biomaterials

Amstutz HC (ed): *Academic, Industry and Federal Interactions in Developing and Applying New Technology for Orthopaedics*, ed 1. Rosemont, IL, American

Academy of Orthopaedic Surgeons, 1998. Available at http://www3.aaos.org/technology/techtoc.cfm

Beaule PE, Campbell PA, Walker PS, et al: Polyethylene wear characteristics in vivo and in a knee stimulator. *J Biomed Mater Res* 2002;60:411-419.

Black J: *Biological Performance of Materials: Fundamentals of Biocompatibility*, ed 3. New York, NY, Marcel Dekker, 1999.

Bobyn JD, Tanzer M, Krygier JJ, Dujovne AR, Brooks CE: Concerns with modularity in total hip arthroplasty. *Clin Orthop Relat Res* 1994;298:27-36.

Brown SA, Flemming CA, Kawalec JS, et al: Fretting corrosion accelerates crevice corrosion of modular hip tapers. *J Appl Biomater* 1995;6:19-26.

Burstein AH, Wright TM (eds): *Fundamentals of Orthopaedic Biomechanics*. Baltimore, MD, Williams & Wilkins, 1994.

Cook SD, Renz EA, Barrack RL, et al: Clinical and metallurgical analysis of retrieved internal fixation devices. *Clin Orthop Relat Res* 1985;194:236-247.

Doorn PF, Campbell PA, Worrall J, Benya PD, McKellop HA, Amstutz HC: Metal wear particle characterization from metal on metal total hip replacements: Transmission electron microscopy study of periprosthetic tissues and isolated particles. *J Biomed Mater Res* 1998;42:103-111.

Firkins PJ, Tipper JL, Saadatzadeh MR, et al: Quantitative analysis of wear and wear debris from metal-on-metal hip prostheses tested in a physiological hip joint simulator. *Biomed Mater Eng* 2001;11:143-157.

Gilbert JL, Buckley CA, Jacobs JJ: In vivo corrosion of modular hip prosthesis components in mixed and similar metal combinations: The effect of crevice, stress, motion, and alloy coupling. *J Biomed Mater Res* 1993;27:1533-1544.

Gilbert JL, Buckley CA, Jacobs JJ, Bertin KC, Zernich MR: Intergranular corrosion-fatigue failure of cobalt-alloy femoral stems: A failure analysis of two implants. *J Bone Joint Surg Am* 1994;76:110-115.

Gray RJ: Metallographic examinations of retrieved intramedullary bone pins and bone screws from the human body. *J Biomed Mater Res* 1974;8:27-38.

Jacobs JJ, Gilbert JL, Urban RM: Corrosion of metal orthopaedic implants. *J Bone Joint Surg Am* 1998;80:268-282.

Maloney WJ, Smith RL, Schmalzried TP: Isolation and characterization of wear particles generated in patients who have had failure of a hip arthroplasty without cement. *J Bone Joint Surg Am* 1995;77:1301-1310.

Morita M, Sasada T, Hayashi H, Tsukamoto Y: The corrosion fatigue properties of surgical implants in a living body. *J Biomed Mater Res* 1988;22:529-540.

Muratoglu OK, Perinchief RS, Bragdon CR, O'Connor DO, Konrad R, Harris WH: Metrology to quantify wear and creep of polyethylene tibial knee inserts. *Clin Orthop Relat Res* 2003;410:155-164.

Ratner BD, Hoffman AS, Schoen FJ, Lemons JE (eds): *Biomaterials Science: An Introduction to Materials in Medicine*. San Diego, CA, Academic Press, 1996.

Rimnac CM, Klein RW, Betts F, Wright TM: Post-irradiation aging of ultra high molecular weight polyethylene. *J Bone Joint Surg Am* 1994;76:1052-1056.

Von Recum A, Jacobi JE (eds): *Handbook of Biomaterials Evaluation: Scientific, Technical and Clinical Testing of Implant Materials*, ed 2. Philadelphia, PA, Taylor & Francis, 1999.

Willert HG, Broback LG, Buchhorn GH, et al: Crevice corrosion of cemented titanium alloy stems in total hip replacements. *Clin Orthop Relat Res* 1996;333:51-75.

Williams DF: Titanium as a metal for implantation: Part 1. Physical properties. *J Med Eng Technol* 1977;1:195-198.

Williams S, Butterfield M, Stewart T, Ingham E, Stone M, Fisher J: Wear and deformation of ceramic-on-polyethylene total hip replacements with joint laxity and swing phase microseparation. *Proc Inst Mech Eng [H]* 2003;217:147-153.

Wright TM, Goodman SB (eds): *Implant Wear in Total Joint Replacement: Clinical and Biologic Issues, Materials and Design Considerations*. Rosemont, IL, American Academy of Orthopaedic Surgeons, 2001.

Metallic Materials
Bobyn JD, Toh KK, Hacking SA, Tanzer M, Krygier JJ: Tissue response to porous tantalum acetabular cups: A canine model. *J Arthroplasty* 1999;14:347-354.

Disegi JA, Wyss H: Implant materials for fracture fixation: A clinical perspective. *Orthopedics* 1989;12:75-79.

Long M, Rack HJ: Titanium alloys in total joint replacement: A materials science perspective. *Biomaterials* 1998;19:1621-1639.

Wigfield C, Robertson J, Gill S, Nelson R: Clinical experience with porous tantalum cervical interbody implants in a prospective randomized controlled trial. *Br J Neurosurg* 2003;17:418-425.

Polymers

An YH, Woolf SK, Friedman RJ: Pre-clinical in vivo evaluation of orthopaedic bioabsorbable devices. *Biomaterials* 2000;21:2635-2652.

Baker DA, Bellare A, Pruitt L: The effects of degree of crosslinking on the fatigue crack initiation and propagation resistance of orthopedic-grade polyethylene. *J Biomed Mater Res* 2003;66A:146-154.

Behravesh E, Yasko AW, Engel PS, Mikos AG: Synthetic biodegradable polymers for orthopaedic applications. *Clin Orthop Relat Res* 1999;367:S118-S129.

Bostman O, Pihlajamaki H: Clinical biocompatibility of biodegradable orthopaedic implants for internal fixation: A review. *Biomaterials* 2000;21:2615-2621.

Chang SC, Tobias G, Roy AK, Vacanti CA, Bonassar LJ: Tissue engineering of autologous cartilage for craniofacial reconstruction by injection molding. *Plast Reconstr Surg* 2003;112:793-799.

Cole JC, Lemons JE, Eberhardt AW: Gamma irradiation alters fatigue-crack behavior and fracture toughness in 1900H and GUR 1050 UHMWPE. *J Biomed Mater Res* 2002;63:559-566.

Digas G, Thanner J, Nivbrant B, Rohrl S, Strom H, Karrholm J: Increase in early polyethylene wear after sterilization with ethylene oxide: Radiostereometric analyses of 201 total hips. *Acta Orthop Scand* 2003;74:531-541.

Hopper RH Jr, Young AM, Orishimo KF, Engh CA Jr: Effect of terminal sterilization with gas plasma or gamma radiation on wear of polyethylene liners. *J Bone Joint Surg Am* 2003;85:464-468.

Lewis G: Properties of acrylic bone cement: State of the art review. *J Biomed Mater Res* 1997;38:155-182.

Maher SA, Furman BD, Wright TM: The reduced fracture toughness that accompanies elevated cross-linking of polyethylene is not associated with an increase in pitting and delamination type wear, in Kurtz SM, Gsell R, Martell J (eds): *Crosslinked and Thermally Treated Ultra-High Molecular Weight Polyethylene for Joint Replacements: ASTM STP 1445.* West Conshohocken, PA, ASTM International, 2004.

McGovern TF, Ammeen DJ, Collier JP, Currier BH, Engh GA: Rapid polyethylene failure of unicondylar tibial components sterilized with gamma irradiation in air and implanted after a long shelf life. *J Bone Joint Surg Am* 2002;84-A:901-906.

McKellop H, Shen FW, Lu B, Campbell P, Salovey R: Development of an extremely wear-resistant ultra high molecular weight polyethylene for total hip replacements. *J Orthop Res* 1999;17:157-167.

McKellop H, Shen FW, Lu B, Campbell P, Salovey R: Effect of sterilization method and other modifications on the wear resistance of acetabular cups made of ultra-high molecular weight polyethylene: A hip-simulator study. *J Bone Joint Surg Am* 2000;82:1708-1725.

Muratoglu OK, Bragdon CR, O'Connor DO, Jasty M, Harris WH: A novel method of cross-linking ultra-high-molecular-weight polyethylene to improve wear, reduce oxidation, and retain mechanical properties. *J Arthroplasty* 2001;16:149-160.

Muratoglu OK, Bragdon CR, O'Connor DO, Perinchief RS, Jasty M, Harris WH: Aggressive wear testing of a cross-linked polyethylene in total knee arthroplasty. *Clin Orthop Relat Res* 2002;404:89-95.

Puolakka TJ, Keranen JT, Juhola KA, et al: Increased volumetric wear of polyethylene liners with more than 3 years of shelf-life time. *Int Orthop* 2003;27:153-159.

Ceramic Materials

Dickson KF, Friedman J, Buchholz JG, Flandry FD: The use of BoneSource hydroxyapatite cement for traumatic metaphyseal bone void filling. *J Trauma* 2002;53:1103-1108.

Hamadouche M, Boutin P, Daussange J, Bolander ME, Sedel L: Alumina-on-alumina total hip arthroplasty: A minimum 18.5-year follow-up study. *J Bone Joint Surg Am* 2002;84:69-77.

Hamadouche M, Sedel L: Ceramics in orthopaedics. *J Bone Joint Surg Br* 2000;82:1095-1099.

Kokubo T, Kim HM, Kawashita M: Novel bioactive materials with different mechanical properties. *Biomaterials* 2003;24:2161-2175.

Li P: Bioactive ceramics: State of the art and future trends. *Semin Arthroplasty* 1998;9:165-175.

Urban JA, Garvin KL, Boese CK, et al: Ceramic-on-polyethylene bearing surfaces in total hip arthroplasty: Seventeen to twenty-one-year results. *J Bone Joint Surg Am* 2001;83:1688-1694.

Yoon TR, Rowe SM, Jung ST, Seon KJ, Maloney WJ: Osteolysis in association with a total hip arthroplasty with ceramic bearing surfaces. *J Bone Joint Surg Am* 1998;80:1459-1468.

Chapter 5

Evidence-Based Orthopaedics: Issues in Research Design, Analysis, and Critical Appraisal

Mohit Bhandari, MD

Introduction

The evolution of evidence-based medicine has led to the development of evidence-based nursing, physiotherapy, occupational therapy, podiatry, and specialization. Evidence-based medicine is needed across all disciplines, including obstetrics, gynecology, internal medicine and surgery, and orthopaedic surgery.

What is Evidence-Based Medicine?

The term evidence-based medicine was first mentioned in a 1990 document for applicants to the Internal Medicine residency program at McMaster University. Evidence-based medicine was described as "an attitude of enlightened skepticism towards the application of diagnostic, therapeutic, and prognostic technologies." The evidence-based approach to practicing medicine relies on an awareness of the evidence upon which a clinician's practice is based and the strength of inference permitted by that evidence. The most sophisticated practice of evidence-based medicine requires, in turn, a clear delineation of relevant clinical questions, a thorough search of the literature relating to the questions, a critical appraisal of available evidence and its applicability to the clinical situation, and a balanced application of the conclusions to the clinical problem. The balanced application of the evidence (the clinical decision making) is the central aspect of evidence-based medicine and involves, according to evidence-based principles, integration of clinical expertise and judgment with patient and societal values, and with the best available research evidence.

There are more than 3,800 journals and 7,300 papers published each week. Health care providers, to accommodate their busy schedules, need to develop the skills to efficiently identify the highest quality information to guide their practices. However, evidence-based medicine involves more than just critical appraisal of the literature. Finding evidence requires search skills, and appraising evidence requires an understanding of the hierarchy of research design. An evaluation of evidence-based curricula using focus group and survey data showed that learners appreciated the skills and knowledge gained in devising guidelines in an evidence-based manner but were uncertain that their searches were complete. The clinical evaluation of the guideline implementation showed improvement in several clinical markers of diabetes care, for example. How does evidence-based medicine differ from the traditional approaches to health care provision? According to the traditional paradigm, clinicians may evaluate and solve clinical problems by reflecting on their own clinical experience, by evaluating the underlying biology and pathophysiology of the disorder, or by consulting a textbook or local expert. For many practitioners, time constraints often limit in-depth reviews of published papers. Thus, they often trust that the conclusions of a paper are accurate. Ultimately, their observations from day-to-day clinical experience become a common means of building and maintaining knowledge about patient prognosis, the value of diagnostic tests, and the efficacy of treatment. Because this paradigm places high value on traditional scientific authority and adherence to standard approaches, traditional medical training and common sense provide an adequate basis for evaluating new tests and treatments. Content expertise and clinical experience are sufficient to generate guidelines for clinical practice.

Evidence-based practice posits that although pathophysiology and clinical experience are necessary, they alone are insufficient guides for practice. These evidence sources may lead to inaccurate predictions about the per-

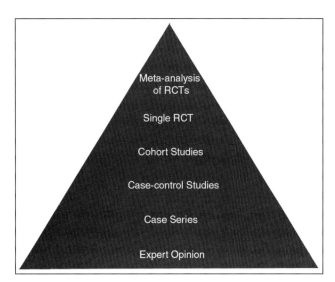

Figure 1   Hierarchy of research design. RCT = randomized clinical trial.

formance of diagnostic tests and the efficacy of treatments. Like the traditional approach to health care, the evidence-based health care paradigm also assumes that clinical experience and the development of clinical instincts (particularly with respect to diagnosis) are crucial elements of physician competence. However, the evidence-based approach includes several additional steps. These steps include using experience to identify important knowledge gaps and information needs, formulating answerable questions, identifying potentially relevant research, assessing the validity of evidence and results, developing clinical policies that align research evidence and clinical circumstances, and applying research evidence to individual patients with their particular experiences, expectations, and values.

Over the past several years the concepts and ideas attributed to and labeled collectively as evidence-based medicine have become more familiar, with terms such as evidence-based guidelines, evidence-based care paths, and evidence-based questions and solutions becoming more common. The controversy has shifted from whether to implement the new concepts to how to do so sensibly and efficiently, while avoiding potential conflicts associated with several misconceptions about what evidence-based medicine is and what it is not. The evidence-based medicine-related concepts such as hierarchy of evidence, meta-analyses, confidence intervals (CIs), and study design are so widespread that clinicians willing to have a better understanding of today's medical literature have no choice but to become familiar with the principles and methodologies of evidence-based medicine.

Critics of evidence-based medicine have mistakenly suggested that it equates evidence with results of randomized trials, statistical significance with clinical relevance, evidence (of whatever kind) with decisions, and lack of evidence of efficacy with the evidence for the lack of efficacy. Other critics argue that evidence-based medicine is not a tool for providing optimal patient care, but merely a cost-containment tool. All these statements are fundamental mischaracterizations. Although evidence-based medicine is sometimes perceived as a strict adherence to the findings of randomized trials, it more accurately involves informed and effective use of all types of evidence, but particularly evidence from the medical literature, in patient care. With the ever-increasing amount of available information, a paradigm shift from traditional practice to one that involves question formulation, validity assessment of available studies, and appropriate application of research evidence to individual patients must be considered.

This chapter presents an overview of the principles of research design, important statistical issues, basics of critical appraisal, and practical guidelines to the development of a research proposal.

Finding Evidence

The most commonly used biomedical database produced by the National Library of Medicine is Medline. Free Medline access is available on the internet as PubMed. Medline indexes more than 4,000 biomedical journals (11 million citations) with coverage from 1966 to present.

Only a small portion of articles in Medline report evidence that can be applied directly to clinical practice. A method of improving the retrieval of high-quality studies applicable to clinical practice is to include search terms that select studies at advanced stages of testing for clinical application.

PubMed has a special feature called Clinical Queries, which automatically filters searches on questions of therapy, diagnosis, etiology, or prognosis by looking at the highest levels of evidence in the literature. The Clinical Queries search filter can be accessed at the PubMed internet Website (www.pubmed.gov) by selecting "clinical queries." Once in the Clinical Queries site, the type of study can be selected (therapy or diagnosis), and then "systematic reviews" selected. Key words can be entered to identify relevant studies.

Study Design
Hierarchy of Research Study Design

Among various study designs, a hierarchy of evidence exists, with randomized controlled trials at the top, controlled observational studies in the middle, and uncontrolled studies and opinion at the bottom (Figure 1). Sackett has proposed a grading system that categorizes the hierarchy of research designs as levels of evidence. Each level is associated with a corresponding grade of recommendations: (1) grade A, consistent level I studies; (2) grade B, consistent level II or level III studies; (3) grade C, level IV studies; and (4) grade D, level V evidence (Table 1).

Table 1 | Levels of Evidence and Grades of Recommendation

Level of Evidence		Grade of Recommendations
Level I:	Large randomized trials with clear-cut results, and low risk of error, or meta-analyses of randomized trials with homogenous (similar) study results and narrow CIs	A
Level II:	Randomized trials with uncertain results and/or moderate to high risk of error; prospective cohort studies of high quality	B
Level III:	Case-control studies or meta-analyses of case-control studies	B
Level IV:	Case series with no controls	C
Level V:	Expert opinion without explicit critical appraisal, or based on physiology or bench research	D

Understanding the association between study design and level of evidence is important. The *Journal of Bone and Joint Surgery*, as of January 2003, has published the level of evidence associated with each published scientific article to provide readers with a gauge of the validity of the study results. Level I studies may be deemed appropriate for the application to patient care, whereas level IV studies will be interpreted with caution. For example, readers should be more confident about the results of a high-quality multi-center randomized trial of reamed versus nonreamed femoral intramedullary nailing on pulmonary function and union rates (level I study) than two separate case series evaluating either reamed or unreamed femoral nailing on the same outcomes (level IV studies). However, when randomized trials are not feasible or ethical, other forms of evidence such as case series become important in providing guides to practice.

Why are grades of recommendation important? Levels of evidence grading for a particular study tell about that specific article but nothing about the complete body of evidence for a particular clinical question. No single study will ultimately provide all the answers. Clinicians need to see the results of a single study replicated in other studies and across different nations. Levels of evidence have limitations. For example, two randomized trials (both labeled as level I evidence) evaluating an orthopaedic therapy with completely opposing conclusions raise a dilemma for clinicians. Grades of recommendations consider all the highest quality literature on this specific therapy and provide an overall recommendation (**Table 1**). There is no consensus on the optimal grading system. Several grading systems have been proposed but none has been validated.

The types of study designs used in clinical research can be classified broadly according to whether the study focuses on describing the distributions or characteristics of a disease or elucidating its determinants (**Figure 2**). Descriptive studies describe the distribution of a disease, particularly what type of people have the disease, in what locations, and when. Cross-sectional studies, case reports, and case series represent types of descriptive studies. Analytic studies focus on determinants of a disease by testing a hypothesis with the ultimate goal of judging whether a particular exposure causes or prevents disease. Analytic

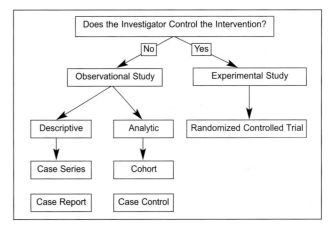

Figure 2   Research designs.

design strategies are typically grouped into two types: observational studies, such as case-control studies, and experimental studies, also called clinical trials. The difference between the two types of analytic studies is the role that the investigator plays in each of the studies. In the observational study, the investigator simply observes the natural course of events, whereas in the clinical trial the investigator assigns the intervention or treatment.

Types of Study Design
Meta-Analysis (Level I Evidence; Grade A Recommendation)
Although not considered to be primary study design, meta-analysis deserves mention because it is frequently used in the surgical literature. A meta-analysis is a systematic review that combines the results of multiple studies (of small sample size) to answer a focused clinical question. By its title as a review, a meta-analysis is retrospective in nature. The main advantage of meta-analysis is the ability to increase the total sample size of the study by combining the results of many smaller studies. When well-designed studies are available on a particular question of interest, a meta-analysis can provide important information to guide clinical practice. However, discrepancies between meta-analysis of small trials and single large trials have been reported. **Figure 3** outlines how the results of many small randomized trials can be statistically com-

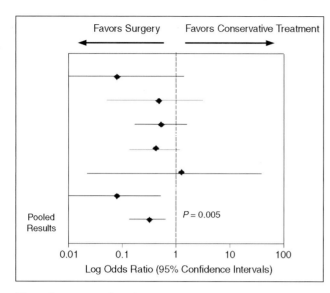

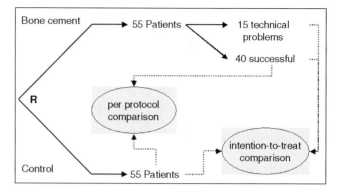

Figure 4   A comparison of a per protocol and intention-to-treat protocol in the evaluation of the results of a randomized trial comparing the use of bone cement versus controls in patients with distal radius fractures is shown.

Figure 3   Forest plot of surgery versus casting for Achilles tendon rupture. The pooled results from six randomized trials suggest that surgery significantly reduces the risk of re-rupture when compared with nonsurgical treatment.

bined to provide a summary estimate of the overall effect of surgical versus nonsurgical management of Achilles tendon ruptures on rates of re-rupture in younger patients. All of the trials, except one, have a wide CI (crosses odds = 1.0 equivalence); however, when the study results are combined statistically, the pooled result reveals a significant advantage to surgical repair in reducing re-ruptures (that is, the CI is narrower and no longer crosses the equivalence point of 1.0). The key issue with meta-analysis is the understanding that the quality of the primary studies is directly related to the quality of the meta-analysis results. For this reason, some investigators argue that meta-analysis of nonrandomized studies should never be conducted.

Randomized Controlled Trials

Randomized controlled trials (level I evidence, grade A recommendation) are considered to provide the highest level of evidence because randomization is the only method for controlling for known and unknown prognostic factors between two comparison groups. Concealed treatment allocation and blinding (outcome assessors, patients, data analysts, and surgeons) limit bias in this design. Lack of randomization predisposes a study to potentially important imbalances in baseline characteristics between two study groups. Investigators can randomize patients using a random numbers table (or computerized random number generators). This randomization ensures an equal probability of patients being allocated to either treatment or control groups. Randomization should be concealed—that is, investigators involved in the study should not be able to determine the treatment allocation of the next enrolled patient. Concealment is best achieved

by having investigators call a 24-hour telephone or internet-based randomization system. It may also be achieved by using opaque envelopes that contain the random allocation of treatments. The use of even-odd days, patient birthdates, or hospital chart identification numbers does not constitute concealed randomization and should be avoided. Surgeons randomizing patients (even/odd days) to receive a bone graft substitute for a distal radius fracture could easily introduce a selection bias by knowing that the next patient in their study was going to receive the substitute. They may preferentially identify (or exclude) patients who would be ideal (or not so ideal) for the product based on their beliefs of its efficacy.

Outcomes in a randomized trial should be tabulated based on the treatment to which patients were allocated, and not necessarily to the treatments they actually received. For example, a patient with a distal radius fracture randomized to a calcium phosphate bone cement who receives a cast only because of technical problems should still be grouped with the bone cement group in the analysis. The principle of analyzing the results in terms of a patient's original treatment allocation is called the intention-to-treat principle and is important in preserving the original balance of prognostic factors achieved by randomization (**Figure 4**).

In addition to the most common parallel group design, randomized trials can use a crossover design. In this design, patients receive both placebo and active drug separated by a break (washout period). Patients are blinded to treatment. This design is efficient in reducing the overall sample size requirements of a study (**Figure 5**). The evaluation of a new drug for patients with chronic diseases (such as rheumatoid arthritis) is ideally suited for a crossover trial design.

The disadvantage of randomization in surgical trials is that individual surgeons may not have equal experience or skill in performing the two treatments to be studied. This situation presents an ethical dilemma when two beneficial treatment options for a musculoskeletal condition exist.

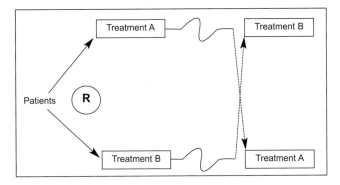

Figure 5   Crossover design for a randomized trial.

Table 2	Critical Appraisal Guide for Orthopaedic Randomized Trials

Guide for Study Validity (Methodology)

Step 1: Did experimental and control groups begin the study with a similar prognosis?
  Were patients randomized?
  Was randomization concealed?
  Were patients analyzed in the groups to which they were randomized?
  Were patients in the treatment and control groups similar with respect to the known prognostic factors?

Step 2: Did experimental and control groups retain a similar prognosis after the study started?
  Blinding?
  Did investigators avoid effects of patient awareness of allocation—were patients blinded?
  Were aspects of care that affect prognosis similar in the two groups—were clinicians blinded?
  Was outcome assessed in a uniform way in experimental and control groups—were those assessing outcome blinded?

Step 3: Was follow-up complete?

Results

Step 4: How large was the treatment effect?

Step 5: How precise was the estimate of the treatment effect?

Applicability

Step 6: Can the results be applied to my patient?

Step 7: Were all patient-important outcomes considered?

Step 8: Are the likely treatment benefits worth the potential harms and costs?

(Reproduced with permission from Bhandari M, Guyatt GH, Swiontkowski MF: User's guide to the orthopaedic literature: How to use an article about a surgical therapy. J Bone Joint Surg Am 2001;83-A:916-926.)

Although two surgical treatments may be beneficial, patients may not always have the same opportunity to receive the best care in both treatment arms. In addition, high-quality randomized trials are expensive to conduct and their results are often not available for several years until follow-up is complete. However, it is not only the trial's design that needs to be satisfactory but also the actual conduct of the trial as it affects each individual patient. Ultimately, it is up to the clinical investigators to ensure that patients do not suffer as a result of their clinical research. The power of randomization is that treatment and control groups are far more likely to be balanced with respect to both the known and the unknown determinants of outcome.

Most surgical interventions have inherent benefits and associated risks. Before implementing a new therapy, the benefits and risks of the therapy should be ascertained, and it should be confirmed that the resources consumed in the intervention will not be exorbitant. A three-step approach to using an article from the medical literature is suggested to guide patient care (Table 2). It is recommended that the physician ask whether the study can provide valid results (internal validity), review the results, and consider how the results can be applied to patient care (generalizability).

Observational Study

It is usually impossible or unethical to randomize patients to different prognostic factors. For example, if smoking is known to negatively affect fracture healing, it would clearly be difficult to randomize consecutive patients to smoking versus no smoking. The best study design to identify the presence of and determine the increased risk associated with a prognostic factor is a cohort study. The role of such nonrandomized (observational) studies in evaluating treatments is an area of continued debate. Deliberate choice of the treatment of each patient implies that observed outcomes may be caused by differences among people being given the two treatments, rather than the treatments alone. Table 3 provides a structured approach to appraising observational studies.

Unrecognized confounding factors can interfere with

attempts to correct for identified differences between groups. Nevertheless, physicians require studies of patient prognosis–examining the possible outcomes of a disease or surgical procedure, and the probability with which they can be expected to occur. To estimate patient prognosis, outcomes are examined in groups of patients with a similar clinical presentation; for example, patients who present with an ankle fracture. A patient's prognosis may then be refined by looking at subgroups, and deciding into which subgroup the patient falls. These subgroups may be defined by demographic variables such as age (younger patients may fare better than older ones), disease-specific variables (patient outcome may differ if the fracture was open or closed), or comorbid factors (those with underlying diabetes may fare badly). When these variables or factors really predict which patients do better or worse, they are called prognostic factors.

Authors often distinguish between prognostic factors and risk factors, those patient characteristics associated with the development of the disease in the first place. For example, low bone density is an important risk factor for the development of a hip fracture in an elderly patient, but is not as important a prognostic factor in determining

Table 3 | Critical Appraisal Guide for Orthopaedic Observational Studies (Prognosis)

I Guides for Validity (Study Methodology)

Step 1: Assess primary guides:
   Was there a representative sample of patients?
   Were the patients sufficiently homogeneous with respect to prognostic risk? If not, did investigators provide estimates for all clinically relevant subgroups?

Step 2: Assess secondary guides:
   Was follow-up sufficiently complete?
   Were objective and unbiased outcome criteria used?

II Understanding the Results (Study Results)

Step 3: Identify how likely are the outcomes over time

Step 4: Identify the precision of the estimates of likelihood

III Using the Results in Patient Care (Applying the Results to Your Patient)

Step 5: Ask yourself whether the study patients and their management are similar to your own

Step 6: Ask yourself whether the follow-up was sufficiently long

Step 7: Ask yourself if you can use the results in your patient management

(Reproduced with permission from Bhandari M, Guyatt GH, Montori V, Swiontkowski MF: User's guide to the orthopaedic literature: How to use an article about a diagnostic test. Bone Joint Surg Am 2003;85-A:1133-1140.)

survival after hip fracture. Issues in assessing the validity of studies of prognostic factors and risk factors, and using the results in patient care, are identical. Risk factors may also be considered as one particular kind of prognostic factor.

A cohort study can be conducted by following one or more groups (cohorts) of individuals who have not yet experienced an adverse event and monitoring the number of outcome events over time. Follow-up in this design is considered "active" in contrast to the 'passive' follow-up (with charts) in retrospective studies. An ideal cohort study consists of a well-defined sample of individuals who are representative of the population of interest, and uses objective outcome criteria. A potential cohort study may document the smoking status of all consecutive patients with a tibial shaft fracture and compare rates of nonunion (or time to fracture union).

Prospective Cohort Study (Level II Evidence; Grade B Recommendation)

Cohort studies may be prospective in that they begin at a specified point in time (time of onset of symptoms, or time of fracture) and move forward in time to evaluate the effect a potential prognostic factor (for example, surgical versus nonsurgical treatment) on specified outcomes at a predetermined length of follow-up. Such studies have the advantage of ensuring that all the relevant data are collected at the start of the study, but are often time-

consuming to conduct.

Case-Control Study (Level III Evidence; Grade B Recommendation)

To study prognostic factors, surgeons can use an alternative study design in which individuals who have already experienced the outcome event are compared with control patients who have not. In these case-control studies, surgeons can count the number of individuals with each prognostic factor in both groups (that is, were patients who had aseptic loosening of their hip replacement more likely to have decreased bone density than those who did not?). Case-control studies are limited by the retrospective nature of the data collection, often relying on the hospital chart or a patient's memory. Moreover, case-control studies do not provide information about the absolute risk of an adverse event, but only about the relative odds. Despite these limitations, case-control studies can be useful when the outcome of interest is very rare or duration of follow-up needed to detect the outcome of interest is long.

Retrospective Cohort Study (Level IV Evidence; Grade C Recommendation)

Studies may also be retrospective in that they begin at a specified point in time and move backward in time to collect data on potential risk factors for an undesirable outcome (for example, risk factors for fracture nonunion) or compare the results of two treatments. The obvious advantage of this approach is the efficiency in time required to collect the data. However, the major drawback to this approach is the investigator's inability to ensure the quality of the data collected because the investigator is often reliant on patient records for information. In most instances, the variability of reporting in patients' hospital charts may inhibit the collection of all relevant data.

Statistical Issues

Critical to the conduct or appraisal of clinical or experimental research is a fundamental understanding of statistics. This does not mean that all investigators or consumers of research findings need to be statisticians. It does, however, imply an appreciation for the principles of hypothesis testing, errors in hypothesis testing, basic summary statistics, sample size determination, and common statistical tests.

Hypothesis Testing

The essential paradigm for statistical inference in the medical literature has been that of hypothesis testing. The investigator starts with what is called a null hypothesis that the statistical test is designed to consider and possibly disprove. Typically, the null hypothesis is that there is no difference between treatments being compared. In a randomized trial in which investigators compare an experimental treatment with a placebo control, the null hypothesis can be stated as follows: the true difference in effect on the outcome of interest between the experimental and control treatments is zero. The assumption can be made that the treatments are equally effective, and this position is adhered to unless data make it untenable.

In this hypothesis-testing framework, the statistical analysis addresses the question of whether the observed data are consistent with the null hypothesis. The logic of the approach is as follows: even if the treatment truly has no positive or negative impact on the outcome (that is, the effect size is zero), the results observed will seldom show exact equivalence; that is, no difference will be observed between the experimental and control groups. As the results diverge farther and farther from the finding of "no difference," the null hypothesis that there is no difference between treatment effects becomes less and less credible. If the difference between results of the treatment and control groups becomes large enough, clinicians must abandon belief in the null hypothesis. The underlying logic of these principles will be further developed by describing the role of chance in clinical research.

In a hypothetical experiment, a coin is tossed 10 times and on all 10 occasions, the result is heads. How likely is this event to have occurred if the coin was indeed unbiased? Most people would conclude that it is highly unlikely that chance could explain this extreme result. The hypothesis that the coin is unbiased (the null hypothesis) could be rejected, and it could be concluded that the coin is biased. Statistical methods allow more precision by ascertaining just how unlikely the result is to have occurred simply as a result of chance if the null hypothesis is true. According to the law of multiplicative probabilities for independent events (where one event in no way influences the other), the probability of 10 consecutive heads can be found by multiplying the probability of a single head (1/2) 10 times over; that is, $1/2 \cdot 1/2 \cdot 1/2$, and so on. The probability of getting 10 consecutive heads is then slightly less than 1 in 1,000. In a journal article, this probability is expressed as a P value, such as $P < .001$.

P Value

What is the precise meaning of P value? Statistical convention calls results that fall beyond this boundary (that is, P value < 0.05) statistically significant. The setting of the P value threshold for significance is arbitrary but has been set to 0.05 by convention. The meaning of statistically significant, according to Guyatt and associates, therefore, is "sufficiently unlikely to be due to chance alone that we are ready to reject the null hypothesis." In other words, the P value is defined as the probability, under the assumption of no difference (null hypothesis), of obtaining a result equal to or more extreme than what was actually observed.

Errors in Hypothesis Testing

Any study that compares two or more treatments (such as a comparative study: randomized trial, observational study with control group, case-control) can be subject to errors in hypothesis testing. For example, when investigators conduct studies to determine whether two treatments have different outcomes, there are four potential outcomes (Table 4). These outcomes are: (1) a true positive result (the study correctly identifies a true difference between treatments); (2) a true negative result (the study correctly identifies no difference between treatment); (3) a false-negative result-type II (β) error (the study incorrectly concludes no difference between treatments when a difference really exists); and (4) a false-positive result-type I (α) error (the study incorrectly concludes a difference between treatments when no difference exists).

Type II Error (β Error)

It is perceived that trials of surgical therapies may be sufficiently undersized to have a meaningful impact on clinical practice. Such trials of small sample size are subject to type II errors: the probability of concluding that no difference between treatment groups exists, when, in fact, there is a difference (Table 4). Investigators will accept a type II error rate of 20% (β = 0.20), which corresponds with a study power of 80%. Most investigators agree that type II error rates greater than 20% (study power less than 80%) are subject to unacceptably high risks of false-negative results.

Type I Error (α Error)

Most are familiar with the concept of type II errors as the risk of concluding no difference between two treatments when a difference actually exists. Less appreciated by investigators is the risk of concluding that the results of a particular study are true, when, in fact, they are really caused by chance (or random sampling error). This erroneous false-positive conclusion is designated as a type I or α error (Table 4). By convention, most studies in orthopaedics adopt a type I error rate of 0.05. Thus, investigators can expect a false-positive error about 5% of the time.

A review of recently published randomized trials (within the past 2 years) was conducted to determine the risk of type I errors among surgical trials that did not explicitly state a primary outcome. A manual search of four orthopaedic journals, six general surgery journals, and five medical journals was done to identify recently published randomized trials. Information on outcomes and statistical adjustment for multiple outcomes was recorded for each study. The risk of a type I error was calculated for each study that did not explicitly state a primary outcome measure for the main statistical comparison. A total of 159 studies met the inclusion criteria for the study—60 from orthopaedic journals, 49 from nonorthopaedic surgical journals, and 50 from medical journals. In orthopaedic surgical journals, only 33.3% of the trials provided

Table 4 | Errors in Hypothesis Testing

		Truth	
		Difference	No Difference
Results of the Study	Difference	Correct conclusion $(1-\beta)$	False positive (α error or type I error)
	No Difference	False negative (β error or type II error)	Correct conclusion $(1-\alpha)$

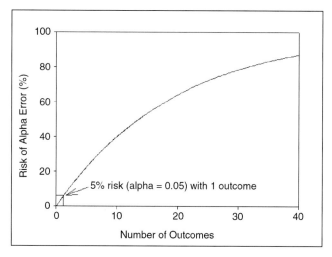

Figure 6   Graph showing multiple outcomes and α error risk.

an explicit statement of the primary outcomes, whereas 44.8% of the nonorthopaedic surgical journals and 56.0% of the randomized trials in the medical journals provided an explicit statement of the primary outcomes. Of those trials that did not state a primary outcome measure, the risk of type I errors (false-positive results) in orthopaedic and nonorthopaedic surgery journals (mean: 37.3 % ± 13.3% and 37.6 % ± 10.5%, respectively) were significantly greater than medical journals (10.1 % ± 1.9%) ($P < 0.05$). It was concluded that the reporting of primary outcomes in trials was inadequate; 1 in 3 trials in surgery and 1 in 10 trials in medicine risked false-positive results. Few trials in surgery and medicine consider adjustment for multiple comparisons.

Most readers are intuitively skeptical when 1 in a list of 20 outcomes measured by an investigator is significant ($P < 0.05$) between two treatment groups. This situation typically occurs when investigators are not sure what they are looking for and therefore test several hypotheses hoping that one may be true. Statistical aspects of the multiple testing issue are straightforward. If the number (n) of independent associations are examined for statistical significance, the probability that at least one of them will be found statistically significant is $1-(1-\alpha)^n$ if all n of the individual null hypotheses are true (**Figure 6**). Therefore, it can be argued that studies that generate a large number of measures of association have markedly greater probability of generating some false-positive results because of random error than does the stated α level for individual comparisons. For example, with $\alpha = 0.05$ and n = 20, the probability of at least one statistically significant finding by random chance is 64% (assuming that all the null hypotheses are true). If an investigator chooses to examine 50 separate associations, the probability of at least one statistically significant result is 92%. In the review of randomized trials, the number of tests of association ranged from 2 to 35. Therefore, these studies risked a false-positive finding from 9.8% to 83% of the time.

Various procedures (Bonferroni correction) require the establishment of a smaller critical P value for rejecting the null hypothesis on each individual test in light of the multiple tests to preserve the α level for the entire study. This approach is simple and practical but can lead to some

potentially unsatisfactory situations. For instance, if an investigator plans to conduct 10 tests of significance on 10 different outcome measures and report significance at the $P < 0.05$ level, the effective P value is not 0.05 but rather can be approximated by a rule of thumb (10 outcomes × 0.05 = 0.5). Using this rule of thumb, there is a 50% chance of having a false-positive result among the 10 outcome measures. To limit such incorrect conclusions (α errors), the α level of significance can be adjusted from 0.05 to 0.005. Therefore, only those P values that fall less than 0.005 are considered statistically significant in this model.

Descriptive Statistics
Measures of Central Tendency and Spread
Investigators will often provide a general summary of data from a clinical or experimental study. Several measures can be used. These include measures of central tendency (mean, median, and mode) and measures of spread (standard deviation, range, percentiles). The sample mean is equal to the sum of the measurements divided by the number of observations. The median of a set of measurements is the number that falls in the middle. The mode, however, is the most frequently occurring number in a set of measurements. Continuous variables (such as blood pressure or body weight) can be summarized with a mean if the data are normally distributed. If the data are not normally distributed, then the median may be a better summary statistic. Categorical variables (pain grade: 0 through 5) can be summarized with a median.

Along with measures of central tendency, investigators will often include a measure of spread. The standard deviation is derived from the square root of the sample variance. The variance is calculated as the average of the squares of the deviations of the measurements about their mean. The range of a dataset reflects the smallest value and largest value.

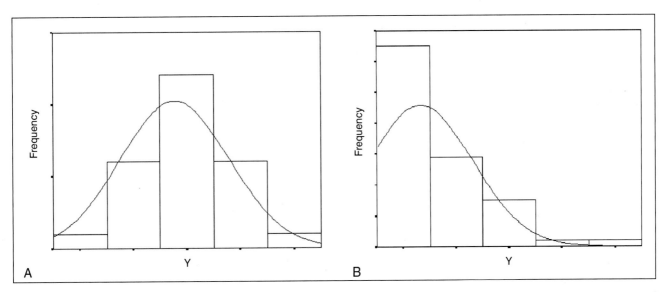

Figure 7   **A,** Normal probability distribution. The horizontal axis depicts the variable Y and the vertical axis is the frequency of observations. The peak of the normality probability curve corresponds to the mean of the distribution. **B,** Skewed distribution.

Normal Distribution

A large number of continuous variables possess a frequency distribution with many values near the mean and progressively fewer values toward the extremes. If the number of observations is large, the curve that is formed is bell-shaped and approximates the normal distribution (**Figure 7, A**). Several statistical tests assume a normal distribution (Student's *t* test). Prior to conducting a statistical test, a simple histogram plot of the data can provide insight into the distribution of the sample. A skewed sample is one in which the mean is not in the center of the distribution (**Figure 7, B**). Statistical tests that can assist in assessing for normality include the Kolmogorov-Smirnov test and the Shapiro-Wilk (W) statistic. If a sample is not normally distributed, a separate set of statistical tests should be applied. These tests are referred to as nonparametric tests because they do not rely on parameters such as the mean and standard deviation. An alternative approach is to transform a nonnormal distribution to a normal distribution by a transformation. For instance, data can be log-transformed to reduce skewness. Interpretation of results can be difficult after such transformations.

Measures of Treatment Effect (Dichotomous Variables)

Information comparing the outcomes (dichotomous—mortality, reoperation) of two procedures can be presented to patients as an odds ratio, a relative risk, a relative risk reduction, an absolute risk reduction, and the number needed to treat (**Table 5**). Both reduction in relative risk and reduction in absolute risk have been reported to have the strongest influences on patient decision-making in nonsurgical therapies.

Table 5	Presentation of Results		
	Infection	**No Infection**
Treatment Group	10 A	90 B
Control Group	50 C	50 D

Treatment event rate (TER): A/A + B = 10/100 = 10%
The incidence of infection in the treatment group

Control event rate (CER): C/C + D = 50/100 = 50%
The incidence of infection in the control group

Relative risk (RR): TER/CER = 10/50 = 0.2
The relative risk of infection in the treatment group relative to the control group

Relative risk reduction (RRR): 1- RR = 1-0.2 = 0.8 or 80%
Treatment reduces the risk of infection by 80% compared with controls

Absolute risk reduction (ARR): CER-TER = 50%-10% = 40%
The actual numerical difference in infection rates between treatment and controls

Number needed to treat (NNT): 1/ARR = 1/0.40 = 2.5
For every 2.5 patients who received the treatment, 1 infection can be prevented.

Odds ratio (OR): AD/BC = (10)(50)/(90)(50) = 500/4500 = 0.11
The odds of infection in treatment compared with controls is 0.11

95% Confidence Interval

Investigators usually (though arbitrarily) use the 95% CI. The 95% CI can be considered as defining the range that includes the true difference 95% of the time. In other words, if the investigators repeated their study 100 times, it would be expected that the point estimate of their result would lie within the CI 95 of those 100 times. The true

Table 6	Common Statistical Tests*			
Data Type and Distribution Samples		Categorical	Ordered Categorical or Continuous and Nonnormal	Continuous and Normal
Two samples	Different individuals	χ^2 test Fisher's exact test	Mann-Whitney U test Wilcoxon rank sum test	Unpaired t test
	Related or matched samples	McNemar's test	Wilcoxon signed rank test	Paired t test
Three or more samples	Different individuals	χ^2 test Fisher's exact test	Kruskal-Wallis statistic	ANOVA
	Related samples	Cochran Q-test	Friedman statistic	Repeated measures ANOVA

*Consult a statistician when planning an analysis or planning a study. ANOVA = analysis of variance, χ^2 = chi-square
(Adapted with permission from Griffin D, Audige L: Common statistical methods in orthopaedic clinical studies. Clin Orthop Rel Res 2003;413:70-79.)

point estimate will lie beyond these extremes only 5% of the time, a property of the CI that relates closely to the conventional level of statistical significance of $P < 0.05$. The 95% CI is preferred over P values for determining the significance of a finding because P values tell us nothing about the magnitude or direction of a treatment effect.

Statistical Analysis

Common statistical tests include those that examine differences between two or more means, differences between proportions, and associations between two or more variables (Table 6).

Comparing Two Independent Means

When testing the null hypothesis that the means of two independent samples of normally distributed continuous data are the same, the appropriate test statistic is called t, hence the t test. The author of the original article describing the distribution of the t-statistic used the pseudonym Student, leading to the common attribution Student's t test. When the data are nonnormally distributed, a nonparametric test such as the Mann-Whitney U or Wilcoxon rank sum test can be used. If the means are paired, such as left and right knees, a paired Student's t test is most appropriate. The nonparametric correlate of this test is the Wilcoxon signed rank test.

Comparing Multiple Independent Means

When three or more different means have to be compared (for example, hospital stay among three tibial fracture treatment groups—plate fixation, intramedullary nail, and external fixation), single factor analysis of variance is a test of choice. If the test yields statistical significance, investigators can conduct post hoc comparison tests (usually a series of pairwise comparisons using Student's t tests) to determine where the differences lie. It should be recalled that the P value (α level) should be adjusted for multiple post hoc tests. One rather conservative method is the Bonferroni correction factor that simply divides the α level ($P = 0.05$) by the number of tests performed.

Comparing Two Proportions

A common situation in the orthopaedic literature is that two proportions are compared. For example, these may be the proportion of patients in each of two treatment groups who experience an infection. The chi-square (χ^2) test is a simple method of determining whether the proportions are really different. When samples are small the χ^2 test becomes approximate because the data are discrete, but the χ^2 distribution from which the P value is calculated is continuous. A Yates correction is a device that is sometimes used to account for this, but when cell counts in the contingency table become very low (say, less than five) the χ^2 test becomes unreliable and a Fisher's exact test is the test of choice.

Determining Association Between One or More Variables Against One Continuous Variable

When two variables are associated, it may be logical to try to use one variable to predict the other. The variable to be predicted is called the dependent variable, and that to be used for prediction the independent variable. For such a linear relationship, the equation $y = a + bx$ is defined as the regression equation (a is a constant and b the regression coefficient). Fitting the regression equation, generally using a software package, is the process of calculating values for a and b which allow the regression line represented by this equation to best fit the observed data. The P value reflects the result of a hypothesis test that x and y are in fact unrelated, or in this instance that b is equal to zero.

Correlation

The strength of the relationship between two variables (such as age versus hospital stay in patients with ankle fractures) can be summarized in a single number, the correlation coefficient. The correlation coefficient, which is denoted by the letter r, can range from −1.0 (representing the strongest possible negative relationship, in which the person who scores the highest on one variable scores the lowest on the other variable) to 1.0 (representing the strongest possible positive relationship, in which the person who is older also has the longest hospital stay). A correlation coefficient of zero denotes no relationship between the two variables.

The Research Proposal
The design of a study in orthopaedics needs to incorporate all of the concepts already presented. The validity of a clinical study can be ensured with a careful research protocol before it begins.

Step 1: Formulating the Question
The question formulation typically includes a description of the population, intervention, and outcomes. The question will also determine the most appropriate study design. For example, the following question may be posed: What is the effect of internal fixation versus arthroplasty (intervention) on revision surgery rates (outcome) in patients older than 65 years with displaced femoral neck fractures (population)? This question may best be answered with a randomized trial.

Step 2: Conducting a Systematic Review of the Literature
Prior to committing large amounts of time, personnel, and funding to a project, investigators must ensure that their proposed study is novel and advances the current understanding of a problem. A careful and systematic review of the available literature can inform investigators about the current evidence to date. A well-conducted meta-analysis is invaluable because it is unusual for single studies to provide definitive answers to clinical questions. Moreover, a well-conducted quantitative review may resolve discrepancies between studies with conflicting results. Guiding principles in the conduct of meta-analyses include a specific health care question, a comprehensive search strategy, the assessment of the reproducibility of study selection, the assessment of study validity, evaluation of heterogeneity (differences in effect across studies), and inclusion of all relevant and clinically useful measures of treatment effect.

Step 3: Deciding on the Study Design
As stated, the question informs the study design. If an investigator wishes to compare the results of two or more treatment strategies, a randomized controlled trial is the best option; however, if the goal is to identify predictors of mortality in patients treated for hip fractures, a case-control study may be designed to compare prognostic variables in patients who died compared with those who lived. If an investigator plans to compare outcomes following surgical versus conservative treatment of spinal fractures, a prospective cohort may be best. Randomizing patients in this circumstance may be deemed unethical.

Step 4: Eligibility Criteria
Investigators should be explicit about the criteria for including patients in their study. A large and comprehensive list of eligibility criteria will limit the generalizability (external validity) of the study results beyond the specific group of included patients. Thus, one strategy to improve the external validity of a randomized trial is to be inclusive in enrolling a diverse group of patients. Alternatively, in a cohort study where the risk of imbalances between patient groups is high, having a comprehensive list of criteria (inclusion and exclusion) may improve the degree to which patient groups are similar. Pilot studies of eligibility can be helpful in determining patient enrollment rates in a particular center or setting.

Step 5: Identification of Subjects
Strategies to identify and enroll patients into a study need to be defined before the start of a study. Considerations may include whether to enroll patients from a single center (academic versus community), multiple centers, and single city, state, or country versus multiple cities, states, and countries. The decision may also include whether to enroll an entire population or a sample of a population. In most instances, investigators will include either a random sample, a systematic random sample (taking every x^{th} patient from a list) or a convenience sample (those who present to the fracture clinic) of a population.

Step 6: Defining the Intervention
The details of the intervention need to be clarified before the study begins. In surgical interventions, surgeons may require additional training or education in a surgical technique they infrequently perform. Protocols for patient management should be reviewed by all investigators and standardized to limit cointervention biases (that is, differential applications of additional interventions that may influence patient outcomes).

Step 7: Choosing the Primary/Secondary Outcomes
The choice of the outcome measure has important implications on the required sample size. Continuous outcome measures (hospital stay, blood loss, functional scores) have been found to require smaller samples of patients to achieve adequate study power than dichotomous outcome variables (mortality, infection rates, reoperation rates). Study power was reviewed in published studies with 50 patients or less to examine the effect of outcome variable. There were 76 trials with a sample size of 50 patients or less (29 trials, continuous outcomes; 47 trials, dichotomous outcomes). Studies that reported continuous outcomes had significantly higher mean power than those that reported dichotomous variables (power = 49% versus 38%, $P = 0.042$). Twice as many trials with continuous outcome variables reached acceptable levels of study

power (for example, > 80% power) when compared to trials with dichotomous variables (37% versus 18.6%, $P = 0.04$).

Step 8: Avoiding Type II Errors: Sufficient Sample Size and Study Power

The power of a study is the probability of concluding a difference between two treatments when one actually exists. Power $(1-\beta)$ is simply the complement of the type II error (β). Thus, if a 20% chance of an incorrect study conclusion is accepted $(\beta = 0.20)$, it must also be accepted that the correct conclusion will be drawn 80% of the time. Study power should be used before the start of a clinical trial to assist with sample size determination.

The power of a statistical test is typically a function of the magnitude of the treatment effect, the designated type I error rate (α), and the sample size (N). When designing a trial, investigators can decide on the desired study power $(1-\beta)$ and calculate the necessary sample to achieve this goal. If investigators are conducting a post hoc power analysis after the completion of the study, they will use the actual sample size obtained to calculate the study's power.

The magnitude of the effect is, for example, the difference between the mean functional score of the surgically treated group and that of the nonsurgically treated group. To compensate for the variability of the functional scores in each group (variance or standard deviations about the mean scores), the difference can be divided by the standard deviation of the control group. This resultant value is termed the 'effect size.' Interpretation of the 'effect size' is largely a clinical one. It should represent the point at which a change in practice will be made if the results are true. Cohen has reported broad guidelines to the interpretation of effect sizes, with 0.2 a small effect, 0.5 a moderate effect, and 0.8, a large effect.

Sample size plays an important role in power analyses. The smaller the difference an investigator wishes to detect the larger the sample size needed for the study. Extreme examples of large sample sizes for relatively small treatment effects are evident from trials of cardiovascular disease. The recent trial of angiotensin-converting enzyme-inhibitor therapy in patients at high risk for cardiovascular events recruited 9,297 patients to identify a 0.5% difference $(P = 0.02)$ in myocardial infarction between treatment and placebo groups.

Given the prevalence of type II errors in orthopaedic trauma trials, future investigators should endeavor to pre-plan estimated sample size requirements based on conventionally accepted standards for study power (80%) and type I errors $(\alpha = 0.05)$. Small pilot studies on a topic of interest or previously reported literature can be helpful in determining the likely treatment effect.

For example, in planning a trial of alternate strategies for the treatment of tibial shaft fractures, an investigator may identify a systematic review of the literature that reports time to fracture healing with treatment A is 120 ± 45 days, whereas time to healing with treatment B (control group) can be expected to be up to 140 ± 40 days. The expected treatment difference is 20 days and the effect size is 0.5 (20/40). According to Cohen's study, this is a moderate effect and is likely clinically significant if it is indeed true. The anticipated sample size for this continuous outcome measure is determined by the following equation:

$$N = 2 \left\{ \frac{(Z\alpha + Z\beta)\sigma}{\delta} \right\}^2$$

where $Z\alpha = 1.96$, $Z\beta = 0.84$, $\sigma = 40$, and $\delta = 20$

This study will require approximately 63 patients to have sufficient power to identify a difference of 20 days between treatments, if it occurs. An investigator may then audit the number of patients treated at their center during the prior year to determine if enough patients will present to the center to meet the sample size requirements.

The assumption can be made that this same investigator chooses nonunion as the primary outcome instead of time to union. Based on the previous literature, the investigator believes that treatment A will result in an 95% union rate and treatment B (control group) will result in an 90% union rate. A different sample size calculation for dichotomous variables is presented below:

$$N = \frac{PA (100-PA) + PB(100-PB) \times f(\alpha,\beta)}{(PB-PA)^2}$$

where PA = 95, PB = 90, and $f(\alpha,\beta) = 7.9$

Now, 869 patients are required for the study to identify a 5% difference in nonunion rates between treatments. An investigator may realize that this number is sufficiently large to prohibit conducting this trial at one center, and may elect to gain support at multiple sites for this trial.

Step 9: Planning the Analysis

As discussed, the research question, study design, and proposed outcome measures will define the analysis procedures (see Statistical Analysis section).

Step 10: Ensuring Completeness of Follow-up

Incomplete follow-up can seriously threaten the validity of a clinical study. When patients are lost to follow-up, how serious is the threat to validity? So-called rules of thumb (thresholds such as 20%) are misleading. Consider a hypothetical randomized trial that enters 1,000 patients into both treatment and control groups of whom 200 (20%) are lost to follow-up (100 in the treatment group and 100 in the control group). Treated patients have adverse outcomes at half the rate of the control group (200 versus 400), a reduction in relative risk of 50%. To what extent does losing patients to follow-up potentially threaten the inference that treatment reduces the complication rate in half? If the worst assumption is made, that all treated patients lost to follow-up had the worst outcome, the number of adverse outcomes in the treatment group would be 300 (30%). If there were no adverse outcomes among the control patients who were lost to follow-up, the best estimate of the effect of treatment in reducing the risk of complications drops from (1 − 200/400) or 50% to (1 − 300/400) or 25%. Thus, the worst assumption does change the estimate of the magnitude of the treatment effect. If assuming a worst-case scenario does not change the inferences arising from study results, then losing patients to follow-up is not a problem.

Step 11: Data Management
Investigators must plan in advance the strategies they will use to ensure the quality of data and the storage of data in preparation for analysis. Large studies often employ full-time database managers and research assistants to prepare and collect data forms, ensure that data forms are complete, and enter data into computerized databases for later analysis.

Step 12: Ethics and Confidentiality
Currently in North America, strict guidelines for the ethical conduct of clinical and experimental research exist. Investigators must be familiar with local ethics and institutional review processes. Consent forms must be prepared in advance and approval for research must be obtained before the study begins. The Health Insurance Portability and Accountability Act (HIPAA) has encouraged the development of a health information system through the establishment of standards and requirements for the electronic transmission of certain health information. More information can be found at http://www.hhs.gov/ocr/hipaa/bkgrnd.html.

Step 13: Developing the Research Team
A successful research project is supported by a motivated, cooperative, and competent research team. The optimal team is greater than the sum of its parts. Each member should provide specific skills to ensure all competencies are maintained. Typically, a team for a large study should have clinical experts, biostatisticians, methodologists/epidemiologists, administrative personnel, and research coordinators/assistants. The principal investigator is key in the overall supervision and organization of a trial. In a multicenter trial, the principal investigator at each site is responsible for ensuring study compliance, patient recruitment, follow-up, and timely completion of data forms.

Step 14: Providing a Timeline
The conduct of a well-designed study requires a large time commitment. Often, in a large study, the planning phase will require almost as much time as the conduct phase. As a rule of thumb, it can be assumed that a study that will take 1 year to conduct will likely take 1 year to plan (literature search, protocol development and revision, obtaining funding).

Moving Toward Evidence-Based Orthopaedic Practice
Resources for the Practitioner
The practice of evidence-based medicine means integrating individual clinical expertise with the best available external clinical evidence from systematic research. The User's Guide to the Medical Literature that has appeared in the *Journal of the American Medical Association* and the recent installments of the User's Guide to the Orthopaedic Literature in the *Journal of Bone and Joint Surgery* provide clinicians with the tools to critically appraise the methodologic quality of individual studies and apply the evidence.

To provide clinicians with easy access to the best available evidence, several specialized sources include summaries of individual studies, systematic reviews, and evidence-based clinical guidelines. One such example is the *Cochrane Database*, which is an extensive database of systematic reviews on various topics in musculoskeletal disease. Additionally, the *Cochrane Database* contains a controlled clinical trial registry, which provides a comprehensive list of randomized clinical trials in orthopaedics and other subspecialty areas. The *Canadian Journal of Surgery*, *The Journal of Bone and Joint Surgery*, and the *Journal of Orthopaedic Trauma* all provide evidence summaries on a variety of topics.

Incorporating Patient Values in Decision-Making
Because there are always advantages and disadvantages to an intervention, evidence alone cannot determine the best course of action. Most would agree that the values and preferences that the clinician must use to balance risks and benefits should be those of the patient. Given the variability in patient values, the physician should proceed with great care; it is easy to assume that the patient's and physician's values are similar, yet this assumption may well be incorrect. The challenge, then, is to integrate the evidence with the patient's values. When benefits and risks are balanced more precariously and the best choice may differ across patients, clinicians must attend to the variability in patients' values. One fundamental strategy for integrating evidence with preferences involves communicating the benefits and risks to patients, thus permitting them to incorporate their own values and preferences in the decision.

Summary

The purpose of evidence-based medicine is to provide health care practitioners and decision makers (physicians, nurses, administrators, regulators) with tools that allow them to gather, access, interpret, and summarize the evidence required to make informed decisions and to explicitly integrate this evidence with the values of patients. In this sense, evidence-based medicine is not an end in itself, but rather a set of principles and tools that help clinicians distinguish ignorance of evidence from real scientific uncertainty, distinguish evidence from unsubstantiated opinions, and ultimately provide better patient care.

Selected Bibliography

What Is Evidence-Based Medicine?

Bhandari M, Guyatt GH, Montori V, Devereaux PJ, Swiontkowski MF: User's guide to the orthopaedic literature: How to use a systematic literature review. *J Bone Joint Surg Am* 2002;84:1672-1682.

Bhandari M, Guyatt GH, Montori V, Swiontkowski MF: User's guide to the orthopaedic literature: How to use an article about a diagnostic test. *J Bone Joint Surg Am* 2003;85-A:1133-1140.

Bhandari M, Guyatt GH, Swiontkowski MF: User's guide to the orthopaedic literature: How to use an article about a surgical therapy. *J Bone Joint Surg Am* 2001;83-A:916-927.

Bhandari M, Guyatt GH, Swiontkowski MF: User's guide to the orthopaedic literature: How to use an article about prognosis. *J Bone Joint Surg Am* 2001;83-A: 1555-1564.

Brighton B, Bhandari M, Tornetta P III, Felson DT: Hierarchy of evidence: From case reports to randomized controlled trials. *Clin Orthop Relat Res* 2003;413:19-24.

Epling J, Smucny J, Patil A, Tudiver F: Teaching evidence-based medicine skills through a residency-developed guideline. *Fam Med* 2002;34:646-648.

Guyatt GH: Evidence-based medicine. *ACP J Club* 1991;114:A16.

Haynes RB, Hayward RS, Lomas J: Bridges between health care research evidence and clinical practice. *J Am Med Inform Assoc* 1995;2:342-350.

Finding Evidence

Bhandari M, Guyatt GH, Siddiqui F, et al: Operative versus non-operative treatment of achilles tendon rupture: A systematic overview and meta-analysis. *Clin Orthop Relat Res* 2002;400:190-200.

Sackett DL, Richardson WS, Rosenberg WM, Haynes RB: *Evidence-Based Medicine: How to Practice and Teach EBM*. New York, NY, Churchill Livingstone, 1997.

Statistical Issues

Bhandari M, Lochner H, Tornetta P III: The effect of continuous versus dichotomous variables on statistical power in orthopaedic randomized trials with small sample sizes. *Arch Orthop Trauma Surg* 2002;122:96-98.

Bhandari M, Morrow F, Kulkarni A, Tornetta P III: Meta-analyses in orthopaedic surgery: A systematic review of their methodologies. *J Bone Joint Surg Am* 2001;83-A:15-24.

Bhandari M, Whang W, Kuo JC, Devereaux PJ, Sprague S, Tornetta P III: The risk of false positive results in orthopaedic surgical trials. *Clin Orthop Relat Res* 2003;413:63-69.

Cohen J: A power primer. *Psycological Bulletin* 1992; 112:155-159.

Concato J, Shah N, Horwitz RI: Randomized, controlled trials, observational studies, and the hierarchy of research designs. *N Engl J Med* 2000;342:1887-1892.

Dorrcy F, Swiontkowski MF: Statistical tests: What they tell us and what they don't. *Adv Ortho Surg* 1997; 21:81-85.

Freedman KB, Back S, Bernstein J: Sample size and statistical power of randomized, controlled trials in orthopaedics. *J Bone Joint Surg Br* 2001;83:397-402.

Guyatt GH, Jaeschke R, Heddle N, Cook DJ, Shannon H, Walter SD: Basic statistics for clinicians: Hypothesis testing. *Can Med Assoc J* 1995;152:27-32.

Guyatt GH, Jaeschke R, Heddle N, Cook DJ, Shannon H, Walter SD: Basic statistics for clinicians: Interpreting study results and confidence intervals. *Can Med Assoc J* 1995;152:169-173.

Lochner H, Bhandari M, Tornetta P: Type II error rates in randomized trials in orthopaedic trauma. *J Bone Joint Surg Am* 2001;83-A:1650-1655.

Moher D, Dulberg CS, Wells GA: Statistical power, sample size, and their reporting in randomized controlled trials. *JAMA* 1994;272:122-124.

Pocock SJ: *Clinical Trials: A Practical Approach*. Toronto, Ontario, John Wiley and Sons, 1983, pp 123-140.

Streiner DL: Sample size and power and psychiatric research. *Can J Psychiatry* 1990;35:616-620.

The Research Proposal
Sackett DL, Haynes RB, Guyatt GH, Tugwell P: *Clinical Epidemiology: A Basic Science for Clinical Medicine*. Boston, MA, Little Brown, 1991.

Moving Toward Evidence-Based Orthopaedic Practice
Guyatt GH, Rennie D (eds): *User's Guides to the Medical Literature: A Manual for Evidence-Based Clinical Practice*. Chicago, IL, American Medical Association Press, 2001.

Section 2

Physiology of Musculoskeletal Tissues

Chapter 6

Thromboembolism and Pulmonary Distress in the Setting of Orthopaedic Surgery

Augustine H. Conduah, MD
Jay R. Lieberman, MD

Introduction

Episodes of hypoxia and acute respiratory insufficiency often occur after orthopaedic trauma and specific orthopaedic procedures, including total hip and total knee arthroplasty. Furthermore, patients with major injury to the pelvis or long bones and those who have undergone a total knee or hip arthroplasty are particularly prone to thromboembolic complications and fat embolism syndrome (FES), which have potentially life-threatening complications. This chapter focuses on the pathophysiology, diagnosis, and treatment of thromboembolic disease and respiratory insufficiency syndromes related to conditions in the musculoskeletal system.

Thromboembolic Disease

Venous thromboembolism (VTE) is a significant cause of morbidity and mortality, especially among patients undergoing major orthopaedic surgery involving the pelvis, hip, or knee. VTE is a term that encompasses deep venous thrombosis (DVT) and pulmonary embolism (PE). The incidence of DVT and PE in a variety of clinical situations is outlined in Table 1. VTE is an important condition to diagnose and prevent because acute PE causes over 150,000 deaths per year in the United States. Furthermore, patients who undergo total joint arthroplasty are at the highest risk for the development of VTE. Without either mechanical or pharmacologic prophylaxis, asymptomatic DVT will develop in 40% to 60% of patients undergoing total hip and knee arthroplasty. Proximal DVT will develop in 15% to 25% and a fatal PE in 0.5% to 2% of these patients. Symptomatic and fatal PE is less common after total knee than total hip arthroplasty. Patients having hip fracture surgery are also at significant risk for development of VTE. Based on results of contrast venography, the rates of total and proximal DVT are approximately 60% and 27%, respectively, without prophylaxis, and the rate of fatal PE is reported to be approximately 3.5% within 3 months after hip fracture surgery. DVT is a common complication, especially in trauma patients. For example, for patients with pelvic trauma, the incidence of DVT is 20% to 60%. Factors generally acknowledged to pose a risk for VTE in surgical patients include advanced age, history of thromboembolic disease, immobility, smoking, obesity, hypercoagulable states, stroke, and cancer.

Within the hemostatic system a delicate, well-regulated balance exists between maintaining the blood in a fluid state and converting blood into an insoluble state. VTE is an important example of the pathologic consequences of unchecked thrombus formation. Thromboembolic disease that originates in the lower extremity has significant clinical sequelae, especially in the setting of major orthopaedic surgery.

Coagulation

The coagulation system is a complex enzyme cascade in which the components are activated by proteolysis, and the final product of the cascade is fibrin, which forms the basis of blood clots. Each reaction in the pathway results from the assembly of a complex composed of an activated coagulation factor, a proenzyme form of another coagulation factor, and a reaction accelerator (Figure 1). The blood coagulation cascade is divided into extrinsic and intrinsic pathways, converging downstream in a shared pathway. The extrinsic pathway is initiated when tissue damage, such as a fracture or soft-tissue injury, results in

Table 1 | Frequency of Fatal PE and DVT (Diagnosed by Venography)

Unprotected Patients	DVT	Fatal PE
Total hip arthroplasty	70%	0.5% to 2%
Total knee arthroplasty	80%	< 1%
Open meniscectomy	20%	?
Hip fracture	60%	3.5%
Spine trauma with paralysis	100%	1%
Multiple-trauma patients	35% to 58%	?
Pelvic fracture	20% to 60%	?

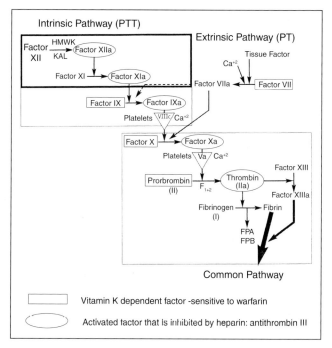

Figure 1   The coagulation pathway. Important features include the contact activation phase, vitamin K dependent factors (affected by warfarin), and the activated serine proteases that are inhibited by heparin-antithrombin III. Prothrombin measures the function of the extrinsic and common pathways; the partial thromboplastin time measures the function of the intrinsic and common pathways. PT = prothrombin time, PTT = partial thromboplastin time, HMWK = high molecular weight kallikrein, KAL = kallikrein, FPA = fibrinopeptide A, FPB = fibrinopeptide B. *(Adapted with permission from Stead RB: Regulation of hemostasis, in Goldhaber SZ (ed): Pulmonary Embolism and Deep Venous Thromboembolism. Philadelphia, PA, WB Saunders, 1985, p 32.)*

exposure of tissue factor to activated factor VIIa. This complex forms in the presence of calcium and phospholipids to catalyze the activation of factors IX and X. Factor Xa can also be generated through the intrinsic pathway by the contact of factor XII in the plasma with collagen fibrils exposed in damaged vessel walls. Both pathways lead to the formation of thrombin, which is the most important enzyme in the cascade. Thrombin is essential for normal hemostasis, directly promoting the conversion of fibrinogen to fibrin. Thrombin also activates circulating factor XIII, which in turn stabilizes fibrin. In addition, thrombin is a potent agonist of platelets through a protease-activated receptor-glycoprotein complex.

Once activated, the clotting cascade must be restricted to the local site of vascular injury to prevent clot propagation. The fibrinolytic system provides a balance to the coagulation system. It is composed of three groups of naturally occurring anticoagulants: antithrombins, proteins C and S, and the plasmin-plasminogen system. Activated by binding to heparin-like molecules, antithrombins inhibit the activity of thrombin. Proteins C and S are characterized by their ability to inactivate the cofactors Va and VIIIa. However, the most crucial element of the fibrinolytic system is the plasminogen-plasmin system, which directly breaks down fibrin and interferes with fibrin polymerization.

Pathogenesis of Venous Thromboembolism

Three primary influences predispose a patient to venous thrombosis formation, the so-called Virchow's triad: (1) endothelial injury, (2) venous stasis or turbulence of blood flow, and (3) hypercoagulability.

Endothelial injury is a dominant influence, and by itself can lead to thrombosis. It is particularly important in thrombus formation during hip surgery. For example, it has been documented that endothelial injury can occur secondary to kinking of the femoral vein during positioning and manipulation of the lower extremity. Investigators have demonstrated that this kinking can lead to both local trauma and adjacent, excessive venodilation that disrupts

the endothelium, exposing the subendothelium to potent platelet activators. Furthermore, direct damage to the endothelium can occur from thermal injury caused by bone cement. These events provide a nidus for formation and propagation of clots. Regardless of the cause of endothelial damage, the end results include exposure of subendothelial collagen, adherence of platelets, release of tissue factor, and local depletion of plasminogen activators.

Venous stasis may occur secondary to the positioning of the limb during hip surgery, localized postoperative swelling, and reduced mobilization of the patient after surgery. The use of a tourniquet during total knee arthroplasty promotes venous stasis. Stasis results from impeded venous flow and brings platelets into contact with the endothelium, prevents dilution of activated clotting factors by fresh-flowing blood, and retards the inflow of clotting factor inhibitors, permitting the buildup of thrombi. Tissue thromboplastin and other clotting factors also are released during the course of surgery, and they can aggregate in regions of venous stasis.

Hypercoagulability, the remaining component of the triad, is a poorly understood cause of venous thrombosis.

In the normal physiologic state, there is a delicate balance between the coagulation system and the fibrinolytic system. A hypercoagulable state results from an alteration of the coagulation pathways that predisposes a patient to thrombosis. Primary causes include genetic conditions such as factor V Leiden mutation, protein C and protein S deficiency, and antiphospholipid syndromes. Secondary causes of hypercoagulability include trauma and surgery. A relative hypercoagulable state can develop during any surgical procedure because blood loss can result in reduction in antithrombin III and inhibition of the endogenous fibrinolytic system, which further promotes thrombus generation. A total joint arthroplasty is a potent stimulus for thrombus formation. Measuring markers of thrombosis and fibrinolysis including fibrinopeptide A, prothrombin F1.2, and thrombin-antithrombin complexes during different phases of total hip arthroplasty demonstrates that the most pronounced thrombogenic stimulus occurs during preparation of the femoral canal and insertion of a cemented femoral component. It has been hypothesized that manipulation of the femoral canal leads to release of thromboplastin, which leads to the thrombogenic stimulus. Minimal activation of thrombosis occurs during femoral neck osteotomy and preparation of the acetabulum.

Platelets also play a critical role in thrombus generation. After trauma or vascular injury, there may be decreased blood flow, often at valve cusps or the soleal vein, and exposure of the subendothelium, which is associated with local platelet activation and aggregation. Activated platelets secrete nucleotides and expose surface complexes that further promote both platelet aggregation and the intrinsic coagulation pathway, leading to thrombin generation and subsequent fibrin deposition about the platelet plug.

Natural History of Thrombosis and Embolization

If a patient survives the immediate effects of a thrombotic vascular occlusion, the natural history is variable: (1) the thrombus may accumulate more platelets and fibrin, eventually obstructing a critical vessel; (2) the thrombus may dislodge and be transported to other sites in the vasculature; (3) the thrombus may be removed by fibrinolytic activity; or (4) the thrombus may induce inflammation and fibrosis (organization) and may eventually become recanalized. At approximately 1 week after thrombus formation there will be 10% vessel patency, and by 3 months there will be 50% to 70% patency.

Most DVTs that occur with lower extremity orthopaedic procedures usually form in the deep veins of the calf, often originating in the valve cusps. Leg scanning and venographic studies have shown that such thrombi often begin intraoperatively. Most of these thrombi are small and clinically insignificant. Less commonly, thrombi can occur de novo in the proximal veins of the thigh. This situation is noted more frequently in patients who undergo total hip arthroplasty. These thrombi may be nonocclusive and asymptomatic, and some of these thrombi will resolve without adverse effects. However, proximal thrombi are clearly more dangerous than those that occur more distally because they are more likely to result in symptomatic or fatal PE. Approximately 80% of symptomatic DVT involves the proximal veins

Thrombosis of the veins of the calf is generally an asymptomatic, self-limiting process that resolves spontaneously, usually within 72 hours. These thrombi are associated with a low risk of chronic venous insufficiency. However, approximately 15% of unsuppressed thrombi of the calf have the potential to propagate proximally, which leads to an increased risk of PE. In fact, 80% of symptomatic DVT involve the proximal veins.

Diagnosis of Thromboembolic Disease

The clinical signs of DVT include pain and tenderness in the calf or thigh, erythema, unilateral swelling, low-grade fever, tachycardia, and a positive Homans' sign. A positive Homans' sign is calf pain with forceful dorsiflexion of the ankle with the knee in a flexed position. Pain is elicited as the calf muscles compress the inflammatory tissue surrounding the DVT. However, Homans' sign has a very poor predictive value for the presence or absence of DVT, like any other symptom or clinical sign of this disease. Homans' sign, swelling, and erythema have sensitivities of 60% to 88% and specificities of 30% to 72% in well-designed studies for the diagnosis of DVT (using venography as the reference standard). However, in more than 50% of patients, the diagnosis is not apparent by physical examination. In addition, no laboratory test has been developed that can definitively diagnose DVT. However, there is interest in using D-dimer testing as an adjunct to noninvasive testing because it has a high negative predictive value. D-dimer is a degradation product of fibrin, and D-dimer levels can be elevated in the presence of acute DVT or PE, pregnancy, or malignancy. Some investigators believe the combination of a negative ultrasound and a negative D-dimer assay can safely rule out an acute DVT.

Screening studies appear to be the most effective method of determining the presence of DVT after total joint arthroplasty in symptomatic patients. The proper choice in screening options must be made based on the ability to detect proximal deep vein thrombi because they are the major source of pulmonary emboli. The various screening studies have differing rates of sensitivity, specificity, and accuracy. Furthermore, the validity of these studies can be operator dependent. Current modalities that can be considered as screening studies after total joint arthroplasty include contrast venography, venous ultrasonography, iodine 125-fibrinogen scanning, and impedance plethysmography.

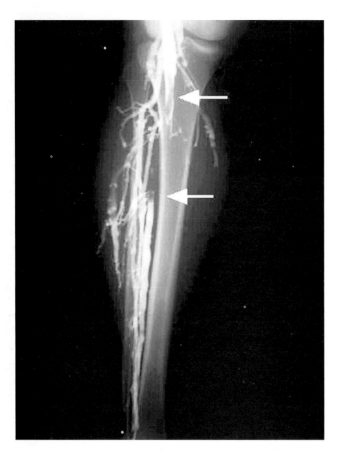

Figure 2   A venogram revealing a large thrombus in the popliteal region (*arrows*).

Iodine 125-fibrinogen scanning and impedance plethysmography have accurately identified the presence of DVT in symptomatic patients. However, in asymptomatic but high-risk total hip replacement patients, these methods have a combined sensitivity of only 23%; therefore, these tests are not used routinely.

Contrast venography remains the gold standard for identifying DVT (**Figure 2**). With contrast venography, thrombosis can be simultaneously identified in the venous system proximal and distal to the popliteal space. Although sensitive and reproducible, the contrast venogram is technically challenging to use and expensive. In addition, the venogram may be painful, is potentially thrombogenic, and is associated with hypersensitivity reactions.

Venous ultrasonography has become the most popular noninvasive screening modality for use in the detection of symptomatic DVT. It is painless and offers a two-dimensional cross-sectional representation of tissue and direct visualization of the thrombus. With venous ultrasonography, thrombi can be detected in the proximal veins of symptomatic patients, especially those having total joint arthroplasty. However, its use as a screening tool for asymptomatic patients has been questioned by some investigators. For example, in a randomized trial of 1,024 patients, venous ultrasonography was not effective as a

screening tool after total hip arthroplasty. Furthermore, the reliability of venous ultrasonography depends directly on the experience of the technician. In general, in institutions where ultrasound DVT surveillance is not performed routinely, this technique's sensitivity is inadequate for routine screening. Overall, it appears safer and more cost-effective to continue DVT prophylaxis after hospital discharge than to develop and maintain a screening program.

Pulmonary Embolism

PE is the major complication of DVT; it ranges from incidental, clinically unimportant thromboembolism to massive embolism with sudden death. Once a thromboembolus travels to the lungs, several events occur in concert. Initially, an embolus lodges in the pulmonary vasculature. Subsequent pulmonary arterial obstruction and the release by platelets of vasoactive agents such as serotonin elevate pulmonary vascular resistance. The resulting increase in alveolar dead space (ventilation of nonperfused lung) and redistribution of blood flow impair gas exchange and lead to hypoxemia. Hypoxemia and stimulation of irritant receptors cause alveolar hyperventilation, which leads to hypocapnia. Furthermore, reflex bronchoconstriction augments airway resistance, and lung edema decreases pulmonary compliance. Severe PE can cause right ventricular failure, shock, and pulmonary infarction.

Diagnosis

PE has a wide spectrum of clinical presentations, ranging from subtle clinical signs to hemodynamic instability resulting in death within 1 hour of acute onset. In most instances, PE goes undetected and is a silent killer identified only at autopsy. Dyspnea is the most frequent symptom of PE, and tachypnea is the most frequent sign. Whereas the presence of dyspnea, syncope, or cyanosis can indicate a massive PE, a finding of pleuritic pain, cough, or hemoptysis can often suggest a small embolism near the pleura. However, because of the lack of sensitivity and specificity associated with the aforementioned clinical findings, they cannot solely be relied on to confirm the presence of PE.

Evaluation of the arterial blood gas (ABG) for hypoxemia and the presence of an alveolar to arteriolar gradient consistent with intrapulmonary shunting is important in the initial workup of a suspected PE. A low Pao_2 is usually associated with respiratory dysfunction. However, a normal ABG does not definitely rule out a PE. Studies have shown that from 8% to 23% of patients with a normal alveolar to arteriolar gradient had an angiographically documented PE. Therefore, evaluation of ABG is not useful as a diagnostic tool for suspected PE but is usually helpful during treatment. Chest radiography and electrocardiography must also be incorporated into the diagnostic workup for PE. Abnormal findings on the chest film may include a peripheral wedge-shaped density above the diaphragm (the classic Hampton's hump), focal oligemia (Westermark's sign), and an enlarged right descending pulmonary artery (Palla's sign). Electrocardiogram findings often associated with an acute PE include acute right heart overload: right bundle branch block, right axis deviation, and, rarely, atrial fibrillation. The most frequent abnormal finding on electrocardiogram is T-wave inversion, especially leads V1 to V4. These findings are seen in only about 25% of patients following an acute PE.

The primary method of confirming the presence of PE is with imaging studies. The most useful and commonly used imaging modalities include ventilation-perfusion (V/Q) lung scanning, pulmonary angiography, and spiral CT. However, investigators have discovered that the predictive values of these tests rely heavily on the pretest probability of having a PE.

Pulmonary angiography is the gold standard diagnostic test for PE. This imaging modality allows direct visualization of acute obstructions or filling defects in pulmonary vessels. However, it is an invasive test and is associated with a 1% to 2% risk of major complications that include death, renal failure, cardiac arrhythmias, and adverse reactions to the contrast dye. Current recommendations state that pulmonary angiography is the reference standard but should be reserved for patients in whom noninvasive tests have proved inconclusive. A normal angiogram can safely be assumed to rule out suspected PE.

V/Q scanning has been the most frequently used imaging modality for establishing the diagnosis of acute PE. This test tracks the perfusion of a radioactive isotope throughout the pulmonary vasculature along with the dispersion of radioactive aerosols to the peripheral bronchial tree. A mismatch occurs when an area of the lung is being ventilated but not perfused and vice versa. In approximately 90% of patients, this scan detects mismatches of V/Q in the setting of PE. V/Q scanning is an appropriate initial study unless the patient has an abnormal chest radiograph.

In the Prospective Investigation of Pulmonary Embolism Diagnosis (PIOPED) study, almost all patients with PE had abnormal V/Q scans of high, intermediate, or low probability, but so did most patients without PE (sensitivity, 98%; specificity, 10%). Results of the PIOPED study revealed that there was a high percentage of indeterminate V/Q scans (73% of all studies performed). Indeterminate V/Q scans create a diagnostic dilemma, because 30% of all patients with such a result have an angiographically proven PE. Therefore, further investigations, either by pulmonary angiography, spiral CT, or Doppler ultrasound or contrast venography of the lower extremities, are currently recommended in such patients to establish a definitive diagnosis.

The combination of a high rate of indeterminate scans and a lack of intraobserver agreement inherent in V/Q scans makes contrast-enhanced spiral CT scanning an attractive option for the diagnosis of PE in certain patients.

Recent studies have advocated spiral CT as the next test for patients with an indeterminate V/Q scan or as an alternative to the V/Q scan. Spiral CT scans are minimally invasive, widely available, and offer the advantage of imaging any emboli directly within the pulmonary arteries. Pooled data indicate a sensitivity of approximately 70% and a specificity of 88%. A spiral CT scan appears to be more accurate in diagnosing central or lobar PE than segmental PE. Spiral CT is more sensitive and specific for the detection of PE than V/Q scanning. However, to date few studies have compared spiral CT scanning and pulmonary angiography; concerns exist that this technology will detect small emboli that are not clinically relevant.

Treatment

Once a diagnosis of PE has been made, immediate treatment is necessary. For years intravenous heparin had been the cornerstone of management in patients with PE, but low-molecular-weight heparins (LMWHs) have recently become available. Heparin accelerates the action of antithrombin III, thereby preventing formation of an additional thrombus and allowing dissolution of some of the clot via endogenous fibrinolysis. Heparin affects the intrinsic pathway of the coagulation cascade, which is monitored by the partial thromboplastin time. A bolus of unfractionated heparin followed by a continuous infusion usually results in a therapeutic partial thromboplastin time of 60 to 80 seconds. However, to avoid bleeding, a bolus of heparin should not be administered in patients who have had major surgery less than 1 week before the diagnosis of the PE. LMWH is an effective alternative to heparin. Several studies have confirmed that LMWH is as effective and safe as unfractionated heparin in the acute treatment of PE. The major advantages of this therapy are that no monitoring is required, and if the patient is stable from a respiratory standpoint, outpatient treatment can be instituted.

Heparin or LMWH therapy (usually 5 to 10 days) should be bridged by treatment with oral warfarin. In general, the International Normalized Ratio (INR) value should be at 2.0 for 2 days before heparin therapy is discontinued. Warfarin affects the extrinsic pathway, and its dosing is determined by measuring the prothrombin time. However, the anticoagulant effect associated with a particular prothrombin time has varied considerably among different institutions, depending on the thromboplastin sensitivity. The INR represents the prothrombin time ratio that would have been obtained if the international reference thromboplastin had been used instead of the local thromboplastin sensitivity. The INR ratio is defined as the observed prothrombin time ratio raised to the power of the international sensitivity index of the specific thromboplastin used. A normal INR is 1.0. The target INR value for prophylaxis is 2.0 and the target value to treatment is 3.0, but this target level may be decreased if there are concerns about bleeding. The optimal duration of anticoagulation after PE remains uncertain. However, the most current guidelines state that 3 to 6 months of anticoagulant therapy is ideal for preventing recurrences of PE.

Fat Embolism Syndrome

FES, a serious manifestation of the phenomenon of the migration of fat emboli to the lungs, is a collection of respiratory, hematologic, neurologic, and cutaneous symptoms and signs associated with trauma and other serious surgical and medical conditions. The orthopaedic procedures most commonly associated with FES are intramedullary (IM) nailing of long-bone fractures and total hip and knee arthroplasty, all of which involve instrumentation of the medullary canal. Other orthopaedic procedures that have been associated with FES include femoral lengthening, closed femoral osteotomy, and spinal fusion. Nontraumatic conditions that have been associated with FES include diabetes mellitus, chronic pancreatitis, and fatty liver disease.

FES is defined as fat in the circulation associated with an identifiable clinical pattern of symptoms and signs. It includes the clinical triad of progressive respiratory insufficiency, deteriorating mental status, and skin petechiae. Reports in the literature show that FES usually develops within 48 hours after skeletal injury. Fat embolism, a clinical entity different from FES, is defined as fat in the circulation, most often occurring after major trauma or long-bone fractures, that can produce embolic phenomena with or without clinical sequelae. It is an almost inevitable consequence of long-bone fractures with an estimated incidence of 90%. However, fat embolism rarely causes clinically significant signs and symptoms.

The clinical prevalence of FES in patients who have fractures has been reported to range from 0.25% (11 of 4,530 patients) to 1.2% (92 of 7,701 patients), and it occurs in fewer than 1% of patients undergoing total hip or knee arthroplasty. The overall mortality rate of patients who develop classic FES is approximately 5% to 15%; however, morbidity from posttraumatic FES remains high. Although FES may occur at any age, it is most common in the second or third decade of life, when long-bone fractures are frequent.

Pathophysiology

The pathophysiology of FES is not fully understood, but excessive and uncontrolled activation of the coagulation, fibrinolytic, and inflammatory pathways and hemodynamic changes within the lung parenchyma have been implicated. Over the past 20 years, two main theories have emerged: the biochemical theory and the mechanical theory. It generally is agreed that the source of fat emboli as a result of trauma is the bone marrow of long bones at the site of injury. Pulmonary injury may occur after a long-bone fracture in association with intravasation of marrow fat into the systemic circulation. Furthermore, a multiple trauma activates a systemic inflammatory response that produces elevated levels of mediators such as fibrinogen, tissue thromboplastin, prostacyclins, cytokines, and elastase. These mediators play an important role in lung injury.

The biochemical theory of FES suggests that circulating free fatty acids directly affect pneumocytes. Once the neutral fat (derived from bone marrow) emboli are trapped in the lung microvasculature, the lung responds by secreting lipase that hydrolyzes the nontoxic neutral fat into chemically toxic free fatty acids. These free fatty acids trigger a severe inflammatory reaction that leads to complement-mediated leukocyte aggregation that releases chemotoxins from these cells. The chemotoxins cause endothelial and lung surfactant damage, alveolar architecture injury, and increased capillary permeability. These events often induce adult respiratory distress syndrome. Other humoral factors such as serotonin, catecholamines, and 5-hydroxytryptamine can cause further lung injury. When released, these factors trigger pulmonary vasospasm, bronchospasm, and vascular endothelial injury.

The mechanical theory suggests that fat droplets are physically forced into the venous system during trauma. These droplets from the violated medullary canal gain access to the vasculature via nearby torn veins and are then transported to the pulmonary vascular bed where they embolize in the lung capillaries. Initially, the effect of the fat emboli on the lung is mechanical, causing increased perfusion pressure, that if severe enough could lead to right heart failure secondary to pulmonary hypertension. This mechanical obstruction is worsened by the accumulation of activated platelets that adhere to the fat droplets causing a plug. Smaller fat droplets ranging from 7 to 10 μm in diameter may circulate through the pulmonary capillaries and into the systemic circulation, causing embolization in the brain, kidney, and other organs. The presence of fat alone does not produce FES and acute pulmonary injury, but it can lead to hypoxemia and impaired pulmonary gas exchange. Many autopsy studies have shown that there is little correlation between the presence and amount of intravascular fat and the severity of clinical manifestations, supporting the notion that FES is caused by more than just mechanical obstruction.

The increase in IM pressure in the long bones is the most decisive pathogenic factor for the development of FES. The normal marrow pressure in the femur is 30 to 50 mm Hg, and this pressure must be exceeded for marrow fat to enter the circulation. Reaming of the femoral canal and implantation of IM rods and hip and knee prostheses can generate peaks in IM pressure, ranging from 600 to 1,400 mm Hg, leading to release of fat droplets into the circulation. Sampling of blood from the femoral vein has localized the origin of these fat droplets to the involved extremity, and intraoperative transesophageal echocardiograms have demonstrated migration of emboli to the

Table 2 | Clinical Features of Fat Embolism

Major	1) Petechial rash
	2) Respiratory symptoms plus bilateral signs with positive radiographic changes
	3) Cerebral signs unrelated to head injury or any other condition
Minor	1) Tachycardia
	2) Pyrexia
	3) Retinal changes (fat or petechiae)
	4) Urinary changes (anuria, fat globules)
	5) Sudden drop in hemoglobin level
	6) Sudden thrombocytopenia
	7) High erythrocyte sedimentation rate
	8) Fat globules in the sputum

(Reproduced with permission from Gurd AR: Fat embolism: An aid to diagnosis. J Bone Joint Surg Br 1970;52:732-737.)

lungs during these procedures. IM devices are associated with higher pressures within the marrow cavity and more fat embolism than extramedullary fixation. Ultrasound monitoring reveals that most emboli develop during opening and manipulation of the IM cavity. Fat embolism can also be induced experimentally by reaming and pressurizing the IM space with polymethylmethacrylate cement.

Diagnosis

FES is a diagnosis of exclusion that depends on the clinician's index of suspicion. Patients who are most at risk for FES often have multiple fractures or placement of a long cemented prosthesis in the femoral canal. Laboratory, radiologic, electrocardiographic, and other findings are either too sensitive or not specific enough to be pathognomonic for FES, which may reflect the multisystem pathology of FES. Therefore, clinical findings are the cornerstone for the diagnosis of FES. Gurd described major and minor features for diagnosing FES (Table 2). The diagnosis of FES requires at least one major and four minor criteria. The classic pathologic triad for FES is respiratory insufficiency, neurologic derangement, and petechial rash. Pulmonary insufficiency is always present and is usually the first manifestation of the syndrome. Neurologic decompensation occurs in up to 86% of patients with FES; signs range from drowsiness and confusion to coma. A petechial rash is typical of FES and is present in up to 60% of patients, usually on the conjunctiva, oral mucous membranes, and skin folds of the neck and axillae. Factors that may contribute to the rash include stasis, loss of clotting factors and platelets, and endothelial damage from free fatty acids leading to rupture of thin-walled capillaries.

Laboratory findings in patients with FES include hypoxemia, thrombocytopenia, anemia, and hypocalcemia. The most useful diagnostic test is ABG analysis. The presence of fat emboli in the lung can lead to hypoxemia. Although Pao_2 may be normal on admission, development of FES causes Pao_2 to decrease to 50 mm Hg or less within 72 hours. Thrombocytopenia and unexplained anemia are common (37% and 67%, respectively) but rarely are they difficult to treat. Plasma free fatty acid levels rise after trauma, and this increase may result in hypocalcemia because of the affinity of free fatty acids for calcium. Many laboratory test findings have been considered characteristic of FES; however, these findings are nonspecific and occur in trauma patients both with and without FES. Examples of such findings include fat globules in the blood and urine and elevated serum lipase levels. Furthermore, findings on the chest radiograph usually are normal in patients with mild FES. In severe FES, when radiographic changes occur, the most common finding is a diffuse, bilateral infiltrate that can be interstitial or alveolar. When present, electrocardiographic findings reveal signs of right heart strain or failure.

The role of pulmonary catheterization and bronchoalveolar lavage has been investigated. Reports in the literature advocate their potential use for detecting FES. Pulmonary artery catheterization has been advocated for the diagnosis of fat embolism either by detecting a rise in mean pulmonary arterial blood pressure or by sampling pulmonary artery blood for fat. A handful of studies have shown this test to be useful when the cause of respiratory failure is equivocal. Bronchoscopy and bronchoalveolar lavage have been used to reveal the presence of lipids within alveolar macrophages. However, bronchoalveolar lavage seems to be unreliable in the actual detection of fat embolism because healthy control subjects have fat-containing alveolar macrophages in 5% to 95% of alveolar samples. Because these more invasive studies involve small numbers of patients, additional investigation is required to determine their usefulness.

Prevention and Treatment

Because the pathophysiologic pathway of FES is still obscure, it is clear that full attention should be given to preventive measures. In the orthopaedic literature, timing of fracture fixation and reamed versus unreamed IM nailing are key issues related to reducing the risk of developing FES. Inadequate or delayed fixation of long-bone and pelvic fractures is associated with a higher incidence of FES. Most of the comparative studies performed over the past 20 years have shown a reduction in the risk of FES after early definitive stabilization of fractures, both in patients with isolated fractures and in those with injury to multiple systems. Furthermore, immediate open reduction and internal fixation within 24 to 48 hours decreases the development of FES compared with conservative treatments such as traction or casting. There are several controversies regarding the type of fracture fixation, particularly the timing of surgical intervention and the use of IM devices in patients with a significant chest injury. Overall, the data suggest that early fracture fixation will reduce the prevalence of pulmonary complications. Surgical techniques may have a significant effect on the severity of fat embolization. Findings of clinical studies have both supported and rebutted the claim that there is an increase in FES and adult respiratory distress syndrome after IM nailing of femoral fractures in patients who have concomitant pulmonary injuries.

Concerns regarding the relationship between elevated IM pressure and FES may influence fracture fixation. Reaming increases the patient's risk of developing FES. Compared with IM fixation, plate fixation and external fixation result in less insult to the lungs; however, these types of fixation may not be optimal for management of a particular fracture. The surgeon must weigh the risks and benefits of each type of treatment.

Bone marrow intravasation is directly proportional to a rise in IM pressure. For example, after reaming, the pressure generated during nail insertion is greater than that produced by an unreamed nail, and the incidence of fat embolism has been shown to be lower when unreamed nails are used. However, it has not been established in clinical studies that unreamed nails are safer for patients with chest injuries. IM pressures can be reduced by using sharp-tipped rather than blunt reamers, and hollow nails produce far lower pressures than solid ones. Repeatedly pushing and pulling the reamer may also result in high pressure peaks.

Treatment of FES often is supportive. Of paramount importance is early resuscitation and stabilization of patients to minimize the stress response and hypovolemia. The most common manifestation of FES is pulmonary dysfunction and, for this reason, any patient who is at risk should be monitored closely with continuous pulse oximetry or ABG analysis. At the first sign of respiratory compromise, oxygen should be administered. For patients with severe pulmonary dysfunction, such as adult respiratory distress syndrome, mechanical ventilation is urgently required. A review of the literature reveals that from 10% to 44% of these patients require mechanical ventilation. However, pulmonary dysfunction caused by FES usually resolves in 3 to 5 days. Furthermore, because hypovolemia is considered to be a cornerstone in the development of FES, prevention of circulatory instability with intravenous fluid administration is also critical.

Because the specific pathophysiology of FES has not been confirmed, the administration of medication and/or special types of infusion fluid has been controversial. Heparin, for example, is known to clear fat globules in the serum by stimulating lipase activity. However, the use of heparin has been rejected by various investigators because of the potential for increased free fatty acids in the circulation. In addition, there is a risk of bleeding in patients with multiple injuries. Corticosteroids have been studied in prospective randomized trials, and these agents clearly limit the development of FES and pulmonary distress. Possible beneficial effects include stabilizing the pulmonary capillary membrane, blunting inflammatory responses caused by free fatty acids in the lung, stabilizing complement system activation, and retarding platelet aggregation. However, corticosteroids have the disadvantage of increasing the risk of septic complications in multiply injured patients and, in some instances, contributing to the development of fat emboli.

Unraveling the basic molecular and cellular pathogenic processes of FES will lead to improved therapeutic strategies for the treatment of this condition. A review of the current literature indicates that early and appropriate treatment of fractures in most instances protects against the development of posttraumatic respiratory insufficiency. Currently, the best and most effective therapeutic tool for the practicing orthopaedic surgeon is prevention.

Selected Bibliography
Thromboembolic Disease

Geerts WH, Pineo GF, Heit JA, et al: Prevention of venous thromboembolism. *Chest* 2004;126:338S-400S.

Goldhaber SZ: Venous thrombosis: Prevention, treatment, and relationship to paradoxical embolus. *Cardiol Clin* 1994;12:505-516.

Kearon C: Duration of venous thromboembolism prophylaxis after surgery. *Chest* 2003;124:386S-392S.

Lieberman JR, Hsu WK: Prevention of venous thromboembolism after total hip and knee arthroplasty. *J Bone Joint Surg Am* 2005;87:2097-2112.

Mitchell RN: Hemodynamic disorders, thrombosis, and shock, in Kumar V, Cotran RS, Robbins SL (eds): *Basic Pathology*, ed 6. Philadelphia, PA, WB Saunders, 1997, pp 60-80.

Montgomery KD, Geerts WH, Potter HG, Helfet DL: Thromboembolic complications in patients with pelvic trauma. *Clin Orthop Relat Res* 1996;329:68-87.

Robinson KS, Anderson DR, Gross M, et al: Accuracy of screening compression ultrasonography and clinical examination for the diagnosis of deep vein thrombosis after total hip or knee arthroplasty. *Can J Surg* 1998; 41:368-373.

Sharrock NE, Go G, Harpel PC, Ranawat CS, Sculco TP, Salvati EA: Thrombogenesis during total hip arthroplasty. *Clin Orthop Relat Res* 1995;319:16-27.

White RH, Henderson MC: Risk factors for venous thromboembolism after total hip and knee replacement surgery. *Curr Opin Pulm Med* 2002;8:365-371.

Deep Venous Thrombosis and Pulmonary Embolism

Gefter WB, Hatabu H, Holland GA, Gupta KB, Henschke CI, Palevsky HI: Pulmonary thromboembolism: Recent developments in diagnosis with CT and MR imaging. *Radiology* 1995;197:561-574.

Goldhaber SZ: Pulmonary embolism. *N Engl J Med* 1998;339:93-104.

Kakkar VV, Howe CT, Flanc C, Clarke MB: Natural history of postoperative deep-vein thrombosis. *Lancet* 1969;2:230-232.

Kearon C: Natural history of venous thromboembolism. *Circulation* 2003;107:I22-30.

Merli GJ: Pulmonary embolism in medical patients: Improved diagnosis and the role of low-molecular-weight heparin in prevention and treatment. *J Thromb Thrombolysis* 2004;18:117-125.

Paiement GD, Desautels C: Deep vein thrombosis: Prophylaxis, diagnosis, and treatment: Lessons from orthopedic studies. *Clin Cardiol* 1990;13:VI19-VI22.

Rahimtoola A, Bergin JD: Acute pulmonary embolism: An update on diagnosis and management. *Curr Probl Cardiol* 2005;30:61-114.

Rosenthal I, Herba MK, Leclerc JR: Diagnosis of pulmonary embolism, in Leclerc JR (ed): *Venous Thromboembolic Disorders*. Philadelphia, PA, Lea Febiger, 1991, pp 229-266.

The PIOPED Investigators: Value of the ventilation/perfusion scan in acute pulmonary embolism: Results of the prospective investigation of pulmonary embolism diagnosis. *JAMA* 1990;263:2753-2759.

The Task Force on Pulmonary Embolism: Guidelines on the diagnosis and management of acute pulmonary embolism. *Eur Heart J* 2000;21:1301-1336.

Fat Embolism Syndrome

Bulger EM, Smith DG, Maier RV, Jurkovich GJ: Fat embolism syndrome: A 10-year review. *Arch Surg* 1997;132:435-439.

Chan KM, Tham KT, Chiu HS, Chow YN, Leung PC: Post-traumatic fat embolism: Its clinical and subclinical presentations. *J Trauma* 1984;24:45-49.

Fabian T: Unraveling the fat embolism syndrome. *N Engl J Med* 1993;329:961-963.

Gurd AR: Fat embolism: An aid to diagnosis. *J Bone Joint Surg Br* 1970;52:732-737.

Hofmann S, Huemer G, Salzer M: Pathophysiology and management of fat embolism syndrome. *Anaesthesia* 1998;53(suppl 2):35-37.

Johnson MJ, Lucas GL: Fat embolism syndrome. *Orthopedics* 1996;19:41-49.

Levy D: The fat embolism syndrome. *Clin Orthop Relat Res* 1990;261:281-286.

Robinson CM: Current concepts of respiratory insufficiency syndromes after fracture. *J Bone Joint Surg Br* 2001;83:781-791.

Schemitsch EH, Jain R, Turchin DC, et al: Pulmonary effects of fixation of a fracture with a plate compared with intramedullary nailing: A canine model of fat embolism and fracture fixation. *J Bone Joint Surg Am* 1997;79:984-996.

Talucci RC, Manning J, Lampard S, Bach A, Carrico CJ: Early intramedullary nailing of femoral shaft fractures: A cause of fat embolism syndrome. *Am J Surg* 1983;146:107-111.

Chapter 7

Growth and Development of the Skeleton

R. Tracy Ballock, MD, PhD
Regis J. O'Keefe, MD

Introduction

Paired human limbs reach the same adult length and proportions through a highly regulated series of biologic events involving both intramembranous and endochondral ossification pathways. This remarkable achievement is the culmination of a finely orchestrated signaling program executed at the cellular and molecular level that begins with formation of the limb bud, progresses through the development of the primary and secondary ossification centers of a long bone, and ends with the closure of the growth plate at skeletal maturity.

Over the past decade, the understanding of the molecular signals required for successful progression through each stage of limb growth and development has increased dramatically. Many of these advances have resulted from molecular genetic studies of families with inherited mutations affecting the musculoskeletal system. This genetic approach has resulted in the elucidation of the underlying molecular defect in nearly all forms of human chondrodysplasia.

This chapter reviews the current state of knowledge of human limb growth and development, focusing on how this new information applies to the diagnosis and treatment of children with disorders of the growth plate.

Embryonic Skeletal Development

Spine Development

The spinal column originates from organized pairs of mesodermal structures known as somites, which organize from a cranial to caudal direction on either side of the developing notochord and neural tube. This formation of somites does not occur in the absence of the *paraxis* gene, which encodes a helix-loop-helix DNA transcription factor. Each somite further condenses into three layers: the sclerotome, which will become the vertebral bodies and vertebral arches; the myotome, which will become myoblasts; and the dermatome, which will become skin. Sclerotomal condensation appears to be dependent on expression of the *Pax1* gene. Each sclerotome further divides itself into cranial and caudal regions, an event that is regulated by *Mox1*. Caudal regions of the sclerotome fuse with the adjacent cranial regions of the neighboring sclerotome to form the precartilage models of the vertebrae. This so-called metameric shift allows the spinal nerves, which originally passed through the center of the sclerotome between the cranial and caudal portions, to exit between the newly formed vertebrae at each level to innervate the myotomes of each segment.

In the cervical spine, the cranial portion of the first cervical sclerotome contributes to formation of the occiput, whereas the caudal region of the eighth cervical sclerotome helps form the first thoracic vertebra. The first cervical nerve therefore exits between C1 and the occiput, whereas the eighth cervical nerve exits between C7 and T1. This metameric shift explains why eight cervical nerves are associated with only seven cervical vertebrae.

Limb Development

The appendicular skeleton forms between the fourth and eighth weeks of gestation. The limb bud begins as an outpouching from the lateral body wall and initially consists of both ectodermal and mesodermal layers. This initial outgrowth appears to be under control of the fibroblast growth factor (FGF) family of signaling molecules because FGF-1, FGF-2, and FGF-4 all are able to induce the formation of ectopic limb buds on the flanks of chick embryos. The progressive enlargement of the limb bud results from biochemical signaling between the layer of ectodermal cells at its distal layer (apical ectodermal ridge) and the rapidly proliferating mesodermal cells (progress zone) adjacent to this ectodermal layer. The function of

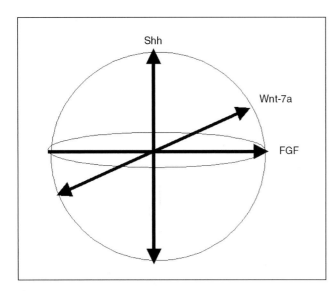

Figure 1   Three-dimensional regulatory axis of limb bud pattern formation. FGF regulates proximal-distal outgrowth, whereas *Wnt-7a* controls dorsal-ventral fate, and *Shh* regulates anterior-posterior patterning.

the apical ectodermal ridge (AER) is to promote the outgrowth of the limb bud in the proximal-distal direction by maintaining the mesodermal cells in an undifferentiated state, whereas the role of the progress zone is to secrete a factor that maintains the AER. If the AER is experimentally removed in chick embryos, the cells immediately subjacent to the AER undergo massive cell death, and limb formation is truncated at a variable proximal-distal level, depending on the timing of the AER removal. The severe transverse phocomelic birth defects caused by thalidomide exposure during the first trimester of pregnancy have been postulated to involve damage to the progress zone. Surgical replacement of the AER in chick embryos or implantation of a bead loaded with FGF-4 prevents this cell death and restores the normal proximal-distal sequence of limb formation. The proximal-distal axis of limb formation is therefore under control of the FGF family of signaling molecules.

Similar gain and loss of function experiments performed primarily in chick limb buds have established that a three-dimensional regulatory axis controls pattern formation of the limb (**Figure 1**). As the limb bud enlarges, its constituent cells acquire a positional identity with respect to each of these three axes (proximal-distal, anterior-posterior, and dorsal-ventral) that ultimately specifies cell fate and sculpts the mesenchymal condensations that form the precursors of the skeletal elements of the limb. This positional identity is acquired as cells pass through the progress zone beneath the AER.

Digit formation is determined along the anterior-posterior axis of the limb bud. Cells located in the zone of polarizing activity in the posterior aspect of the limb bud direct both the number and type of digits formed. This

organizing activity of the zone of polarizing activity has been traced to the product of the Sonic hedgehog (*Shh*) gene. *Shh* controls the formation of digits by activating the expression of homeobox (*HOX*) genes. *HOX* genes encode DNA-binding transcription factors that propagate a cascade of molecular events that pattern digit formation along the anterior-posterior axis.

Limb formation along the dorsal-ventral axis of the limb bud is under the control of a member of the *Wnt* gene family, *Wnt-7a*. This regulatory molecule is expressed in a restricted area on the dorsal aspect of the limb bud and specifies dorsal-ventral patterning. Misexpression of *Wnt-7a* on the ventral aspect of the limb bud in mice results in digits that flex in the dorsal direction and extend in the ventral direction.

The formation of skeletal elements in the limb bud is heralded by the condensation of mesenchymal cells into shapes that serve as models of the developing bones. During the sixth week of embryonic development, these mesenchymal condensations undergo chondrogenesis as the cells begin to synthesize a cartilage extracellular matrix. The cartilage matrix elaborated by the chondrocytes of the skeletal anlagen allows the anlagen to expand by interstitial growth (growth from within) as this extracellular matrix accumulates between the cells. This transformation into cartilage tissue is regulated by the activity of members of the *SOX* gene family, specifically *SOX5*, *SOX6*, and *SOX9*. These DNA transcription factors regulate the expression of genes encoding many of the extracellular matrix proteins of cartilage, including collagen II, collagen IX, collagen XI, and aggrecan. Chimeric mice containing cells with no functional *SOX9* genes fail to achieve chondrocyte differentiation because of a block at the stage of mesenchymal condensation, indicating that in addition to regulating the synthesis of cartilage extracellular matrix proteins, *SOX9* may also control the expression of cell surface proteins involved in the condensation process. Mutations in *SOX9* have been linked to the human skeletal malformation syndrome, camptomelic dysplasia.

Endochondral and Intramembranous Ossification

The cartilage model of the skeleton is converted into bone during development through a combination of endochondral and intramembranous bone formation. Endochondral ossification involves formation of a cartilage model of bone that becomes mineralized. The mineralized cartilage is used by osteoblasts as a template for subsequent bone formation. The series of cellular events that comprise the process of endochondral ossification consist of chondrocyte proliferation, chondrocyte hypertrophy, matrix mineralization, apoptosis, vascular invasion, ossification, and remodeling to lamellar bone. These same cellular processes are also recapitulated during longitudinal growth of the skeleton at the growth plate and during the

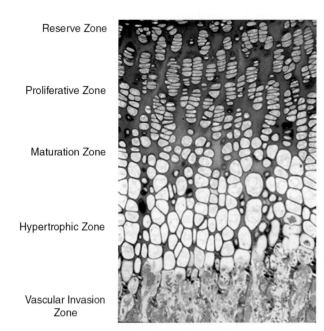

Reserve Zone

Proliferative Zone

Maturation Zone

Hypertrophic Zone

Vascular Invasion Zone

Figure 2   Photomicrograph shows the growth plate structure and zones, x220. *(Adapted with permission from Farnum CE, Nixon A, Lee AO, Kwan DT, Belanger L, Wilsman NJ: Quantitative three-dimensional analysis of chondrocytic kinetic responses to short-term stapling of the rat proximal tibial growth plate. Cells Tissues Organs 2000;167:247-258.)*

healing of fractures by callus formation. The most dramatic example of longitudinal growth by endochondral ossification that can be found in nature is the growth of deer antlers, which can grow as long as 2 to 3 feet within a period of 9 months every year.

Intramembranous ossification involves the direct elaboration of bone matrix by osteoblasts without a calcified cartilage template. The process of intramembranous ossification is responsible for the formation of flat bones, such as the calvaria, and is also the process by which long bones grow in width (appositional growth). It is important to note that in its final form, the bone formed by the endochondral route is histologically and biochemically indistinguishable from bone formed by the intramembranous route.

Development of the Primary and Secondary Centers of Ossification

During the seventh week of embryonic life, the chondrocytes located in the center of the cartilage anlagen hypertrophy by increasing their intracellular volume by nearly a factor of 10 and begin to mineralize their surrounding matrix in preparation for eventual ossification. As matrix mineralization is completed, the hypertrophic chondrocytes undergo programmed cell death (apoptosis). Mesenchymal cells in the periosteum surrounding this calcified cartilage core simultaneously differentiate into osteoblasts and begin to elaborate a collar of intramembranous bone around the middle of the developing bone. By the eighth

week of embryonic life, blood vessels from the periphery invade the empty chondrocyte lacuna, followed by osteoblasts that secrete bone matrix onto the calcified cartilage surfaces to form primary spongiosa. These primary spongiosa are known as mixed spicules because they consist of both calcified cartilage and bone. These primary spongiosa are subsequently remodeled to true lamellar bone by removal of the calcified cartilage by chondroclasts and continued deposition of bone matrix by osteoblasts to form secondary spongiosa.

As the primary center of ossification expands and advances toward the ends of the long bone, the cellular events of endochondral ossification are repeated at the ends of the bone to form the secondary center of ossification. The major long bones each have two secondary centers of ossification located at opposite ends of the growing bone, whereas metacarpals and metatarsals have only one center of ossification. The secondary center of ossification expands radially to convert the entire chondroepiphysis to lamellar trabecular bone with the exception of the thin layer of hyaline articular cartilage that constitutes the surface of the adjacent joint.

Structure, Function, and Biochemistry of the Growth Plate

The growth plate initially forms as the leading edge of the primary center of ossification as it expands toward the ends of the bone. As the secondary center of ossification enlarges to fill the chondroepiphysis, the growth plate (physis) becomes a narrow disk of cartilage located between the epiphysis and metaphysis of the growing bone.

The growth plate can be divided into a series of anatomic zones that distinguish unique morphologic and biochemical stages during the process of chondrocyte differentiation (**Figure 2**). In the reserve zone, the ratio of extracellular matrix to cell volume is quite high, and the cells are in a relatively quiescent state. In the proliferative zone, chondrocytes assume a flattened appearance, begin to divide, and become organized into columns. In the zone of maturation, the synthesis of extracellular matrix allows the recently divided cells to separate from each other. This extracellular matrix consists predominantly of collagens and proteoglycans as well as other noncollagenous proteins. Type II collagen is the primary collagen species in the growth plate, although type IX and type XI collagen also are highly expressed. Type IX collagen molecules decorate the surface of the type II collagen fibrils to which they are covalently cross-linked. It is postulated that type IX collagen mediates the interaction of type II collagen with other extracellular matrix components in cartilage. Mutations in type II collagen are associated with a number of skeletal dysplasias in humans, including spondyloepiphyseal dysplasia, Kniest dysplasia, and Stickler's syndrome. *COL9* mutations have been identified in a subset of patients with multiple epiphyseal dysplasia, whereas muta-

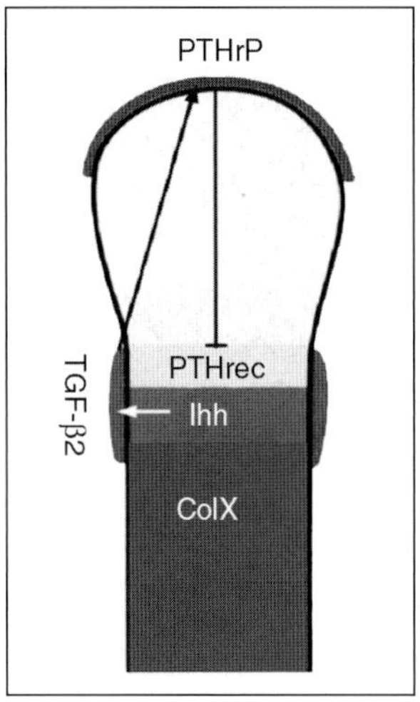

Figure 3   Graphic representation of the PTHrP-Ihh-TGF-β2 regulatory loop. PTHrec = PTHrP receptor. *(Reproduced with permission from Ballock RT, O'Keefe RJ: Current concepts review: The biology of the growth plate. J Bone Joint Surg Am 2003;85:715-726.)*

tions in *COL11* have been linked to some forms of Stickler's syndrome.

Aggrecan, the large aggregating proteoglycan of cartilage, is the principal proteoglycan molecule in the cartilage matrix and provides the osmotic resistance necessary for cartilage to resist compressive loads. Decorin and biglycan, two smaller proteoglycan molecules, also may serve important functions. Decorin, for example, coats the outside of the collagen fibrils and may play a role in regulating collagen fibrillogenesis.

Cartilage oligomeric protein (COMP) is a critical noncollagenous protein also found in the extracellular matrix. COMP is an extracellular calcium-binding glycoprotein belonging to the thrombospondin family. The COMP molecule is composed of five flexible arms with a large globular domain at the end of each arm, resembling a bouquet of flowers. Mutations in COMP have been linked to pseudoachondroplasia as well as some forms of multiple epiphyseal dysplasia.

In the hypertrophic zone, cell division ceases and the chondrocytes begin to terminally differentiate. This terminal differentiation process is associated with a large increase in intracellular cell volume as well as sharp increases in alkaline phosphatase enzymatic activity and synthesis of type X collagen, a unique short-chain collagen found only in the hypertrophic zone of the growth plate. Although the exact function of type X collagen in the growth plate remains unclear, mutations in the *COLX* gene have been found to cause Schmid metaphyseal chondrodysplasia. Surprisingly, transgenic mice lacking type X collagen show only subtle alterations in hematopoiesis and growth plate architecture, but no obvious skeletal phenotype.

Matrix vesicles, formed by budding of the chondrocyte plasma membrane, are deposited into the surrounding extracellular matrix in the hypertrophic zone and serve as a nidus for matrix mineralization. Mineralization of the cartilage extracellular matrix occurs in a somewhat directional pattern, with the longitudinal septa of carti-

lage matrix between the columns of hypertrophic chondrocytes being the favored sites of mineral deposition. The deposited mineral consists primarily of poorly crystallized hydroxyapatite.

In the zone of vascular invasion, invading capillary loops from the metaphysis break through the last transverse septum of mineralized cartilage to enter the hypertrophic chondrocyte lacuna. Approximately two thirds of these transverse septa are actively resorbed by chondroclasts, whereas the remaining one third serve as a template for deposition of bone matrix by osteoblasts. These mixed spicules, containing both mineralized cartilage and bone matrix, are known as primary trabeculae and are subsequently remodeled in the metaphysis to trabeculae of lamellar bone, or secondary trabeculae.

A peripheral ring of fibrocartilage encircles these growth plate zones to provide structural support and to provide for increasing width of the physis. The ossification groove of Ranvier is a wedge-shaped area of chondrocyte progenitor cells that contributes reserve zone cells to allow the physis to expand its width as the bone grows longer. The perichondrial fibrous ring of LaCroix is a band of fibrous tissue that merges with the periosteum of the bone and provides mechanical support in response to compression, tension, or shear loads on the physis.

Cell Proliferation

Proliferation in the growth plate occurs in a narrow band of cells located in the proliferating region of the growth plate. Histomorphometric studies in rats show that one layer of hypertrophic cells is eliminated from the growth plate every 3 hours. This means that eight new cells in each chondrocyte column must be produced by cell proliferation every day to maintain the width of the growth plate. The progression of chondrocytes through the resting, proliferating, and hypertrophic stages of differentiation that culminates in matrix calcification and programmed cell death occurs within 24 hours in growth plates of rapidly growing animals.

The proliferation of chondrocytes in the growth plate is under the control of a local feedback loop that primarily involves three signaling molecules synthesized by growth plate chondrocytes: parathyroid hormone–related peptide (PTHrP), Indian hedgehog (Ihh), and transforming growth factor-beta (TGF-β). This feedback loop acts to regulate the rate at which the growth plate cells leave the proliferative zone of the physis and irreversibly commit to terminally differentiated hypertrophic cells (**Figure 3**).

Cells in the periarticular region of the long bone produce PTHrP; however, the PTHrP receptor is found primarily in the cells of the lower proliferative zone and prehypertrophic zone. PTHrP delays hypertrophic differentiation in these lower proliferative zone cells by maintaining cells in a prehypertrophic phenotype. Growth plate cells that are beginning to undergo hypertrophic dif-

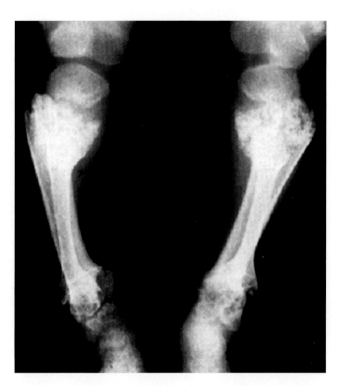

Figure 4   Tibial radiograph of a patient with Jansen's metaphyseal chondrodysplasia. *(Reproduced with permission from Ballock RT, O'Keefe RJ: Physiology and pathophysiology of the growth plate.* Birth Defects Res C Embryo Today *2003;69:123-143.)*

ferentiation secrete Ihh, which relays a signal back through the perichondrium to increase the production of PTHrP. This perichondrial relay involves the receptors for Ihh, Patched and Gli, which are located primarily in the cells of the perichondrium, as well as TGF-β produced by perichondrial cells in response to Ihh. TGF-β acts on the perichondrial and periarticular cells to increase PTHrP synthesis, and can also act directly on chondrocytes to inhibit hypertrophy. This increase in PTHrP synthesis in the periarticular cells is transmitted to the late-proliferating cells expressing the PTHrP receptor, which slow the production of Ihh-producing cells, thereby controlling the pace of hypertrophic differentiation.

Genetic experiments in mice confirm this primary role of PTHrP in controlling the transition between chondrocyte proliferation and differentiation. Transgenic mice lacking either PTHrP or the PTH/PTHrP receptor show evidence of dwarfism resulting from accelerated differentiation and premature hypertrophy. Conversely, mice in which PTHrP is overexpressed in the growth plate also exhibit dwarfism, but this dwarfism is caused by the marked slowing of the rate of differentiation. In humans, mutations in the PTH/PTHrP receptor that result in a constitutively active PTHrP signal have been identified as the cause of Jansen's metaphyseal chondrodysplasia, a dwarfing condition associated with delays in growth plate mineralization and hypercalcemia (Figure 4) .

Although this PTHrP-Ihh-TGF-β feedback loop currently appears to be the primary regulator cell of proliferation in the growth plate, it is also likely that this regulatory network is modulated by other systemic and local signaling molecules that have been previously shown to have effects on cell proliferation in the growth plate. For example, genetic disruption of the murine fibroblast growth factor receptor-3 (FGFR-3), which binds at least nine members of the fibroblast growth factor family, results in prolonged endochondral bone growth with expansion of the proliferating and hypertrophic zones of the growth plate. An activating mutation in this FGFR-3 receptor has been identified as the cause of the markedly reduced proliferation of growth plate cells in achondroplasia, the most common dwarfing condition in humans (Figure 5) . It is therefore likely that FGF signaling is able to modulate the PTHrP-Ihh-TGF-β regulatory loop.

Another important growth factor is insulin-like growth factor-I (IGF-I), which is an autocrine factor that stimulates increased rates of cell division. In addition to its effects on circulating levels of IGF-I, growth hormone increases the local synthesis of IGF-I in growth plate cells, which then leads to increased rates of cell division. IGF-I produced locally by growth plate chondrocytes in response to growth hormone is the source for maintenance of normal postnatal skeletal growth. Mutations in the growth hormone receptor result in Laron syndrome, a hereditary dwarfism associated with truncal obesity and low serum IGF-I levels.

Chondrocyte Hypertrophy

As chondrocytes hypertrophy, intracellular volume is increased fivefold to tenfold. Chondrocyte hypertrophy is not a passive swelling of the cell, but reflects an active process marked by an increase in the number of intracellular organelles, including mitochondria and endoplasmic reticulum. The factors that stimulate cellular enlargement are not clear, but likely involve alterations in ion channels that lead to an ingress of water.

Chondrocyte hypertrophy has an important role in the longitudinal growth of the skeleton. It has been shown that the increase in chondrocyte height is responsible for 44% to 59% of long bone growth, with the remainder caused by matrix synthesis and chondrocyte proliferation. Furthermore, the differential growth of various bones appears to be highly related to differences in the cell size of hypertrophic chondrocytes. Chondrocytes in bones with more rapid growth, such as the femur, undergo a larger increase in size than chondrocytes in growth plates in bones with slower growth, such as the radius. The factors that control these local differences in chondrocyte hypertrophy have not been defined, but likely involve an interaction of both local and systemic factors.

Both in vitro and in vivo models of chondrocyte differentiation show that in the absence of inhibitory factors

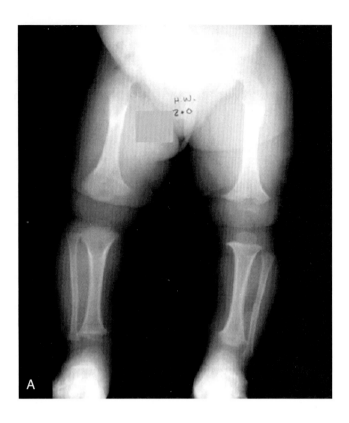

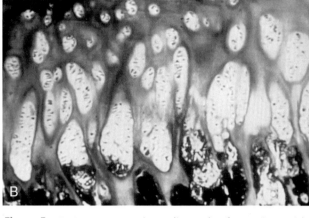

Figure 5   **A,** Lower extremity radiograph of a patient with achondroplasia. Note the retardation of longitudinal bone growth with normal appositional growth. *(Reproduced with permission from Ballock RT, O'Keefe RJ: Physiology and pathophysiology of the growth plate.* Birth Defects Res C Embryo Today *2003;69:123-143.)* **B,** Histologic features of achondroplasia. *(Reproduced from Iannotti JP, Goldstein S, Kuhn J, et al: The formation and growth of skeletal tissues, in Buckwalter JA, Einhorn TA, Simon SR (eds):* Orthopaedic Basic Science: Biology and Biomechanics of the Musculoskeletal System, *ed 2. Rosemont, IL, American Academy of Orthopaedic Surgeons, 2000, pp 78-109.)*

chondrocytes undergo hypertrophy spontaneously. Autocrine signaling from bone morphogenetic proteins (BMPs) expressed by growth plate chondrocytes appears to be responsible for this spontaneous completion of maturation.

Other factors that induce chondrocyte maturation also appear to act through BMP signaling. Thyroxine induces type X collagen synthesis and other maturational characteristics in growth plate chondrocytes in culture through induction of BMP-2, an effect that can be blocked by addition of the BMP antagonist noggin. Similarly, the induction of chondrocyte differentiation by retinoic acid appears to be related to effects on BMP signaling. Retinoic acid has recently been shown to induce the expression of the BMP-signaling molecules SMAD-1 and SMAD-5 in chondrocytes, making retinoic acid-treated chondrocytes more sensitive to BMP-mediated signaling events.

Similar to the role of *SOX9* in chondrogenesis, the transcription factor core binding factor alpha-1 (cbfa-1, also known as runx2) appears to have a critical role during the process of chondrocyte hypertrophy and terminal differentiation. Although cbfa-1 is able to induce terminal differentiation in chondrocytes, mice without cbfa-1 have an absence of hypertrophic chondrocytes in some growth plates, whereas in other growth plates hypertrophy proceeds normally, suggesting that other transcription factors are involved in this process. The transcription factors in the BMP-signaling pathway, SMAD-1, SMAD-5, and SMAD-8 have recently been shown to interact with cbfa-1

at the type X collagen promoter to induce the expression of this gene. Mutation in the human *cbfa-1* gene results in cleidocranial dysplasia, a disorder manifested by abnormalities in the clavicles, the facial bones, skull and pelvis, emphasizing the importance of *cbfa-1* in osteogenesis and also the intramembranous ossification pathway.

Apoptosis

Growth and development in all organisms requires the proliferation, differentiation, and subsequent removal of cells. Apoptosis is the mechanism by which cells undergo programmed cell death, a process necessary for the homeostasis of most organs, including the growth plate. The cells in the growth plate that undergo apoptosis are terminally differentiated hypertrophic chondrocytes. The role of terminally differentiated chondrocytes is to prepare the matrix for calcification, which then acts as a template for primary bone formation. Death and removal of terminally differentiated hypertrophic chondrocytes provides space for the ingress of vascular channels and osteoblasts into the chondrocyte lacunae. Although it was initially thought that hypertrophic chondrocytes died through a passive process caused by depletion of nutrients and oxygen tension in the hypertrophic region of the growth plate, it is now recognized that the process is an actively regulated event. The morphologic events result from activation of a set of caspase enzymes that target and metabolize important intracellular structures. Morphologic findings in cells undergoing programmed cell death include condensation of the nuclear chromatin, cell shrinkage, and plasma membrane blebbing. In contrast to necrotic cells, which lyse and release degradative enzymes into the local environment, apoptotic cells are rapidly recognized by and taken up by neighboring or phagocytic cells, but do not induce inflammation as necrotic cells do.

The mechanisms regulating physiologic cell death in the growth plate have not been well defined. Mineralization of the matrix is associated with the release of phosphate ions. In vitro work demonstrates that chondrocytes have increased apoptosis in the presence of increased phosphate levels and that the effect is dependent on the maturational state of the cells; differentiated chondrocytes are more sensitive to increased phosphate levels than less differentiated cells. The increase in phosphate concentration is associated with abnormalities in mitochondrial function; chondrocytes have loss of mitochondria membrane potential and greater reliance on glycolysis with progression through hypertrophy. It is hypothesized that Pi triggers apoptosis in these energy-compromised cells by promoting a mitochondrial membrane transition, leading to the release of cytochrome c and other proapoptotic factors, thereby inducing the death process. Conversely, abnormally low levels of pyrophosphate, as occurs during hypophosphatemia associated with rickets, inhibit apoptosis of hypertrophic chondrocytes and result in widening of the growth plate.

Matrix Mineralization

The mineralization of cartilage is primarily limited to matrix between distinct hypertrophic chondrocyte columns. Matrix vesicles are the initial sites of mineralization in the hypertrophic region of the growth plate. Matrix vesicles are 100 nm in diameter, extracellular membrane-invested particles that are released by budding from the surfaces of chondrocytes, osteoblasts, and odontoblasts. Matrix vesicle accumulation of calcium appears to be dependent on a family of calcium-channel molecules referred to as annexins. Annexin II, V, and VI are present within the lipid bilayer of matrix vesicles and are involved in and necessary for accumulation of calcium in these structures. Calcium-channel blockers specific for annexins block their uptake of calcium. The incorporation of calcium into matrix vesicles, which are then shed into the extracellular space, appears to occur, in part, intracellularly.

Matrix vesicles also contain enzymes that increase dramatically in activity during endochondral bone formation, including alkaline phosphatase and matrix metalloproteinases (MMPs). The role of alkaline phosphatase in matrix mineralization is not certain, but likely involves the important step of metabolism of pyrophosphate to yield molecules of orthophosphate. Whereas pyrophosphate is a known inhibitor of hydroxyapatite crystal formation, pyrophosphate stimulates mineralization.

MMPs are responsible for catabolism and turnover of the matrix, and this activity is induced during the process of chondrocyte hypertrophy. MMP-2, MMP-9, and MMP-13 are present in matrix vesicles, and mineralization of the matrix is associated with a marked increase in the cleavage of type II collagen by collagenase. Matrix vesicles also contain TGF-β, which is present in a latent form but is activated by MMP-13. The increased levels of active TGF–β present in the growth plate at the onset of mineralization is believed to be the result of, at least in part, the presence of MMP-13 in matrix vesicles. Additionally, MMPs are critical for angiogenesis in the growth plate and thus are necessary for normal calcification and bone formation. The effects of the MMPs on angiogenesis may be related to a decrease in catabolism of the matrix, release of important growth factors, or other effects, but these effects have not yet been elucidated.

Proteoglycans are major components of the extracellular matrix in cartilage. As with articular cartilage, the growth plate contains large aggregating proteoglycans and is thus characterized as hyaline cartilage. Although it was initially believed that the content of aggregating proteoglycans is reduced in the hypertrophic region, it has now been established that there are increased concentrations of aggregating proteoglycans at the onset of calcification. However, there are changes in the relative content of the proteoglycan monomers, their degree of sulfation, and size during maturation that are likely important.

Cartilage also contains components that inhibit calcification of the extracellular matrix. The best characterized is matrix Gla protein (MGP), a 14-kD extracellular matrix protein of the mineral-binding Gla protein family. MGP is expressed by proliferative and late hypertrophic chondrocytes, but not by the intervening chondrocytes. MGP inhibits calcification both in vitro and in vivo. MGP-deficient mice have inappropriate calcification of the growth plate that leads to short stature, osteopenia, and fractures.

Vascular Invasion

The blood supply to the developing secondary center of ossification is delivered through epiphyseal arteries that enter the bone from the periphery. Prior to skeletal maturity, these epiphyseal vessels are the sole source of vascularization of the epiphysis. These vessels also contribute branches to the reserve zone of the growth plate and terminate at the uppermost proliferative zone cell, but do not extend further into the proliferative or hypertrophic zones.

The growth plate itself is therefore essentially an avascular structure that relies on diffusion of both oxygen and nutrients for cell metabolism from vascular arcades located on the metaphyseal side of the growth plate. The metaphyseal vascular channels are found in compartments bounded by calcified cartilage beneath the last row of hypertrophic chondrocytes. These vascular channels are aligned along the longitudinal axis of the bone and

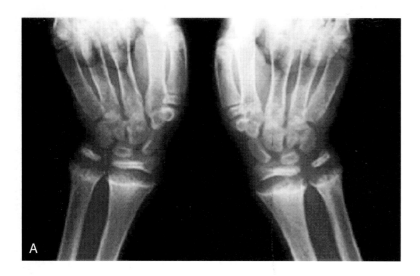

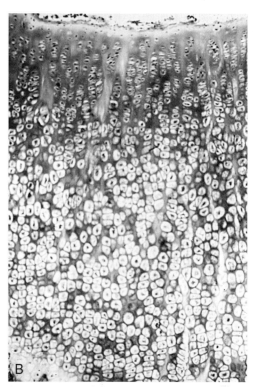

Figure 6   **A,** Wrist radiograph of a child with rickets. Note the widened physes and the flaring and cupping of the metaphyses. *(Reproduced with permission from Ballock RT, O'Keefe RJ: Physiology and pathophysiology of the growth plate.* Birth Defects Res C Embryo Today *2003;69:123-143.)* **B,** Histologic features of rickets. The zone of proliferation is largely unaffected, but the hypertrophic zone is markedly widened. *(Reproduced courtesy of Henry J. Mankin, MD.)*

contain an ascending and descending capillary system. It has been recognized in recent years that vascular invasion is a pivotal event in the regulation of endochondral ossification and is necessary for normal bone formation.

Vascular endothelial growth factor (VEGF) appears to be the factor responsible and necessary for vascular ingrowth into the growth plate. VEGF is a 44-kDA protein that targets vascular endothelial cells and stimulates their proliferation, migration, and ultimately vessel formation. VEGF is expressed by hypertrophic chondrocytes in the growth plate, but is absent in resting and proliferating chondrocytes. In animals, loss of function of VEGF, with use of an oral agent or an injected, genetically engineered protein that blocks activation of the receptor for VEGF, leads to loss of vascular invasion.

Physeal Closure

As skeletal maturity approaches, the rate of longitudinal bone growth diminishes as growth plate chondrocytes decrease their proliferation. This decreased growth rate is associated with structural changes in the physis, including a gradual decline in growth plate width because of the reduced height of the proliferative and hypertrophic zones as well as reduced hypertrophic cell size and column density. In humans and in some other mammals, the growth plate is completely resorbed following puberty, resulting in fusion of the epiphysis to the metaphysis.

Recently, it has become evident that this process of physeal closure is primarily under the control of estrogen in both sexes. In patients with genetic mutations in either

the gene encoding the aromatase enzyme that converts androgen to estrogen or in the gene encoding the estrogen receptor-α, the physes fail to close at the time of sexual maturation and show evidence of increased height resulting from longitudinal bone growth well into adulthood. Conversely, in patients with precocious puberty who are exposed to estrogen prematurely, the physes close earlier than predicted.

The molecular mechanisms involved in estrogen-mediated physeal closure remain incompletely characterized. Experiments in rabbits, which as with humans resorb their growth plates following sexual maturation, suggest that estrogen may exert its effect by promoting a process of programmed replicative senescence in growth plate chondrocytes rather than accelerating vascular invasion or ossification. Once the proliferative potential of the growth plate cells is exhausted, epiphyseal fusion may occur spontaneously.

Pathologic States Affecting the Growth Plate
Rickets

It is well known that vitamin D deficiency results in defective mineralization and widening of the growth plate **(Figure 6)**. Mice lacking the vitamin D receptor develop classic signs of rickets, including thickening of the growth plate and decreased mineralization. However, if mineral ion homeostasis is normalized in vitamin D receptor-ablated mice, growth plate morphology and width return to normal. Recently, it has been demonstrated that the specific cause of the widened hypertrophic zone in mice with rickets is inhibition of apoptosis of hypertrophic chondrocytes caused by the resultant secondary hyperparathyroidism and hypophosphatemia.

Hypophosphatasia

Hypophosphatasia is a heritable disease that is characterized by deficient activity of the tissue nonspecific isoenzyme of alkaline phosphatase and results in rickets because of decreased calcification of the matrix (**Figure 7**). Electron microscopic studies have shown that matrix vesicles in patients with rickets maintain the ability to concentrate calcium and phosphate internally and to initiate mineral formation. However, in the absence of alkaline phosphatase, there is retarded extravesicular calcium-hydroxyapatite crystal propagation.

Irradiation

Radiation injury to the growth plate may occur during radiation therapy of juxta-articular tumors of bone. Irradiation of chondrocytes results in premature apoptosis of proliferative chondrocytes and subsequent inhibition of longitudinal growth.

Scurvy

Scurvy is a condition resulting from deficiency of ascorbic acid (vitamin C) that is rarely encountered today. Ascorbic acid is necessary for hydroxylation of proline during collagen synthesis and also stimulates matrix mineralization in growth plate chondrocytes through its positive effects on alkaline phosphatase activity and type X collagen synthesis. The net result of ascorbic acid deficiency in vivo is abnormal type I collagen accumulation in the metaphysis with osteopenia.

Lead Poisoning

Clinical data in human populations suggest that the growth plate is an important target tissue. Both the Second and Third National Health and Nutrition Examination Survey (NHANES II and NHANES III) demonstrated decreased skeletal growth in children who were exposed to lead. The negative association between stature and lead levels is present even at concentrations as low as 4 µg/dL. This concentration of lead is typically not associated with measurable pathologic effects in other tissues, which demonstrates the sensitivity of the developing skeleton to lead.

Recent work has shown that the inhibition of skeletal growth in children exposed to lead along with associated growth plate morphologic abnormalities may be caused by an alteration in chondrocyte responses to PTHrP and TGF-β. Lead interferes with the inhibitory effect of PTHrP and TGF-β on chondrocyte differentiation, and thus alters the normal regulatory events that control the rate of chondrocyte hypertrophy.

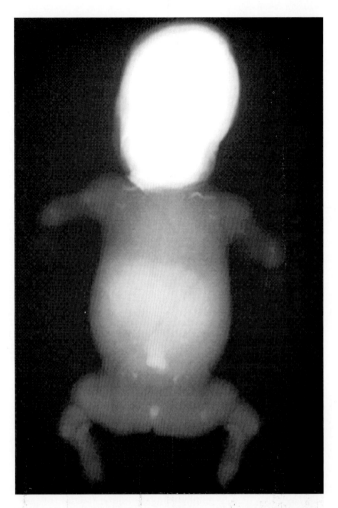

Figure 7 Radiograph of a patient with severe hypophosphatasia. Note the nearly complete absence of detectable bone mineralization. *(Reproduced with permission from Ballock RT, O'Keefe RJ: Physiology and pathophysiology of the growth plate. Birth Defects Res C Embryo Today 2003;69:123-143.)*

Response of the Growth Plate to Mechanical Loading
The Heuter-Volkman Law

It has been appreciated for more than a century that increasing compression forces across the growth plate slow longitudinal growth from the physis (Heuter-Volkman Law), whereas increasing tension forces have the opposite effect (Delpech Law). This observation has been frequently invoked to explain the progression of angular deformities of the lower extremities such as genu varum and genu valgum as the mechanical axis shifts from the center of the knee to the medial or lateral compartments, respectively. Despite this long-standing appreciation of the role of mechanical forces on physeal growth, the cellular and molecular basis of the Heuter-Volkman law remains largely uninvestigated. Finite element modeling of the proximal tibial physis has suggested that a 10° increase in varus deformity at the knee results in an increase in forces

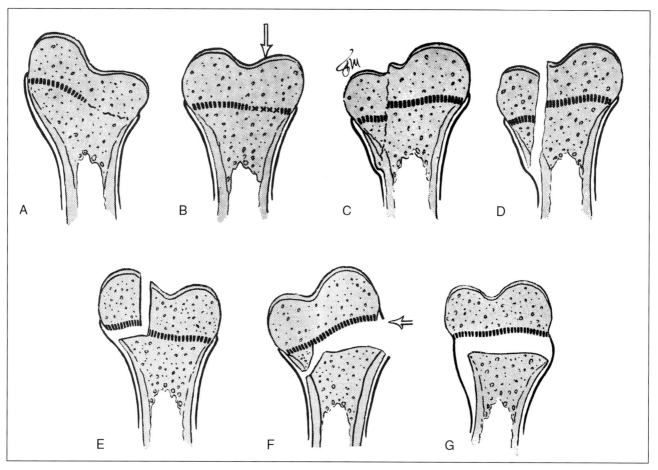

Figure 8   **A,** Type I epiphyseal plate injury: separation of the epiphysis. **B,** Type II epiphyseal plate injury: fracture-separation of the epiphysis. **C,** Type III epiphyseal plate injury: fracture of part of the epiphysis. **D,** Type IV epiphyseal plate injury: fracture of the epiphysis and epiphyseal plate. **E,** Bone union and premature closure. **F,** Type V epiphyseal plate injury: crushing of the epiphyseal plate. **G,** Premature closure. *(Reproduced with permission from Salter RB, Harris WR: Injury involving the epiphyseal plate.* J Bone Joint Surg Am *1963;45:587-622.)*

of two to three times body weight over the medial compartment.

Growth Plate Injury and Repair

The growth plate resists shear stresses by virtue of the strength of the perichondrial ring of LaCroix as well as the presence of undulations in the physis. These undulations create a series of ridges and valleys that resist horizontal displacement. When these restraints are exceeded, a fracture occurs through the physis. Fractures of long bones in children involve the growth plates in approximately 20% of patients. Because fractures involving the physis may result in growth arrest and/or deformity, these injuries present special management challenges.

Salter-Harris Classification of Growth Plate Injury

Previous studies of physeal injuries indicate that the likelihood of developing a growth abnormality depends on the pattern of growth-plate fracture that occurs. Salter and

Harris classified growth plate injuries into five types according to the mechanism of injury and the relationship of the fracture line to the growth plate (Figure 8). Type I injuries are a result of shearing or avulsion forces and produce a transverse fracture through the growth plate without involving the surrounding bone. Type II injuries are also a result of shearing or avulsion forces and produce a fracture that extends through the physis for a variable distance before exiting through the bony metaphysis, leaving a triangular metaphyseal fragment. Type III fractures involve the surface of the adjacent joint and occur as a result of intra-articular shearing forces. The fracture line traverses the bony epiphysis from the joint surface to the growth plate and then extends along the growth plate to the periphery. In type IV injuries, the shear force is slightly more vertically oriented, and the fracture line extends from the joint surface completely across the epiphysis and the growth plate before exiting obliquely through the metaphysis. Type V injuries are caused by vertical compression to the epiphysis and result in a crushing of growth plate tissue.

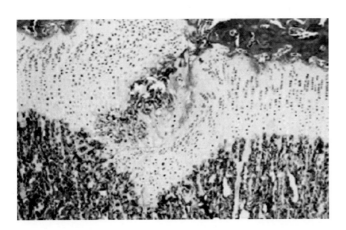

Figure 9   Photomicrograph of the early stage formation of a bony bridge across the growth plate after physeal fracture. Note that the growth plate is wider at the site of injury and bone formation is occurring at the site of the growth plate defect. *(Reproduced with permission from Wattenbarger JM, Gruber HE, Phieffer LS: Physeal fractures, part I: Histologic features of bone, cartilage and bar formation in a small animal model. J Ped Orthop 2002;22:703-709.)*

Growth disturbances following physeal fracture are rare in type I or type II injuries, but occur commonly following type III, IV, and V injuries. If the growth arrest is complete, no further longitudinal growth will occur from the involved growth plate. This will often result in development of a significant limb-length discrepancy. A complete growth arrest is particularly devastating around the knee, where the growth plates contribute approximately 80% of the entire growth of the limb. A partial growth arrest produces both a deficiency of longitudinal growth and angular deformity. The angular deformity occurs as a result of a difference in growth rates between the central and peripheral regions of the physis.

Pathophysiology of Growth Arrest
Various animal models of physeal injury have been studied in an effort to understand the pathophysiology of growth disturbance following growth-plate fracture. In type I and II injuries, the separation occurs primarily through the hypertrophic region of the growth plate in the transverse plane. Although the physis may widen and growth may slow temporarily, by 25 days after injury the physis appears histologically normal. In type III and IV injuries, the defect passes through all layers of the growth plate, thereby creating a potential conduit between the bone of the epiphysis and the bone of the metaphysis. Invasion of new blood vessels into this gap from both the epiphyseal and metaphyseal sides of the growth plate creates a focal vascular anastomosis across the relatively avascular physis (**Figure 9**). Osteoblasts migrate into the gap behind the invading blood vessels to form a bony bridge or bar across the physis. This bone bridge acts as a tether to further longitudinal growth.

Once a bone bridge forms across the physis and growth is affected, surgical excision of the bridge may be attempted if the bridge constitutes less than 20% of the cross-sectional area of the physis. This is a technically demanding procedure that requires removal of surrounding normal growth plate cartilage and leaves a large defect in the physis that is filled with an interposition material to prevent reformation of the bridge. Materials that have been historically used for interposition include autogenous fat grafts, silastic, and methylmethacrylate (bone cement). Of these three materials, fat is the most widely used because it is both readily available and biologically inert.

Unfortunately, the success rates of physeal bar excision and interposition grafting in terms of restoration of longitudinal growth are highly variable. Failure is often the result of migration of the interposition material out of the defect with reformation of the bone bridge. Even when bridge reformation does not occur, surgery is frequently required to correct limb-length inequality or deformity that occurs prior to bridge excision (this occurred in 48 of 58 children studied in one of the largest series reported to date).

Physeal bridges occupying more than 20% of the cross-sectional area of the growth plate cannot be treated successfully by bridge excision and interposition grafting. In these patients, the remaining normal physis is insufficient to restore normal longitudinal growth even if the bar is excised. These patients must have the remaining normal portion of the physis surgically ablated to prevent an angular deformity from developing, which will result in a complete growth arrest and limb-length discrepancy.

Summary
The development and growth of the skeleton occur as a result of a finely orchestrated molecular signaling program that regulates the formation of the limb bud, the primary and secondary centers of ossification, and the process of endochondral ossification at the growth plate. Molecular genetic studies of both transgenic mice and families with inherited disorders of the musculoskeletal system are identifying many of the key regulators of skeletal growth and development. This new information is improving the understanding of the pathophysiology of human skeletal growth disorders and will eventually translate into novel treatments of these musculoskeletal diseases in the future.

Selected Bibliography
Embryonic Skeletal Development

Alvarez J, Horton J, Sohn P, Serra R: The perichondrium plays an important role in mediating the effects of TGF-β1 on endochondral bone formation. *Dev Dyn* 2001;221:311-321.

Anderson HC, Hsu HH, Morris DC, Fedde KN, Whyte MP: Matrix vesicles in osteomalacic hypophosphatasia bone contain apatite-like mineral crystals. *Am J Pathol* 1997;151:1555-1561.

Ballock RT, Heydemann A, Wakefield LM, Flanders KC, Roberts AB, Sporn MB: TGF-β1 prevents hypertrophy of epiphyseal chondrocytes: Regulation of gene expression for cartilage matrix proteins and metalloproteases. *Dev Biol* 1993;158:414-429.

Bi W, Deng JM, Zhang Z, Behringer RR, Crombrugghe BD: *Sox9* is required for cartilage formation. *Nat Genet* 1999;22:85-89.

Bilezikian JP, Morishima A, Bell J, Grumbach M: Increased bone mass as a result of estrogen therapy in a man with aromatase deficiency. *N Engl J Med* 1998; 339:599-603.

Carani C, Qin K, Simoni M, et al: Effect of testosterone and estradiol in a man with aromatase deficiency. *N Engl J Med* 1997;337:91-95.

Colvin JS, Bohne BA, Harding GW, McEwen DG, Ornitz DM: Skeletal overgrowth and deafness in mice lacking fibroblast growth factor receptor-3. *Nat Genet* 1996;12:390-397.

Deere M, Sanford T, Francomano CA, Daniels K, Hecht JT: Identification of nine novel mutations in cartilage oligomeric matrix protein in patients with pseudoachondroplasia and multiple epiphyseal dysplasia. *Am J Med Genet* 1999;85:486-490.

Gerber HP, Vu TH, Ryan AM, Kowalski J, Werb Z, Ferrara N: VEGF couples hypertrophic cartilage remodeling, ossification and angiogenesis during endochondral bone formation. *Nat Med* 1999;5:623-628.

Hogan BL: Morphogenesis. *Cell* 1999;96:225-233.

Holden P, Canty EG, Mortier GR, et al: Identification of novel pro-α2(IX) collagen gene mutations in two families with distinctive oligoepiphyseal forms of multiple epiphyseal dysplasia. *Am J Hum Genet* 1999;65: 31-38.

Hunziker EB, Schenk RK, Cruz-Orive LM: Quantitation of chondrocyte performance in growth-plate cartilage during longitudinal bone growth. *J Bone Joint Surg Am* 1987;69:162-173.

Kirsch T, Harrison G, Golub EE, Nah HD: The roles of annexins and types II and X collagen in matrix vesicle-mediated mineralization of growth plate cartilage. *J Biol Chem* 2000;275:35577-35583.

Lanske B, Karaplis AC, Lee K, et al: PTH/PTHrP receptor in early development and Indian hedgehog-regulated bone growth. *Science* 1996;273:663-666.

Laron Z, Pertzelan A, Mannheimer S: Genetic pituitary dwarfism with high serum concentration of growth hormone: A new inborn error of metabolism? *Isr J Med Sci* 1966;2:152-155.

Mansfield K, Rajpurohit R, Shapiro IM: Extracellular phosphate ions cause apoptosis of terminally differentiated epiphyseal chondrocytes. *J Cell Physiol* 1999; 179:276-286.

Ohlsson C, Nilsson A, Isaksson O, Lindahl A: Growth hormone induces multiplication of the slowly cycling germinal cells of the rat tibial growth plate. *Proc Natl Acad Sci USA* 1992;89:9826-9830.

Schipani E, Langman CB, Parfitt AM, et al: Constitutively activated receptors for parathyroid hormone and parathyroid hormone-related peptide in Jansen's metaphyseal chondrodysplasia. *N Engl J Med* 1996;335:708-714.

Shapiro F, Holtrop ME, Glimcher MJ: Organization and cellular biology of the perichondrial ossification groove of Ranvier: A morphological study in rabbits. *J Bone Joint Surg Am* 1977;59:703-723.

Sirko-Osadsa DA, Murray MA, Scott JA, Lavery MA, Warman ML, Robin NH: Stickler syndrome without eye involvement is caused by mutations in COL11A2, the gene encoding the α2(XI) chain of type XI collagen. *J Pediatr* 1998;132:368-371.

Smith EP, Boyd J, Frank GR, et al: Estrogen resistance caused by a point mutation in the estrogen receptor gene in a man. *N Engl J Med* 1994;331:1056-1061.

Vortkamp A, Lee K, Lanske B, Segre GV, Kronenberg HM, Tabin CJ: Regulation of rate of cartilage differentiation by Indian hedgehog and PTH-related protein. *Science* 1996;273:613-622.

Vu TH, Shipley JM, Bergers G, et al: MMP-9/gelatinase B is a key regulator of growth plate angiogenesis and apoptosis of hypertrophic chondrocytes. *Cell* 1998;93: 411-422.

Warman ML, Abbott M, Apte SS, et al: A type X collagen mutation causes Schmid metaphyseal chondrodysplasia. *Nat Genet* 1993;5:79-82.

Weise M, De-Levi S, Barnes KM, Gafni RI, Abad V, Baron J: Effects of estrogen on growth plate senescence and epiphyseal fusion. *Proc Natl Acad Sci USA* 2001;98:6871-6876.

Wilsman NJ, Farnum CE, Leiferman EM, Fry M, Barreto C: Differential growth by growth plates as a function of multiple parameters of chondrocytic kinetics. *J Orthop Res* 1996;14:927-936.

Pathologic States Affecting the Growth Plate
Amling M, Priemel M, Holzmann T, et al: Rescue of the skeletal phenotype of vitamin D receptor-ablated mice in the setting of normal mineral ion homeostasis: Formal histomorphometric and biomechanical analyses. *Endocrinology* 1999;140:4982-4987.

Gonzalez-Riola J, Hernandez ER, Escribano A, Revilla M, Villa LF, Rico H: Effect of lead on bone and cartilage in sexually mature rats: A morphometric and histomorphometry study. *Environ Res* 1997;74:91-93.

Pateder DB, Eliseev RA, O'Keefe RJ, et al: The role of autocrine growth factors in radiation damage to the epiphyseal growth plate. *Radiat Res* 2001;155:847-857.

Schwartz J, Angle C, Pitcher H: Relationship between childhood blood lead levels and stature. *Pediatrics* 1986;77:281-288.

Zuscik MJ, Pateder DB, Puzas JE, Schwarz EM, Rosier RN, O'Keefe RJ: Lead alters parathyroid hormone-related peptide and transforming growth factor-β1 effects and AP-1 and NF-κB signaling in chondrocytes. *J Orthop Res* 2002;20:811-818.

Response of the Growth Plate to Mechanical Loading
Bonnel F, Peruchon E, Baldet P, Dimeglio A, Rabischong P: Effects of compression on growth plates in the rabbit. *Acta Orthop Scand* 1983;54:730-733.

Farnum CE, Nixon A, Lee AO, Kwan DT, Belanger L, Wilsman NJ: Quantitative three-dimensional analysis of chondrocytic kinetic responses to short-term stapling of the rat proximal tibial growth plate. *Cells Tissues Organs* 2000;167:247-258.

Mankin KP, Zaleske DJ: Response of physeal cartilage to low-level compression and tension in organ culture. *J Pediatr Orthop* 1998;18:145-148.

Chapter 8

Form and Function of Bone

Joshua D. Miller, MD, PhD
Barbara R. McCreadie, PhD
Andrea I. Alford, PhD
Kurt D. Hankenson, DVM, PhD
Steven A. Goldstein, PhD

Introduction

The structure and composition of bone provides it with a remarkable set of properties. Bone has excellent resistance to failure or fracture while maintaining relatively low mass, making it ideally suited for a structural role in a mobile organism. Although commonly viewed as an inert material, bone is a dynamic tissue that possesses cellular sensory and response systems that allow it to adjust its gross and microscopic structure in response to changing physiologic and mechanical environmental cues. These properties provide bone with a significant capacity for self-renewal, allow it to mechanically optimize its structural role and its role in mineral homeostasis, and give it the unique ability among tissues to heal without scarring. As such, bone can be characterized as a "smart" material, with the ability to monitor its local environment and, when necessary, effect alterations in the organization of its mass to accommodate functional demand.

This chapter discusses gross bone anatomy, tissue organization and structure, extracellular matrix (ECM), and the various cells and cellular activities found in bone. The way in which the function of these different components is integrated into the composite that makes bone a mechanically and biologically optimized organ will then be described in the subsequent sections on remodeling of bone, mechanical regulation of bone structure, and bone mechanics, the ultimate macroscopic determinant of how bone properties are manifested clinically.

Bone Structure

Bone has a specific organization at different size scales enabling its primary functions: mechanical support (providing physical protection of vital organs and acting as a structural framework that allows for motion, power, grasp, and ambulation), housing the marrow, and participation in mineral homeostasis.

Whole Bone Structure
Anatomy

Whole bone structure encompasses the overall shape of the bone as well as the organization of the bone tissue at a macroscopic level. The three types of bone shapes (long, flat, and short) are formed through one of two developmental pathways. Long bones and short bones arise from a cartilage model, through a process called endochondral ossification, whereas flat bones form in loose condensations of mesenchymal tissue, through intramembranous ossification. This section primarily addresses the anatomy of long bones, but the concepts are also applicable to other bone types.

Long bones, such as the femur, tibia, and humerus, are divided into three sections: diaphysis, metaphysis, and epiphysis (**Figure 1**). These regions are distinguished by their geometry and by the type of bone structure present. The epiphysis and metaphysis consist primarily of a loosely organized network of bony struts known as trabecular or cancellous bone. This trabecular network is surrounded by a thin layer of very densely organized cortical bone. The growth plate (physis) makes a distinct separation between the epiphysis and metaphysis in growing animals. Following the closure of the growth plate, the physeal scar or epiphyseal line (visible because of altered density and/or orientation of trabecular struts) marks this separation. The

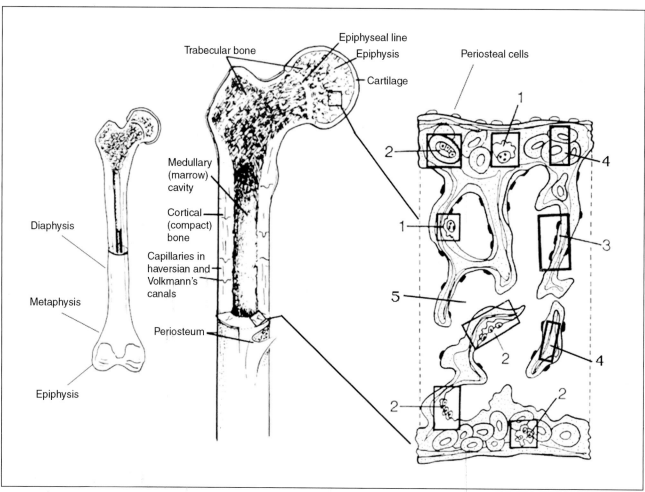

Figure 1   Schematic diagram of cortical and trabecular bone showing the different structures and cell types. 1 = osteoclasts, 2 = osteoblasts, 3 = bone lining cells, 4 = osteocytes, 5 = marrow space. *(Reproduced with permission from Hayes WC: Biomechanics of cortical and trabecular bone: Implications for assessment of fracture risk, in Basic Orthopaedic Biomechanics. New York, NY, Raven Press, 1991, pp 93-142 and Bostrom MPG, Boskey A, Kaufman JK, Einhorn TA: Form and function of bone, in Buckwalter JA, Einhorn TA, Simon SR (eds): Orthopaedic Basic Science: Biology and Biomechanics of the Musculoskeletal System, ed 2. Rosemont, IL, American Academy of Orthopaedic Surgeons, 2000, pp 320-369.)*

diaphysis is roughly a tube of very thick cortical bone surrounding a thin layer of trabecular bone with a hollow central area, the intramedullary canal. The inner surface of cortical bone is continuous with individual trabecular struts and is defined as the endosteal surface (**Figure 2**). The outer surface of the nonarticular regions of the bone is referred to as the periosteal surface. At the ends of long bones, just below the articular cartilage, is the specialized region of the subchondral bone.

All bone surfaces are covered by specialized tissues or cells. The periosteal membrane covers the periosteal surface. It is composed of an outer layer of fibrous connective tissue and an inner osteogenic layer of undifferentiated progenitor cells that can form bone during growth or fracture healing (**Figure 2**). Cartilage cells cover the subchondral bone. The endosteal and trabecular surfaces are covered with a single cell layer, which consists primarily of a flat, inactive cell type known as a bone lining cell. In ar-

eas of active bony metabolism the surfaces are lined with either bone-forming osteoblast cells or bone-resorbing osteoclast cells (**Figure 1**).

Flat bones, including the skull, scapula, pelvis, and mandible, vary from being purely cortical in thin regions to having a cortical shell with an internal layer of trabecular bone in thicker regions. Short bones such as the vertebrae, sternum, carpal bones, and tarsi are composed primarily of trabecular bone. The vertebrae have a thin shell of "compact" bone, which consists solely of densely packed trabeculae with no true cortical structure. The other short bones have a thin shell of true cortical bone.

Neurovascular Supply
Blood supply is critical to bone maintenance and bone healing as well as bone marrow function. Long bones receive nutrition from several arteries. Nutrient arteries pass obliquely through a foramen in the diaphyseal cortex to

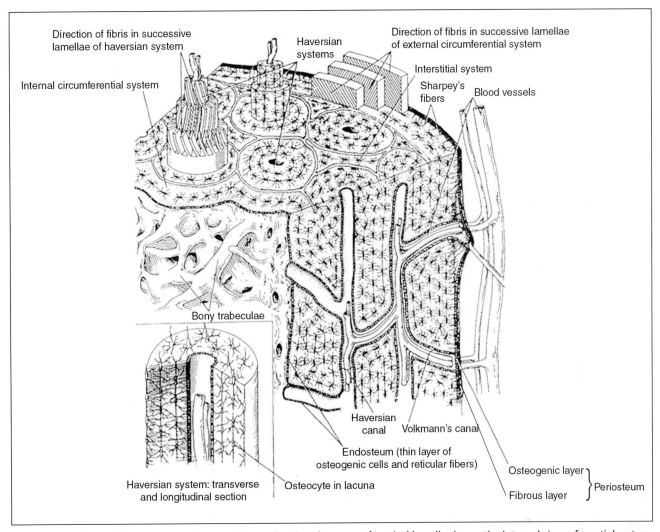

Figure 2   Diagram of the structure of cortical bone, showing the types of cortical lamellar bone: the internal circumferential system, interstitial system, osteonal lamellae, and outer circumferential system. The diagram also shows the intraosseous vascular system that serves the osteocytes and connects the periosteal and medullary blood vessels. The haversian canals run primarily longitudinally through the cortex, whereas the Volkmann's canals create oblique connections between the haversian canals. Cement lines separate each osteon from the surrounding bone. Periosteum covers the external surface of the bone and consists of two layers: an osteogenic (inner) cellular layer and a fibrous (outer) layer. *(Reproduced with permission from Kessel RG, Kardon RH: Tissues and Organs: A Text-Atlas of Scanning Microscopy. New York, NY, WH Freeman, 1979, p 25.)*

enter the intramedullary canal. They branch after entering the intramedullary canal to supply the inner two thirds of the diaphyseal cortex. This endosteal blood supply is at risk of injury during intramedullary reaming. The nonarticular surfaces of bone are covered by a tissue layer known as the periosteal membrane. Arteries from the periosteal membrane enter the body of the bone at various points and supply the outer third of the cortex of the diaphysis. These arteries arise from the nutrient artery before passing into the cortex, and from vessels in the muscle surrounding the bone. The periosteal blood supply may be damaged by periosteal stripping from fracture or in exposing the bone during surgery. The periarticular plexus primarily supplies the ends of the bone through metaphyseal and epiphyseal arteries. Blood vessels supply cortical

bone through channels in the bone tissue known as haversian and Volkmann's canals, but do not enter the hard tissue of the trabecular bone. Trabecular bone receives nutrition from the blood supply in the marrow space by diffusion through the tissue. Nerves from the periosteum enter the bone alongside arteries, and are found alongside blood vessels in the haversian and Volkmann's canals.

Trabecular Bone Structure

Trabecular bone tissue is organized into a network of plates and/or rods. Plates are generally flat, thin, and wide whereas rods are cylindrical. Collectively, the rods and plates are called struts. Both of these structures have a maximum thickness of approximately 200 microns, which approximates twice the maximum distance that nutrients can diffuse into the bone tissue. The macroscopic spaces between the struts make trabecular bone quite porous (greater porosity means fewer or thinner struts). The spaces between the struts are filled with the contents of the bone marrow as described in subsequent paragraphs. The macroscopic porosity of trabecular bone varies from about 30% to 90%, depending on anatomic location and health of the bone. For example, in osteoporosis bone resorption leads to thinning of the trabecular struts and a resulting increase in macroscopic porosity

The organization of trabecular bone into plates and rods and their orientation to one another creates a distinctive architecture. As discussed in the mechanical properties section, this architecture has important implications for the mechanical properties of the trabecular bone in both health and disease. For example, the unique architecture of trabecular bone may make it ideally suited to act as a "shock absorber" around joints to protect the articular cartilage. Trabecular bone architecture can be quantified using such important clinical measures as the bone volume fraction (volume of mineralized tissue per total volume of marrow and bone space), trabecular number (average number of trabecular struts in an area or volume), trabecular thickness (average thickness of the trabecular struts), and anisotropy (the degree of orientation of the trabecular struts in three-dimensional space). Although bone volume fraction cannot be measured without biopsy, bone mineral density (such as a dual-energy x-ray absorptiometry measurement) is a surrogate measure used clinically to define osteoporosis. The number of trabecular struts and their thickness decrease in osteoporosis, contributing to weaker bone. In addition, patients with osteoporosis who have femoral neck fractures have increased anisotropy of the trabecular bone in the femoral neck region compared with that found in the corresponding region in osteoporosis patients without fracture.

Cortical Bone Structure

Cortical bone is a type of compact bone. In contrast to trabecular bone, compact bone is extremely dense with no macroscopic spaces and, therefore, has very low porosity. Other examples of compact bone are the vertebral compact bone shell previously described and subchondral bone, which is a thin, perforated compact bone plate. Both of these bone types differ from cortical bone in their structure as well as their tissue organization, which will be described in the next section. The macrostructure of cortical bone varies by anatomic location. The cortical bone in the diaphysis is organized as a thick-walled cylinder surrounding the intramedullary canal and acts as a load-bearing segment. There is relatively little trabecular bone. In the metaphysis and epiphysis (and in flat bones), the cortical bone acts as a shell serving as a thin constraining border to the trabecular bone which, in turn, carries the majority of the load. The cortical shell carries only a small

fraction of the load, but because it allows mechanical forces to be spread more evenly across the trabecular bone it makes a very large contribution to the mechanical function of this region.

Tissue Organization

Trabecular and cortical bone differ not only in their gross/macroscopic structure, but also, at the microscopic level, in the organization of the tissue making up the cortical bone and trabecular struts. Bone tissue is primarily ECM, which is a composite of organic molecules such as collagen and inorganic mineral. Osteocytes are cells embedded within the substance of the matrix. In addition, the spaces in the matrix for the osteocytes and their cell processes have important effects on the tissue structure and function. These components are organized in various ways to create discrete bone tissue types.

Woven Bone Tissue

Initial bone tissue, or primary bone, is formed de novo, where there previously was no bone. Examples include the initial bone formation in the embryo, bone growth, fracture callus, heterotopic ossification, and bone formed by tumors. Primary bone is usually composed of woven bone tissue. The exception occurs with the circumferential bone growth described in the next paragraph. In microscopic evaluation of woven bone, the collagen and mineral appear randomly oriented, and there is no clear organization of the osteocytes. Woven bone is subsequently remodeled into an organized tissue by the removal of primary bone and deposition of secondary bone. This new, remodeled bone has a very different organization than woven bone and is referred to as lamellar bone.

Lamellar Bone Tissue

In contrast to the poorly organized woven bone, lamellar bone is organized into layers, called lamellae. Lamellae are 3 to 7 microns thick and are visible by imaging modalities such as polarized light microscopy. The reasons for this layered appearance remain somewhat controversial, but appear to be related to differences in the density or orientation of collagen fibers or other ECM components. Lamellae are usually formed as a result of the remodeling process by removal of a region of bone and subsequent addition of layers of new bone. Secondary bone tissue, thus, is always lamellar. Primary bone, on the other hand, is usually woven, but can sometimes be lamellar. For example, as a bone grows circumferentially, circumferential lamellae are formed around the outer surface of the bone by cells from the periosteal membrane (**Figure 2**). The differences in woven and lamellar bone tissue impart them with distinct, physiologically important functions. Woven bone is formed rapidly, an important attribute during growth and fracture healing. In addition, woven bone is less mineralized with smaller crystals than lamellar bone, which may make it easier to remove in the remodeling

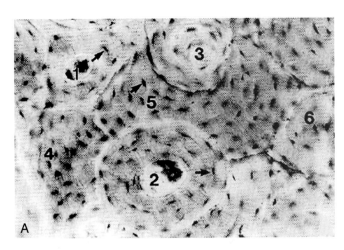 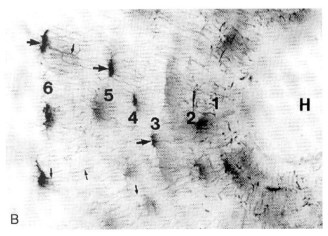

Figure 3   Electron photomicrographs of cortical bone. **A,** A thin-ground cross section of human cortical bone in which osteocyte lacunae (arrows) and canaliculi have been stained with India ink. Osteocytes are arranged around a central vascular channel to constitute haversian systems. Active haversian systems (1, 2, and 3) have concentric lamellae in this plane. Older haversian systems (4, 5, and 6) have had parts of their original territories invaded and remodeled. This is seen most clearly where 2 and 3 have invaded the territory originally occupied by 5. (Original magnification: X185.) **B,** Higher magnification of part of a haversian system showing the successive layering (numbers) of osteocytes (large arrows) from the central core (H) that contains the vasculature. Small arrows identify the canaliculi that connect osteocyte lacunae in different layers. (Original magnification: X718.) *(Reproduced with permission from Marks SC, Odgren PR: Structure and development of the skeleton, in Bilezikian JP, Raisz LG, Rodan GA (eds):* Principles of Bone Biology, ed 2. *San Diego, CA, Academic Press, 2002, pp 3-15.)*

process. Lamellar bone is formed more slowly than woven bone, but its organized structure imparts improved mechanical properties, which are critical for mature bone tissue function.

Cortical Lamellar Bone

Lamellar tissue has a distinctly different geometry in cortical versus trabecular bone. Secondary cortical bone is organized into osteons (also called haversian systems) that are cylindrical structures of concentric lamellae (**Figures 2 and 3**). Osteons are generally 3 to 6 mm long, and approximately 150 to 200 microns in diameter. At the center of the osteon is a small cylindrical space called the haversian canal, through which blood vessels and poorly myelinated nerve fibers pass. Volkmann's canals are similar, but run approximately perpendicular to the haversian canals and connect haversian canals to each other or to the bone surface. The haversian and Volkmann's canals contribute a small amount of porosity (5% to 10%) to the cortical bone tissue. Osteons have a specific orientation, reflective of the mechanical demand on the bone. Their orientation is aligned along axes of load most frequently experienced in a given area of the bone in question, generally along the mechanical axis.

Each osteon is bounded by a "cement line" (described below) that separates it from adjacent osteonal or nonosteonal tissue such as circumferential and interstitial lamellae. Interstitial lamellae appear as sections of lamellar bone between fully formed osteons. They are the remnants of osteons that remain after a region of cortical bone has been remodeled. Circumferential lamellae, an example of primary lamellar bone that does not arise

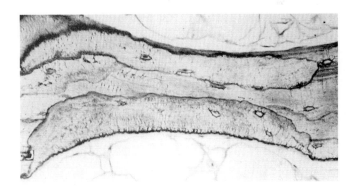

Figure 4   A part of a trabecula showing two packets (hemiosteons) separated by scalloped cement lines with the intervening interstitial lamellae. *(Reproduced with permission from Fleisch H:* Bisphosphonates in Bone Disease: From the Laboratory to the Patient. *New York, NY, Parthenon Publishing Group, 1997.)*

from remodeling, are formed on the periosteal surface of bone, and encircle the bone.

Trabecular Lamellar Bone

As in cortical lamellar tissue, trabecular lamellar bone is organized into lamellae bounded by cement lines. The geometry of the lamellae, however, is quite different and reflects the differences in the way trabecular and cortical bone are remodeled. The cortical lamellae are organized into concentric rings, whereas the trabecular lamellae are relatively flat structures that lie roughly parallel to the trabecular strut surface. Trabecular lamellae form discrete "packets" of bone tissue (**Figure 4**). The region defined as a trabecular packet is the structure resulting from a localized cycle of remodeling initiated at the surface of a trabecular strut. Like the osteon, the trabecular packet is separated from adjacent bone tissue by a cement line, and on average is approximately 1 mm long and 50 microns thick.

Lacunae/Canaliculi

The spaces in bone tissue make an important contribution to the mechanical properties and behavior of the tissue. All bone tissue, be it woven or lamellar, contains numerous cells, known as osteocytes, embedded within the mineralized matrix (Figures 1 through 3). They reside in ellipsoidal spaces in the bone tissue called lacunae. Lacunae are small but numerous, approximately 15,000 per mm^3 of bone and comprise 1% of the bone volume. They are distributed throughout the bone tissue and recent studies suggest that their size and number may vary as a function of anatomic location and health state of the bone. Many cracks have been found to end in lacunae, so it is possible that they may act as crack arrestors, contributing to the prevention of crack propagation. Lacunae are connected to each other by canaliculi, which are minute channels through the bone tissue (Figure 3, B). Canaliculi also extend to bone surfaces and haversian canals (Figure 2, inset). Osteocyte cell processes travel through the canaliculi to interconnect with other osteocytes and cells on the bone surfaces. This network allows the transport of oxygen and nutrients to the osteocytes, and removal of wastes. This process is critical because the mineralized matrix is impermeable to the diffusion of nutrients.

Cement Lines

Cement lines, also called "reversal" lines (described in the remodeling section), appear in both cortical and trabecular secondary bone. They are 1 to 2 microns thick, and are believed to be low in collagen content compared with adjacent bone. Cement lines form the border of remodeled lamellar bone. Their purpose is unclear, although there is evidence to suggest that, like lacunae, cement lines may stop crack propagation. Osteocyte processes (and canaliculi) rarely cross the cement line, meaning that nutrients and chemical signals may not be efficiently transferred from one osteon or trabecular packet to another. This concept has significant implications for the bone tissue that is cut off from a vascular supply during remodeling (or pathologic processes such as fracture or infection), because death of the osteocytes may occur because of lack of nutrients.

Although it is clear that the bone tissue in trabecular and cortical bone is arranged differently, the actual ECM itself appears to be the same. The ECM of bone is fascinating in that it not only plays a structural role as one of the primary determinants of the unique material properties of bone, but also plays a critical role in regulating the biologic behavior of bone.

Extracellular Matrix
Bone Matrices

Bone is relatively less cellular than other tissues and is primarily composed of ECM. Bone ECM is a composite material of mineral, protein, water, salts, lipids, glycoproteins, and proteoglycans. It is formed primarily by osteoblasts (bone-forming cells). As an organ, bone is composed of a mixture of distinct types of extracellular matrices that include the mineralized bone ECM, osteoid (similar to bone but unmineralized), and lacunar ECM (the matrix that surrounds the osteocytes). The lacunar matrix presumably extends through the canalicular network of the osteocytes.

Osteoid is the provisional matrix that subsequently becomes mineralized to form bone. A small percentage of total bone volume is osteoid except in disorders of undermineralization, such as osteomalacia. Osteoid is generally found in areas of new bone formation as well as in a very thin layer over mature bone surfaces where it may play a critical role in regulating remodeling. The lacunar matrix is poorly characterized because of the technical difficulty in directly separating this specific matrix from mineralized bone. Lacunar-canalicular ECM is rich in proteoglycans and unmineralized, and its contribution to the mechanical as well as the biologic environment of osteocytes may be an important regulator of their function.

Mineralized Bone ECM Components
Overview

The mineralized bone matrix comprises most bone matrix and largely defines the bone tissue material properties. In contrast to the lacunar and osteoid matrices, mature bone ECM contains a significant inorganic mineral component in addition to the organic component. The mineral makes up 60% to 70% of the tissue. It is primarily calcium, phosphate, and other associated ions, including sodium, magnesium, and carbonate. The ions are found as salts in the form of hydroxyapatite and tricalcium phosphate. The organic matrix comprises approximately 20% to 25% of the tissue; 90% of this organic ECM is type I collagen and 5% is noncollagenous proteins. There are other minor collagen types present as well, including types III and V. Numerous noncollagenous proteins have either been purified from bone or are produced by osteoblasts in culture, including osteocalcin, bone sialoprotein, proteoglycans, and matricellular proteins. Bone morphogenetic proteins (BMPs) and other growth factors also are incorporated into the mineralized matrix. The remaining tissue volume is occupied by water. All mineralized bone surfaces are overlaid with a thin layer of unmineralized osteoid.

ECM has a distinct structural and biologic contribution to bone form and function. It has long been recognized that the mineralized matrix provides the material properties required for the mechanical function of bone.

More recently it has become apparent that the ECM also plays a dynamic role in regulating bone cell behavior and that there is cross talk between bone matrix and bone cells. Because the effect of bone matrix on bone cell biology is an important determinant of the structure and mechanical behavior of bone, the structural and biologic roles of the ECM are linked. It is now recognized that ECM plays a role in tissue development, acts as a scaffold for cells, regulates osteoblast, osteocyte, and osteoclast behavior, regulates diffusion of other macromolecules and ions, and can bind to and modulate the activity of growth factors and proteases. In the subsequent sections, components of the bone matrix will be discussed in the context of the structural and/or modulatory roles they play in skeletal physiology.

Collagen

Collagen is the most abundant protein in mammals. There are more than 20 types of collagens with a fascinating array of structures and functions. Most of the collagen found in bone is type I. Immature woven bone, and to a lesser degree lamellar bone, also contain small amounts of type III and type V collagen. Type X collagen is associated with hypertrophic chondrocytes in mineralizing cartilage such as in the growth plate. Type I collagen is a fibril-forming collagen with a triple helical structure as are types III and V. The assembly of type I collagen into fibrils contributes tremendous tensile strength to the bone ECM. Nonfibrillar collagens also exist. Some of these collagen types have short triple helical regions, whereas others form very different structures such as sheets. Some of these are fibril-associated collagens and serve to regulate the assembly, structure, and/or function of the fibrillar collagens. Others act independently of the fibrillar collagens. The fibrillar collagens themselves can also interact. Type V is generally found in association with type I collagen and is believed to regulate the size of the fibrils it forms. Type V collagen mutations in mice result in disorganization of the type I collagen fibrils. The exact function of type III collagen is not known but it seems to localize near soft-tissue attachments to bone. Mutations in humans cause a severe form of Ehlers-Danlos syndrome.

All fibrillar collagens are trimeric, composed of three α chains arranged in a helical structure. The molecule can exist as a homotrimer or as a heterotrimer – composed of different types of α chains. Type I collagen, for example, is composed of two α1 chains and one α2 chain. They are coded for by different genes but have similar protein structure. The individual collagen chains have a very unusual composition and structure. Most of each α chain is a repeating triplet of amino acids of the sequence (glycine-X-Y)n, where X is often proline and Y is often hydroxyproline, such that approximately one third of the amino acids are proline and every third is glycine. These repeating triplets are located centrally in the molecule, and are flanked by nonhelical domains at the amino and

carboxyl termini. The high proline content confers a completely unique primary protein structure to the collagen monomer. Because of stearic repulsion from the many prolines, an extended chain is formed that is elongated and rigid compared with the α helical motifs found commonly in proteins. This chain is one of the longest but smallest diameter proteins known. Ultimately three of these chains will wrap together to form procollagen, a central triple helix flanked by globular domains called propeptides. Because of the extended nature of the individual α chains there is very little space in the center of the triple helix. In fact, glycine, which is the smallest amino acid, is the only amino acid that can be accommodated in this region. Thus, every third amino acid residue of each chain must be a glycine.

Another unusual feature of the type I collagen that is critical for its structure and function is that it becomes posttranslationally modified in a unique way. For the collagen molecule to reach the ECM where it functions, it must pass through the secretory pathway of the cell. As an α chain is being synthesized it is translocated across the membrane and into the lumen of the endoplasmic reticulum, an intracellular organelle. In this compartment, enzymes begin to modify the amino acids of the protein. These modifications include hydroxylation of proline and lysine as well as the addition of unusual sugar groups. Collagen is the only protein containing significant amounts of hydroxyproline, and urinary detection of this molecule is a specific marker of collagen breakdown that can be used clinically. The hydroxylation modifications contribute greatly to the stability of the triple helix. The enzymes prolyl hydroxylase and lysyl hydroxylase require ascorbate (vitamin C) to catalyze the hydroxylation of proline and lysine. In the absence of ascorbate the collagen helix has a lower melting point, and extreme fragility of the connective tissues results in the disease called scurvy.

The modification process is terminated when three α chains wind into a helix such that the modification enzymes can no longer access the proper areas of the amino acids. The amount of modification is dependent on the speed with which the helix forms. In the bone fragility disorder osteogenesis imperfecta, there is often a mutation of a glycine residue in type I collagen to a larger amino acid. This mutation slows the folding of the α chains into the triple helix so that the resulting procollagen molecule becomes overmodified. The cell recognizes this as an abnormal molecule and retains it in the cell for degradation. As a result, there is decreased collagen secreted into the ECM, weaker bone matrix, and severely decreased mechanical integrity of bone.

Normal procollagen molecules continue through the secretory pathway to reach the extracellular space. There the nascent collagen propeptides are cleaved by specific propeptidases to yield the collagen molecule also known as tropocollagen. Outside of the cell, many collagen triple helices then spontaneously assemble into large complexes

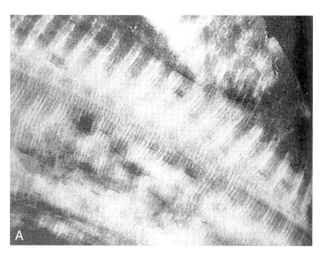
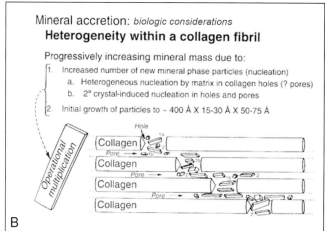

Figure 5 Collagen and mineralization. **A,** Electron photomicrograph of collagen fibrils. **B,** Diagram describing mineral accretion. *(Reproduced from Bostrom MPG, Boskey A, Kaufman JK, Einhorn TA: Form and function of bone, in Buckwalter JA, Einhorn TA, Simon SR (eds):* Orthopaedic Basic Science: Biology and Biomechanics of the Musculoskeletal System, *ed 2. Rosemont, IL, American Academy of Orthopaedic Surgeons, 2000, pp 320-369.)*

called collagen fibrils (**Figure 5**). This process was prevented from occurring prematurely inside the cell by the propeptides on either end of the triple helix. In some types of Ehlers-Danlos syndrome, absence of one of the procollagen peptidases results in retention of one of the propeptides on the triple helix and disorganized fibril assembly, leading to the characteristic loss of connective tissue integrity found in this disorder.

Collagen fibrils are intrinsically stable because of noncovalent lateral interactions between helices, but are strengthened further by interchain, covalent cross-links that form between lysine residues. The resulting cross-linked collagen fibrils have tensile strength on the order of steel. The cross-linking is catalyzed by the enzyme lysyl oxidase. This process can be regulated to vary the rigidity of the fibrils in different tissues. A mutation in lysyl oxidase causes another type of Ehlers-Danlos syndrome, and urinary detection of pyridinoline breakdown products of the cross-links is a useful clinical marker of bone resorption. Collagen fibrils can be quite large, up to 50 nm in diameter and 1 micron in length, and easily seen on electron microscopy. Many fibrils combine to form collagen fibers that are several microns in diameter and are visible by light microscopy. In osteogenesis imperfecta, because less collagen is secreted, the diameter of the fibrils and fibers is reduced.

Inorganic Matrix and Mineralization
As previously described, the ECM is approximately 70% mineralized and the mineral is responsible for the compressive strength of bone. The inorganic mineral component of bone is closely associated with the collagen fibrils. The tropocollagen helices in the fibrils are organized in a regular, quarter-staggered arrangement that creates empty regions between their ends every 680 Å (**Figure 5,** *B).* These

hole zones give rise to the banded appearance of the fibrils on electron microscopy (**Figure 5,** *A).* The hole zones communicate with pore regions running lengthwise between the collagen molecules. The mineral crystals are found in the pores and holes created by the quarter-staggered arrangement of the collagen fibril. The calcium phosphate compound hydroxyapatite is an analog of the predominant form of mineral in bone. Its chemical formula is $Ca_{10}(PO4)_6(OH)_2$. There are various substitutions possible in bone, such as fluoride for the hydroxide groups and strontium for calcium. These substitutions can have significant effects on bone quality.

The mineralization process itself is not completely understood but it is initiated by the nucleation of ions into a stable crystal, a relatively energetically unfavorable process. The high energy barrier of initiation is overcome by creating a favorable environment for nucleation in or around the hole zones by the presence of promoters of initiation such as biglycan and phosphoproteins such as bone sialoprotein (also known as bone sialoprotein 2). An alternative theory is that matrix vesicles produced by osteoblasts facilitate the nucleation process; however, they are found more remotely to the collagen than most of the mineral. Secondary nucleation then ensues from the surface of the initial crystals followed by crystal growth, which takes place in a multidirectional and branching manner along the pores of the collagen fibril, and agglomeration or fusion into larger crystals. This accretion of mineral mass is a much more energetically favorable reaction than formation of the initial crystal and is the means by which most of the mineral is deposited. The various steps in accretion of mineral are likely regulated by factors such as the local concentrations of ions, the mineralization promoters, and mineralization inhibitors in the ECM and possibly the osteoblasts.

Noncollagenous ECM Proteins

Vitamin K-Dependent Proteins

Osteocalcin is the most prevalent noncollagenous protein in bone. Because of its high expression by mature osteoblasts, and absence in most other cell types, osteocalcin is a good marker of osteoblast differentiation. It is detectable in the urine and can be elevated with increased bone formation or conversely with increased bone resorption, which liberates the protein from the bony matrix. Osteocalcin (also known as bone gamma-carboxyglutamic acid-containing protein or bone Gla protein) is a member of a family of proteins that undergo posttranslational modification through gamma carboxylation of glutamic acid residues in a vitamin K-dependent step. Osteocalcin null mice have an increase in bone mass secondary to enhanced bone formation. The nature of this defect is not completely understood, but these null mice seem to have excessively mineralized bones with abnormally small crystals, giving rise to the theory that osteocalcin is involved in mineral maturation. In this regard, it is believed that the heavy net negative charge of osteocalcin from the carboxylation allows it to interact with positively charged mineral ions such as calcium. The other primary vitamin K-dependent protein is matrix Gla protein (MGP). MGP is not expressed exclusively in bone and the most significant phenotype of the MGP knockout mouse is severe vascular calcification. The MGP null mice are also osteopenic.

Adhesive Proteins

Adhesive proteins, such as fibronectin and vitronectin, facilitate the interaction of cells with the ECM. Adhesive proteins not only facilitate cell attachment but they can also promote a de-adhesion process that is important for cell migration. Both osteoclasts and osteoblasts must migrate to and along bone surfaces to carry out their respective functions. Adhesive ECM proteins interact with bone cells by binding to transmembrane protein receptors called integrins. These interactions have been shown to be important for both osteoblast and osteoclast cell function. Integrin receptors are heterodimeric proteins composed of a single α and a single β chain. Integrins mediate many ECM-cell interactions by binding to arginine-glycine-aspartic acid (RGD) domains on extracellular proteins. Intracellularly, they communicate directly with the cell's cytoskeleton through complexes called focal adhesions.

Fibronectin is a multidomain protein cross-linked by disulfide linkages. The molecule contains RGD domains that interact with cell surface integrin receptors, as well as domains that bind other ECM proteins, and domains for interchain cross-linking. Fibronectin is found throughout the body in various tissue matrices, and is also found in a soluble form in plasma. Fibronectin is found in bone and is likely involved in the interaction of osteoblasts with the osteoid matrix. Mice with a disrupted fibronectin gene die early in embryonic development, so the importance of fibronectin in bone has been demonstrated indirectly by targeting expression of a dominant-negative β-1 integrin receptor to bone cells. In this transgenic mouse, bone mass is significantly decreased. In cultures, osteoblasts from these mice show a failure to adhere to the substratum. Because other ECM proteins also interact with β-1 integrin, this is only indirect evidence about the importance of fibronectin. However, blocking of fibronectin in cell culture results in a failure of osteoblasts to survive. Thus, fibronectin is likely important for both osteoblast adhesion to bone surfaces as well as osteoblast survival.

Although fibronectin and β-1 integrin interactions appear to be crucial for osteoblast function, vitronectin is believed to play a role in the adhesion of osteoclasts to bone through the α-v/β-3 integrin receptor. Studies have clearly shown that blocking α-v/β-3 integrin inhibits osteoclast resorption of bone and this may be a clinically important drug target.

Matricellular Proteins

Matricellular proteins are a functional group of proteins that mediate cell-matrix interactions but are not required purely for adhesion and in many cases are de-adhesive. In addition, they are not primarily structural. Rather, matricellular proteins mediate and modulate signaling from the matrix to the cells. These molecules are characterized by gene disruptions in mice that have subtle but interesting phenotypes. Generally, these knockout bone phenotypes are more pronounced during tissue remodeling, such as during the healing process. This group includes thrombospondins (TSPs), osteopontin (OPN), tenascin, the CCN family of proteins, and secreted-protein acidic and rich in cysteine (SPARC), which is also known as osteonectin. Osteonectin and OPN are also phosphoproteins and may play a role in mineralization.

OPN, also known as bone sialoprotein 1, is a bone ECM protein that is expressed in high levels in bone, but is also present in many actively remodeling tissues. Because of its enhanced expression during tissue remodeling, OPN is believed to play an important role in the function of phagocytic cells such as macrophages and osteoclasts. Like all matricellular proteins, OPN has multiple domains, including an RGD. Like vitronectin, OPN binds to α-v/β-3 integrin through its RGD domain. Several studies of OPN null mice suggest that OPN likely functions in regulating osteoclast function. Osteoclasts purified from OPN null mice are less active in bone resorption. This is believed to be secondary to altered adhesion to α-v/β-3 integrin. In addition, OPN is a chemotactic factor for osteoclasts in culture. In animal models, estrogen depletion and decreased weight bearing stimulate bone resorption. OPN null mice show a decrease in bone resorption under these conditions, consistent with an osteoclast defect.

TSPs are a family of five proteins that have a broad tissue distribution including bone. TSP1 and TSP2 are produced by both osteoblasts and osteoblast precursors. TSP1 overexpression has been shown to increase osteoclast activity. Mice lacking TSP2 have increased bone mass because of an increase in the number of osteoblast progenitor cells and increased mineralization. TSP5 mutations are not associated directly with defects in bone, but mutations in the human TSP5 gene result in a dwarfing syndrome, pseudoachondroplasia.

SPARC (osteonectin) is abundant in bone but, like TSP1 and TSP2, SPARC has a broad tissue distribution and is not bone specific. The protein binds both collagen and mineral so it may play a role in mineralization. Mice with a gene disruption of SPARC have an increase in age-associated osteopenia and a decrease in the number of osteoblast progenitors. Thus, it may play a regulatory role in osteoblast differentiation as well as in mineralization.

Phosphoproteins

Some of the ECM proteins such as bone sialoprotein 2 (BSP), OPN, and SPARC are phosphorylated. Because the phosphate-derived negative charge can interact with calcium and because some of these proteins, like BSP, are localized to the hole zones in collagen fibers, they are believed to play a role in initiation, specifically nucleation, of mineralization. Consistent with this idea, BSP protein has been shown to nucleate crystal formation in vitro.

Growth Factors and Cytokines

ECM contains small quantities of biologically active molecules including growth factors such as BMPs, transforming growth factor-β (TGF-β), basic fibroblast growth factor (bFGF), and insulin-like growth factor (IGF), as well as cytokines such as interleukins (ILs), leukotrienes, and prostaglandins. The exact role these factors play in the ECM is not clear but they are potent regulators of bone cell differentiation and activity and may play a role in integration of bone cell function during bone remodeling. Therefore, the activity of these factors is discussed in more detail in the bone cell and remodeling sections.

Proteoglycans

Proteoglycans are found throughout the bone ECM and in the pericellular matrices surrounding the various bone cell types. Proteoglycans are molecules that are hybrids of protein and sugar. They are composed of a linear protein core that undergoes extensive posttranslational modification through the addition of glycosaminoglycan (GAG) side chains. GAGs are repeating disaccharide units composed of modified sugars. Proteoglycans differ from glycoproteins in that they are heavily modified by long chains of GAG, as opposed to having the short sugar residues found in glycoproteins. Different proteoglycans can have several different functions. They can act as selective sieves, provide tissue structure, bind to growth factors including TGF-β and bFGF, regulate cellular proliferation,

bind to cells, and act as receptors on the surface of cells.

The best characterized proteoglycan is aggrecan, which is an important structural component of articular cartilage. Proteoglycans are much less abundant in bone than in cartilage and play more of a regulatory role than a structural one. The proteoglycans that have been shown to be the most important in bone function include perlecan, decorin, biglycan, and syndecan. Perlecan, decorin, and biglycan are found in bone matrix and syndecan is a cell surface proteoglycan found on osteoblasts. Perlecan is a large proteoglycan that binds to bFGF and regulates the activity and formation of osteoblasts. Perlecan knockout mice have skeletal developmental defects that are characterized by a reduction in skeletal mass. Decorin and biglycan are members of a family of small leucine-rich proteoglycans. Decorin is primarily found in skin, but also is present in bone, whereas biglycan is found predominantly in bone. Decorin decorates collagen molecules and may play a role in fibril assembly. Biglycan is believed to promote initiation of mineralization and binds TGF-β. Biglycan-deficient mice have an age-associated osteopenia that seems to be associated with a decrease in the number of mesenchymal progenitor cells and may be caused by an alteration in TGF-β signaling.

In summary, the ECM is composed of a variety of different components. Some, typified by collagen and mineral, make a large structural contribution to the mechanical and structural integrity of bone. Others play more of a regulatory role, likely exerting their influence through effects on the cells of the bone. Because the bone cells synthesize/remove the bone tissue in such a way as to create its structural organization, matrix modulation of cellular behaviors such as attachment, mobility, proliferation, and signaling is an important determinant of bone structure and function. The following section will discuss the various bone cells and their respective roles in this process.

Bone Cells
Overview

The cells intimately associated with the bone matrix are the osteocytes, osteoblasts, osteoclasts, and the "bone lining cells" (**Figure 1**). They reside directly on the bone matrix or within its substance and regulate and/or carry out the synthesis and degradation of this matrix. Many other cell types, however, also reside in and around the bone proper. Internally, these constitute the cells of the bone marrow. Externally, along the periosteal bone surface, they constitute the cells of the periosteal membrane. The marrow contains numerous different cell types including marrow stromal cells (some of which can give rise to the cells of the osteoblast linage), the cells of the hematopoietic system (some of which can act as osteoclast precursors), and adipocytes or fat cells. This section will focus on the bone-forming cells (osteoblasts), the bone resorbing cells (osteoclasts), and the cells that live within the substance of the mineralized matrix itself (osteocytes). New concepts regarding the potential importance of other cell types to bone form and function will be discussed briefly at the end of this section.

Osteoblast Lineage
Osteoblasts

Osteoblast Morphology and Function

The mature osteoblast is a cuboidal cell with an eccentrically placed nucleus that resides on the bone surface. It is characterized by a variety of molecular "markers" that help distinguish it from other cell types. Alkaline phosphatase is highly expressed in mature osteoblasts as well as some precursors. It is also found in many other cells and many other tissue types, but a cell on a bone surface that stains strongly for alkaline phosphatase can be considered to be an osteoblast. Osteocalcin is the most specific marker of the osteoblast phenotype and is expressed only in mature osteoblasts. Other markers include cell surface receptors for the hormones that act on osteoblasts, such as the parathyroid hormone (PTH) receptor, as well as transcription factors and the molecules that osteoblasts secrete, such as type I collagen. The matrix proteins osteocalcin, osteonectin, and OPN are other markers of the osteoblast phenotype.

The osteoblast has two clearly distinct roles: to form bone matrix and to regulate the activity of bone removal by osteoclasts to balance or couple the processes of bone formation and resorption. This critical function will be discussed in detail in the remodeling section. With respect to bone formation, the osteoblast is an efficient synthetic machine, able to synthesize and secrete large quantities of the macromolecules found in the organic part of the matrix. In order for these macromolecules to reach the extracellular space, they must pass through the series of membranous intracellular organelles that comprise the secretory apparatus. This pathway begins in the rough endoplasmic reticulum and leads through the Golgi complex and secretory vesicles. This system is highly developed in the osteoblast. Osteoblasts are polarized cells with an eccentrically located nucleus. They sense hormones and other signaling molecules at their apical surface and secrete matrix at their basal surface. This allows for vectorial discharge of secreted molecules onto the bony surface upon which the cell is sitting, and results in the lamellar pattern of matrix deposition seen in secondary or remodeled bone.

Recent work has determined that signaling through low-density lipoprotein receptor-related protein 5 (LRP5) is a critical regulator of osteoblast matrix production. LRP5 is a critical component of the Wnt/Frizzled signal transduction pathway known to be important in a variety of processes such as cancer, metastasis to bone, apoptosis, and cellular proliferation. LRP5 is a transmembrane protein found on the surface of osteoblasts. It plays an important role in regulating osteoblast proliferation as well as regulating the amount of bone matrix synthesized by the mature osteoblast. Signaling through LRP5 appears to be required for maintenance of normal bone mass. Complete loss of LRP5 function results in the disease osteoporosis-pseudoglioma, which is characterized by low bone mass with extreme skeletal fragility and deformity. Alternatively, mutations in LRP5 that increase signaling through this pathway have been isolated from families that carry a trait for abnormally high bone mass. This high bone mass seems to protect affected individuals from fractures even with very advanced age. Other factors also seem to help regulate activity of the mature osteoblast. For example, IGF-1 is a growth factor that enhances osteoblast differentiation, but also seems to stimulate bone formation by the mature osteoblast.

In addition to secreting the components of the organic matrix, osteoblasts are believed to play a role in matrix mineralization. During this process, granules of calcium phosphate are visible in the mitochondria of the osteoblast as well as in structures called matrix vesicles that form from the plasma membrane surface of the cell. As previously described, initiation of mineralization is energetically unfavorable compared with the subsequent growth of the mineral crystals. Matrix vesicles may facilitate this process and make it more energetically favorable by concentrating calcium and phosphate in an appropriate environment containing phosphatases such as alkaline phosphatase as well as calcium binding proteins and by excluding mineralization inhibitors.

Osteoblast Differentiation

Osteoblasts are part of a developmental continuum including the bone lining cells and the osteocytes. These three cell types arise from cells of mesenchymal origin residing in the marrow that are known as marrow stromal cells (MSCs). In humans, these cells are characterized by the presence of the STRO-1 antigen. MSCs have the capacity to give rise to a variety of mesenchymally derived cells, in addition to those of the osteoblast lineage, including fibroblasts, adipocytes, myocytes, and chondrocytes. For this reason, they are also referred to as mesenchymal stem cells (also abbreviated MSC) and have tremendous therapeutic potential. Unlike a true stem cell, MSCs lose their capacity for differentiation, as well as for proliferation, over time. It is presumed that a true stem cell, with unlimited capacity for self renewal, exists upstream of MSCs; however, this is unknown.

Osteoblasts on the periosteal surfaces arise from the cells of the periosteal membrane. The periosteal membrane lines the external surfaces of the bone, except for the articular portions. It has an inner, cellular layer and an outer, fibrous layer (**Figure 2**). The inner or cambial layer of the periosteum contains cells that have bone-forming potential. This periosteal bone-forming activity gives rise

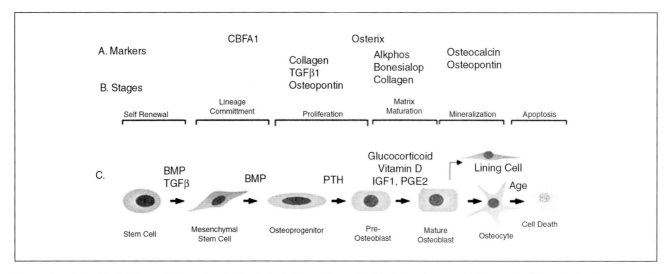

A. Markers

CBFA1   Osterix

Collagen   Alkphos   Osteocalcin
TGFβ1   Bonesialop   Osteopontin
Osteopontin   Collagen

B. Stages

Self Renewal   Lineage Committment   Proliferation   Matrix Maturation   Mineralization   Apoptosis

C.

BMP TGFβ   BMP   PTH   Glucocorticoid Vitamin D IGF1, PGE2   Lining Cell   Age

Stem Cell   Mesenchymal Stem Cell   Osteoprogenitor   Pre-Osteoblast   Mature Osteoblast   Osteocyte   Cell Death

Figure 6   Osteoblast differentiation. An idealized depiction of the osteoblast developmental lineage to illustrate the key concepts of early proliferation versus terminal phenotypic differentiation, the temporal onset of molecular markers, and important regulators of this process as well as the different fates possible for cells of the osteoblastic lineage. *(Adapted with permission from Lian JB, Stein GS, Aubin JE: Bone formation: Maturation and functional activities of osteoblast lineage cells, in Favus MJ (ed): Primer on the Metabolic Bone Diseases and Disorders of Mineral Metabolism, ed 5. Washington, DC, American Society for Bone and Mineral Research, 2003, pp 13-28.)*

to the circumferential lamellae (**Figure 2**) formed during radial growth of the bone and is important in fracture healing. The relationship of the cambrial layer cells to the previously described MSCs and osteoprogenitor cells is unknown, but they do have the ability to differentiate into other cell types besides osteoblasts, such as chondrocytes. This characteristic may be important for the periosteal contribution to fracture healing

For precursor cells to begin osteoblastic differentiation, there must be an induction step to initiate the process. Subsequently there must be a commitment toward the osteoblastic phenotype as opposed to these cells developing into adipocytes or chondrocytes.

A cell committed to osteoblastic differentiation is referred to as an osteoprogenitor cell. These cells go through a temporally programmed sequence of molecular events, causing them to progress from osteoprogenitor to preosteoblast to the fully synthetically active osteoblast itself (**Figure 6**). The proliferative potential of cells early in the lineage is high, but decreases as differentiation progresses, so that mature osteoblasts do not divide. LRP5, TGF-β, and IGF-1 play a role in regulation of proliferation. Each stage of differentiation is characterized by molecular markers such as cell surface receptors, transcription factors, or secreted matrix proteins. Cellular morphology changes from the spindle-shaped MSCs to the progressively larger and more cuboidal mature cells (**Figure 7**). In addition, the spatial localization of the cells changes such that the immature cells in the marrow move progressively closer to the bone surface as they progress along their lineage toward mature osteoblasts (**Figure 7**).

The factors that induce MSCs to begin differentiation

toward any given fate are not completely understood. This process may be regulated in part by the BMPs. The BMPs are members of the TGF-β super family of proteins, and are important in many aspects of skeletal development. The importance of BMPs in osteoblast differentiation is demonstrated by the finding that they can induce bone formation when injected into animals and greatly stimulate osteoblastic differentiation of MSC and other precursors in tissue culture. In addition, alterations in BMP function have been identified in human bone diseases. An activating mutation in the BMP receptor ACVR1 causes the disease fibrodysplasia ossificans progressiva, in which excess bone formation takes place heterotopically. In a mouse model, the BMP antagonist Noggin blocks the disease phenotype. Furthermore, genetic loss of another such antagonist, sclerostin (SOST), causes the disease sclerosteosis, characterized by massive overgrowth of both trabecular and cortical bone, which causes gigantism, distortion of the facies, and nerve entrapment. The properties of BMP that drive osteoblast differentiation and bone formation give it great potential for applications in orthopaedics and tissue engineering. BMP is now used clinically to promote bone formation in spine fusions and fracture nonunions.

The factors that control commitment by a differentiating cell to one of the specific cell type lineages (such as bone, fat, or cartilage) are also unknown. BMP does not lead to commitment to the osteoblastic lineage as it also promotes differentiation of MSC into other cell types such as chondrocytes. TGF-β stimulates osteoblastic differentiation because it promotes proliferation of early precursor cells. Like BMP, TGF-β does not direct cells to

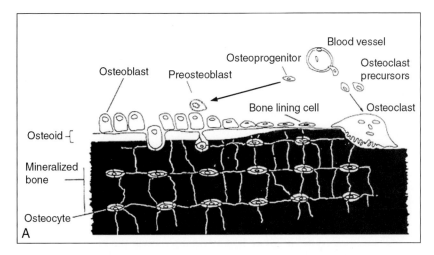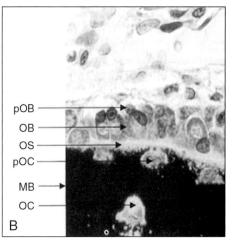

Figure 7   Bone cell organization and activities. **A,** The origins and locations of bone cells. *(Adapted with permission from Marks SC Jr, Popoff SN: Bone cell biology: The regulation of development, structure, and function in the skeleton. Am J Anat 1988;183:1-44.)* **B,** Cellular organization of bone formation: pOB, preosteoblast; OB, osteoblasts; OS, osteoid; pOC, preosteocytes; MB, mineralized bone matrix; OC, osteocyte. *(Adapted with permission from Lian JB, Stein GS, Aubin JE: Bone formation: Maturation and functional activities of osteoblast lineage cells, in Favus MJ (ed): Primer on the Metabolic Bone Diseases and Disorders of Mineral Metabolism, ed 5. Washington, DC, American Society for Bone and Mineral Research, 2003, pp 13-28.)*

commit to the osteoblast lineage, however, because later in the differentiation process, it actually inhibits osteoblast differentiation and drives cells toward the chondroblast lineage.

Following commitment to the osteoblast lineage, differentiation is driven by several factors that regulate cell division (early) and differentiation (late). Recent work on osteoblast differentiation has identified two factors essential to this process. Runx 2 (formerly called Cbfa 1) and Osterix are transcription factors that control the expression of genes that are required for a cell to function as an osteoblast. Their function is so critical that mice deficient in the production of either of these transcription factors have skeletons completely composed of cartilage, representing a defect in both intramembranous and endochondral ossification. Runx 2 seems to act upstream of Osterix and is required for Osterix expression. As such, Runx 2 is considered a "master regulator" of osteoblast differentiation. In humans, loss of a single copy of Runx 2 leads to a defect of intramembranous bone formation resulting in the disease cleidocranial dysostosis, which is characterized by pubic diastasis, coxa vara, absence of the clavicle, and defects in cranial bone formation. Other factors such as IGF-1 are not essential for osteoblast differentiation but seem to be important in the efficiency of the process.

The mature osteoblast has a limited lifespan with a half-life of approximately 100 days, during which it will continue to synthesize osteoid under the global control of hormonal and mechanical influences. Ultimately, the mature osteoblast has several potential fates (Figure 6). It can remain on the bone surface and transform into a bone lining cell. It can become embedded in the matrix that it has synthesized and become an osteocyte. Alternatively, it can

die by apoptosis (programmed cell death). Regulation of apoptosis is an important factor in determining the balance between bone formation and resorption. Bone-forming activity can be enhanced by factors such as IGF-1 and PTH that prolong osteoblast survival. Because the mature osteoblast cells do not divide, new osteoblasts to replace those with alternate fates must arise in another fashion. These new osteoblasts can arise through the differentiation of precursor cells into new osteoblasts, or from activation of bone lining cells.

Bone Lining Cells

Osteoblasts that do not undergo apoptosis or become embedded as osteocytes go on to become what are referred to as "bone lining cells". As mentioned previously, all bone surfaces are lined with cells. In areas of active bone formation the surface is lined with osteoblasts. In areas of bone resorption the bone surface is lined with osteoclasts. Most trabecular and endosteal bone surfaces, however, are not metabolically active and these are covered by the bone lining cells. They are thin, flattened cells adhering closely to the surface of the bone (Figure 8). They are much less metabolically active than the osteoblast and have lost the cell volume, polarization, and synthetic machinery of their osteoblastic precursors. The function of bone lining cells remains unknown. They likely have the ability to become "reactivated" as functional osteoblasts and thus act as a reservoir for bone-forming potential. In addition, by covering bone surfaces the bone lining cells may physically control the ability of osteoclasts to initiate resorption in bone remodeling. They may also play a role in remodeling by cleaning out resorption pits left by osteoclasts so that new bone can be deposited.

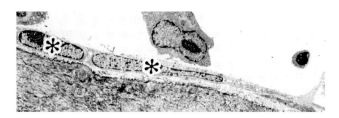

Figure 8   Transmission electron micrograph of bone lining cells (asterisks). These flat cells have few organelles and form a thin cellular layer on inactive bone surfaces that is often hard to resolve by light microscopy. (Original magnification: X3000.) *(Reproduced with permission from Marks SC, Odgren PR: Structure and development of the skeleton, in Bilezikian JP, Raisz LG, Rodan GA (eds): Principles of Bone Biology, ed 2. San Diego, CA, Academic Press, 2002, pp 3-15.)*

Osteocytes

Approximately one third of the actively secreting osteoblasts will become embedded in the mineralizing matrix to become osteocytes. It is not known what causes osteoblasts to become embedded or how this process takes place. Osteocytes are the most numerous of the classic bone cells (approximately 90%) and reside in the lacunar spaces within the mineralized matrix of both cortical and trabecular bone. The terminal differentiation from osteoblasts into osteocytes results in both morphologic and biochemical changes in the cells. The osteocyte cell body is smaller than that of the osteoblast. It is neither polarized nor replete with the components of the secretory system. Unlike the osteoblast, the osteocyte is not highly synthetically active, although it does produce small amounts of some matrix proteins such as BSP, OPN, and osteocalcin. Biochemically, osteocytes can be distinguished from osteoblasts by an osteocyte-specific monoclonal antibody, as well as in the absence of alkaline phosphatase expression in the osteocyte.

The most striking morphologic feature of the osteocyte is its numerous tiny, narrow cell processes that extend throughout the bone substance via the canaliculi (Figure 3, B). Osteocyte cell processes are highly reminiscent of the dendrites of nerve cells. Just as nerve cells communicate with one another via synapses, osteocytes are connected by their cell processes. Signaling between cells is mediated by specialized protein complexes called gap junctions. These complexes form small pores in the cell surface, which allow small (approximately 1-kD cutoff) molecules such as ions and sugars and signaling molecules such as cyclic adenosine monophosphate or inositol derivatives to pass between the connected cells. In this way, each osteocyte is connected to many of its neighbors, forming a syncytium that resembles a neuronal network. It remains to be seen if there are functional similarities to neural networks in addition to these structural ones. The extensive connections formed between osteocytes and other cells via these processes include not only neighboring osteocytes, but also bone lining cells and osteoblasts on the bone surface. Re-

cent work has shown that these processes also can extend into the marrow space. Thus it is possible that osteocytes can communicate directly with osteoclast and/or osteoblast precursors or, potentially, any of the other bone resident cell types.

The function of osteocytes remains a mystery. Postulated roles tend to focus on the canalicular network. The canalicular network comprises a huge surface area in which the cell processes are in intimate contact with the bone matrix and are bathed in the extracellular fluid of bone. Thus, the osteocytes could possibly sense/monitor the condition of the matrix as well as the levels of calcium, phosphate oxygen, other nutrients, or signaling molecules in the tissue fluid. By far, the prevailing theory regarding osteocyte function is that they participate in the mechanosensing process. The massive intracellular connection network would seem ideally situated to monitor mechanical strain levels within the matrix as well as actual damage to the matrix in different parts of the bone and to integrate all of these signals via the osteocyte syncytium. In addition, these cells are biologically responsive to a variety of mechanical stimuli. This response will be discussed further in the section on mechanical regulation.

Unlike osteoblasts, osteocytes can live for decades. Osteocyte death is at least partially regulated by apoptosis and this may constitute an important signal that allows osteoclasts to target resorption to an area of damaged bone or to areas experiencing an abnormal strain environment. Thus, osteocytes may help to integrate the bone-forming activity of osteoblasts just described with the bone-resorbing activity of osteoclasts.

Osteoclast Lineage
Osteoclast Morphology and Function

Bone resorption is mediated by the multinucleated giant cells referred to as osteoclasts. Mature osteoclasts, like osteoblasts and bone lining cells, are found on bone surfaces. They function to resorb mineralized bone matrix. Interestingly, osteoclasts are unable to resorb unmineralized osteoid matrix such as overlies mineralized bone surfaces. This characteristic may be important in remodeling as discussed in the following section. Osteoclastic removal of bone from a bone surface results in the formation of a pit known as a Howship's lacuna. Osteoclasts are very large cells (20 to 100 microns in diameter) with from 3 to 20 nuclei because they are formed from the fusion of multiple mononuclear cells. They contain large numbers of mitochondria and lysosomal vesicles, intracellular organelles that house degradative enzymes. Osteoclasts have a ruffled border adjacent to the bone surface on electron microscopy (Figure 9, A). Besides these characteristic morphologic features, osteoclasts are readily identifiable by staining for the enzyme tartrate-resistant acid phosphatase. Other important molecular markers of osteoclasts include calcitonin receptor, receptor activator of nuclear

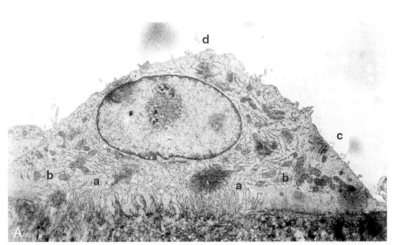
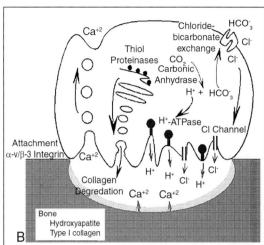

Figure 9   Osteoclast structure and function. **A,** A transmission electron microscopic image of a bone-resorbing osteoclast. a, ruffled border; b, sealing zone; c, basal membrane; d, functional secretory domain. Original magnification: X2500. *(Reproduced with permission from Marks SC, Odgren PR: Structure and development of the skeleton, in Bilezikian JP, Raisz LG, Rodan GA (eds): Principles of Bone Biology, ed 2. San Diego, CA, Academic Press, 2002, pp 3-15.)* **B,** The osteoclast acid degradation mechanism. A vacuolar-like H^+-ATPase, carbonic anhydrase II, and CIC-7 chloride channel electrically coupled to the electrogenic ATPase are, along with a Cl^-/HCO_3^- exchanger that maintains pH balance, mediators of acid secretion. Osteoclasts also secrete acid phosphatase and thiol proteinases. The extracellular compartment is formed by processes including α-v/β-3 integrin binding. Degraded calcium and collagen fragments are removed by vacuolar transcytosis. *(Adapted with permission from Blair HC, Zaidi M, Schlesinger PH:Mechanisms balancing skeletal matrix synthesis and degradation.* Biochem J 2002;364:329-341.)

factor-kappaβ (NF-κβ) (RANK) and the α-v/β-3 integrin on the surface of the cell.

To resorb bone the osteoclast adheres tightly to the surface through a ring-like "sealing zone" that is rich in the cytoskeletal protein actin (Figure 9, *A*). This situation creates a closed space over the bone surface into which the cell secretes acid as well as degradative enzymes (Figure 9). Intracellularly, carbon dioxide is converted to carbonic acid by the enzyme carbonic anhydrase II. The acid is pumped across the ruffled border into the resorptive space in an adenosine triphosphate-dependent manner, hence the large number of mitochondria found in the cell. The acidic environment is clinically important as carbonic anhydrase mutations cause some forms of the disease osteopetrosis in humans. Bone density in this disorder is pathologically high because of poor osteoclast function. This paradoxically results in bone fragility caused by accumulation of damaged bone (remodeling is discussed later in this chapter). Like the osteoblast, the osteoclast synthesizes a large amount of secretory protein. Instead of secreting matrix, however, osteoclasts produce matrix-degrading enzymes that are optimized to work in the acid environment of the resorption space. This finding is clinically important because a deficiency of one of these enzymes, cathepsin K, causes the human disease pyknodysostosis, which is characterized by acroosteolysis, skull deformities, and short stature. Cathepsin K inhibitors are being clinically evaluated as potential antiresorptive drugs.

Resorption of bone generates fragments of matrix macromolecules as well as calcium and phosphate ions in the resorption space. These resorption products undergo endocytosis at the basal membrane. They are then transported either to the lysosome for further degradation, or to the apical membrane by transcytosis where they are released into the extracellular space. Both the secretion of acid and enzymes as well as the resorption of degradation products take place through the basal membrane. Because the ruffled border increases the surface area of the basal membrane inside the sealing zone, it greatly increases the resorptive capacity of the osteoclast. This is clinically significant because bisphosphonate drugs result in loss of the ruffled border, thus inhibiting the resorptive activity of osteoclasts.

The osteoclast half-life is approximately 10 days. They can likely move from one resorption site to another during this time. There is little known about what happens to these cells at the end of life. They may die via apoptosis or revert to mononuclear cells. Recent data suggest that, in addition to causing loss of the ruffled border, bisphosphonates also induce osteoclast apoptosis, thus reducing the number of resorbing osteoclasts.

Osteoclast Differentiation

Osteoclasts are closely related to macrophages and arise from cells of the hematopoietic lineage as opposed to the mesenchymal precursors of the osteoblast lineage. Like osteoblasts, osteoclasts undergo an ordered differentiation process, passing through a succession of intermediate states before becoming mature osteoclasts. Also like osteoblasts, each of these steps is highly regulated and abnormalities at any of these steps can lead to human disease. Osteoclast precursors come from either the marrow space or arise from the circulation via marrow capillaries that closely parallel bone surfaces (**Figure 7,** *A*). They develop into mononuclear "preosteoclasts" that eventually fuse to form the mature multinuclear osteoclast cell. The regulation of this process is highly linked to the process of bone remodeling and will be discussed in more detail in the next section.

Other Bone Cell Types

As noted above, there are a large number of other cells residing in bone besides those typically believed of as bone cells. It has long been believed that bone simply provided a structural residence for these other cell types with no functional interactions occurring between these cells and the bone. Recently, however, there has been great interest in the possibility that cells in the marrow regulate activity of "bone" cells and vice versa. The presence of osteoblast and osteoclast precursors in the marrow was discussed above. There appears to be a direct interaction between osteoblast precursors and hematopoietic cells that controls hematopoietic differentiation. The hematopoietic cells, in turn, may regulate differentiation of osteoblast precursors. There is increased osteoblast formation in the "red marrow," which contains hematopoietic elements, versus the predominantly fatty "yellow marrow." This finding suggests that hematopoietic cells may support osteoblastic differentiation, but could also represent adipocytic suppression of osteoblast differentiation.

The best studied relationship between cells of the marrow and cells of the bone lineage is between osteoblasts and adipocytes. They arise from the same MSC precursor cell and their differentiation pathways are more similar initially than those of the other cell types, such as muscle, fibrous/tendon, and cartilage cells, which can arise from MSCs. In fact, a newly emerging paradigm is that there is a reciprocal relationship between osteoblastic and adipogenic differentiation. Several factors have been identified that drive osteoblastic differentiation while suppressing adipocytic differentiation and visa versa. These factors may play an important clinical role in the development of osteoporosis, as decreased bone mass with aging is correlated with increased marrow fat content. In addition, fat seems to directly regulate bone mass through a molecule called leptin. Leptin is produced by adipose tissue and negatively regulates bone mass. Leptin acts both directly on osteoblasts via leptin receptors and indirectly through the central nervous system. This intriguing pathway involves circulating leptin binding to cells in the hypothalamus, which in turn stimulate the sympathetic nervous system to release the beta-adrenergic compound noradrenalin. Noradrenalin works directly on osteoblasts to decrease bone formation. This finding not only strengthens the intriguing connection between fat and

bone but also identifies a connection between bone and the central nervous system. This is clinically relevant as it raises the possibility that beta blockers could be used clinically to increase bone mass.

Other interesting cells in the marrow are the endothelial cells and pericytes of capillary blood vessels, and the megakaryocytes. Endothelial cells are metabolically active and participate in several signaling events. Pericytes are modified smooth muscle cells that support the endothelium and may have the potential to undergo osteoblastic differentiation. Megakaryocytes have been implicated as regulators of bone mass through effects on osteoclast activity.

All the different cellular activities described in this section function together to control bone formation and bone resorption in a tightly regulated manner. This highly orchestrated process allows bone to change its shape and material properties to optimally meet the demands placed on it as well as to modulate serum calcium levels as needed. This process is known as bone remodeling.

Regulation of Bone Form and Function

The hard, mineralized nature of bone, which allows it to be cut, cemented, nailed, and to hold screws, has led it to be viewed as an inert substance. In fact, bone is a dynamic, metabolically active tissue that continuously renews itself and is able to modulate its shape and its ultrastructure to accommodate its functional demands. As described in the following sections, this dynamic nature of bone allows it to maintain its structural integrity, to adapt to changes in its mechanical environment, and to heal without a scar. These qualities are made possible because of the different cellular activities described in the previous section, which cooperate to orchestrate a remarkably coordinated integration of bone resorption and bone formation. This concept is clinically important because the processes of bone formation and resorption are abnormal in diseases such as osteoporosis and osteopetrosis and are targets for therapies such as bisphosphonates and PTH.

A variety of factors (physiologic, pharmacologic, or pathologic) control levels of bone resorption and formation. The net effect controls overall bone mass as well as the location of this mass. Physiologic regulators can be either systemic or local, arising within the bone itself. An in-depth discussion of the systemic regulation of bone mass is beyond the scope of this chapter, but the local cellular effects of some of these factors are discussed in the following sections.

The role of systemic factors in regulation of bone resorption through the modulation of osteoclast activity is relatively well understood, especially with regard to the regulation of serum calcium levels. Osteoclastic resorption and release of calcium from the bone is increased by circulating molecules such as vitamin D and PTH, and decreased by molecules such as calcitonin. Systemic regulation of bone formation is less well understood. PTH may be an important positive regulator of bone formation. Central regulation through leptin was discussed in the cell section. At a local level, recent breakthroughs have identified important pathways, such as Wnt signaling through LRP5 and growth factors such as BMP and IGF-1, as important positive regulators of formation. Other molecules such as IL-10 can decrease bone formation. Abnormal or ectopic expression of these physiologic regulators can cause them to act pathologically to inappropriately resorb bone, such as with metastatic tumors, or inappropriately form bone, such as in fibrodysplasia ossificans progressiva.

Clinically, some pharmacologic regulators of bone resorption and formation are important therapeutic agents for bone disease whereas others actually induce bone disease as an unwanted side effect. Steroid medications decrease bone formation and increase bone resorption leading to dramatic osteopenia with chronic use. The bisphosphonates are used to inhibit osteoclastic bone resorption and are used to treat osteoporosis, lytic metastatic bone disease, and Paget's disease. Until recently, there was no good way of increasing bone formation. PTH is classically thought of as a stimulus to bone resorption through stimulation of osteoclast formation. Although this observation is true for continuous administration of PTH as would be seen with a parathyroid gland tumor, intermittent dosing of PTH actually results in stimulation of bone formation. The reasons behind this surprising observation are unclear; however, the recent clinical introduction of intermittent PTH to increase bone formation provides clinicians with the first proformation drug.

The following sections describe the normal coordinated cycle of bone removal and replacement known as remodeling and discuss the molecular interactions between the bone forming and bone resorbing cells that mediate this process, the physiologic and pathologic ways that the process can be modulated, and the important role that mechanical influences play in guiding the balance and spatial localization of bone resorption and formation.

Remodeling

The removal and replacement of bone tissue in the same location is referred to as remodeling. The remodeling process is so active that it results in a complete turnover of an individual's bone mass every 4 to 20 years. The rate of turnover in adult bone is approximately 5% per year, but this rate varies with patient age and in different bone sites. Bone in children turns over at a rate much higher than that in adults, with trabecular bone turnover of approximately 25% per year and cortical bone turnover of 2% per year. This turnover is absolutely critical to the function of bone as a structural element. As bone tissue ages it become progressively more brittle because of changes in its mineral phase. In addition, the continuous mechanical demands placed on bone can cause damage to its structure that, in the absence of remodeling, would accumulate over time and degrade its mechanical integrity. This damage could eventually lead to catastrophic failure of bone as seen in osteopetrosis where osteoclast activity, and thus remodeling, is greatly reduced. The baseline remodeling process allows this damaged bone as well as the brittle, older bone to be removed and replaced with new, structurally sound bone. In a similar way, the woven bone of fracture callus is remodeled into stronger lamellar bone with a normal histologic anatomy, thus healing without a scar.

The Remodeling Cycle

Trabecular Bone

Remodeling begins with the initiation of osteoclastic resorption on a bone surface. As described below, the signal to begin resorption in a given area of a bone surface is unknown, but may involve the localized retraction of bone lining cells to allow access of osteoclasts to the underlying bone. Bone removal in this area by the osteoclasts creates a pit known as a Howship's lacuna. After the osteoclasts have completed bone resorption, they leave the pit and osteoblasts appear on the eroded surface where they begin to secrete and mineralize new matrix. This phase of the remodeling cycle is called "reversal" and the junction at which the resorption of old bone stopped and new bone formation began is marked by the cement line (discussed in the first section). The osteoblasts then lay down new bone, replacing that which was removed. As described previously, some of the osteoblasts become encased in ECM and phenotypically become osteocytes. Others probably undergo apoptosis, whereas a final group may become bone lining cells on the new surface. Once the resorption pit is refilled with new bone, the new surface becomes covered with quiescent bone lining cells (**Figure 10**).

The net effect of the remodeling cycle is that one "quantum" of bone is resorbed followed by the replacement or reformation of that quantum of bone. In trabecular bone this quantum represents a trabecular packet. In cortical bone it represents an osteon. All of the cells that are necessary to participate and control this process are referred to as a "basic multicellular unit" or BMU. The resorption phase lasts approximately 10 days, which is on the order of the half-life of the osteoclast. The formation phase lasts a few months, again consistent with the half-life of the osteoblast.

Cortical Versus Trabecular Bone

As the remodeling cycle is initiated by osteoclastic removal of bone from a bone surface, it is clear that the re-

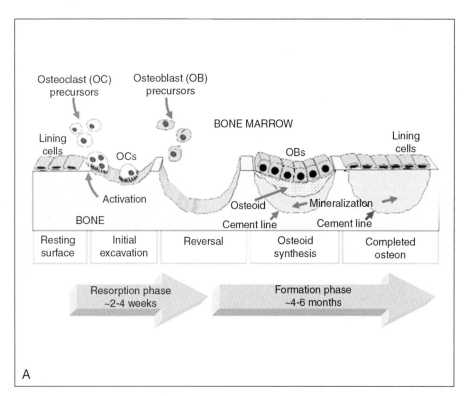
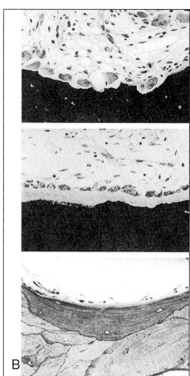

Figure 10   The remodeling cycle. **A,** An illustration of a bone marrow unit showing the various stages of cellular activity that it passes through temporally from the resorption of old bone by osteoclasts and the subsequent formation of new bone by osteoblasts. For simplicity, the illustration shows remodeling in only two dimensions, whereas in vivo it occurs in three dimensions, with osteoclasts continuing to enlarge the cavity at one end and osteoblasts beginning to fill it in at the other end. *(Adapted with permission from Riggs BL, Parfitt AM: Drugs used to treat osteoporosis: The critical need for a uniform nomenclature based on their action on bone remodeling.* J Bone Miner Res *2005;20:177-184.)* **B,** Cancellous bone remodeling to form a trabecular packet or hemiosteon. Upper panel: the resorption phase with osteoclasts eroding a parcel of bone (black); Middle panel: formation phase with osteoblasts and osteoid seam; and Lower panel: completed trabecular packet or hemiosteon showing bone lining cells and scalloped cement line. *(Reproduced with permission from Schenk RK, Felix R, Hofstetter W: Morphology of connective tissue: Bone, in Royce PM, Steinmann BL (eds):* Connective Tissue and Its Heritable Disorders: Molecular, Genetic, and Medical Aspects. *New York, NY, Wiley-Liss, 1993, pp 85-101.)*

modeling process is a surface phenomenon. The porous architecture of trabecular bone creates a high bone surface area that lends itself well to remodeling. Cortical bone, being thick and nonporous, has a relatively low surface area for resorption. Cortical bone, therefore, requires a special adaptation to allow remodeling to occur. This consists of osteoclasts tunneling through the cortical bone to form a structure known as a cutting cone (**Figure 11**). Osteoclastic resorption likely initiates on a cortical bone surface (either on the endosteal surface or within a haversian or Volkmann's canal) with the organization of a group of osteoclasts that then penetrate into the bone tissue. A blood vessel forms within the resorbed space, followed by osteoblast recruitment. The cutting cone then tunnels through the cortical bone by osteoclastic bone resorption at its leading edge. There is subsequent deposition of matrix on the eroded surfaces created by the osteoblast that fills the resorption space surrounding the trailing blood vessel. The end result is the deposition of bone in a circumferential pattern around a blood vessel, thus creating the histologic entity known as an osteon. The

vessel space is denoted as a haversian canal. The osteonal organization of cortical bone is easily visualized by microscopy. Complete osteons (recognized as concentric lamellae around a haversian canal) represent the more recently remodeled regions of the bone. Partial osteons or interstitial regions of bone (called interstitial lamellae) reflect areas that were deposited earlier and subsequently had portions remodeled, thus disrupting the original osteonal architecture (**Figure 3,** *A*).

Measures of Bone Formation and Resorption

Both bone formation and resorption can be assayed using straightforward assays of urine or serum. These assays are used for continuous monitoring for dynamic changes, for instance, in osteoporosis to verify that an anticatabolic (such as a bisphosphonate) treatment is effectively reducing resorption. Bone formation can be measured most effectively by assaying the production of osteocalcin or the release of products associated with collagen production. Excess osteocalcin is released into the systemic circulation during bone formation. Because osteoblasts are the pri-

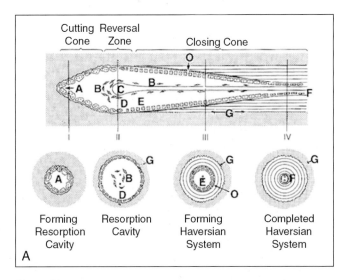

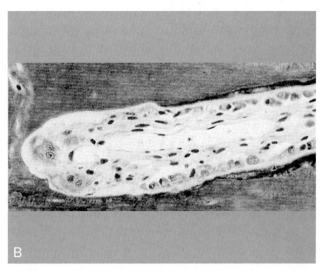

Figure 11   Cortical remodeling. **A,** Diagram showing a longitudinal section through a cortical remodeling unit with corresponding transverse sections below. A – Multinucleated osteoclasts in Howship's lacunae advancing longitudinally from right to left and radially to enlarge a resorption cavity. B – Perivascular spindle-shaped precursor cells. C – Capillary loop delivering osteoclast precursors and pericytes. D – Mononuclear cells (osteoblast progenitors) lining reversal zone. E – Osteoblasts apposing bone centripetally in radial closure and its perivascular precursor cells. F – Flattened cells lining the haversian canal of completed haversian system or osteon. Transverse sections at different stages of development: (I) resorption cavities lined with osteoclasts; (II) completed resorption cavities lined by mononuclear cells, the reversal zone; (III) forming haversian system or osteons lined with osteoblasts that had recently apposed three lamellae; and (IV) completed haversian system or osteon with flattened bone cells lining canal. Cement line (G); osteoid (stippled) between osteoblast (O) and mineralized bone. (*Reproduced with permission from Parfitt AM: The actions of parathyroid hormone on bone: Relation to bone remodeling and turnover, calcium homeostasis, and metabolic bone diseases. II. PTH and bone cells: Bone turnover and plasma calcium regulation.* Metabolism *1976;25:909-955.*) **B,** Cortical cutting cone. Osteoclasts resorbing a tunnel and osteoblasts filling it. (*Reproduced with permission from Schenk RK, Felix R, Hofstetter W: Morphology of connective tissue: Bone, in Royce PM, Steinmann BL (eds):* Connective Tissue and Its Heritable Disorders: Molecular, Genetic, and Medical Aspects. *New York, NY, Wiley-Liss, 1993, pp 85-101.*)

mary source of osteocalcin in the body, osteocalcin is relatively specific for bone. Because osteocalcin is liberated from the matrix by osteoclastic activity, it also increases with bone resorption and is, therefore, not specific for formation. During collagen production, both N-terminal and C-terminal propeptide portions of the collagen molecule are released into the circulation and can be assayed from either urine or serum. Assays of bone resorption typically measure collagen breakdown products or by-products of osteoclast metabolism. The most commonly used measure of bone resorption is called NTX. It is a cross-linked breakdown product of an N-terminal region of the mature type I collagen fibril called a telopeptide. NTX can be measured in serum or urine. Pyridinoline compounds are a breakdown product of collagen cross-links and are sensitive for the detection of collagen catabolism. Because hydroxyproline is found only in collagen, urinary hydroxyproline is the most specific measure of bone resorption. The products of osteoclast metabolism that can be used to measure bone resorption are tartrate-resistant acid phosphatase and cathepsin K.

Initiation and Targeting of Remodeling

The remodeling cycle begins with bone resorption but it remains unknown what events initiate this process and

what factors determine where this should take place. As described previously, all bone surfaces are covered with a layer of cells, primarily the bone lining cell, which may be a key factor in the regulation of remodeling activity. It is believed that the bone lining cell prevents the access of osteoclasts or osteoclast precursors to the surface of the bone, thus suppressing the initiation of remodeling. In addition, osteoclasts need a mineralized surface and cannot begin resorption on the thin layer of unmineralized osteoid that exists between the cell and the deeper mineralized bone. Therefore, it is believed that resorption likely begins with a signal to the bone lining cell to resorb the underlying osteoid and retract to provide access for osteoclasts to the mineralized matrix. The signal(s) that promotes these changes in bone lining cell activity are not completely defined. PTH has been shown to promote osteoid resorption and retraction from the bone surface by the bone lining cell, and it is possible that other proresorptive agents also may act on bone lining cells. An alternative hypothesis is that osteocytes, through their direct connections to bone lining cells, may be able to regulate this process.

It is believed that in the continuously occurring base line remodeling, initiation of resorption may occur in a random, stochastic pattern, resulting in generalized turn-

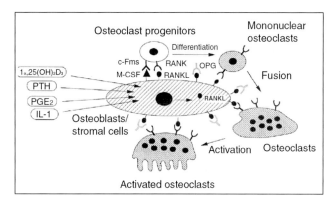

Figure 12   Schematic representation of osteoclast differentiation and function regulated by RANKL and M-CSF. Osteoclast progenitors and mature osteoclasts express RANK, the receptor for RANKL. Osteotropic factors such as $1\alpha,25(OH)_2D_3$, PTH, and IL-1 stimulate expression of RANKL in osteoblasts/stromal cells. Membrane- or matrix-associated forms of both M-CSF and RANKL expressed by osteoblasts/stromal cells are responsible for the induction of osteoclast differentiation in the coculture. RANKL also directly stimulates fusion and activation of osteoclasts. Mainly osteoblasts/stromal cells produce OPG, a soluble decoy receptor of RANKL. OPG strongly inhibits the entire differentiation, fusion, and activation processes of osteoclasts induced by RANKL. *(Reproduced with permission from Takahashi N, Udagawa N, Takami M, Suda T: Osteoclast generation, in Bilezikian HP, Raisz LG, Rodan GA (eds): Principles of Bone Biology, ed 2. San Diego, CA, Academic Press, 2002, pp 109-126.)*

over of bone tissue on a regular basis. Other elements of remodeling are targeted in a specific location. Some bones and regions of bone are remodeled at a higher rate than others. One theory suggests that microdamage to the bone matrix in the area of an osteocyte generates a signal to the nearby bone lining cells, causing initiation of remodeling at that site. This damage may cause the osteocytes to undergo apoptosis, which may be a key part of the signaling event. Mechanical stimuli are also a powerful influence on the sites at which bone formation and resorption occur. It is possible that local matrix mechanical strains detected by the osteocyte syncytium could provide important signals to either promote or inhibit initiation of resorption locally.

Coupling of Resorption and Formation
To maintain a constant bone mass, the resorption and formation of bone in the remodeling cycle must be balanced or coupled so that the same amount of bone that is removed is replaced. The integration of the formation and resorption processes is critical to this coupling and implies a connection between the bone-forming osteoblasts and the bone-resorbing osteoclasts. Studies of osteoclast differentiation have uncovered an elegant interaction between osteoblasts and osteoclasts that has advanced the field and generated concepts for new therapies.

Osteoclast Differentiation
In contrast to osteoblasts, which come from the mesen-

chymal cell lineage, osteoclasts arise from hematopoietic stem cell precursors, in a common pathway with macrophages. The multipotent hematopoietic stem cells become more lineage specific under the influence of the transcription factor PU.1 (analogous to Runx-2 and Osterix in osteoblast differentiation), differentiating into myeloid precursors. Macrophage colony stimulating factor (M-CSF) is critical for these cells to proliferate and to survive so they may progress down either the macrophage or osteoclast pathway. Gene disruption of either PU.1 or M-CSF in mice results in loss of both macrophages and osteoclasts. The factors c-Fos and NFκB drive osteoclast commitment and suppress macrophage differentiation. Committed osteoclast precursors express a cell surface receptor called receptor activator of NFκB (RANK). Binding of RANK to the extracellular protein RANK ligand (RANKL) promotes several of the steps leading to the development of mature, multinucleated, bone-resorbing osteoclasts. Purified M-CSF and RANKL alone are sufficient to drive osteoclast formation from purified osteoclast progenitor cells.

Molecular Mechanisms of Coupling
Systemic signals that cause bone resorption, such as PTH, do so by increasing the number of actively resorbing osteoclasts. Osteoclasts, however, do not have PTH receptors on their cell surface and cannot respond to the hormone directly. Osteoblasts, on the other hand, do have PTH receptors. They respond to PTH by synthesizing factors that are critical for osteoclast development, M-CSF and RANKL. Thus, physiologic signals such as PTH, which act to increase bone resorption activity, must be processed through the bone-forming osteoblast cells. The bone-forming cells then secrete the proresorptive, osteoclastic factors, appropriately ensuring coupling of resorption and formation (**Figure 12**).

It is presumed that there is communication directed from the osteoclast to the osteoblast as well. This is not fully understood but an intriguing hypothesis is that osteoclastic bone resorption releases factors such as BMP, TGF-β, and IGF-1 from the organic matrix that act as potent stimulators of osteoblast differentiation and would act locally to drive bone formation in areas of bone resorption, thus coupling the two processes (**Figure 13**). Other experiments suggest that a direct cell-to-cell interaction takes place. Actively resorbing osteoclasts express a transmembrane protein on their surface called ephrinB2. This protein can bind to a tyrosine kinase receptor on osteoblasts called EphB4, creating a direct interaction between the osteoclast and the osteoblast. This interaction stimulates differentiation and new bone formation in the osteoblastic cell. Thus, osteoclasts in a resorption pit may signal osteoblasts to begin bone formation to fill in the Howship's lacuna.

As noted above, osteoblasts and osteoclasts are generally found in close proximity to each other, as in a resorp-

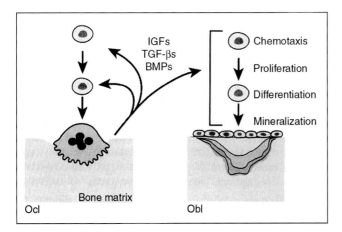

Figure 13   Growth factor concept of coupling. This concept suggests that coupling of osteoblast (Obl) differentiation and bone formation is caused by growth factors such as TGF-β and related family members and other growth factors such as IGF-1 and the FGFs being released from bone in active form as a consequence of osteoclastic (Ocl) resorption. *(Adapted with permission from Mundy GR, Chen D, Oyajobi BO: Bone remodeling, in Favus MJ (ed): Primer on the Metabolic Bone Diseases and Disorders of Mineral Metabolism, ed 5. Washington, DC, American Society for Bone and Mineral Research, 2003, pp 46-58.)*

tion pit, and thus a spatial coupling exists. Although RANKL exists and can function in a soluble form, it is also localized to the surface of osteoblasts and, thus, direct contact between osteoblasts and osteoclasts may be mediated through the RANKL/RANK interaction (**Figure 12**). Spatial coupling is also facilitated by the secretion of proteins by the osteoblast, such as monocyte chemotactic protein and OPN, that act as chemoattractants for osteoclast and osteoclast precursors.

Recent evidence demonstrates that, like osteoclasts, osteoblasts also express RANK on their surface and respond to RANKL by increasing bone formation. This finding suggests an additional method of coupling by which osteoclastic signals increase not only bone resorption but also osteoblast activity. PTH actions on the osteoblast cause an increase in survival and bone formation as well as the secretion of proresorptive factors. Thus, by fostering both osteoblast function and osteoclast differentiation, PTH activity ensures that bone formation is linked to resorption.

A further level of regulation takes place through osteoblast secretion of the protein osteoprotegerin (OPG). This is a soluble homologue of the receptor RANK. It binds to RANKL and inactivates it (**Figure 12**). This protein blocks the steps in osteoclastogenesis that are promoted by RANKL. OPG synthesis is upregulated by factors acting on the osteoblast—both osteoclastic signals such as PTH as well as promoters of bone formation such as estrogen, calcium, and BMP. Thus, osteoblasts can temper the osteoclast formation in response to PTH stimulation by secretion of antiresorptive factors such as OPG in addition to the proresorptive factors such as RANKL.

Modeling—Uncoupled Resorption and Formation

In the steady state situation of the mature skeleton, the resorption and formation of bone are coupled and bone mass is held constant. There are several instances, however, both normal as well as pathologic, in which formation and resorption are not balanced. The nomenclature for bone remodeling is complex. For the purposes of this chapter, bone "remodeling" is defined as the coupled actions of resorption and formation, removing and replacing the same amount of bone at the same site so that bone mass and shape are maintained. In contrast, bone "modeling," which occurs during growth and repair as well as bone response to mechanical load, is defined as bone formation or resorption in excess of the other and in different sites, resulting in a change in bone shape and mass.

An example of uncoupling of resorption and formation occurs to liberate calcium when systemic calcium levels are low, or to increase calcium deposition when systemic calcium levels are high. The relative balance of bone resorption and bone formation also changes with age. In children, formation exceeds resorption and therefore uncoupled modeling occurs, resulting in bone growth. In the young adult, resorption and formation are coupled so that constant bone mass is maintained. In older individuals there is decreased bone formation resulting in a gradual loss of bone mass at approximately 0.3% to 0.5% per year. In postmenopausal women, this loss of bone mass increases dramatically to 3% to 5% per year. The eventual result of this imbalance is progressive bone loss, leading to osteoporosis and increased risk of fracture.

Other pathologic and clinically important examples of uncoupling are osteopetrosis (decreased bone resorption from lack of osteoclast function), fibrodysplasia ossificans progressiva (excess bone formation), and Paget's disease (increased bone formation and bone resorption). Tumors that are metastatic to bone need to create a lytic lesion to survive there. These tumors do not resorb bone but secrete factors such as IL-1 and parathyroid hormone-related protein (PTHrP) that stimulate osteoclast differentiation. They also secrete factors such as the Wnt antagonist SFRP and the LRP5 inhibitor Dkk1, which inhibit bone formation by osteoblasts. Intra-articular T cells and synovial fibroblasts in rheumatoid arthritis secrete RANKL, causing the juxta-articular bone erosions seen in that disease. RANKL levels are also increased in fluid around loose prostheses and osteolytic lesions in total joint arthroplasties. The secretion of these factors bypasses the osteoblast and directly stimulates osteoclast differentiation resulting in pathologic, uncoupled resorption. In pathologies where this mechanism exists, OPG as well as antibodies that block RANKL function are promising antiresorptive therapies.

Mechanical influences are also important regulators of modeling and remodeling. The mechanical environment not only helps determine the original shapes of bones but

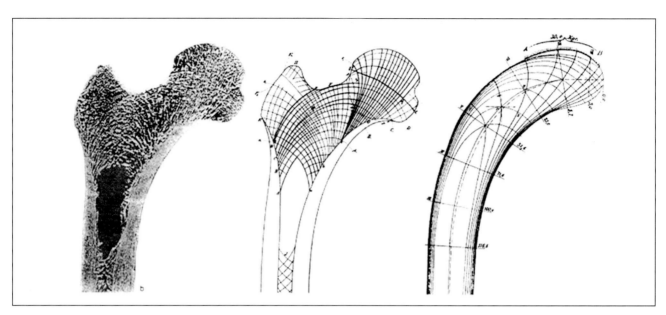

Figure 14   The basis of Wolff's trajectorial theory. On the left is a midfrontal section of the proximal femur, showing trabecular architecture; in the middle a schematic representation drawn by Meyer (1967); and on the right, the stress trajectories in a model analyzed by Culmann, using graphical statics. Stress trajectories are curves representing the orientations of the maximal and minimal principal stresses in the material under load. The maximal and minimal stress trajectories always intersect perpendicularly. *(Reproduced with permission from Huiskes R: If bone is the answer, then what is the question? J Anat 2000;197:145-56.)*

is also critical for maintenance of bone mass and general mechanical optimized organization of bone tissue. The shape or structure of a bone can change as it grows or as it responds to changing mechanical demands. In order for this to happen, bone formation and resorption must occur such that one occurs in excess of the other or in different locations. An example of this is the modeling of pediatric fracture malunions to return the bones to a normal or mechanically optimal shape. The mechanical regulation of bone formation and resorption is the subject of the next section.

Mechanical Regulation of Structure
Wolff's Law
It is widely assumed that bone structure, organization, and mechanical properties are factors that directly reflect patterns of habitual functional demand. This assumption was originally based on observations made by anatomists in the late 1800s that the orientation of trabecular bone structure coincides with lines of principal stresses (**Figure 14**). Combining these observations with insights from the emerging field of static mechanics led to the description of the trajectorial theory of trabecular bone architecture. The trajectorial theory hypothesizes that trabeculae are aligned in an optimal way to withstand the major stresses associated with usual/habitual mechanical demand across the bone.

These concepts were the foundation for Wolff's Law, which states that every change in the form and/or the function of a bone is followed by certain definite changes

in its internal architecture, and secondarily in its external conformation, in accordance with mathematical laws. This law is often summarized as: bone is deposited and resorbed in accordance with the stresses placed upon it. An example of this process occurs when a fracture heals in a malunited position. This changes the bone's form or shape, resulting in a change in the mechanical environment of the bone. In response, the pattern of bone removal and deposition is altered. This leads initially to changes in the internal architecture of the bone because the inner trabecular bone is more readily modeled and remodeled. Subsequently, and more slowly, the external cortical bone changes its shape resulting in a normalization of the mechanical environment of the bone. In this way, bone adapts to changes in either its own shape or changes in the environment to remain a mechanically optimized structure.

Adaptation
Wolff's law explains how bone structure, growth, and repair are influenced by its functional demands and how bone responds to a variety of pathologic conditions. This process of altering bone structure in response to mechanical influences is called adaptation. Examples of adaptation include the increased bone mass seen with load bearing exercise (as in the hypertrophy of the bones in the dominant forearm of the tennis player), normalization of fracture malunions in children, and the bone response to space-filling tumors. There is also an important mechanical contribution to the maintenance of bone mass typified by the bone loss seen with decreased load such as in space

flight or in extended periods of no weight bearing often necessary in fracture treatment. Decreased mechanical input or decreased sensitivity to mechanical stimulation may also play a role in the loss of bone mass with aging and osteoporosis as described below. The clinically important mechanical effects on bone have been reproduced in many analytical and experimental studies. For example, loading an animal bone leads to increased bone formation.

Mechanical Signals in Bone

The process regulating bone adaptation to mechanical load has been likened to the function of a household thermostat, a concept known as the "mechanostat" theory. If the house gets too cold, the thermostat causes the furnace to heat the house to bring the temperature back to a set point. If the house gets too warm, the thermostat causes the air conditioner to bring the temperature back down to a set point. Likewise, when the mechanical conditions in a region of bone change, the process of adaptation results in an alteration in the amount and organization of bone tissue in that region, to bring the perceived mechanical conditions back to a given set point.

In the analogy of the thermostat, temperature is the relevant modality upon which the set point is based. In bone, the specific characteristics of mechanical signals in the bone that affect adaptation remain unknown. Although definitive proof is lacking, many investigators believe that local strain is the key sensory parameter associated with mechanical regulation of bone. As such, many consider the "set point" to represent the typical maximum strain seen in normal bone across species, which is approximately 2,000 to 3,000 microstrain (1,000 microstrain is equivalent to 0.1% strain or 10^{-3} mm/mm). Strains greater than 2,000 to 3,000 microstrain in a region of bone would lead to bone accumulation, whereas strains less than 2,000 to 3,000 microstrain would lead to bone loss.

Candidates for parameters other than local strain have included strain magnitude, strain rate, strain frequency, and strain energy density, as well as local accumulation of matrix failure or damage. It is also possible that multiple factors, or possibly interacting factors, are important for generating a response or affecting the magnitude of a response. For example, in some experimental systems both strain magnitude and strain rate combine to modulate the adaptation response. In these experiments, a few cycles of loading per day at high strain levels generate a given mechanical response. Conversely, very low magnitude strains applied at a very high frequency seem to have the same effect. This is a clinically important concept because a device that applies low magnitude, high frequency loads has been shown to increase bone mass in humans and could become an important treatment modality in the future.

One unproven, but intriguing, theory is that bone experiences constant high frequency/low magnitude loads

that occur at baseline in all individuals, even in the absence of activity. An extension of this theory is that the bone loss seen with aging may be caused by the normal age-associated loss of muscle mass, and the concomitant loss of the fasciculation stimulus to bone. If this is the case, exercise may help prevent loss of bone mass in aging by helping to maintain muscle mass as well as by direct mechanical stimulation of the bone.

Cellular Mechanisms of Response

Just as it remains to be determined what mechanical signals in the bone control adaptation, the cellular responses to these signals, which result in the alteration of bone structure, are also unknown. Several key questions in this area remain unresolved: (1) Which of the myriad number of cell types found in bone generates a response to load that is physiologically important to adaptation? (2) What characteristic of load at the cellular level triggers a response in the mechanically responsive cells? (3) How is load sensed by the cells and converted into an intracellular signaling cascade?

To answer the first question, it is the bone-forming and bone-resorbing cells that ultimately are the effectors of the mechanical stimulus to bone. These cells must receive a signal that in turn regulates their respective activities, resulting in appropriate adaptation responses. The osteoblast and osteoclast cells, however, are not necessarily the primary load sensors. In theory, any of the cell types in bone, including the marrow cells, could be a primary load sensor that then generates a biochemical signal that is transmitted to the effector cells. This could happen either in a paracrine fashion or by some of the direct connections that have been discussed previously in the bone cell section. It is also possible that multiple cells play an important mechanosensing role. Many of the different cell types found in bone have been shown to be mechanically responsive in tissue culture systems and, thus, could potentially fulfill this role in vivo.

Regarding the second question, local strain in a region of bone may control the adaptation response in this area. The type of load the bone cells in this area experience, however, may be quite different than those measured at the tissue/whole bone level. Strain is not homogeneous throughout bone tissue. Strain magnitude depends on the load applied to the bone, but also on the exact location where it is measured. The variability in strain magnitude increases as more microscopic scales are studied. This variability is perhaps most easily seen in trabecular bone. At the whole bone level, trabecular bone strain is assessed in volumes of bone approximately 8 mm to 1 cm on a side, whereas strain in the trabecular struts is assessed in volumes of bone tissue of approximately 10 to 200 microns on a side. Strain at this level is not similar to the whole bone strain because the struts do not deform in a homogeneous way. Regardless of how the overall trabecular bone is loaded, some of the struts will be loaded in bending, some in tension, and others in compression. The strain magnitudes in the struts also tend to vary more widely than the overall strain in the trabecular bone at the whole bone level. Strain is higher in tissue surrounding porosities such as osteocyte lacunae than the strain in the overall tissue.

A compressive load at the whole bone level can also induce secondary mechanical events, such as hydrostatic pressure and fluid flow. Fluid flow has been demonstrated to take place throughout the bone including along the canaliculi, and increases with compressive load applied at the whole bone level. Several different loading modalities have been demonstrated to induce a response in cells loaded in culture. For example, fluid flow over cells in culture generates shear forces at the cell surfaces and is a potent stimulus for generating a biologic response to loading. It remains to be determined which cells in which regions of the bone experience which types of loads in mechanically loaded bone.

In response to the third question, for cells to respond to mechanical load they must first sense a mechanical stimulus, then convert this mechanical signal into a biochemical signal, which must then generate a biologic response (for example, matrix secretion). This process is referred to as mechanotransduction by analogy to standard biochemical signaling processes that are referred to as signal transduction. There seem to be molecular pathways that are common to both hormonal and mechanical regulation of bone resorption and formation. For example, osteoblasts loaded in culture sense the mechanical stimulus and in turn modulate internal signaling pathways to decrease the secretion of RANKL. This decreases the formation of osteoclasts grown in coculture. If this mechanism holds true in vivo, it provides a mechanism for how loading leads to bone modeling. Mechanical loading of osteoblasts increases bone formation, but downregulates RANKL expression, and hence osteoclast differentiation. Therefore, loaded areas of bone will increase formation and also decrease resorption, resulting in increased bone in the mechanically stimulated region.

How load is sensed by cells is not fully understood. There may, in fact, be multiple mechanisms of mechanosensing and response. The integrin molecules described in the previous sections seem to be important in the mechanotransduction process. Mechanical strains may be transmitted from the ECM through integrins directly to the cytoskeleton and then activate biochemical signaling pathways. Alternatively, direct connections to the nucleus could trigger transcriptional responses leading to a biologic response. There is also evidence that strain-gated channels can play a role in mechanotransduction.

Currently, the prevailing theory regarding these three issues is that osteocytes are a primary mechanosensor. As described before, their location within the bony matrix and their extensive network of interconnections make them ideally positioned to monitor and integrate levels of mechanical strain from different areas of the bone, and then directly modulate the function of the bone lining and bone forming cells through their gap junction connections. It is believed that whole bone loading generates fluid flow over the osteocyte cell bodies and cell processes and that osteocytes responding to shear generated by this flow generate the critical mechanical or mechanotransduction response leading to modulation of effector cell activity. Fluid flow throughout the bone, including along the canaliculi connecting the osteocytes, has been demonstrated and increases with mechanical loading. Purified osteocytes and osteocyte-like cells in culture are, in fact, extremely sensitive to fluid shear forces. They respond to these types of loads by the activation of a variety of signaling pathways.

A clinically relevant illustration of the interplay between mechanical and biologic response of bone can be observed from evaluating the response of proximal femoral bone to the femoral component of a hip arthroplasty. Often, proximal stress shielding is observed with a distally fixed femoral implant. In this setting, the implant, which has a very high stiffness compared with bone, transmits weight-bearing loads directly into the diaphyseal bone, thus bypassing the proximal metaphyseal bone. The proximal bone experiences decreased stress and decreased deformation (strain). Consequently, the cells in this region perceive decreased mechanical stimulus. This, in turn, alters the cellular mechanical response and the biochemical signaling that controls osteoblast and osteoclast activity. Thus, the change in cellular response to this change in mechanical input leads, ultimately, to decreased bone formation and/or increased bone resorption. In this way, the adaptation to the altered mechanical environment creates the proximal bone loss seen radiographically with these implants. Clearly, an understanding of bone adaptation, and methods to alter this process, mechanically or biologically, may lead to new approaches to therapy.

Many of the biochemical signaling pathways activated by mechanical load are the same as those activated by chemical mediators of signal transduction, such as hormones. This may provide an important route for integrating the effects of mechanical and biologic signals on bone. In general, biologic signals such as hormones have a larger effect on overall bone mass, but may be fine tuned by mechanical influences. For example, PTH may dictate resorption of bone, but the mechanical environment may dictate where and how that bone is removed. The net result of the hormonal and mechanical modulation of bone structure is a mechanically optimized structure whose material and mechanical properties are the keys to bone function as a structural skeletal element. These critical mechanical properties of bone will be described in the following section.

Mechanical Properties of Bone

Understanding the structural and material properties of bone is critical for assessment of its mechanical and physiologic role. Familiarity with the biomechanical properties of bone is critical for the orthopaedic surgeon to understand the ramifications of bone loss, fracture mechanics, stability of fracture constructs, and implant fixation. With knowledge of bone biomechanical properties, the impact of bone disease and changes with age and other conditions on the ability of the skeleton to support the body in normal or overloaded situations can be evaluated.

Bone is characterized mechanically in the same way as other materials (such as steel and concrete). Bone mechanical properties can be directly measured at several size scales, from the level of bone ECM to the whole bone. Mechanical properties are determined by the structure and the material comprising it. The structural properties of the whole bone are dependent on its shape, size, and architecture. The material properties of bone are dependent on the specific organic and inorganic constituents of the matrix and how they are organized. Measurements of bone tissue characterize the properties of a composite structure that includes the ECM and its cells and geometry. For example, trabecular tissue is considered to be a composite of material composed of multiple lamellae, cement lines, lacunae, and cells, which make up the composition of the trabecular struts. Cortical tissue is a composite of material that includes multiple lamellae, cement lines, lacunae, and cells with either an osteonal or interstitial bone geometry.

The following section discusses generalized matrix and tissue mechanical properties, the specific tissue and structural properties of cortical bone and trabecular bone, and how these two tissue types integrate in a long bone.

Bone Matrix/Tissue
Preyield Properties
In general, the two major components of bone tissue, mineral and organic matrix, contribute differently to the material properties of the ECM and thereby to the tissue. In terms of the elastic or preyield properties of bone, the mineral dominantly provides stiffness to the tissue and resistance to compressive load. The organic matrix, primarily the collagen, provides resistance in tension. Tissue mineralization can be affected by bone tissue age and type (such as woven versus lamellar). Newly formed bone has less mineral than "older" bone. In this context, "old" bone is defined by the length of time since it was formed. From the time it is formed, bone tissue will become increasingly more mineralized as it "ages" until it is removed by remodeling. As a result of the increased mineral, both trabecular and cortical bone tissue become stiffer, resulting in improved preyield mechanical properties of the bone.

An example of the influence of tissue type on bone properties is the effect of replacing woven bone with lamellar bone. In contrast to lamellar bone, the collagen matrix of woven bone has a highly disorganized architecture, which results in mineral that also is more disorganized. The combined effect of the disorganized collagen and mineral is to render woven tissue less stiff and less strong than lamellar tissue. On the other hand, woven bone can be very rapidly formed, an advantage that can rapidly increase the structural integrity in the early stages of healing fractures. In addition, woven bone can become more highly mineralized than lamellar bone, which can help improve its relative lack of stiffness. In nonpathologic cases, woven bone is replaced with lamellar bone through remodeling, which improves the mechanical characteristics of the bone tissue by depositing a very well-organized matrix and subsequently more effectively organized mineral crystals.

Postyield Properties
The organic matrix plays a dominant role in the postyield behavior of the tissue (the energy absorption after yield and before failure). For example, in osteogenesis imperfecta, the abnormalities in the type I collagen component of the organic matrix result in reduced postyield behavior (increased brittleness), whereas the stiffness of the bone (most influenced by mineral) is relatively normal. Although the organic matrix is, in general, the greatest determinant of postyield behavior of bone, the mineral component also can have an effect on brittleness. This effect is important in individuals who are taking drugs such as bisphosphonates to reduce osteoclast activity and decrease bone resorption. Under these conditions, when remodeling is inhibited, bone tissue continues to mineralize and becomes stiffer as previously noted. Experiments have demonstrated, however, that the increased mineral content also leads to the tissue becoming more brittle. There is concern that this increase in brittle postyield behavior will result in tissue that cannot absorb as much energy before failure. In other words, toughness decreases. Clinically, however, these concerns seem offset by the improved mechanical properties gained by the improvement in bone mass and stiffness.

Fatigue Properties
Fatigue damage of trabecular bone tissue degrades its material properties (making the tissue less stiff and less strong), and may be important in osteoporotic and stress fractures. Linear microcracks and diffuse damage are generated when tissue is repetitively loaded, either at relatively high strains or for a large number of cycles. These damage-inducing mechanical conditions can occur even during normal activities. Because bone is able to remodel, a process that replaces the microcracks and diffuse damage, fatigue damage generally does not lead to failure of the bone. However, if the bone is loaded enough, or remodeling is impaired, the cracks can coalesce and result

in failure of the bone, seen clinically as stress fractures. In osteoporosis, the decreased structural/whole bone properties make the tissue at higher risk for fatigue damage because increased deformation and strain occurs with normal loads. Indeed, increased microdamage is seen with increasing age. With extensive damage, individual cracks may coalesce into large cracks that may lead to fracture under normal loading conditions. This occurrence is seen in some osteoporotic vertebral compression fractures where there is no overt trauma. Extensive cracks may also induce a large region of remodeling that may become vulnerable to failure during the time when large amounts of tissue have been resorbed by osteoclasts or before the new bone is fully mineralized.

Cement lines, formed during remodeling, and osteocyte lacunae are believed to play a role in the mechanical behavior of bone tissue. Cement lines contain less collagen and mineral. Because the tissue in the cement lines is less stiff and more deformable than the adjacent lamellar bone, the growth of cracks is halted in the bone tissue between osteons or Howship's lacunae. This allows the tissue as a whole to become tougher (able to absorb more energy before overt failure). Similar to cement lines, lacunae, as small holes in the bone tissue, also act as crack arrestors.

Cortical Bone

The material properties of cortical bone vary with loading direction, type of loading (compression versus tension), species, age, and anatomic location. Typical stiffness values for cortical bone are approximately 10 to 20 GPa, whereas ultimate strength is generally 50 to 200 MPa when tested at a macroscopic scale. Longitudinal specimens (obtained parallel to the long axis of the bone) of diaphyseal cortical bone are stronger than those obtained in a transverse direction (perpendicular to the axis of the bone). Likewise, the stiffness (Young's modulus) of longitudinal specimens is greater than the stiffness of transverse specimens. This is an example of transverse isotropy, where properties measured in any direction within a given plane are the same, but properties measured in a direction perpendicular to that plane are different from those in the plane. These variations in properties are related to the organization of the cortical bone, most importantly, the orientation, size, and number of osteons. In cortical bone, maximum strength and stiffness are generally obtained in the direction of the osteons, which are oriented longitudinally, in the primary loading direction of the bone. Thus, the tissue organization of the diaphyseal cortical bone is optimized for the axial loads it usually sees. This tissue organization also results in minimum strength and stiffness in the plane perpendicular to this direction. Cortical bone tissue is stronger in compression than tension. Therefore, cortical bone is strongest in longitudinal compression and weakest in transverse tension. This is clinically important because press-fit hip stems generate hoop stresses that load the bone transversely in tension and can lead to intraoperative femur fracture.

Although fracture patterns are complex, some generalities based on bone mechanical properties can be made. In tension a transverse fracture is generated. Compression tends to result in an oblique fracture, likely with a butterfly fragment. In bending there is a combination of tensile and compressive loads. Fractures generally start on the tensile side with a transverse fracture line that then deviates obliquely from about the center. Diaphyseal cortical bone also experiences torsional loads. These are clinically important because these torsional loads generate shear stress in the bone tissue, which can lead to spiral fractures. Shear stress can be broken down into equivalent tension and compression components that can be used to predict fracture patterns.

Under polarized light, cortical bone sectioned perpendicular to the osteons demonstrates variability in the appearance of the osteons. Some osteons are dark, some are bright, and some have lamellae that alternate dark and light bands. These patterns are believed to be caused by variations in the density or orientation of the collagen fibers. The patterns seen under the polarized microscope have been found to correspond to specific variations in mechanical properties. The observed variations are believed to be reflective of morphologic adaptation to habitual loading conditions to the region. These variations are evidence of bone being adapted at a local level to the mechanical requirements placed on it by daily activities.

Cortical bone is a viscoelastic material because its mechanical properties are strain rate-dependent. Strain rate dependency means that the measured properties differ depending on how quickly the material is loaded. Bone has a higher stiffness and strength at higher loading rates. Thus, bone can sustain higher loads in high-speed impacts than it can with slow loading rates. Postyield behavior is also affected by strain rate. Cortical bone is somewhat ductile at normally experienced strain rates, even up to those seen with vigorous running. At very high rates of loading, however, such as a high-speed motor vehicle accident, the bone becomes quite brittle and will actually resist less energy to failure. The viscoelastic nature of bone may provide an advantage, enabling it to withstand larger forces if they occur at higher velocities. The downside is that, because the bone will be more brittle when loaded at very high rates, if it reaches the fracture threshold it will fail more catastrophically (resulting in a comminuted fracture).

Trabecular Bone

Although trabecular and cortical bone tissue have similar material properties, trabecular bone as an organized collection of struts has lower stiffness and strength than cortical bone, with an elastic modulus of approximately 10 to

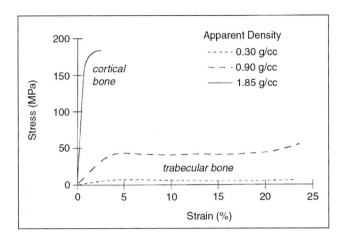

Figure 15   Stress-strain behavior for cortical and trabecular bone. Example of typical compressive stress-strain behaviors of trabecular and cortical bone for different apparent densities. *(Reproduced with permission from Keaveny TM, Hayes WC: Mechanical properties of cortical and trabecular bone, in Hall BK (ed): Bone. Boca Raton, FL, CRC Press, 1993, vol 7, pp 285-344.)*

2,000 MPa (**Figure 15**). Also in contrast to cortical bone, the stiffness and strength of trabecular bone appears to be similar in tension and compression. The compressive strength (σ) of trabecular bone is often estimated based on a power law function:

$$\sigma = A\rho^B$$

where A is a constant, B is a constant between 2 and 3, and ρ is the apparent density (defined as the mass of the bone tissue divided by the total volume of the test specimen, including marrow spaces). Because of the exponent B, this equation demonstrates that small changes in bone density can result in large changes in the mechanical properties of trabecular bone. This information is important when considering drug therapies that combat low bone mass. Even small increases in density significantly increase bone strength. Likewise, small decreases in density lead to large changes in strength. Therefore, sensitive measures of density are needed to evaluate changes in bone strength.

Yield of trabecular bone occurs at 1% to 4% strain, regardless of its bone volume fraction (BVF) (**Figure 15**). In other words, a trabecular bone specimen yields when it is deformed a specific amount, independent of its mass (or BVF) or the applied load. Because the stiffness of trabecular bone is strongly dependent on BVF, the stress at yield is also dependent on BVF. Thus osteoporotic trabecular bone (low BVF) and normal trabecular bone (high BVF) will deform the same amount before they yield, but normal bone is much stiffer so it takes greater load or stress to make it deform to the yield point.

A unique characteristic of trabecular bone is that it is able to absorb a large amount of energy through large deformations before failure. This is equivalent to saying that

trabecular bone is very tough (as opposed to strength, which is load to failure). After yield, trabecular bone deforms at a relatively constant stress, and then the stress increases as the bone specimen compacts and becomes increasingly dense. These properties of trabecular bone make it more compliant than cortical bone, a property important for its function around joints. The architecture (organization) of trabecular bone in large part determines its mechanical properties. Trabecular bone with a higher bone volume fraction (volume of mineralized tissue per total volume of marrow and bone space) is generally stiffer and stronger. Trabecular bone is anisotropic. The direction in which the trabecular struts are primarily oriented has the greatest stiffness and strength, and is generally the same direction in which the bone is habitually loaded. It is important to understand anisotropy because not all loading occurs in the preferential loading direction. For example, falls on the hip will result in loads applied in a different direction than those habitually applied during normal ambulation. Aging has been shown to result in significant loss of trabecular bone mass and often a change in overall orientation through preferential loss of struts in a direction not associated with habitual loads. Consequently, while the resistance of the bone to loads delivered in the direction of habitual use is relatively maintained, the resistance to loads in an unusual direction (as might occur in a fall) is significantly reduced. When comparing individuals with osteoporotic fractures to individuals with similar BVF and age, it was found that anisotropy was greater in those with fracture. This likely caused decreased mechanical properties in the direction that was not habitually loaded. This situation may cause few problems until an individual falls, loading the bone in a nonhabitual direction and resulting in fracture.

Trabecular bone samples taken from different anatomic regions, age groups, and individuals have different mechanical properties. Clinically, understanding the variance between these samples would improve the ability to predict fracture risk. A variety of conditions cause substantial effects on trabecular orientation as well as mass (BVF). Using mass alone, the predictions of mechanical properties can be underestimated. Both the mass and the orientation of the struts (direction and proportion in a specific direction of orientation) can independently be used to predict the mechanical properties of volumes of trabecular bone (about 60% to 70% of variance explained). Combining information from both the mass and measures of orientation can explain 90% of the variance in trabecular bone properties. From a clinical perspective, BVF is difficult to measure (bone biopsy is required). Bone mineral density is relatively easy to measure noninvasively using dual-energy x-ray absorptiometry. Good estimates of mechanical properties (stiffness and modulus) can be made using bone mineral density as a substitute for BVF. Orientation cannot be determined using clinical imaging modalities. In the future, improved imaging techniques may allow more precise determination of bone mass and orientation.

Whole Bone Properties

Although the mechanical behavior of bone tissue, trabecular bone, and cortical bone has been discussed separately, it is important to consider their interdependencies in providing a structural framework for the body. For example, stiffer tissue leads to stiffer trabecular or cortical bone, all other factors being equal. When whole bone properties change, this must be related to changes in the tissue properties and/or geometry of the structure.

Because all bones have different geometries and shape, there are no ways to describe their individual mechanical properties other than through individual experimental studies. However, there are a few general principles to consider. The size and shape of the bones play a large role in their response or resistance to load. Cross-sectional area, moments of inertia, and material properties of the included tissue (cortical and trabecular) all contribute to the whole bone properties. The details of how size and geometry contribute to structural properties can be reviewed in chapter 3. In general, the geometric attributes of a whole bone (size, shape) contribute the greatest to the structural integrity.

In addition, although trabecular and cortical bone have been discussed separately, they actually work in combination in such a way as to make specialized use of their unique tissue and whole bone properties. In the shaft of long bones, a tube of cortical bone is an ideal structural element for several reasons. Because long bones have a slight curvature, the cortical bone is generally loaded with a small amount of bending superimposed on relatively large axial compression. Torsional loads are commonly seen. The thick cortical diaphysis of long bones is well suited to handle these loads. The outer diameter and thickness of the bone determines its ability to sustain bending loads as characterized by the bending moment of inertia (proportional to the radius cubed). Being hollow allows it to house the marrow and also to remain as light as possible without sacrificing much strength. In the hollow cylinder, bending properties are improved because the bone tissue is located farther from the neutral axis. The ability of cortical bone tissue to sustain axial loads is proportional to its cross-sectional area. The thick, strong cylinder is excellent for resisting axial compressive loads. The ability of cortical bone tissue to sustain torsional loads is characterized by the polar moment of inertia, which is proportional to the radius cubed. There is little trabecular bone in the diaphysis except along the periosteum, where it could play a role in providing surface for remodeling.

Thus, the diaphysis is really an optimized structure for its habitual loads. Near the surface of joints, however, the diaphyseal structure would be too stiff to provide a good support for the delicate articular cartilage. The specialized structure of the metaphysis/epiphysis at the ends of the long bones, however, acts as a shock absorber to protect the joint surface. Additionally, the broad surface for weight bearing decreases the loads on the articular cartilage. As discussed previously, the metaphysis and epiphysis are primarily trabecular bone with only a thin shell of cortical bone. The cortical bone is very thin, but has a very important contribution to the mechanical function of the trabecular bone because it acts as a constraining rim or border, allowing mechanical forces to be spread more evenly across the trabecular bone. The important role of the constraining rim of cortical bone demonstrates how cortical and trabecular bone augment the function of the other and work together to provide an optimized structure for weight bearing. A further specialization in this area is the subchondral bone. This compact bone layer underlying the articular cartilage is perforated, which maintains a flexible support for the cartilage. This flexibility is lost in osteoarthritis, where there is stiffening and sclerosis of the subchondral bone that worsens the mechanical environment for the cartilage, possibly hastening disease progression.

Aging

In early life bone mass steadily increases and peaks in the third decade of life. Subsequently, there is a slow and steady decline in bone mass. This process occurs in both men and women and in both trabecular and cortical bone. In menopause, trabecular bone loss is accelerated to a much greater degree than cortical loss. Osteoporosis is defined as a bone mineral density (by dual x-ray absorptiometry) of 2.5 standard deviations below that of a young normal population mean. This is the best clinically available correlate of fracture risk.

As discussed in the remodeling section, the differences in macroscopic porosity between cortical and trabecular bone are reflected in the available surface area for cellular activity. From a clinical perspective, the large surface area of trabecular bone makes it far more "vulnerable" to resorption and therefore trabecular bone has much greater loss of mass during aging. With trabecular bone loss, the rods become thinner and the plates perforate, thus becoming rods. Therefore, there is an increase of the number of rods relative to plates in aging. This situation changes the way the bone can resist loads. This bone loss creates increased porosity and decreased BVF. There is also a change in overall orientation of struts through preferential loss of struts in a direction not associated with habitual loads. This loss of struts results in increased anisotropy. Consequently, while the resistance of the bone to loads delivered in the direction of habitual use is relatively maintained, the resistance to loads in an unusual direction (as might occur in a fall) is significantly reduced.

In aging, cortical bone becomes somewhat less stiff, less strong, and more brittle. The bone in the cortex generally becomes thinner and often has an increase in intracortical porosities, both of which contribute to a decrease in mechanical properties. However, cortical bone changes with age are generally not as substantial as those seen in trabecular bone. A typical geometric change occurs in the long bone shafts with aging. The inner diameter and outer diameter both increase, with an overall loss in bone mass. Despite the loss in bone mass and decreased tissue strength, the whole bone properties remain similar because both the bending and polar moments of inertia are relatively unchanged because of the increase in the radius. This adaptation does seem to be protective as the incidence of femoral shaft fracture does not markedly increase with age-related bone loss as it does with hip and spine fractures.

Summary

The skeleton provides mechanical support to the body, allowing for motion as well as protection of vital organs. It also participates in mineral homeostasis and houses the bone marrow. The bones comprising the skeleton are optimized in their shape and mechanical properties to carry out their specific roles while remaining light but resistant to fracture. This is achieved through organization of the bone mineral, organic matrix, and cells into tissue motifs that are, in turn, combined in different ways to create different whole bone structures. This optimization of bone's structure-function is an active process, possible because of sensory mechanisms that allow it to monitor its tissue integrity as well as its mechanical and physiologic environments. These sensory inputs result in defined biologic responses that regulate the functions of bone resorption and bone formation. These precisely balanced processes result in optimization of bone form and function in health, while imbalances in aging and disease are manifested as skeletal disease.

Selected Bibliography
Bone Structure
Crock HV: *An Atlas of the Vascular Anatomy of the Skeleton and Spinal Cord*. St. Louis, MO, Mosby, 1996, pp 131-303.

Eriksen EF, Axelrod DW, Melsen F: *Bone Histomorphometry*. New York, NY, Raven Press, 1994, pp 3-12.

Fawcett DW: *Bloom and Fawcett: A Textbook of Histology*, ed 12. New York, NY, Chapman and Hall, 1994, pp 194-204.

Hancox NM: *Biology of Bone*. London, England, Cambridge University Press, 1972, pp 18-35.

Jee WS: The skeletal tissues, in Weiss L (ed): *Cell and Tissue Biology: A Textbook of Histology*. Baltimore, MA, Urban and Schwarzenberg, 1988, pp 211-254.

McCarthy ID: Blood flow and transport in bone, in Hughes S, McCarthy ID (eds): *Sciences Basic to Orthopaedics*. London, England, WB Saunders, 1998.

Stewart C, Reid RW: *Holden's Human Osteology*. Philadelphia, PA, Blakiston Son and Company, 1887, pp 1-22.

Extracellular Matrix
Anderson HC: Molecular biology of matrix vesicles. *Clin Orthop Relat Res* 1995;314:266-280.

Bennett JH, Moffatt S, Horton M: Cell adhesion molecules in human osteoblasts: Structure and function. *Histol Histopathol* 2001;16:603-611.

Bonadio J, Byers PH: Subtle structural alterations in the chains of type I procollagen produce osteogenesis imperfecta type II. *Nature* 1985;316:363-366.

Boskey AL: Matrix proteins and mineralization: An overview. *Connect Tissue Res* 1996;35:357-363.

Globus RK, Doty SB, Lull JC, Holmuhamedov E, Humphries MJ, Damsky CH: Fibronectin is a survival factor for differentiated osteoblasts. *J Cell Sci* 1998; 111:1385-1393.

McKee MD, Addison WN, Kaartinen MT: Hierarchies of extracellular matrix and mineral organization in bone of the craniofacial complex and skeleton. *Cells Tissues Organs* 2005;181:176-188.

Sykes B: Genetics cracks bone disease. *Nature* 1987; 330:607-608.

Tsipouras P, Ramirez F: Genetic disorders of collagen. *J Med Genet* 1987;24:2-8.

Young MF: Bone matrix proteins: Their function, regulation, and relationship to osteoporosis. *Osteoporos Int* 2003;14(suppl 3):S35-S42.

Bone Cells
Abe E: Function of BMPs and BMP antagonists in adult bone. *Ann N Y Acad Sci* 2006;1068:41-53.

Bianco P, Robey PG: Diseases of bone and the stromal cell lineage. *J Bone Miner Res* 1999;14:336-341.

Bianco P, Robey PG: Stem cells in tissue engineering. *Nature* 2001;414:118-121.

Blair HC: How the osteoclast degrades bone. *Bioessays* 1998;20:837-846.

Franz-Odendaal TA, Hall BK, Witten PE: Buried alive: How osteoblasts become osteocytes. *Dev Dyn* 2006; 235:176-190.

Levasseur R, Lacombe D, deVernejoul MC: LRP5 mutations in osteoporosis-pseudoglioma syndrome and high-bone-mass disorders. *Joint Bone Spine* 2005;72: 207-214.

Mackie EJ: Osteoblasts: Novel roles in orchestration of skeletal architecture. *Int J Biochem Cell Biol* 2003;35: 1301-1305.

Nakashima K, Zhou X, Kunkel G, et al: The novel zinc finger-containing transcription factor osterix is required for osteoblast differentiation and bone formation. *Cell* 2002;108:17-29.

Noble BS, Reeve J: Osteocyte function, osteocyte death and bone fracture resistance. *Mol Cell Endocrinol* 2000;159:7-13.

Otto F, Thornell AP, Crompton T, et al: Cbfa1, a candidate gene for cleidocranial dysplasia syndrome, is essential for osteoblast differentiation and bone development. *Cell* 1997;89:765-771.

Shore EM, Xu M, Feldman GJ, et al: A recurrent mutation in the BMP type I receptor ACVR1 causes inherited and sporadic fibrodysplasia ossificans progressiva. *Nat Genet* 2006;38:525-527.

Westendorf JJ, Kahler RA, Schroeder TM: Wnt signaling in osteoblasts and bone diseases. *Gene* 2004;341: 19-39.

Regulation of Bone Form and Function
Blair HC, Zaidi M, Schlesinger PH: Mechanisms balancing skeletal matrix synthesis and degradation. *Biochem J* 2002;364:329-341.

Boyle WJ, Simonet WS, Lacey DL: Osteoclast differentiation and activation. *Nature* 2003;423:337-342.

Ducy P, Schinke T, Karsenty G: The osteoblast: A sophisticated fibroblast under central surveillance. *Science* 2000;289:1501-1504.

Ehrlich PJ, Lanyon LE: Mechanical strain and bone cell function: A review. *Osteoporos Int* 2002;13:688-700.

Harada S, Rodan GA: Control of osteoblast function and regulation of bone mass. *Nature* 2003;423:349-355.

Manolagas SC, Jilka RL: Bone marrow, cytokines, and bone remodeling. *New Engl J Med* 1995;332:305-311.

Mundy GR, Chen D, Oyajobi BO: Bone remodeling, in Favus MJ (ed): *Primer on the Metabolic Bone Diseases and Disorders of Mineral Metabolism*, ed 5. Washington, DC, American Society for Bone and Mineral Research, 2003, pp 46-58.

Mundy GR, Elefteriou F: Boning up on ephrin signaling. *Cell* 2006;126:441-443.

Parfitt AM: Osteonal and hemiosteonal remodeling: The spatial and temporal framework for signal traffic in adult human bone. *J Cell Biochem* 1994;55:273-286.

Roodman GD: Mechanisms of bone metastasis. *N Engl J Med* 2004;350:1655-1664.

Rubin J, Rubin C, Jacobs CR: Molecular pathways mediating mechanical signaling in bone. *Gene* 2006;367:1-16.

Mechanical Properties of Bone
Ammann P, Rizzoli R: Bone strength and its determinants. *Osteoporos Int* 2003;14(suppl 3):S13-S18.

Burr DB: The contribution of the organic matrix to bone's material properties. *Bone* 2002;31:8-11.

Carter DR, Spengler DM: Mechanical properties and composition of cortical bone. *Clin Orthop Relat Res* 1978;135:192-217.

Cullinane DM, Einhorn TA: Biomechanics of bone, in Bilezikian JP, Raisz LG, Rodan GA (eds): *Principles of Bone Biology*, ed 2. San Diego, CA, Academic Press, 2002, pp 17-32.

Currey JD: *Bones: Structure and Mechanics*. Princeton, NJ, Princeton University Press, 2002, pp 54-124, 194-245.

Hayes WC: Biomechanics of cortical and trabecular bone: Implications for assessment of fracture risk, in *Basic Orthopaedic Biomechanics*. New York, NY, Raven Press, 1991, pp 93-142.

Keaveny TM, Morgan EF, Niebur GL, Yeh OC: Biomechanics of trabecular bone. *Annu Rev Biomed Eng* 2001;3:307-333.

Martin RB: Determinants of the mechanical properties of bones. *J Biomech* 1991;24(suppl 1):79-88.

Wang X, Puram S: The toughness of cortical bone and its relationship with age. *Ann Biomed Eng* 2004;32:123-135.

Chapter 9

Articular Cartilage and Osteoarthritis

Henry J. Mankin, MD
Alan J. Grodzinsky, ScD
Joseph A. Buckwalter, MD, MS

Introduction

Articular cartilage is the tissue that lines the joints and makes low friction and painless movement of synovial joints possible throughout life. The tissue consists of a sparse population of highly specialized cells, chondrocytes, that are embedded within a matrix consisting of collagens, proteoglycans, and noncollagenous proteins. The matrix protects the cells from injury caused by normal joint use and also serves as a resilient structure, which allows for flexibility of the joints and provides a lubrication system for frictionless movement. The matrix also limits the ingress of materials from the synovial fluid and the egress of materials from within the cartilage and thus acts as a system that determines the types and concentrations of molecules that reach the cells. Articular cartilage is not only remarkably frictionless in function and self-lubricating but is also self-renewing. Thus, throughout life the cells synthesize matrix macromolecules lost through degradation and maintain the capacity for motion and resiliency. With aging, however, chondrocytes slowly lose their ability to maintain and restore the matrix materials and over time and with recurrent trauma, the cartilage failure leads to the clinical syndrome recognized as osteoarthritis.

Articular Cartilage Composition

The gross and microscopic structure of adult articular cartilage suggests that the tissue is simple in composition and inert. Examining the tissue inside a joint shows that the surface is smooth and resists deformation when probed. Watching cartilage move on cartilage strongly supports the concept that the movement is virtually frictionless. Light microscopic examination shows that articular cartilage consists primarily of extracellular matrix, with a sparse population of cells. Furthermore, there are no blood vessels, lymphatic vessels, and nerves (**Figures 1 and 2**). If the relative metabolic activity of cartilage is com-

pared with that of muscle or bone, there is little doubt that cartilage is limited in its response to alterations in various parameters, except as stated above, the almost frictionless movement in relation to other cartilaginous surfaces. Despite these characteristics, study of the morphology and biology of adult articular cartilage shows that it has an elaborate highly ordered structure and that complex interactions between the chondrocytes and the matrix are essential to maintain the tissue and its function in the synovial joint.

Chondrocytes

There is only one type of cell within cartilage: the highly specialized chondrocyte (**Figure 2**). These cells contribute little to the volume of the tissue, representing approximately 1% of the composition of adult human articular cartilage. Chondrocytes from different cartilage zones and from different joints vary in size, shape, and probably in metabolic activity but all of these cells contain the organelles such as endoplasmic reticulum and Golgi apparatus necessary for matrix synthesis. The cells also frequently contain intracytoplasmic filaments, lipid, glycogen, and secretory vesicles, which are likely necessary for maintenance of the matrix structure. Chondrocytes surround themselves with extracellular matrix and unlike osteocytes do not form cell-to-cell contacts. The chondrocytes in the surface layer are elongated and resemble fibroblasts whereas those in the transitional layer are rounded and appear actively involved in the cartilage chemistry. Deeper layers in adult cartilage show the cells in a radial pattern; below the tidemark the cells are smaller and appear to be nonfunctional (**Figure 1**).

At first glance chondrocytes seem to be observers rather than participants in the function of mature articular cartilage. They appear to remain unchanged in size, location, appearance, and activity for decades and do not seem to participate in water distribution, which is essential for cartilage resiliency and joint lubrication or in the concentrations of collagen and proteoglycans. It is clear, however, that the chondrocytes are in large measure responsible for the maintenance and structural competence of these materials and for allowing them to carry out their required activities and functions. The chondrocytes are responsible for producing and replacing appropriate amounts of macromolecules and assembling them into a highly ordered macromolecular framework. To accomplish these activities, the cells must sense changes in the matrix composition caused by degradation of macromolecules and the mechanical demands placed on the articular surface, and then respond by synthesizing appropriate types and amounts of macromolecules.

Aging profoundly alters chondrocyte function. With aging, the capacity of the cells to synthesize some types of proteoglycans, their proliferative capacity, and their response to anabolic stimuli (including growth factors) decreases. These changes may limit the ability of the cells to maintain and restore the tissue and thereby contribute to the development and progression of articular cartilage degeneration.

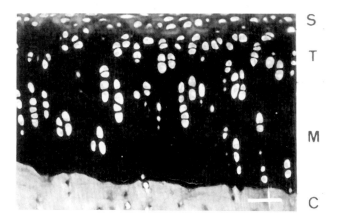

Figure 1   Articular cartilage from the medial femoral condyle of an 8-month-old rabbit. The tissue is organized into four layers or zones: the superficial zone (S), the transitional zone (T), the middle (radial or deep) zone (M), and the calcified cartilage zone (C). Bar = 50 nm. *(Reproduced from Buckwalter JA, Hunziker EB, Rosenberg LC, et al: Articular cartilage: Composition and structure, in Woo SL, Buckwalter JA (eds): Injury and Repair of the Musculoskeletal Soft Tissues. Park Ridge, IL, American Academy of Orthopaedic Surgeons, 1988, pp 405-425.)*

Extracellular Matrix

The articular cartilage matrix consists of two components: the tissue fluid and the framework of structural macromolecules that give the tissue its form and stability. The interaction of the tissue fluid and the macromolecular framework give the tissue its mechanical properties of stiffness and resilience. Water contributes up to 80% of

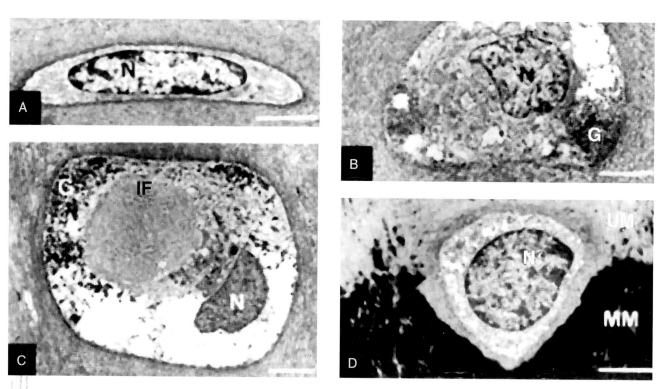

Figure 2   Electron micrographs showing the superficial zone (A), transitional zone (B), middle (radial or deep) zone (C), and calcified cartilage zone (D) of mature articular cartilage chondrocytes from the medial femoral condyle of a rabbit. N = nucleus, G = glycogen, IF = intermediate filaments, MM = mineralized matrix, UM = unmineralized matrix, bar = 3 nm. *(Reproduced from Buckwalter JA, Hunziker EB, Rosenberg LC, et al: Articular cartilage: Composition and structure, in Woo SL, Buckwalter JA (eds): Injury and Repair of the Musculoskeletal Soft Tissues. Park Ridge, IL, American Academy of Orthopaedic Surgeons, 1988, pp 405-425.)*

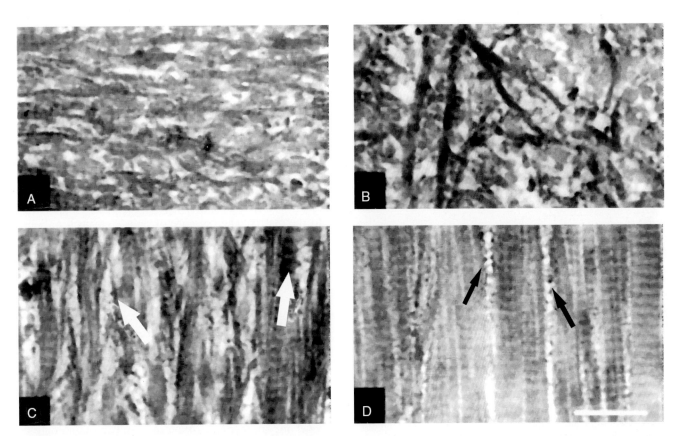

Figure 3   Electron micrographs showing the superficial zone **(A)**, transitional zone **(B)**, upper portion of the middle (radial or deep) zone **(C)**, and lower portion of the middle zone **(D)** of the articular cartilage interterritorial matrix from the medial femoral condyle of an 8-month-old rabbit. Arrows indicate proteoglycans precipitated with ruthenium hexamine trichloride. Bar = 0.5 nm. *(Reproduced from Buckwalter JA, Hunziker EB, Rosenberg LC, et al: Articular cartilage: Composition and structure, in Woo SL, Buckwalter JA (eds): Injury and Repair of the Musculoskeletal Soft Tissues. Park Ridge, IL, American Academy of Orthopaedic Surgeons, 1988, pp 405-425.)*

the weight of articular cartilage and the interaction of water with the matrix macromolecules significantly influences the mechanical properties of the tissue. Some of the water is in the form of a gel and thus with pressure can move freely in and out of the tissue. With pressure on the cartilage the water may move out of the tissue and form a relationship with the cartilage surface, which then serves as the lubrication system for cartilage movement on cartilage. The volume, concentration, and behavior within the tissue depends primarily on its interaction with the structural macromolecules: in particular, the large aggregating proteoglycans that help maintain the fluid within the matrix and the fluid electrolyte concentrations. Because these macromolecules have large numbers of negative charges that attract positively charged ions and repel negatively charged ions, they increase the concentration of positive ions such as sodium and decrease the concentration of negative ions such as chloride. The increase in total inorganic ion concentration increases the tissue osmolarity.

Structural Macromolecules

The cartilage structural macromolecules, collagens, proteoglycans, and noncollagenous proteins contribute 20% to 40% of the wet weight of the tissue. The three classes of

macromolecules differ in their concentrations within the tissue and in their contributions to the tissue properties. Collagens contribute about 60% of the dry weight of cartilage, proteoglycans contribute 25% to 35%, and the noncollagenous proteins and glycoproteins contribute 15% to 20%. Collagens are distributed relatively uniformly throughout the depth of the cartilage, except for the collagen-rich superficial zone ("the skin" of cartilage in which the collagen fibers run parallel the surface). The collagen fibrillar meshwork gives cartilage its form and tensile strength and also is responsible for maintaining the physical location of the chondrocyte. Proteoglycans and noncollagenous proteins bind to the collagenous meshwork or become mechanically entrapped within it, and water fills this molecular framework. Some noncollagenous proteins help organize and stabilize the matrix macromolecular framework whereas others help chondrocytes bind to the macromolecules of the matrix.

Articular cartilage, like most tissues, contains multiple genetically distinct collagen types, the major ones being collagen types II, VI, IX, X and XI. Collagen types II, IX and XI form the cross-banded fibrils seen by electron microscopy (**Figure 3**). The organization of these fibrils into a tight meshwork that extends throughout the tissue provides the tensile stiffness and strength of articular cartilage and contributes to the cohesiveness of the tissue by mechanically entrapping the large proteoglycans. The principal articular cartilage collagen, type II, accounts for 90% to 95% of the cartilage collagen and forms the primary component of the cross-banded fibrils. Type IX collagen molecules bind covalently to the superficial layers of the cross-banded fibrils and project into the matrix where they also can bind covalently to other type IX collagen molecules. Type XI collagen molecules bind covalently to type II collagen molecules and probably form part of the interior structure of the cross-banded fibrils. The projecting portions of type IX collagen molecules may also help bind together the collagen fibril mesh and connect the collagen meshwork with proteoglycans. Type VI collagen appears to form an important part of the matrix immediately surrounding chondrocytes and help chondrocytes attach to the matrix. The presence of type X collagen only near the cells of the calcified cartilage zone of articular cartilage and the hypertrophic zone of growth plate (where the longitudinal cartilage septa begin to mineralize) suggests that it has a role in cartilage mineralization.

Proteoglycans

Proteoglycans consist of a protein core and one or more glycosaminoglycan chains (long unbranched polysaccharide chains) consisting of repeating disaccharides that contain an amino sugar. Each disaccharide unit has at least one negatively charged carboxylate or sulfate group, so the glycosaminoglycans form long strings of negative charges that repel one another and attract cations. Glycosaminoglycans found in cartilage include hyaluronic acid, chondroitin sulfate, keratan sulfate, and dermatan sulfate. The concentration of these molecules varies among sites within articular cartilage and also with age, cartilage injury, and disease.

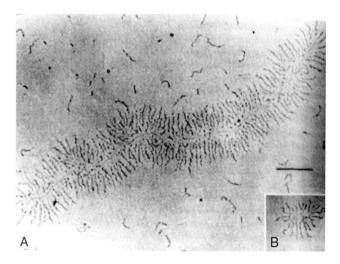

Figure 4   Transmission electron micrograph showing bovine articular cartilage proteoglycan aggregates from a calf **(A)** and steer **(B)** consisting of central hyaluronan filaments and multiple attached aggrecans. Aggregates from older animals have shorter hyaluronan filaments and fewer aggrecans. In addition, the aggrecans are shorter and vary more in length. Bar = 500 nm. *(Reproduced with permission from Buckwalter JA, Kuettner KE, Thonar EJ-M: Age-related changes in articular cartilage proteoglycans: Electron microscopic studies.* J Orthop Res *1985;3: 251-257.)*

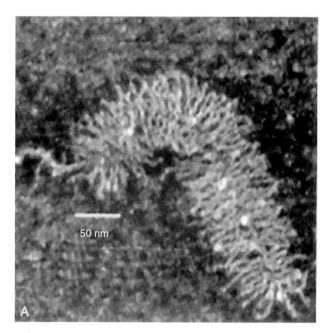
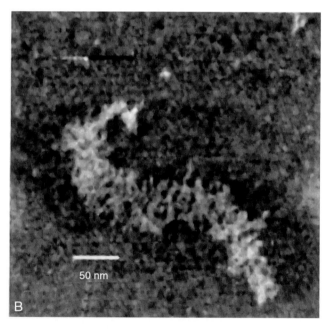

Figure 5   **A,** Atomic force image of aggrecan from fetal bovine epiphyseal cartilage. Note that glycosaminoglycan chains project from the central protein filament of the aggrecan molecule. **B,** Atomic force image of aggrecan from mature bovine nasal cartilage. Note that the aggrecan molecule from a skeletally mature animal is shorter and has shorter glycosaminoglycan chains. *(Reproduced with permission from Ng L, Grodzinsky AJ, Sandy JD, et al: Structure and conformation of individual aggrecan molecules and the constituent GAG chains via atomic force microscopy.* J Struct Biol *2003;143:242-257.)*

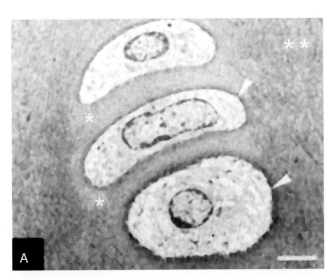
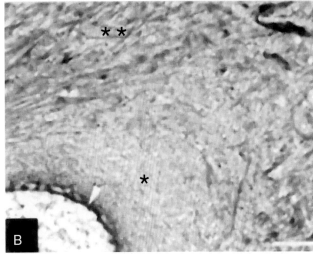

Figure 6   **A,** Electron micrograph showing the articular cartilage matrix compartments of the medial femoral condyle of an 8-month-old rabbit. Arrowheads indicate pericellular matrix, * indicates territorial matrix. Bar = 3 nm. **B,** A higher magnification electron micrograph showing the same matrix compartments and the relationship between the cell membrane and the pericellular matrix. Bar = 1 nm. Notice the short-cell processes that extend through the pericellular matrix. *(Reproduced from Buckwalter JA, Hunziker EB, Rosenberg LC, et al: Articular cartilage: Composition and structure, in Woo SL, Buckwalter JA (eds): Injury and Repair of the Musculoskeletal Soft Tissues. Park Ridge, IL, American Academy of Orthopaedic Surgeons, 1988, pp 405-425.)*

Articular cartilage contains two major classes of proteoglycans: large aggregating molecules or aggrecans (**Figure 4**) and smaller proteoglycans including decorin (d*Eco*-RIn), biglycan, and fibromodulin. Because it may have a glycosaminoglycan component, type IX collagen is also considered a proteoglycan. Aggrecans have large numbers of chondroitin sulfate and keratan sulfate chains attached to a protein core filament (**Figure 5**). Decorin has one dermatan sulfate chain, biglycan has two dermatan sulfate chains, and fibromodulin has several keratan sulfate chains. Aggrecan molecules fill most of the interfibrillar space of the cartilage matrix. They contribute about 90% of the total cartilage matrix proteoglycan mass, whereas large nonaggregating proteoglycans contribute 10% or less and small nonaggregating proteoglycans contribute about 3%.

In the articular cartilage matrix, most aggrecans (**Figure 6**) noncovalently associate with hyaluronic acid (hyaluronan) and link proteins, small noncollagenous proteins, to form proteoglycan aggregates (**Figure 4**). These large molecules have a central hyaluronan backbone that can vary in length from several hundred nanometers to more than 10,000 nanometers. Large aggregates may have more than 300 associated aggrecan molecules. Link proteins stabilize the association between monomers and hyaluronic acid. Aggregate formation helps anchor proteoglycans within the matrix, preventing their displacement during deformation of the tissue, and helps organize and stabilize the relationship between proteoglycans and the collagen meshwork.

The small nonaggregating proteoglycans have shorter protein cores than aggrecan molecules, and unlike aggrecans they do not fill a large volume of the tissue or contribute directly to the mechanical behavior of the tissue. Instead they bind to other macromolecules and probably influence cell function. Decorin and fibromodulin bind with type II collagen and may have a role in organizing and stabilizing the type II collagen meshwork, and biglycan may interact with type VI collagen. The small proteoglycans also can bind transforming growth factor β and may limit healing of cartilage and alter degradative enzyme production.

Noncollagenous Proteins and Glycoproteins

A wide variety of noncollagenous proteins and glycoproteins exist within normal articular cartilage and appear to consist primarily of protein and a few attached monosaccharides and oligosaccharides. Some of these appear to help organize and maintain the macromolecular structure of the matrix. Anchorin CII, a collagen-binding chondrocyte surface protein, may help "anchor" chondrocytes to the matrix collagen fibrils. Cartilage oligomeric protein (COMP), an acidic protein, is concentrated primarily within the chondrocyte territorial matrix and appears to be present only within cartilage and have the capacity to bind to chondrocytes. Fibronectin and tenascin, noncollagenous matrix proteins that are found in a variety of tissues, have also been identified within cartilage but thus far their functions are not well understood.

Zones of Articular Cartilage

The morphologic changes in chondrocytes and matrix from the articular surface to the subchondral bone make it possible to identify four zones, or layers: the superficial zone, the transitional zone, the radial zone, and the zone of calcified cartilage (**Figure 1**). The relative size and appearance of these zones varies among species and among joints within the same species; although each zone has different morphologic features, the boundaries between zones cannot be sharply defined. Nonetheless, recent biologic and mechanical studies have shown that the zonal organization has an important functional significance. The matrices differ in water, proteoglycan and collagen concentrations, and in the size of the aggregates. Cells in different zones not only differ in shape, size, and orientation relative to the articular surface (**Figure 2**), they also appear to differ in metabolic and synthetic activity.

Superficial Zone

The unique structure and composition of the thinnest articular cartilage zone, the superficial zone, give it specialized mechanical and possibly biologic properties. It typically consists of two layers. A sheet of fine fibrils with little polysaccharide and no cells covers the joint surface. This portion of the superficial zone presumably corresponds to the clear film, often identified as the lamina splendens. Deep to this acellular sheet of fine fibrils, flattened ellipsoid-shaped chondrocytes resembling fibroblasts arrange themselves so that their major axes are parallel to the articular surface (**Figure 2**). They synthesize a matrix that has a high collagen concentration and a low proteoglycan concentration relative to the other cartilage zones. The collagen fibers formed by the cells form the "cartilage skin" and limit ingress of materials that might be toxic and limit egress of important components. The superficial zone may thus serve effectively to isolate cartilage from the immune system. Fibronectin and water concentrations are also highest in this zone.

The dense mat of collagen fibrils lying parallel to the joint surface in the superficial zone (**Figure 3**) also give this cartilage zone greater tensile stiffness and strength and probably acts to resist compressive forces generated during joint use. Alterations in this zone may contribute to the development of osteoarthritis by altering the mechanical behavior of the tissue. Thus, disruption of the superficial zone may not only alter the structure and mechanical properties of articular cartilage, it may release cartilage molecules that stimulate an immune or inflammatory response.

Transitional Zone

As the name transitional zone implies, the morphology and matrix composition of the transitional zone is intermediate between the superficial zone and the radial zone. It usually has several times the volume of the superficial zone. The cells have a higher concentration of synthetic organelles, endoplasmic reticulum, and Golgi membranes than superficial zone cells (**Figure 2**). Transitional zone cells assume a spheroidal shape and synthesize a matrix that has larger diameter collagen fibrils and a higher pro-

teoglycan concentration, but lower concentrations of water and collagen than the superficial zone matrix.

Middle (Radial or Deep) Zone

The chondrocytes in the middle zone are spheroidal in shape, and they tend to align themselves in columns perpendicular to the joint surface (**Figures 1 and 2**). This zone contains the largest diameter collagen fibrils, the highest concentration of proteoglycans, and the lowest concentration of water. The collagen fibers of this zone pass into the tidemark, a thin basophilic line seen on hematoxylin and eosin microscopic sections of decalcified articular cartilage that roughly corresponds to the boundary between calcified and uncalcified cartilage. The structure of the collagen fibers in this region are perpendicular to the cartilage structure and hence are presumed to resist shear stress during movement of the cartilage.

Calcified Cartilage Zone

A thin zone of calcified cartilage separates the radial zone (uncalcified cartilage) and the subchondral bone. The cells of the calcified cartilage zone have a smaller volume than the cells of the radial zone and contain only small amounts of endoplasmic reticulum and Golgi membranes (**Figure 2**). In some regions these cells appear to be completely surrounded by calcified cartilage and are considered to be buried in individual "calcific sepulchers." This appearance suggests that they have an extremely low level of metabolic activity and may not be functional. There is no evidence to suggest that nutrients from the underlying bone traverse this zone.

Matrix Regions

Variations in the matrix within zones distinguish three regions or compartments: the pericellular region, the territorial region, and the interterritorial region (**Figure 7**). The pericellular and territorial regions appear to serve the needs of chondrocytes, that is, binding the cell membranes to the matrix macromolecules and protecting the cells from damage during loading and deformation of the tissue. They may also help transmit mechanical signals to the chondrocytes when the matrix deforms during joint loading. The primary function of the interterritorial matrix (**Figures 3 and 7**) is to provide the mechanical properties of the tissue.

Chondrocyte-Matrix Interactions

The interdependence of chondrocytes and the matrix makes possible the maintenance of the tissue throughout life. The relationship between the chondrocytes and the matrix does not end when the cells secrete the matrix macromolecules. The matrix protects the chondrocytes from mechanical damage during normal joint use and it helps maintain their shape and their phenotype. Nutri-

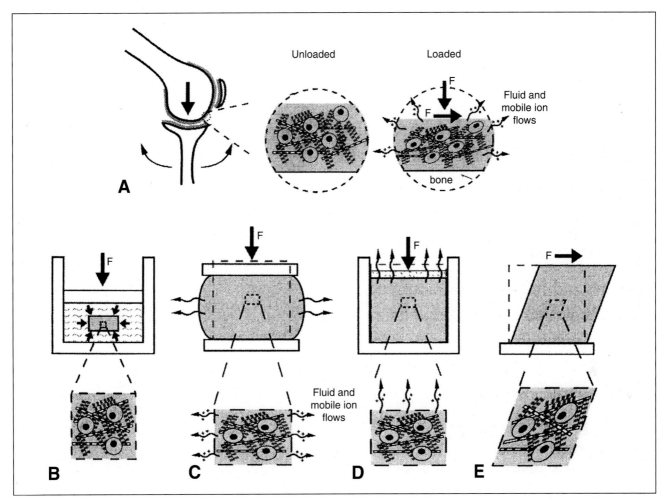

Figure 7   Loading of articular cartilage causes tissue deformation and changes in the cellular microenvironment. During joint motion **(A)**, articular cartilage (gray) is subjected to a complex combination of compression and shear forces, causing deformation of the cells and extracellular matrix as well as fluid and ion flows. Methodologies developed to measure cartilage biomechanical properties under hydrostatic (or osmotic) pressure loading **(B)**, unconfined **(C)** and confined **(D)** compression, shear **(E)**, and tension have been used to quantify the metabolic response of articular cartilage to normal and injurious mechanical loads. *(Adapted with permission from DeMicco M, Kim YJ, Grodzinsky AJ: Response of the chondrocyte to mechanical stimuli, in Brandt K, Doherty M, Lohmander S (eds): Osteoarthritis. Oxford, England, Oxford University Press, 2003.)*

ents, substrates for synthesis of matrix molecules, newly synthesized molecules, degraded matrix molecules, metabolic waste products and molecules that help regulate cell function, such as cytokines and growth factors, all pass through the matrix, and in some instances may be stored in the matrix.

Throughout life, chondrocytes degrade and synthesize matrix macromolecules. The mechanisms that control the balance between these activities remain poorly understood, but cytokines with catabolic and anabolic effects appear to have important roles. For example, interleukin 1 (IL-1) induces expression of matrix metalloproteases that can degrade the matrix macromolecules and interferes with synthesis of matrix proteoglycans at the transcriptional level. Other cytokines such as insulin-dependent growth factor I and transforming growth factor beta oppose these catabolic activities by stimulating matrix synthesis and cell proliferation. In response to a variety of stimuli, chondrocytes synthesize and release these cytokines into the matrix where they may bind to receptors on the cell surfaces (stimulating cell activity either by autocrine or paracrine mechanisms) or become trapped within the matrix. The degradative response, on the other hand, appears to be the result of a complex cascade that includes IL-1, stromelysin, aggrecanase, plasmin, and collagenase being activated or inhibited by factors such as prostaglandins, transforming growth factors beta, tumor necrosis factor, tissue inhibitors of metalloproteases, tissue plasminogen activator, plasminogen activator inhibitor, and other molecules.

Articular Cartilage Biomechanics

Articular cartilage is subjected to a wide range of static and dynamic mechanical loads. Under normal physiologic conditions, in vivo loading can result in peak dynamic mechanical stresses on cartilage as high as 15 to 20 MPa during activities such as stair climbing. These peak stresses occur over very short durations (< 1 second), and therefore lead to small cartilage compressive strains of about 1% to 3%. In contrast, sustained (static) physiologic stresses of approximately 3.5 MPa applied to knee joints for 5 to 30 minutes durations can result in compressive strains of knee cartilages as high as 35% to 45%.

The ability of cartilage to withstand physiologic compressive, tensile, and shear forces depends on the composition and structural integrity of its extracellular matrix. In turn, the maintenance of a functionally intact matrix requires chondrocyte-mediated synthesis, assembly, and degradation of proteoglycans, collagens, noncollagenous proteins and glycoproteins, and other matrix molecules. Measurements have revealed that the equilibrium compressive modulus of adult articular cartilage is on the order of approximately 0.5 to 1 MPa, the shear modulus about 0.25 MPa, and the tensile modulus about 10 to 50 MPa. Although strong rope-like collagen fibrils effectively resist tensile and shear deformation forces (**Figure 3**), the highly charge glycosaminoglycan constituents of aggrecan molecules (**Figure 4**) resist compression and fluid flow within the tissue. Indeed, electrostatic repulsion and osmotic swelling interactions associated with aggrecan contribute more than 50% of the equilibrium compressive stiffness of cartilage.

Studies have shown that joint loading can induce a wide range of metabolic responses in cartilage. Immobilization can cause decreases in matrix synthesis and content and a resultant softening of the tissue. In contrast, aggrecan concentration is higher in areas of loaded cartilage and appears to restore the cartilage structure. More severe impact or strenuous exercise loading can cause cartilage degradation. Acute and chronic injurious compressive overloads can lead to cartilage degeneration. Studies in vitro have demonstrated that static compression within the physiologic range can reversibly inhibit the synthesis of the cartilage matrix. In contrast, cyclically applied intermittent hydrostatic pressure and compressive strain can stimulate aggrecan core protein and protein synthesis.

Thus, mechanical forces in the microenvironment of the chondrocytes can significantly affect the synthesis and degradation of matrix macromolecules. Recent data suggest that there are multiple regulatory pathways by which chondrocytes sense and respond to mechanical stimuli. It also seems that altered pressure can alter not only the rate of matrix production, but the quality and functionality of newly synthesized proteoglycans, collagens, and other molecules. In this manner, specific mechanical loading regimens may either enhance or compromise the long-term biomechanical function of cartilage.

The functional biomechanical properties of cartilage tissue over the long term may be determined in part by the molecular mechanical properties of individual matrix

molecules synthesized by the chondrocytes in the injured cartilage. Thus, the biosynthesis of functionally inferior matrix macromolecules that cannot properly contribute to or assemble into a mechanically functional matrix may be one of the hallmarks of the progression of posttraumatic cartilage degradation.

Articular Cartilage Degeneration and Osteoarthritis

Articular cartilage degeneration, the progressive loss of normal cartilage structure and function, leads to the clinical syndrome of osteoarthritis. Osteoarthritis, also referred to as degenerative joint disease, degenerative arthritis, or hypertrophic arthritis, consists of a generally progressive loss of articular cartilage accompanied by attempted repair of articular cartilage, remodeling and sclerosis of subchondral bone, and in many instances the formation of subchondral bone cysts and marginal osteophytes. In addition to the structural changes in the synovial joint, diagnosis of the clinical syndrome of osteoarthritis requires the presence of symptoms and signs that may include joint pain, restriction of motion, crepitus with motion, joint effusions, and deformity. Osteoarthritis occurs most frequently in the foot, knee, hip, spine, and hand joints, but it can occur in any synovial joint.

Joint degeneration involves all of the tissues that form the synovial joint, including articular cartilage, subchondral and metaphyseal bone, synovium, ligaments, joint capsules, and the muscles that act across the joint; but the primary changes consist of loss of articular cartilage, remodeling of subchondral bone, and formation of osteophytes. The earliest microscopic changes seen in joint degeneration include fraying or fibrillation of the articular cartilage superficial zone extending into the transitional zone, decreased staining for proteoglycans in the superficial and transitional zones, violation of the tidemark by blood vessels from subchondral bone, and subchondral bone remodeling.

The earliest sign of degeneration visible from the articular surface is localized fibrillation or disruption of the most superficial layers of the articular cartilage. As the disease progresses, the surface irregularities become clefts, more of the articular surface becomes roughened and irregular, and fibrillation extends deeper into the cartilage until the fissures reach subchondral bone. As the cartilage fissures grow deeper, the superficial tips of the fibrillated cartilage tear, releasing free fragments into the joint space and decreasing the cartilage thickness. At the same time, enzymatic degradation of the matrix further decreases the cartilage volume. Eventually the progressive loss of articular cartilage leaves only dense and often necrotic eburnated bone.

Many of the mechanisms responsible for progressive loss of cartilage in degenerative joint disease remain unknown, but the process can be divided into three overlapping stages: cartilage matrix damage or alteration, chondrocyte response to tissue damage, and the decline of the chondrocyte synthetic response and progressive loss of tissue.

In the first stage, the matrix macromolecular framework is disrupted and the water content increases. Although the concentration of type II collagen remains constant, decreases in proteoglycan aggregation and aggrecan concentration and decreases in the length of the glycosaminoglycan chains almost invariably accompany the increase in water content. At the same time, alterations in the collagenous framework may allow swelling of the aggrecan molecules. Disruption or decreased organization of the macromolecular framework, decreased aggrecan concentration and aggregation, decreased glycosaminoglycan chain length, and increased water content taken together increase the permeability (that is, the ease with which water and other molecules move through the matrix) and decrease the stiffness of the matrix: alterations that may increase the vulnerability of the tissue to further mechanical damage. This first phase may occur as a result of a variety of mechanical insults including high intensity impact or torsional loading of a joint, accelerated degradation of matrix macromolecules as a result of joint inflammation or similar insults, or as a result of metabolic changes in the tissue that interfere with the ability of chondrocytes to maintain the matrix.

The second stage begins when chondrocytes detect the tissue damage or alterations in osmolarity, charge density, or strain, and release mediators that stimulate a cellular response that is often quite brisk. The response consists of both anabolic and catabolic activity as well as chondrocyte proliferation. Anabolic and mitogenic growth factors presumably have an important role in stimulating synthesis of matrix macromolecules and chondrocyte proliferation; clusters or clones of proliferating cells surrounded by newly synthesized matrix molecules constitute one of the histologic hallmarks of the chondrocytic response to cartilage degeneration. Nitric oxide may have a role in the chondrocyte response because chondrocytes produce this molecule in response to a variety of stresses. The nitric oxide can induce production of the cytokine IL-1, which stimulates expression of metalloproteases that degrade the matrix macromolecules. Fibronectin fragments or other molecules present in damaged tissue may promote continued production of IL-1 and enhanced release of proteases. Degradation of type IX and type XI collagens and other molecules may destabilize the type II collagen fibril meshwork leaving many of the type II fibrils intact initially, but allowing expansion of aggrecan and increased water content. Disruption of the superficial zone, a decline in aggregation, and an associated loss of aggrecan caused by enzymatic degradation would increase the stresses on the remaining collagen fibril network and chondrocytes with joint loading.

In the second stage of osteoarthritis, the repair re-

sponse, increased synthesis of matrix macromolecules, and, to a lesser degree, cell proliferation are noted, which to some extent counters the catabolic effects of the proteases and may stabilize or, in some instances, actually restore the tissue. The repair response may last for years and may in some patients reverse the course of osteoarthritis, at least temporarily. Furthermore, some therapeutic interventions have the potential for facilitating the repair response. For example, study of osteoarthrotic hips and knees following osteotomy shows that altering the joint mechanical environment will stimulate restoration of an articular surface in some instance.

Failure to stabilize or restore the tissue leads to the third stage in the development of osteoarthritis, progressive loss of articular cartilage and a decline in the chondrocytic anabolic and proliferative response. This decline could result from mechanical damage and death of chondrocytes no longer stabilized and protected by a functional matrix, but it also appears to be related to, or initiated by, a downregulation of chondrocyte response to anabolic cytokines. This decline may occur as a result of synthesis and accumulation of molecules in the matrix that bind anabolic cytokines including decorin, insulin-dependent growth factor binding protein, and other molecules that can affect cytokine function. The loss of articular cartilage leads to the clinical syndrome of osteoarthritis: joint pain and loss of joint function. The joint degeneration responsible for osteoarthritis occurs more frequently with increasing age possibly because age-related changes in the cartilage matrix and a decrease in the chondrocyte anabolic response compromise the ability of the tissue to maintain and restore itself.

Alterations of the subchondral bone that accompany the degeneration of articular cartilage include increased subchondral bone density or subchondral sclerosis, formation of cyst-like bone cavities containing myxoid, fibrous, or cartilaginous tissue, and the appearance of regenerating cartilage within and on the subchondral bone surface. This response is usually most apparent on the periphery of the joint where bony and cartilaginous excrescences sometimes form sizable osteophytes. Increased subchondral bone density resulting from formation of new layers of bone on existing trabeculae is usually the first sign of degenerative joint disease in subchondral bone, but in some joints subchondral cavities appear before a generalized increase in bone density. At the end stage of the disease the articular cartilage has been completely lost, leaving thickened dense subchondral bone articulating with a similar opposing denuded bony surface. The bone remodeling combined with the loss of articular cartilage changes joint shape and can lead to shortening of the involved limb, deformity, and instability.

In most synovial joints, growth of osteophytes accompanies the changes in articular cartilage and subchondral and metaphyseal bone. These fibrous, cartilaginous, and bony prominences usually develop around the periphery

Table 1 Causes of Secondary Osteoarthritis	
Cause	**Presumed Mechanism**
Joint injuries	Damage to articular surface and/or residual joint incongruity and instability
Joint dysplasias (developmental and hereditary joint and cartilage dysplasias)	Abnormal joint shape and/or abnormal articular cartilage
Aseptic necrosis	Bone necrosis leads to collapse of the articular surface and joint incongruity
Acromegaly	Overgrowth of articular cartilage produces joint incongruity and/or abnormal cartilage
Paget's disease	Distortion or incongruity of joints resulting from bone remodeling
Ehlers-Danlos syndrome	Joint instability
Gaucher's disease (hereditary deficiency of the enzyme, glucocerebrosidase leading to accumulation of glucocerebroside)	Bone necrosis or pathologic bone fracture leading to joint incongruity
Stickler's syndrome (progressive hereditary arthro-ophthalmopathy)	Abnormal joint and/or articular cartilage development
Joint infection (inflammation)	Destruction of articular cartilage
Hemophilia	Multiple joint hemorrhages
Hemochromatosis (excess iron deposition in multiple tissues)	Mechanism unknown
Ochronosis (hereditary deficiency of enzyme, homogentisic acid oxidase leading to accumulation of homogentisic acid)	Deposition of homogentisic acid polymers in articular cartilage
Calcium pyrophosphate deposition disease	Accumulation of calcium pyrophosphate crystals in articular cartilage
Neuropathic arthropathy (Charcot's joints: syphilis, diabetes mellitus, syringomyelia, meningomyelocele, leprosy, congenital insensitivity to pain, amyloidosis)	Loss of proprioception and joint sensation results in increased impact loading and torsion, joint instability and intra-articular fractures

(Reproduced with permission from Buckwalter JA, Mankin HJ: Articular cartilage II: Degenerationand osteoarthrosis, repair, regeneration and transplantation. J Bone Joint Surg Am 1997;79: 612-632.)

of the joint (marginal osteophytes, usually at the cartilage bone interface, but they may also appear along joint capsule insertions (capsular osteophytes). Intra-articular bony excrescences that protrude from degenerating joint surfaces are referred to as central osteophytes. Most marginal osteophytes have a cartilaginous surface that closely resembles normal articular cartilage and may appear to be an extension of the joint surface. In superficial joints they usually are palpable and may be tender, and in all joints they can restrict motion and contribute to pain with motion. Each joint has a characteristic pattern of osteophyte formation. In the hip they usually form around the rim of the acetabulum and the femoral articular cartilage. A prominent osteophyte along the inferior margin of the humeral articular surface commonly develops in degenerative disease of the glenohumeral joint. Osteophytes presumably represent a response to degeneration of articular cartilage and subchondral bone remodeling including release of anabolic cytokines that stimulate cell proliferation and formation of bony and cartilaginous matrices.

Loss of articular cartilage leads to secondary changes in the synovium, ligaments, and capsules and in the muscles that move the involved joint. The synovial membrane often develops a mild to moderate inflammatory reaction and may contain fragments of articular cartilage and pro-

duce more interleukins that further act to destroy the cartilage. With time the ligaments, capsules, and muscles become contracted. Decreased use of the joint and decreased range of motion leads to muscle atrophy. These secondary changes often contribute to the stiffness and weakness associated with osteoarthritis.

Osteoarthritis develops most commonly in the absence of a known cause; that is, primary or idiopathic osteoarthritis. Less frequently it develops as a result of joint injury, infection, or one of a variety of hereditary, developmental, metabolic, and neurologic disorders: a group of conditions referred to as secondary osteoarthritis (Table 1). The age of onset of secondary osteoarthritis depends on the underlying cause; thus, it may develop in young adults and even children as well as the elderly. In contrast, a strong association exists between the prevalence of primary osteoarthritis and increasing age.

Numerous factors have been suggested as related to the pathogenesis of primary osteoarthritis, including aging, genetic predisposition, hormonal and metabolic disorders, inflammation, and immunologic disturbances.

The incidence and prevalence of osteoarthritis increases rapidly after age 40 years. However, the changes in the chondrocyte and the matrix with age are not those of osteoarthritis. However, changes in articular cartilage caused by aging, in particular the loss of the ability of chondrocytes to maintain and restore the tissue, increase the risk of joint degeneration.

It is evident that some of the disease processes, such as hand and foot deformities, have a genetic and gender-specific origin but there is insufficient evidence to support the frequency and distribution of the process.

There is little doubt that individuals with acromegaly develop the disease quite spectacularly but studies seeking alterations in this and other hormonal influences have failed to locate a single characteristic alteration that could lead to the disease. Similarly, in patients with alkaptonuric ochronosis, osteoarthritis is characteristic and those with Paget's disease often have severe compromise of joints related to variation in structural change on the two sides of the joint. Nevertheless no data support any hormonal, metabolic, or joint disease as an identifiable cause of this widespread disorder.

Recent studies have strongly supported the idea that inflammatory activist agents, principally those of the interleukin series, may be active materials in the development of joint damage. This idea appears to relate principally to the activation of the degradative cascade. The cause of synovial inflammation is not clear but it may develop from the release of materials from damaged cartilage. These ideas suggest that the inflammatory idea is not one of genesis of the disease, but perpetuation.

There is ample evidence to suggest that some of the materials present in articular cartilage are not only unique, but under ordinary circumstances are hidden from the vascular system and the rest of the body. It has often been said of cartilage, which has no blood, nerve, or lymphatic supply and is sealed in a sepulcher with a fibrous membrane at the surface and a tidemark at the bottom, that its chemical or more importantly, immunologic properties are unknown. If this statement is true, if some of the cartilaginous materials "escape" from the sepulcher, they may cause a significant amount of synovial inflammation, which can cause the release of agents that could degrade the cartilage.

Joint Injury and Posttraumatic Osteoarthritis

Injuries to articular surfaces, menisci, joint capsules, and ligaments increase the risk of joint degeneration that leads to a form of osteoarthritis referred to as posttraumatic osteoarthritis. Joint injury is a discrete event, and investigating its effects on articular cartilage could potentially help to understand the pathogenesis of osteoarthritis in general. Despite the development of surgical interventions that can restore mechanical stability and function to a patient's knee joint after ligament damage, these procedures do not appear to greatly reduce the risk for development of osteoarthritis. These developments suggest that in addition to the effects of subsequent functional impairment, the initial traumatic event may have irreversible effects on the joint tissues and resident cells.

Summary

The unique biologic and mechanical properties of articular cartilage depend on the design of the tissue and the interactions between chondrocytes and the matrix that maintain the tissue. Chondrocytes form the tissue matrix macromolecular framework from three classes of molecules: collagens, proteoglycans, and noncollagenous proteins. The matrix protects the cells from injury caused by normal joint use, it determines the types and concentrations of molecules that reach the cells, and it helps maintain the chondrocyte phenotype. Throughout life the tissue undergoes continual internal remodeling as the cells replace matrix macromolecules lost through degradation. The available evidence indicates that normal matrix turnover depends on the ability of chondrocytes to detect alterations in matrix macromolecular composition and organization, including the presence of degraded molecules, and to respond by synthesizing appropriate types and amounts of new molecules. In addition, the matrix acts as a signal transducer for the cells. Loading of the tissue as a result of joint use creates mechanical, electrical, and physicochemical signals that help direct chondrocyte synthetic and degradative activity. Aging leads to alterations in matrix composition and in chondrocyte activity, including the ability of the cells to respond to a variety of stimuli, including growth factors. These alterations may increase the probability of cartilage degeneration. Degeneration of articular cartilage that leads to the clinical syndrome of osteoarthritis is among the most common causes of pain and disability for middle-age and elderly persons. The strong correlation between increasing age and the prevalence of joint degeneration and recent evidence of important age-related changes in chondrocyte function suggest that chondrocyte aging contributes to the development and progression of joint degeneration. Clinical and basic investigations of the pathogenesis of posttraumatic osteoarthritis, the form of osteoarthritis that develops following joint injury, are helping to explain how joint degeneration develops and progresses.

Selected Bibliography
General

Buckwalter JA, Rosenberg LA, Hunziker EB: Articular cartilage: Composition, structure, response to injury, and methods of facilitation repair, in Ewing JW (ed): *Articular Cartilage and Knee Joint Function: Basic Science and Arthroscopy*. New York, NY, Raven Press, 1990, pp 19-56.

Buckwalter JA, Martin J, Mankin HJ: Synovial joint degeneration and the syndrome of osteoarthritis. *Instr Course Lect* 2000;49:481-489.

Martin JA, Buckwalter JA: Aging, articular cartilage chondrocyte senescence and osteoarthritis. *Biogerontology* 2002;3:257-264.

Martin JA, Buckwalter JA: Human chondrocyte senescence and osteoarthritis. *Biorheology* 2002;39:145-152.

Martin JA, Buckwalter JA: The role of chondrocyte senescence in the pathogenesis of osteoarthritis and in limiting cartilage repair. *J Bone Joint Surg Am* 2003;85-A(suppl 2):106-110.

Articular Cartilage Composition

Eyre DR: Collagen structure and function in articular cartilage: Metabolic changes in the development of osteoarthritis, in Kuettner KE, Goldberg VM (eds): *Osteoarthritic Disorders.* Rosemont, IL, American Academy of Orthopaedic Surgeons, 1995, pp 219-227.

Eyre DR, Wu JJ, Woods P: Cartilage-specific collagens: Structural studies, in Kuettner KE, Schleyerbach R, Peyron JG, Hascall VC (eds). *Articular Cartilage and Osteoarthritis.* New York, NY, Raven Press, 1992, pp 119-131, .

Hagiwara H, Schroter-Kermani C, Merker HJ: Localization of collagen type VI in articular cartilage of young and adult mice. *Cell Tissue Res* 1993;272:155-160.

Hedlund H, Mengarelli-Widholm S, Heinegard D, et al: Fibromodulin distribution and association with collagen. *Matrix Biol* 1994;14:227-232.

Heinegard D, Lorenzo P, Sommarin Y: Articular cartilage matrix proteins, in Kuettner KE, Goldberg VM (eds): *Osteoarthritic Disorders.* Rosemont, IL, American Academy of Orthopaedic Surgeons, 1995, pp 229-237.

Hildebrand A, Romaris M, Rasmussen LM, et al: Interaction of the small interstitial proteoglycans biglycan, decorin and fibromodulin with transforming growth factor beta. *Biochem J* 1994;302:527-534.

Lotz M, Blanco FJ, Kempis JV, et al: Cytokine regulation of chondrocyte functions. *J Rheumatol Suppl* 1995;43:104-108.

Marcelino J, McDevitt CA: Attachment of articular cartilage chondrocytes to the tissue form of type VI collagen. *Biochim Biophys Acta* 1995;1249:180-188.

Maroudas A, Schneiderman R: "Free" and "exchangeable" or "trapped" and "non-exchangeable" water in cartilage. *J Orthop Res* 1987;5:133-138.

Martin JA, Buckwalter JA: Effects of fibronectin on articular cartilage chondrocyte proteoglycan synthesis and response to insulin-like growth factor-I. *J Orthop Res* 1998;16:752-757.

Martin JA, Buckwalter JA: The role of chondrocyte-matrix interactions in maintaining and repairing articular cartilage. *Biorheology* 2000;37:129-140.

Martin JA, Miller BA, Scherb MB, et al: Co-localization of insulin-like growth factor binding protein 3 and fibronectin in human articular cartilage. *Osteoarthritis Cartilage* 2002;10:556-563.

Ng L, Grodzinsky AJ, Sandy JD, et al: Structure and conformation of individual aggrecan molecules and the constituent GAG chains via atomic force microscopy. *J Struct Biol* 2003;143:242-257.

Nishida K, Inoue H, Murakami T: Immunohistochemical demonstration of fibronectin in the most superfical layer of normal rabbit articular cartilage. *Ann Rheum Dis* 1995;54:995-998.

Pfaffle M, Borchert M, Deutzmann R, et al: Anchorin CII, a collagen-binding chondrocyte surface protein of the calpactin family. *Prog Clin Biol Res* 1990;349:147-157.

Poole AR, Rosenberg LC, Reiner A, et al: Contents and distribution of the proteoglycans decorin and biglycan in normal and osteoarthritic human articular cartilage. *J Orthop Res* 1996;14:681-689.

Rosenberg LC: Structure and function of dermatan sulfate proteoglycans in articular cartilage, in Kuettner KE, Schleyerbach R, Peyron JG, Hascall VC (eds): *Articular Cartilage and Osteoarthritis.* New York, NY, Raven Press, 1992, pp 45-63.

Roughley PJ, Lee ER: Cartilage proteoglycans: Structure and potential functions. *Microsc Res Tech* 1994;28:385-397.

Sandell LJ: Molecular biology of collagens in normal and osteoarthritic cartilage, in Kuettner KE, Goldberg VM (eds): *Osteoarthritic Disorders.* Rosemont, IL, American Academy of Orthopaedic Surgeons, 1995, pp 131-146.

Sandell LJ, Chansky H, Zamparo O, Hering TM: Molecular biology of cartilage proteoglycans and link protein, in Kuettner KE, Goldberg VM (eds): *Osteoarthritic Disorders*. Rosemont, IL, American Academy of Orthopaedic Surgeons, 1995, pp 117-130.

Tang LH, Buckwalter JA, Rosenberg LC: The effect of link protein concentration on articular cartilage proteoglycan aggregation. *J Orthop Res* 1996;14:334-339.

Articular Cartilage Biomechanics

Buckwalter JA, Grodzinsky AJ: The effects of loading on healing bone, fibrous tissue and muscle: Implications for orthopaedic practice. *J Am Acad Orthop Surg* 1999;7:291-299.

DeMicco M, Kim YJ, Grodzinsky AJ: Response of the chondrocyte to mechanical stimuli, in Brandt K, Doherty M, Lohmander S (eds): *Osteoarthritis*. Oxford, England, Oxford University Press, 2003.

Grodzinsky AJ, Levenston ME, Jin M, Frank EH: Cartilage tissue remodeling in response to mechanical forces. *Annu Rev Biomed Eng* 2000;2:691-713.

Guilak F, Mow VC: The mechanical environment of the chondrocyte: A biphasic finite element model of cell-matrix interactions in articular cartilage. *J Biomech* 2000;33:1663-1673.

Herberhold C, Faber S, Stammberger T, et al: In situ measurement of articular cartilage deformation in intact femoropatellar joints under static loading. *J Biomech* 1999;32:1287-1295.

Morales TI: The role of signaling factors in articular cartilage homeostasis and osteoarthritis, in Kuettner KE, Goldberg VM (eds): *Osteoarthritic Disorders*. Rosemont, IL, American Academy of Orthopaedic Surgeons, 1995, pp 261-270.

Mow VC, Hung CT: Mechanical properties of normal and osteoarthritic articular cartilage and the mechanobiology of chondrocytes, in Brandt K, Doherty M, Lohmander S (eds): *Osteoarthritis*. Oxford, England, Oxford University Press, 2003.

Articular Cartilage Degeneration and Osteoarthritis

Aigner T, Dietz U, Stoss H: Mark Kvd: Differential expression of collagen types I, II, III and X in human osteophytes. *Lab Invest* 1995;73:236-243.

Amin AR, DeCesare PE, Vyas P, et al: The expression and regulation of nitric oxide synthase in human osteoarthritis-affected chondrocytes: Evidence for up-regulated neuronal nitric oxide synthase. *J Exp Med* 1995;182:2097-2102.

Blanco FJ, Ochs RL, Schwarz H, Lotz M: Chondrocyte apoptosis induced by nitric oxide. *Am J Pathol* 1995; 146:75-85.

Buckwalter JA: Articular cartilage injuries. *Clin Orthop Relat Res* 2002;402:21-37.

Buckwalter JA: Sports, joint injury, and posttraumatic osteoarthritis. *J Orthop Sports Phys Ther* 2003;33:578-588.

Buckwalter JA, Lohmander S: Operative treatment of osteoarthrosis: Current practice and future development. *J Bone Joint Surg Am* 1994;76:1405-1418.

Buckwalter JA, Mankin HJ: Articular cartilage: Degeneration and osteoarthrosis, repair, regeneration and transplantation. *Instr Course Lect* 1998;47:487-504.

Chevalier X: Fibronectin, cartilage, and osteoarthritis. *Semin Arthritis Rheum* 1993;22:307-318.

Cs-Szabo G, Roughley PJ, Plaas AH, Glant TT: Large and small proteoglycans of osteoarthritic and rheumatoid articular cartilage. *Arthritis Rheum* 1995;38:660-668.

Dieppe P: The classification and diagnosis of osteoarthritis, in Kuettner KE, Goldberg VM (eds): *Osteoarthritic Disorders*. Rosemont, IL, American Academy of Orthopaedic Surgeons, 1995, pp 5-12.

Farquhar T, Xia Y, Mann K, et al: Swelling and fibronectin accumulation in articular cartilage explants after cyclical impact. *J Orthop Res* 1996;14:417-423.

Felson DT: The epidemiology of osteoarthritis: Prevalence and risk factors, in Kuettner KE, Goldberg VM (eds): *Osteoarthritic Disorders*. Rosemont, IL, American Academy of Orthopaedic Surgeons, 1995, pp 13-24.

Fukui N, Purple CR, Sandell LJ: Cell biology of osteoarthritis: The chondrocyte's response to injury. *Curr Rheumatol Rep* 2001;3:496-505.

Mankin HJ, Dorfman H, Lippiello L, Zarins A: Biochemical and metabolic abnormalities in articular cartilage from osteo-arthritic human hips: II. Correlation of morphology with biochemical and metabolic data. *J Bone Joint Surg Am* 1971;53:523-537.

Marsh JL, Buckwalter J, Gelberman R, et al: Articular fractures: Does an anatomic reduction really change the result? *J Bone Joint Surg Am* 2002;84-A:1259-1271.

Martel-Pelletier J, McCollum R, Fujimoto N, et al: Excess of metalloproteases over tissue inhibitor of metalloprotease may contribute to cartilage degredation in osteoarthritis and rheumatoid arthritis. *Lab Invest* 1994;70:807-815.

Schiller AL: Pathology of osteoarthritis, in Kuettner KE, Goldberg VM (eds): *Osteoarthritic Disorders.*

Rosemont, IL, American Academy of Orthopaedic Surgeons, 1995, pp 95-101.

Testa V, Capasso G, Maffulli M, et al: Proteases and antiproteases in cartilage homeostasis. A brief review. *Clin Orthop Relat Res* 1994;308:79-84.

van Beuningen HM: van der Kraan PM, Arntz OJ, Berg WB: Transforming growth factor-beta 1 stimulates articular chondrocyte proteoglycan synthesis and induces osteophyte formation in the murine knee joint. *Lab Invest* 1994;71:279-290.

Chapter 10

Form and Function of the Meniscus

Scott A. Rodeo, MD
Sumito Kawamura, MD

Introduction

The menisci are fibrocartilaginous tissues composed primarily of an interlacing network of collagen fibers interposed with cells and extracellular matrix. The menisci are an integral component of the knee joint; injury disrupts normal knee mechanics, resulting in progressive articular cartilage degeneration. One factor affecting treatment of meniscal injuries is the limited blood supply of the meniscus. Several studies have evaluated methods to increase the blood supply to this avascular tissue. Recent studies have examined applications of molecular biology to promote meniscal repair and replacement. The ability to design novel treatment strategies depends on a thorough understanding of meniscal structure, function, and physiology. This chapter describes salient basic science aspects of the meniscus, with a focus on clinically relevant basic science studies.

Anatomy

The menisci are C-shaped fibrocartilaginous tissues (Figures 1 and 2). The peripheral border of the meniscus is thick and attached to the capsule of the joint, whereas the inner border tapers to a thin free edge. The anterior and posterior meniscal horns are firmly attached to bone via insertional ligaments. In humans, the anterior horn of the medial meniscus is a flat, fan-shaped structure that inserts into the tibial plateau at the anterior intercondylar fossa, approximately 6 to 7 mm anterior to the insertion of the anterior cruciate ligament (ACL). The posterior horn of the medial meniscus attaches to the posterior intercondylar fossa of the tibia between the posterior attachment of the lateral meniscus and the tibial insertion of the posterior cruciate ligament. The anterior horn of the lateral meniscus attaches to the anterior intercondylar fossa of the tibia, just behind the anterior aspect of the tibial insertion of the ACL. The posterior horn of the lateral meniscus attaches to the tibia posterior to the lateral intercondylar eminence and anterior to the posterior enthesis of the me-

dial meniscus. The two meniscofemoral ligaments (the ligaments of Humphry and Wrisberg) run from the posterior body of the lateral meniscus to the medial femoral condyle, adjacent to the posterior cruciate ligament. An anterior and posterior meniscofemoral ligament has been reported in approximately 50% and 76% of cadaveric knees, respectively.

The medial meniscus is firmly attached to the peripheral joint capsule and is less mobile than the lateral meniscus (Figure 3). The lateral meniscus covers a larger percentage of the articular surface than the medial meniscus. The peripheral portion of the lateral meniscus has a loose attachment to the joint capsule.

Vascular Supply

The menisci are relatively avascular structures with a limited peripheral blood supply that predominantly originates from the lateral and medial genicular arteries. Branches from these vessels give rise to a perimeniscal capillary plexus within the synovial and capsular tissues of the knee joint. During the fetal period, blood vessels have been observed throughout the meniscus, with the greatest density of vessels occurring in the peripheral third of the tissue. From birth through adolescence, the density of meniscal cells and blood vessels decrease. In the adult, anatomic studies have shown that the degree of vascular penetration is 10% to 30% of the width of the medial meniscus and 10% to 25% of the width of the lateral meniscus (Figure 4). A small reflection of vascular synovial tissue (synovial fringe) also extends over the peripheral attachment of the medial and lateral menisci on both the femoral and tibial articular surfaces; however, this tissue does not contribute vessels into the meniscal tissue. Because most of the meniscus is avascular, nutrition must be derived through either diffusion or mechanical pumping; the latter mechanism is generated by intermittent compression of the tissue during weight bearing.

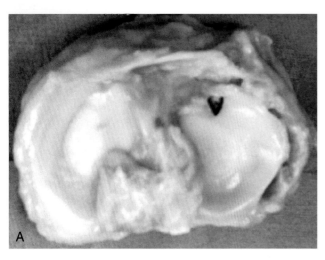

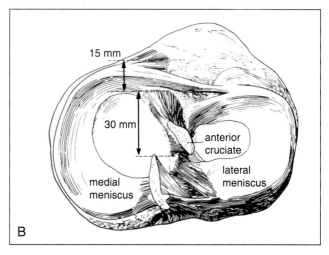

Figure 1   **A,** Human menisci. Right knee joint viewed from above. The tibial tuberosity is on top. The medial (left side of figure) and lateral (right side of figure) menisci are connected by the transverse ligament. **B,** Drawing of a tibial plateau showing the shape and attachments of the medial and lateral menisci. *(B is reproduced with permission from Warren RF, Arnoczky SP, Wickiewicz TL: Anatomy of the knee, in Nicholas JA, Hershman EB (eds):* The Lower Extremity and Spine in Sports Medicine. *St. Louis, MO, Mosby, 1986, pp 657-694.)*

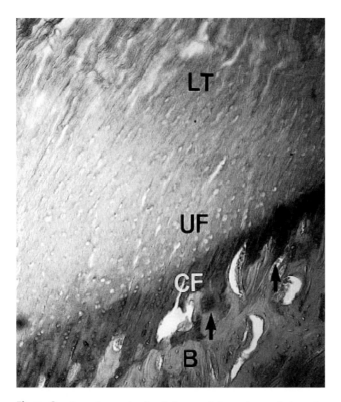

Figure 2   Anterior enthesis of the medial meniscus of the rabbit knee. Four distinct tissue types are identified at the attachment site: ligamentous tissue (LT), uncalcified fibrocartilage (UF), calcified fibrocartilage (CF), and bone (B). The calcified fibrocartilage in the meniscal enthesis interdigitates with the bone at different angles and depths, similar to other ligament entheses. *(Reproduced with permission from Messner K, Gao J: The menisci of the knee joint: Anatomic and functional characteristics, and a rationale for clinical treatment.* J Anat *1998;193: 161-178.)*

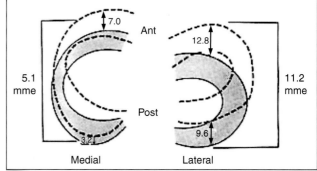

Figure 3   The segmental and mean excursion of meniscus along the tibial plateau. mme = mean meniscal excursion, Ant = anterior, Post = posterior. *(Reproduced with permission from Thomson WO, Thaete FL, Fu FH, Dye SF: Tibial meniscal dynamics using three-dimensional reconstruction of magnetic resonance images.* Am J Sports Med *1991;19:210-215.)*

Nerve Supply

Innervation to the menisci arises mainly from the posterior articular nerve (originating from the posterior tibial nerve in the popliteal fossa), but the medial meniscus also derives partial innervation from branches of the medial articular nerve. It is generally agreed that the nerve supply to menisci is more extensive at the horn attachment sites than the body (somewhat similar to vascularization), but reports vary on the presence of significant innervation in the inner area. However, it is evident that encapsulated end organs with mechanoreceptor function predominate at the horns, and that free nerve endings are found throughout the tissue except for the inner third of the meniscal body.

Histologic studies of human and animal menisci have identified the presence of neural elements within the meniscal tissue; these neural elements were most abundant in the outer portion of the meniscus. Studies of human specimens have identified three morphologically distinct mechanoreceptors within the meniscus: Ruffini-type endings, Golgi-like tension receptors, and pacinian corpuscles. The anterior and posterior horns of the meniscus are well innervated with such mechanoreceptors. The number of nerve endings decreases with increasing age. Nerve filaments also were detected in uncalcified and calcified fibrocartilage and the subchondral bone at the anterior and posterior attachment sites of rabbit medial meniscus. These neural elements are believed to be part of a proprioceptive reflex arc that may contribute to the functional stability of the knee. At the extremes of motion, increased tension at the meniscal horns may activate these neural receptors and provide joint position information to the central nervous system.

Meniscal Cell Biology

There appear to be three cell types in the meniscus: (1) fibrochondrocytes, located predominantly in the inner half; (2) fibroblast-like cells that occupy the outer, more fibrous portion; and (3) superficial zone cells, located on the surface (**Figure 5**).

Fibrochondrocytes are round or oval-shaped cells that synthesize type I collagen as their major form of fibrillar collagen and are surrounded by a pericellular matrix. The

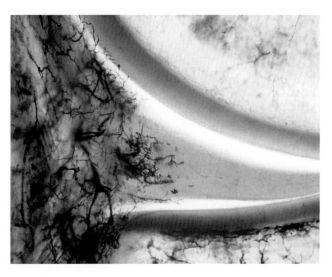

Figure 4   Coronal section of a medial meniscus after vascular perfusion with India ink and tissue clearing with a modified Spalteholz technique. The perimeniscal capillary plexus penetrates into the periphery of the meniscus. (*Reproduced with permission from Arnoczky SP, Warren RF: The microvasculature of the meniscus and its response to injury: An experimental study in the dog. Am J Sports Med 1983;11:131-141.*)

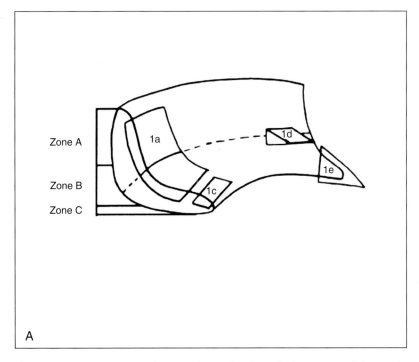

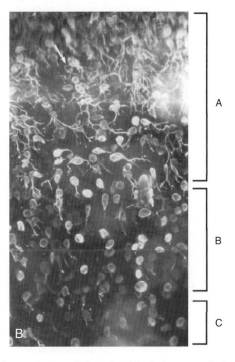

Figure 5   **A,** The schematic diagram shows the three distinct zones of the meniscus (zones A, B, and C). Cells with distinct morphologies are found in each of the three zones. **B,** Montage of an oblique 75 μm section of the meniscus stained with an antibody to vimentin. In the outer margin of the fibrocartilage region (zone A), meniscal cells have numerous long, thin cytoplasmic projections that extend from the cell body. In zone B, meniscal cells have only one or two projections. In contrast, cells in zone C have a round morphology (×600). (*Reproduced with permission from Hellio Le Graverand MP, Ou Y, Schield-Yee T, et al: The cells of the rabbit meniscus: Their arrangement, interrelationship, morphologic variations and cytoarchitecture. J Anat 2001;198:525-535.*)

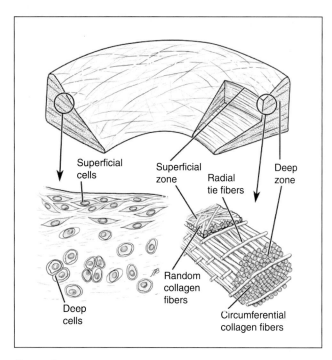

Figure 6 The meniscal cells and collagen ultrastructure. Collagen fibers of the superficial layer are randomly distributed and are predominantly arranged in a circumferential fashion deep in the substance of the tissue. The radial tie fibers are also shown. *(Reproduced with permission from Kawamura S, Lotito C, Rodeo SA: Biomechanics and healing response of the meniscal tissue.* Op Tech Sports Med *2003;11:68-76.)*

pericellular matrix appears in the transmission electron microscope as fine filamentous material with a distinct transition to the fibrous interterritorial matrix. Type VI collagen is a distinct component of the pericellular matrix of the fibrochondrocyte, similar to articular chondrocytes. Fibrochondrocytes are the predominant cell type in the body of the middle and inner meniscus. The location, shape, and properties of the fibrochondrocyte are consistent with this cell functioning in the portion of the meniscus that predominantly experiences compressive forces.

Fibroblast-like cells lack a pericellular matrix. These cells have several long, thin cytoplasmic projections that extend out from the main body of the cell. The location of the cells, with extended projections in the outer portion of the meniscus, enables them to respond to circumferential tensile loads, as opposed to compressive loads. Superficial zone cells have a characteristic fusiform shape, have no cytoplasmic projections, and reside just below the surface of the tissue. The cells in the superficial zone express a smooth muscle actin isoform and appear to migrate into injured meniscal tissue, suggesting a role for these cells in meniscal repair.

Biochemistry

Like bone, cartilage, and ligament, the meniscus consists of scattered cells surrounded by an abundant extracellular matrix. The extracellular matrix contains water, comprising 65% to 70% of the total weight. Most of the water is retained within the tissue in the solvent domains of the proteoglycans. Because of the dense matrix and the small pore size of the meniscus, very large hydraulic pressures are required to overcome the drag of frictional resistance in forcing fluid flow through the tissue. Thus, interactions between water and the macromolecular framework of the matrix significantly influence the viscoelastic properties of the tissue.

The macromolecular framework of the meniscal tissue consists primarily of collagens, which contribute about 60% to 95% of the dry weight of the tissue. Type I collagen accounts for more than 90%, whereas types II, III, V, and VI collagen each may contribute 1% to 2% of the total amount of tissue collagen. Type II collagen fibrils have smaller diameters and are located in the inner third of the meniscus. Little information exists about types III and V collagens in the meniscus. Type VI collagen, classified as a matrix glycoprotein, is a unique type of collagen that can bind to a range of other matrix proteins and may play a role in stabilizing the type I and II collagen framework of the meniscus and in maintaining fibrochondrocyte adhesion to the matrix. The meniscus has a unique collagen structural orientation that is related to its function (**Figure 6**). The superficial layer consists of a thin layer of fine fibrils. Just below the superficial layer is a layer of irregularly aligned collagen bundles. Below this surface layer, large, circumferentially oriented fibers are anchored by a small number of radially oriented fibers. When an axial load is applied to the knee joint, the meniscus is compressed and displaced away from the joint center, resulting in tensile stress (hoop stress) in the circumferential collagen fibers. Biomechanical studies show that the meniscus is much stronger and stiffer in the circumferential direction than the radial direction, and the low circumferential shear strength is believed to be at least partly responsible for the occurrence of longitudinal tears.

The proteoglycan concentration within the meniscus is 1% to 2% of its dry weight. Proteoglycans are composed of polypeptides to which one or more specialized polysaccharides, called glycosaminoglycans (GAGs), are covalently attached. Like other connective tissues, the meniscus contains both large and small proteoglycans. The principal GAG is chondroitin sulfate (40%), with lesser amounts of dermatan sulfate and keratan sulfate. GAGs function to bind water molecules and thus provide the compressive properties of the tissue. The meniscal collagen network and GAGs form a porous-permeable solid matrix. Interstitial fluid flow and solid matrix deformation during loading cause the meniscus to act as a shock absorber during weight bearing. There are significant regional variations in the distribution of different proteoglycans in menisci (**Table 1**). The apparent regional distribution of proteoglycans likely reflects the tissue adaptation to local loads, which is even maintained under

Table 1 Composition of Meniscus by Region

Region	Number	Sulfated Glycosaminoglycan (% Dry Weight)	Water Content	Hydroxyproline (% Dry Weight)
Lateral:				
Anterior	18	1.80 ± 0.50	75.02 ± 2.14	14.3 ± 3.7
Central	18	1.68 ± 0.56	72.99 ± 2.40	13.2 ± 2.0
Posterior	18	1.75 ± 0.45	73.39 ± 2.44	15.2 ± 3.1
Medial:				
Anterior	12	2.20 ± 1.01	72.12 ± 9.73	13.2 ± 3.6
Central	14	2.06 ± 0.68	76.77 ± 2.68	13.9 ± 3.4
Posterior	18	1.94 ± 0.83	74.88 ± 7.32	13.9 ± 3.6

(Reproduced with permission from Fithian DC, Kelly MA, Mow VC: Material properties and structure-function relationship in the menisci. Clin Orthop 1990;252:19-31.)

tissue culture conditions. Specific proteoglycans (aggrecan, biglycan, fibromodulin) seem to accumulate in the inner, compressed region of the meniscus.

Noncollagenous proteins also form part of the macromolecular framework of the meniscus. Two specific noncollagenous proteins, link protein and fibronectin, have been identified in the meniscus. Link protein is required for the formation of stable proteoglycan aggregates capable of forming strong networks or aggregates of GAGs. Fibronectin serves as an attachment protein for cells in the extracellular matrix. Other noncollagenous proteins such as thrombospondin are present in the meniscus and may serve as adhesive proteins, thus contributing to the structure and the mechanical strength of the matrix.

Function

The menisci perform important functional roles in the knee joint, including load bearing, shock absorption, joint stability, and joint lubrication. The biomechanical properties of the meniscus are dependent on its anatomic characteristics and material properties.

Load Bearing

During loading, the meniscus experiences tensile, compressive, and shear stress. The medial meniscus transmits 50% of the joint load in the medial compartment whereas the lateral meniscus transmits 70% of the joint load in the lateral compartment. When one third of the inner meniscus is lost, contact stresses are increased by 65%. This increase in compression stress across the joint causes articular cartilage damage and eventual degeneration. Thus, even partial meniscectomy can affect the ability of the meniscus to function in load transmission across the knee.

When an axial load is applied to the knee joint the meniscus is compressed, but because of its wedge-shaped structure and firm anterior and posterior attachments to the tibia, the axial load is displaced away from the joint center, resulting in tensile stress (hoop stress) in the circumferential collagen fibers (**Figure 7**). Measurements of

tensile stiffness and strength of bovine and human menisci have shown that meniscal tissue is anisotropic and inhomogeneous (**Figure 8**). For the bovine medial meniscus, the posterior specimens are significantly stiffer in tension than the anterior specimens, except at the surface. Biomechanical studies have shown that the meniscus is 100 times stronger and stiffer in the circumferential direction than the radial direction. The meniscus also has unique shear properties because of its ultrastructural construction. The large type I collagen fiber bundles are held together by the radial tie sheaths. When the meniscus is sheared in planes containing the circumferential collagen fibers, the sparse radial tie fibers provide the only resistance to shear. Consequently, the shear modulus of the meniscus is very low and decreases with increasing shear strain. The low circumferential shear strength is believed to be at least partly responsible for the occurrence of longitudinal or horizontal tears.

Shock Absorption

The meniscus can be viewed as a biphasic medium composed of a fluid phase (the interstitial water) and a solid phase (collagen, GAGs, and the other matrix proteins). The collagen network and GAGs form a porous-permeable solid matrix. Interstitial fluid flow and solid matrix deformation during loading cause the meniscus to act as a viscoelastic material. This viscoelasticity determines the creep and stress relaxation behavior of the meniscus. In compression, the meniscus closely resembles articular cartilage, except that the high osmotic swelling pressure is not present in the meniscus because of its low proteoglycan concentration. The meniscal tissue has a compressive stiffness one half that of articular cartilage, and its permeability is one sixth that of articular cartilage because of its microporous collagen-proteoglycan matrix. The combination of the lower compressive stiffness and lower permeability facilitates the role of the meniscus in shock absorption.

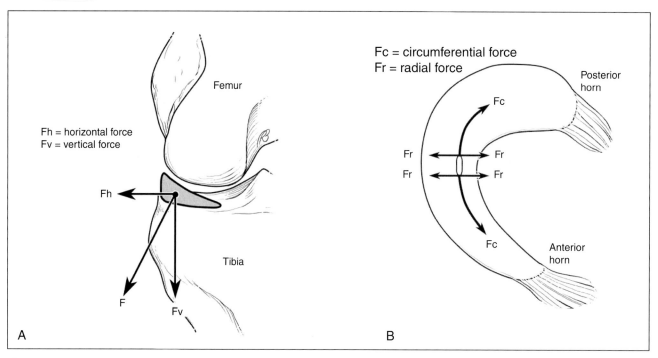

Figure 7   A, The intact meniscus converts axial forces into radial strain. Because of its geometry and anatomic location in the joint, the meniscus is subjected to compressive (vertical force), tensile, and shear stress (horizontal force). **B,** When a load is applied, the meniscus is displaced away from the center, leading to development of tensile stress in the circumferential collagen fibers because of the firm attachments of the anterior and posterior horns. *(Reproduced with permission from Kawamura S, Lotito C, Rodeo SA: Biomechanics and healing response of the meniscal tissue.* Op Tech Sports Med *2003;11:68-76.)*

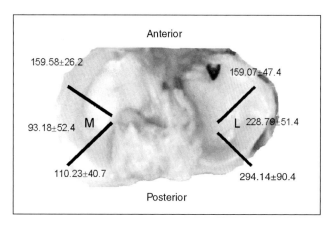

Figure 8   Regional variations in the mean tensile modulus of the menisci in megapascals ± standard deviation. The medial central and the medial posterior menisci are weakest, as measured by tensile stiffness. M = medial; L = lateral. *(Reproduced with permission from Fithian DC, Kelly MA, Mow VC: Material properties and structure-function relationship in the menisci.* Clin Orthop *1990;252:19-31.)*

Joint Stability

The superior concave and inferior flat surface of the meniscus conforms to the femoral and tibial condyles, and the wedge shape of the meniscus contributes to its function in joint stabilization (**Figure 9**). Medial meniscectomy in the ACL-intact knee has little effect on anteroposterior motion; however, in the ACL-deficient knee medial menis-

cectomy results in an increase in anterior tibial translation of up to 58% at 90° of flexion. The posterior horn of the medial meniscus resists an applied anterior tibial force in an ACL-deficient knee. Thus, the force experienced by the medial meniscus in the ACL-deficient knee increased by 52% in full extension and by 197% at 60° of flexion under a 134-N load. In a reciprocal fashion, the resultant force in an ACL graft is increased after medial meniscectomy; this finding supports the importance of preserving the medial meniscus (such as by repair, when possible) in the ACL-deficient knee. Further study is required to determine if the increased stress on the ACL graft in the medial meniscus-deficient knee results in an increased failure rate, and if the long-term results of ACL reconstruction can be improved with medial meniscus transplantation in such knees.

Joint Lubrication

The menisci contribute significantly to joint conformity. It has been suggested that such conformity promotes the viscous hydrodynamic action required for fluid-film lubrication, and this function assists in the overall lubrication of the articular surfaces of the knee joint. Water may be extruded into the joint space during compressive loading, aiding in joint lubrication. The meniscus also may aid in articular cartilage nutrition by helping to maintain a synovial fluid film over the articular surface and by compressing synovial fluid into articular cartilage. However,

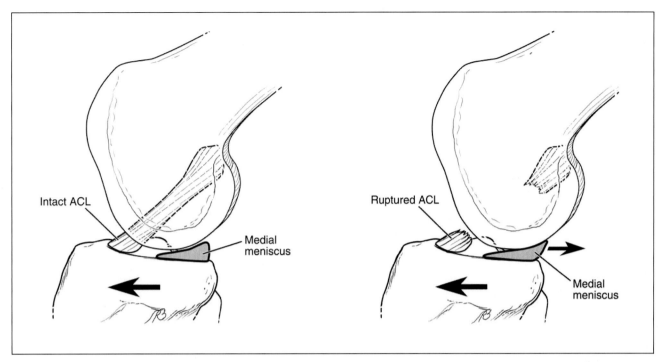

Figure 9   The medial meniscus plays a role in joint stabilization, acting as a restraint to anterior tibial translation in the ACL-deficient knee. *(Reproduced with permission from Kawamura S, Lotito C, Rodeo SA: Biomechanics and healing response of the meniscal tissue. Op Tech Sports Med 2003;11:68-76.)*

the exact contribution of the meniscus to joint lubrication has not been determined.

Healing

Traumatic meniscal tears occur frequently in young, active people, with estimates of 60 to 70 tears per 100,000 persons. Tension, compression, or shear stress that exceeds the strength of the meniscal matrix in any direction will tear the tissue. Intrinsic meniscal degeneration begins at approximately 30 years of age, progresses with increasing age, and occurs in both men and women and in both active and inactive individuals. Degenerative meniscal tears occur in association with age-related degenerative changes in the tissue. Often, these patients do not recall a specific injury, or they recall only a minor load applied to the knee. Degenerative tears often have complex shapes or may appear as horizontal clefts or flaps. Histologic analysis of degenerative meniscal tissue shows mucinous degeneration, hypocellularity, and loss of normal collagen fiber organization. Degenerative meniscal tissue is believed to have a poorer potential for healing; thus, careful attention should be paid to the appearance and consistency of the meniscus at the time of surgery. Although preservation of the meniscus may be more important in a knee with axial malalignment, the rate of healing may be lower because of concomitant degenerative changes in the meniscus. The etiology of such changes is unknown, but may reflect recurrent chronic microtrauma to the meniscus. Studies in animals have demonstrated that alterations in the extracellular ma-

trix of the meniscus (such as an increase in water content) occur following ACL transection. An initial decrease in the concentration of GAGs also has been observed following ACL transection. However, in joints with chronic ACL insufficiency, the concentration of GAGs was found to increase substantially. This occurrence reflects a remarkable ability of meniscal fibrochondrocytes to replenish the lost GAGs. In one study, semiquantitative polymerase chain reaction was used to examine expression of a wide range of genes in the meniscus following ACL transection in rabbits. In the medial meniscus significant increases in the messenger RNA levels for types I and II collagen, tissue inhibitor of metalloproteinase-1, aggrecan, biglycan, and inducible nitric oxide synthase were noted in the pathologic specimens compared with control subjects. A general upregulation of genes for matrix macromolecules, including proteinases (matrix metalloproteinase (MMP)-1, -3, and -13), was evident in other studies. Thus, the meniscus responds to injury by increased expression of genes for matrix protein and enzymes.

Whereas the peripheral regions of the menisci are vascular, the avascular nature of most of the meniscus requires nutrition to be derived via synovial fluid diffusion. A meniscal tear in the vascular periphery has the potential to heal, whereas tears that occur in the avascular zone of the meniscus have poor healing potential. Injury within the peripheral vascular zone of the meniscus results in formation of a fibrin clot at the tear site. This clot acts as a scaffold for the reparative process. Vessels from the peri-

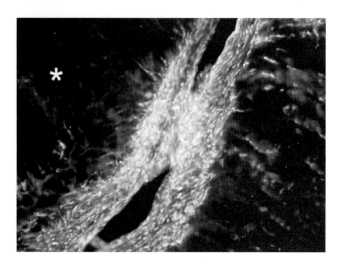

Figure 10   Cells expressing the alpha smooth muscle actin phenotype are identified in the interface between an implanted acellular meniscal plug (asterisk) and the surrounding meniscal tissue. Positively-stained cells were also located on the plug surface. *(Reproduced with permission from Kambic HE, Futani H, McDevitt CA: Cell, matrix changes and alpha-smooth muscle actin expression in repair of the canine meniscus.* Wound Repair Regen *2000;8:554-561.)*

meniscal capillary plexus and synovial fringe proliferate through this fibrin scaffold, accompanied by proliferation of undifferentiated mesenchymal cells. Eventually, the lesion is filled with a fibrovascular scar tissue that bonds the wound edges together and appears continuous with the adjacent normal meniscal fibrocartilage. The exact phenotype of the cells that initiate and regulate the healing process is unknown.

A recent study showed that the cells in the superficial zone appear to play a pivotal role in the repair of a meniscal defect. Examination of the response of cells in an in vivo canine model for meniscal wound healing showed that the superficial zone cells expressed alpha smooth muscle actin and appeared to migrate into the wounds. Smooth muscle actin positive cells were also concentrated at the interface of the wounds and the adjacent meniscus (**Figure 10**). The intriguing possibility arises that the superficial zone contains specialized cells, perhaps progenitor cells, which initiate the wound-healing process. Like other connective tissues, the lesion heals with scar tissue that likely has inferior material properties. In one animal study, the tensile strength of the healed lesion did not reach the strength of normal menisci even after 12 to 16 weeks. Furthermore, the long-term histologic and biomechanical characteristics of the reparative tissue are unknown.

The concept that the meniscus will regenerate following its removal has previously provided the rationale for total meniscectomy. Animal studies have shown that after total meniscectomy there is partial regrowth of a structure that is similar in shape and texture to the removed meniscus. It is hypothesized that bleeding from the perimeniscal

vessels results in an organized clot within the peripheral joint space. However, only the peripheral rim of the meniscus regenerates. Although such regenerated tissues grossly resembled normal peripheral meniscal tissue, the material properties and functional role of this regenerated meniscus is unknown.

Knee range of motion and weight bearing are two important parameters that can affect meniscal healing and should be considered in planning postoperative management. The effect of immobilization has been studied in several animal models. One study using a dog model found that cast immobilization of repaired meniscal lesions in the vascular zone of canine menisci resulted in a decrease in collagen formation after 10 weeks of immobilization compared with nonimmobilized control subjects. Another study examined the effect of knee motion on the tensile properties of the meniscus in a non–weight-bearing sheep model. This study found that the tensile properties of the meniscus (modulus, tensile strength, and ultimate strain) were not significantly affected if even limited range of motion was allowed. These studies suggest that normal mobility of the joint should be restored as soon as possible to promote long-term joint homeostasis. In contrast, there is little information available about the effect of weight bearing on meniscus healing. One study found that immobilization and no weight bearing in a dog model resulted in substantial atrophy of the meniscus (loss of collagen). It is difficult to draw firm conclusions from this study because both knee motion and weight bearing were restricted. The magnitude and type of load (compression, shear, or tension) on the meniscus in commonly used animal models (such as dog, goat, and sheep) likely differs from that of humans because of differences in joint architecture and gait. There is currently little information available about the loads placed on the meniscus during selected activities (such as walking, cycling, and rehabilitation exercises) and about the load magnitudes that are detrimental to healing. Furthermore, the magnitude and type of load that is detrimental to meniscal healing are likely different for various meniscal tear patterns (for example, vertical longitudinal tear versus a radial tear). Further studies are required to determine the optimal type, magnitude, and duration of loading for meniscal healing. At this time, the available evidence indicates that early knee range of motion is the most important parameter to maintain homeostasis of the meniscus.

Repair

The indications for meniscal repair have been well defined. Important factors to consider include the location, type, and length of the tear as well as the quality of tissue and chronicity of the tear, the age of the patient, and the stability of the knee. The most important factor in determining whether the tear is reparable is location of the tear, because tears in the vascular periphery of the meniscus can mount a healing response. The ideal tear for repair is acute, vertical, and longitudinally located in the peripheral third of the meniscus (so-called red-red tear) in a young patient who has a stable knee or who will have concomitant reconstruction of the ACL. Because of the importance of the meniscus, repair can be considered for tears that extend into the central, avascular zone (red-white tear) of the meniscus in young patients. It appears that the rates of healing after repairs of the lateral meniscus are better than those of the medial meniscus, and thus there are broader indications for repair of the lateral meniscus.

Techniques available for meniscal repair include open, outside-in, inside-out, and all-inside arthroscopic methods. Vertical mattress sutures provide superior fixation because of the ability to capture a greater number of the circumferential collagen fibers. There are several commercially available meniscal repair devices for all-inside arthroscopic repair; however, there have been several reports of complications (such as damage to the overlying articular surface). Most of these devices have inferior biomechanical properties, and there is a lack of long-term results compared with the use of suture techniques.

Several techniques have been developed that provide vascularity to the inner, avascular area of the meniscus. Experimental studies have shown that by connecting a lesion in the avascular portion of the meniscus to the peripheral blood supply via vascular channels, these lesions can heal normally. However, the creation of a large vascular channel may disrupt the normal collagen fiber architecture of the peripheral meniscus. Other methods to stimulate vascular ingrowth have been proposed, including synovial abrasion, use of vascular pedicle grafts of synovium, and meniscal rasping. These procedures are intended to produce a vascular pannus, which will migrate from the synovium into the tear site and support a reparative response. An exogenous fibrin clot placed in a stable lesion in the avascular portion of the meniscus supports a reparative response similar to that seen in the vascular area. The clot is presumed to provide chemotactic and mitogenic stimuli for reparative cells and to act as a scaffold for the reparative process.

Recent emphasis has been directed toward applications of cell and molecular biology to promote meniscal healing and regeneration. Numerous growth factors have been identified as signaling molecules that control mitogenic behavior and differentiation of cells. These growth factors have been used on meniscal cells to test their effects on the healing of tears or defects, as well as their effects on extracellular matrix synthesis in tissue and cell culture.

Cells from the peripheral part of the meniscus have an increased ability to synthesize collagen in cell culture compared with cells derived from the inner part of the meniscus. There are other differences in cellular physiology between the cells in the inner and outer regions of the meniscus, including the responsiveness to growth factors and cytokines. Fibroblast growth factor was found to stimulate proliferation of meniscal cells. Transforming growth factor-β increased proteoglycan synthesis of fibrochondrocytes from different regions of the meniscus in a dose-dependent manner. The cells in the inner, central region of the tissue (where the healing capability is diminished) are much less responsive to platelet-derived growth factor-AB than are the cells in the peripheral portion of the tissue. However, one study demonstrated that at optimal concentrations, platelet-derived growth factor-AB, hepatocyte growth factor, and bone morphogenetic protein-2 are equally effective in stimulating DNA synthesis in cells isolated from different zones of the meniscus. Bone morphogenetic protein-2 and insulin-like growth factor-1 stimulated the migration of fibrochondrocytes from the middle zone by 40% to 50%. Interleukin-1 and epidermal growth factor also stimulated migration of meniscal cells. Endothelial cell growth factor was reported to accelerate healing of an allograft to the joint capsule. This information may support the eventual clinical use of cytokines to augment meniscal healing and regeneration.

Other studies reported that hyaluronan and hyaluronic acid improved healing in a cylindrical meniscal defect and stimulated collagen remodeling in the peripheral zone. Intra-articular injections of hyaluronic acid, once a week for 5 weeks, was found to enhance healing of a longitudinal meniscal wound up to 12 weeks after injury compared with saline-injected control subjects. Transection of the ACL in rabbits results in a large production of nitric oxide (NO) by meniscal cells compared with control subjects. Dynamic mechanical stress influences the biologic activity of the meniscal cells by increasing NO production in vivo and ex vivo. Furthermore, the negative effect of interleukin-1 on extracellular matrix turnover is dependent on NO. Administration of hyaluronan produced some reduction in the level of NO, supporting the potential beneficial effect of hyaluronan.

The major challenge for growth factor application at this time is delivery of the selected factor into the target tissue. Because of rapid dilution and short half-lives, single doses of growth factors may not provide adequate local concentrations to induce significant biologic effects. It is evident that a carrier vehicle, such as an absorbable material, will be required to localize the growth factor at the repair site in a biologically relevant concentration. Alternatively, gene therapy techniques may be used to induce local production of the desired protein.

Meniscal Replacement

Although techniques of meniscal repair and partial meniscectomy have limited the number of total meniscectomy procedures performed, there are still instances in which near-total resection of the tissue is the only option. To protect knee joint cartilage from degeneration after these procedures, investigators and surgeons have been exploring several approaches to meniscal tissue replacement.

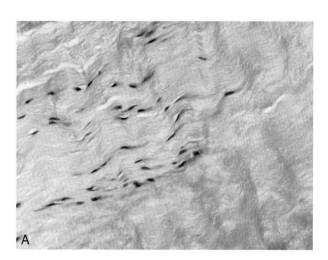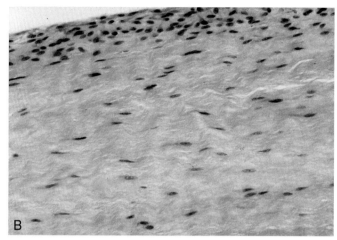

Figure 11   **A,** Biopsy specimen of a human meniscus allograft 16 months after implantation shows incomplete cellular repopulation. **B,** This human meniscus allograft biopsy demonstrates greater cellularity at the surface.

Meniscal Allograft Function

Meniscal transplantation is a useful reconstructive option for patients with loss of the meniscus as a result of previous meniscectomy or an irreparable meniscus tear (**Figure 11**). Laboratory studies have provided the impetus for the clinical use of meniscal allografts, and subsequent clinical and basic science investigations have further refined its application. Clinical studies have demonstrated the effectiveness of this procedure in alleviating pain and swelling and in improving knee function. Results are poor in patients with advanced arthrosis, and this remains the primary contraindication to the use of this procedure. As with any tissue, successful transplantation is dependent on several factors, including tissue preservation, the immunologic compatibility of the donor and host, and the long-term biologic and biomechanical integrity of the transplant.

The goal of meniscal transplantation is to protect the articular cartilage from progressive degeneration following meniscectomy. Although there is sound theoretic evidence to support meniscal replacement in knees with an absent meniscus, there is currently no evidence that meniscal transplantation alters the natural history of cartilage degeneration following meniscectomy. Further studies are required to determine how structural factors such as axial alignment, specific area of cartilage loss in the involved compartment (anterior versus posterior), and changes in joint architecture (such as flattening of the femoral condyle) affect the outcome of meniscal transplantation. Most importantly, randomized clinical trials are required to determine the effectiveness of meniscal transplantation.

The basic biology of meniscal transplantation has been studied in various animal models. Fresh and cryopreserved allografts contain viable cells at the time of transplantation, whereas fresh-frozen and lyophilized tissues are acellular. It is not known what proportion of the cells in a fresh transplant survive after transplantation, and for how long these cells survive in humans. DNA probe analysis in a goat model revealed that all of the donor cells in a fresh meniscal transplant were rapidly replaced by host cells. Experimental studies in goats have suggested that there are no important differences between cryopreserved and deep-frozen grafts. Lyophilized grafts have been found to undergo shrinkage, and thus are not currently recommended. The tissue may be secondarily sterilized using gamma irradiation or ethylene oxide. However, gamma irradiation of more than 3 Mrads adversely affects the material properties of the meniscus. Also, by-products of ethylene oxide sterilization (ethylene chlorhydrin) can induce synovitis following transplantation. Several freeze-thaw cycles do not adversely affect the material properties of the tissue and the freezing process also decreases immunogenicity. Thus, deep-frozen tissue is currently recommended for use in meniscal transplantation.

Animal studies as well as human biopsy studies show incomplete cellular repopulation, with the central core of the graft often remaining acellular. Animal studies demonstrate active collagen remodeling by the cells that repopulate the meniscus. There are alterations in the biochemical composition of the meniscus (proportions of water and proteoglycan) compared with the normal meniscus after transplantation, which are likely to adversely affect the material properties of the tissue.

The process of cellular repopulation requires migration of extrinsic cells into the dense meniscal matrix, resulting in structural remodeling of the matrix. The biomechanical effect of such structural remodeling was studied in a goat model and it was reported that grafts with the greatest degree of cellular repopulation were actually the least effective in load distribution. The long-term ability of the cells that repopulate the allograft to synthesize appropriate matrix proteins and maintain the extracellular matrix is also unknown. The graft undergoes gradual, incomplete revascularization, with new capillaries derived from the capsular and synovial attachment.

Another important aspect of meniscus transplantation is healing of the anterior and posterior horn attachment sites. The meniscus can be transplanted with bone plugs attached to the anterior and posterior horns, or by direct suture of the meniscus horn into bone tunnels. It appears that the healing rates of menisci transplanted with attached bone plugs (fixation by bone-to-bone healing) are better than the healing rates of menisci transplanted with no bone plugs (fixation by meniscus-to-bone healing). This finding supports results from studies of cadaver models that have demonstrated superior load transmission with meniscal horn bone plug fixation compared with no bone plugs. There is very little information available on the healing of meniscus to bone, and no studies have compared healing of bone plugs to healing of meniscal tissue in a bone tunnel. The tensile strength of a healed meniscal attachment after detachment and repair to bone in a rabbit model approached only 20% of the strength of the normal meniscal horn attachment. It is likely that secure fixation of the allograft is critical for initial healing, remodeling of the allograft, and long-term function.

There is very little information available on the histologic characteristics of meniscal transplant in humans. Biopsies of meniscus and synovium from patients with both intact and failed meniscal transplants showed gradual repopulation of the allograft with host cells. Although frank immune rejection is rarely seen clinically, there is histologic evidence of an immune response directed against the graft. It has been demonstrated that the class I and class II histocompatibility antigens are expressed on the meniscal cells, even after freeze-thaw cycles. The presence of these histocompatibility antigens at the time of transplantation indicates the potential for an immune response. The presence of a small number of immunoreactive cells (B-lymphocytes or T-cytotoxic cells) in the meniscus, synovium, or both suggests the possibility of a subtle immune reaction against the transplant. Such an immune reaction may modulate graft healing, graft revascularization, and ultimate graft incorporation. Further studies are required to increase understanding of the process of cell migration into the allograft tissue during cellular repopulation, the resultant phenotype of the repopulating cells, and the effect of an immune response on graft remodeling.

Synthetic Matrix Grafts

Synthetic matrices created from reconstructed collagen, small intestine submucosa, periosteal tissue, or other materials may eventually provide a method to replace lost or damaged meniscal tissue. Initial experimental investigations suggest that synthetic collagen matrices may have the potential to replace menisci. Studies on small intestine submucosa done in dogs have shown some promising results. Although the mechanism of tissue regeneration using small intestine submucosa grafts remains unclear, the presence of collagen types I, III, IV, and VI, GAGs, fibroblast growth factor, and transforming growth factor in small intestine submucosa may contribute to chemotactic, mitogenic, and stimulatory effects on the cells and matrix. Hydrogels (such as polyvinyl alcohols) are a promising class of synthetic materials that may have application as a meniscus prosthesis. The high water content of hydrogels may provide appropriate material properties. However, important issues such as long-term durability, compatibility with the surrounding host tissue, and graft fixation require further investigation.

Tissue Engineering and Gene Therapy

Tissue engineering techniques using absorbable polymer scaffolds seeded with cells and growth factors are also being explored as a means to heal meniscal lesions, as well as to potentially regenerate meniscal tissue. Creating a tissue-engineered meniscus requires that specific biologic considerations such as cell type, matrix scaffold, bioreactor design, and environmental conditions be addressed. Meniscal cells, fibroblasts, chondrocytes, and mesenchymal stem cells have been proposed as potential cell sources and have been grown (both in vivo and in vitro) on various scaffolds.

Gene transfer has emerged as a new approach for local growth factor delivery. Recent studies have demonstrated the ability to transfect meniscal fibrochondrocytes with novel genes using gene therapy techniques, suggesting that bioactive factors could be delivered to meniscus by transferring growth factor genes to meniscal cells. Several investigators have demonstrated the ability to transfer specific genes into meniscal cells using retroviral and adenoviral vectors. An adenoviral suspension with a fibrin clot implanted into experimentally created canine and lapin meniscal lesions demonstrated successful gene delivery, with gene expression lasting the 3-week duration of the experiment. Retrovirally transduced cells transplanted into meniscal defects successfully expressed the transgene for 6 weeks after transplantation. The future ability of gene therapy to treat meniscal injuries depends on precise identification of appropriate growth factors and finding the most effective means for gene delivery. Further study is required to determine the appropriate length of time for gene expression and to develop methods to control the levels of gene expression. Future research in gene therapy will also focus on methods to accelerate meniscal allograft healing and enhance formation of bioengineered meniscal tissue (**Figure 12**).

Radiologic Imaging

Recent technical advances in MRI of the knee have improved the ability to accurately evaluate meniscal pathology. Frequency-selective fat suppression techniques that

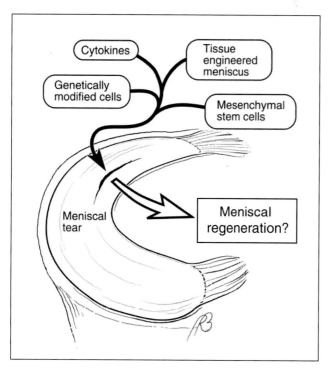

Figure 12   In the future, meniscus repair strategies may include new methods to enhance the cellular response of the meniscus and novel methods to regenerate lost or damaged tissue. *(Reproduced with permission from Kawamura S, Lotito C, Rodeo SA: Biomechanics and healing response of the meniscal tissue. Op Tech Sports Med 2003;11:68-76.)*

can accentuate fluid in the repair site can now be used to accurately distinguish healed tissue from a persistent tear. Such techniques eliminate the need for intra-articular contrast to assess meniscal healing.

MRI provides information about the water, collagen, and GAG components of the matrix. Newer MRI techniques have improved the ability to evaluate the architectural structure and biochemical composition of connective tissue extracellular matrix. Recent advances in MRI techniques for evaluation of hyaline cartilage may eventually have some applicability to the meniscus. For example, because T2 relaxation reflects the content, orientation, and structure of collagen in cartilage, changes in T2 can be monitored over time to monitor matrix damage. Such imaging will eventually prove valuable for noninvasive evaluation of tissue-engineered meniscus.

Summary

The important role of the meniscus in normal knee function is well established. The meniscus plays a role in load bearing, shock absorption, joint lubrication, and in conjunction with the knee ligaments, assists in knee stability. Loss of one or both menisci alters the loading of articular cartilage and increases the probability and the severity of degenerative joint disease. Efforts must be continued to find better methods and techniques to treat meniscal inju-

ries, especially tears through the avascular regions where there is poor intrinsic healing potential. To prevent the degeneration of articular cartilage that results from loss of the meniscus, attempts should be made to preserve or repair the menisci when possible. In the near future, meniscal repair strategies may include new methods to enhance the cellular response of the meniscus and novel methods to regenerate lost or damaged tissue. Meniscal transplantation has emerged as a useful treatment option for selected patients with meniscal deficiency. Further studies are required to increase understanding of the process of cell migration into the meniscus, the resultant phenotype of these cells, and the effect of an immune response on graft remodeling. This information will also be applicable to synthetic matrices, created from reconstructed collagen and other materials, or tissue-engineered meniscal replacements. The addition of growth factors or mesenchymal cells to the synthetic matrices may produce even better results. Tissue-engineered menisci will provide a valuable treatment alternative, but further investigations are required before this option will become a clinical reality.

Selected Bibliography

Anatomy

Arnoczky SP, Warren RF: The microvasculature of the human meniscus. *Am J Sports Med* 1982;10:90-95.

Arnoczky SP, McDevitt CA: The meniscus: Structure, function, repair, and replacement, in Buckwalter JA, Einhorn TA, Simon SR (eds): *Orthopaedic Basic Science*, ed 2. Rosemont, IL, American Academy of Orthopaedic Surgeons, 2000, pp 531-545.

Arnoczky SP, Warren RF: The microvasculature of the meniscus and its response to injury: An experimental study in the dog. *Am J Sports Med* 1983;11:131-141.

Dye SF, Vaupel GL, Dye CC: Conscious neurosensory mapping of the internal structures of the human knee without intraarticular anesthesia. *Am J Sports Med* 1998;26:773-777.

Hellio Le Graverand MP, Ou Y, Schield-Yee T, et al: The cells of the rabbit meniscus: Their arrangement, interrelationship, morphologic variations and cytoarchitecture. *J Anat* 2001;198:525-535.

Henning CE, Lynch MA, Clark JR: Vascularity for healing meniscus repairs. *Arthroscopy* 1987;3:13-18.

Kennedy JC, Alexander IJ, Hayes KC: Nerve supply of the human knee and its functional importance. *Am J Sports Med* 1982;10:329-335.

McDevitt CA, Mukherjee S, Kambic H, Parker R: Emerging concept of the cell biology of the meniscus. *Curr Opin Orthop* 2002;13:345-350.

Messner K, Gao J: The menisci of the knee joint: Anatomical and functional characteristics, and a rationale for clinical treatment. *J Anat* 1998;193:161-178.

Biochemistry
Adams ME, Billingham MEJ, Muir H: The glycosaminoglycans in menisci in experimental and natural osteoarthritis. *Arthritis Rheum* 1983;26:69-76.

Bhargava MM, Attia ET, Murrell GAC, et al: The effect of cytokines on the proliferation and migration of bovine meniscal cells. *Am J Sports Med* 1999;27:636-643.

Fithian DC, Kelly MA, Mow VC: Material properties and structure-function relationship in the menisci. *Clin Orthop* 1990;252:19-31.

McDevitt CA, Webber RJ: The ultrastructure and biochemistry of meniscal cartilage. *Clin Orthop* 1990;252:8-18.

Proctor CS, Schmidt MB, Whipple RR: Material properties of the normal medial bovine meniscus. *J Orthop Res* 1989;7:771-781.

Spindler KP, Mayes CE, Miller RR, et al: Regional migration response of the meniscus to platelet-derived growth factor (PDGF-AB). *J Orthop Res* 1995;13:201-207.

Spindler KP, Miller RR, Andrish JT, et al: Comparison of collagen synthesis in the peripheral and central region of the canine meniscus. *Clin Orthop* 1994;303:256-263.

Function
Allen CR, Wong EK, Livesay GA, et al: Importance of the medial meniscus in the anterior cruciate ligament-deficient knee. *J Orthop Res* 2000;18:109-115.

Allen PR, Denham RA, Swan AV: Late degenerative changes after meniscectomy: Factors affecting the knee after operation. *J Bone Joint Surg Br* 1984;66:666-671.

Anderson DR, Woo SL, Kwan MK, et al: Viscoelastic shear properties of the equine medial meniscus. *J Orthop Res* 1991;9:550-558.

Baratz ME, Fu FH, Mengato RL: The effect of meniscectomy and of repair on intra-articular contact areas and stress in the human knee. *Am J Sports Med* 1986;14:270-275.

Fairbank TJ: Knee joint changes after meniscectomy. *J Bone Joint Surg Br* 1948;30:664-670.

Levy IM, Torzilli PA, Gould JD, Warren RF: The effect of lateral meniscectomy on motion of the knee. *J Bone Joint Surg Am* 1989;71:401-406.

Levy IM, Torzilli PA, Warren RF: The effect of medial meniscectomy on anterior-posterior motion of the knee. *J Bone Joint Surg Am* 1982;64:883-888.

Markolf KL, Kochan A, Amstutz HC: Measurement of knee stiffness and laxity in patients with documented absence of the anterior cruciate ligament. *J Bone Joint Surg Am* 1984;66:242-252.

Papageorglou CD, Gill JE, Kanamori A, et al: The biomechanical interdependence between the anterior cruciate ligament replacement graft and the medial meniscus. *Am J Sports Med* 2001;29:226-231.

Proctor CS, Schmidt MB, Whipple RR, et al: Material properties of the normal medial bovine meniscus. *J Orthop Res* 1989;7:771-782.

Shin SJ, Fermor B, Weinberg JB, Pisetsky DS, Guilak F: Regulation of matrix turnover in meniscal explants: The role of mechanical stress, interleukin 1, and nitric oxide. *J Appl Physiol* 2003;95:308-313.

Shoemaker SC, Markolf KL: The role of the meniscus in the anterior-posterior stability of the loaded anterior cruciate ligament deficient knee: Effects of partial versus total excision. *J Bone Joint Surg Am* 1986;68:71-79.

Tissakht M, Ahmed AM: Tensile stress-strain characteristics of the human meniscal material. *J Biomech* 1995;28:411-422.

Healing and Repair
Albrecht-Olsen P, Kristensen G, Burgaard P: The arrow versus horizontal suture in arthroscopic meniscus repair: A prospective randomized study with arthroscopic evaluation. *Knee Surg Sports Traumatol Arthrosc* 1999;7:268-273.

Arnoczky SP, Warren RF, Spivak JM: Meniscal repair using an exogenous fibrin clot: An experimental study in dogs. *J Bone Joint Surg Am* 1988;70:1209-1217.

Barrett GR, Richardson K, Koenig V: T-Fix endoscopic meniscal repair: Technique and approach to different types of tears. *Arthroscopy* 1995;11:245-251.

Collier S, Ghosh P: Effects of transforming growth factor beta on proteoglycan synthesis by cell and explant cultures derived from the knee joint meniscus. *Osteoarthritis Cartilage* 1995;3:127-138.

Dowdy PA, Miniaci A, Arnoczky SP, Fowler PJ, Boughner DR: The effect of cast immobilization on meniscal healing: An experimental study in the dog. *Am J Sports Med* 1995;23:721-728.

Hashimoto J, Kurosaka M, Yoshiya S, et al: Meniscal repair using fibrin sealant and endothelial cell growth factor: An experimental study in dogs. *Am J Sports Med* 1992;20:537-541.

Hellio Le Graverand MP, Vignon E: Early changes in lapine menisci during osteoarthritis development: Part II: molecular alterations. *Osteoarthritis Cartilage* 2001; 9:65-72.

Kambic HE, Futani H, McDevitt CA: Cell, matrix changes and alpha-smooth muscle actin expression in repair of the canine meniscus. *Wound Repair Regen* 2000;8:554-561.

Kawamura S, Lotito C, Rodeo SA: Biomechanics and healing response of the meniscal tissue. *Op Tech Sports Med* 2003;11:68-76.

Klein L, Player JS, Heiple KG, Bahniuk E, Goldberg VM: Isotopic evidence for resorption of soft tissues and bone in immobilized dogs. *J Bone Joint Surg Am* 1982;64:225-230.

Noyes FR, Barber-Westin SD: Arthroscopic repair of meniscal tears extending into the avascular zone in patients younger than twenty years of age. *Am J Sports Med* 2002;30:589-600.

Port J, Jackson DW, Lee TQ, Simon TM: Meniscal repair supplemented with exogenous fibrin clot and autogenous cultured marrow cells in the goat model. *Am J Sports Med* 1996;24:547-555.

Rodeo SA: Arthroscopic meniscal repair with use of the outside-in technique. *Instr Course Lect* 2000;49: 195-206.

Sonoda M, Harwood FL, Amiel ME: The effects of hyaluronan on tissue healing after meniscus injury and repair in a rabbit model. *Am J Sports Med* 2000;28:90-97.

Suzuki Y, Takeuchi N, Sagehashi Y: Effects of hyaluronic acid on meniscal injury in rabbits. *Arch Orthop Trauma Surg* 1998;117:303-306.

Sweigart MA, Athanasiou KA: Toward tissue engineering of the knee meniscus. *Tissue Eng* 2001;7:111-129.

Takahashi K, Hashimoto S, Kudo T, et al: Hyaluronan suppressed nitric oxide production in the meniscus and synovium of rabbit osteoarthritis model. *J Orthop Res* 2001;19:802-808.

Van Trommel MF, Simonian PT, Potter HG: Different regional healing rates with the outside-in technique for meniscal repair. *Am J Sports Med* 1998;26:446-452.

Meniscal Replacement and Tissue Engineering

Arnoczky SP, DiCarlo EF, O'Brien SJ, et al: Cellular repopulation of deep-frozen meniscal autografts: An experimental study in the dog. *Arthroscopy* 1992;8:428-436.

Cole BJ, Carter TR, Rodeo SA: Allograft meniscal transplantation: Background, techniques, and results. *J Bone Joint Surg Am* 2002;84-A:1236-1250.

Cook JL, Tomlinson JL, Arnoczky SP, et al: Kinetic study of the replacement of porcine small intestinal submucosa grafts and the regeneration of meniscal-like tissue in large avascular meniscal defects in dogs. *Tissue Eng* 2001;7:321-334.

Fabbriciani C, Lucania L, Milano G, Schiavone Panni A, Evangelisti M: Meniscal allografts: Cryopreservation vs deep-frozen technique: An experimental study in goats. *Knee Surg Sports Traumatol Arthrosc* 1997;5: 124-134.

Gao J, Wei X, Messner K: Healing of the anterior attachment of the rabbit meniscus to bone. *Clin Orthop* 1998;348:246-258.

Goto H, Shuler FD, Lamsam C, et al: Transfer of lacZ marker gene to the meniscus. *J Bone Joint Surg Am* 1999;81:918-925.

Jackson DW, McDevitt CA, Simon TM, et al: Meniscal transplantation using fresh and cryopreserved allografts: An experimental study in goats. *Am J Sports Med* 1992;20:644-656.

Jackson DW, Whelan J, Simon TM: Cell survival after transplantation of fresh meniscal allografts: DNA probe analysis in a goat model. *Am J Sports Med* 1993;21:540-550.

Khoury MA, Goldberg VM, Stevenson S: Demonstration of HLA and ABH antigens in fresh and frozen human menisci by immunohistochemistry. *J Orthop Res* 1994;12:751-757.

Kobayashi M, Toguchida J, Oka M: Preliminary study of polyvinyl alcohol-hydrogel (PVA-H) artificial meniscus. *Biomaterials* 2003;24:639-647.

Lu L, Zhu X, Valenzuela RG: Tissue Engineering, cells, scaffolds, and growth factors: Biodegradable polymer scaffolds for cartilage tissue engineering. *Clin Orthop* 2001;391:251-270.

Martinek V, Usas A, Pelinkovic D, et al: Genetic engineering of meniscal allografts. *Tissue Eng* 2002;8:107-117.

Rodeo SA: Meniscal allografts: Where do we stand? *Am J Sports Med* 2001;29:246-261.

Rodeo SA, Seneviratne A, Suzuki K, et al: Histological analysis of human meniscal allografts: A preliminary report. *J Bone Joint Surg Am* 2000;82-A:1071-1082.

Rodkey WG, Steadman JR, Li ST: A clinical study of collagen meniscus implants to restore the injured meniscus. *Clin Orthop Relat Res* 1999;(suppl 367):S281-S292.

Wada Y, Amiel M, Harwood F, et al: Architectural remodeling in deep frozen meniscal allografts after total meniscectomy. *Arthroscopy* 1998;14:250-257.

Radiologic Imaging
Van Trommel MF, Potter HG, Ernberg LA, Simonian PT, Wickiewicz TL: The use of noncontrast magnetic resonance imaging in evaluating meniscal repair: Comparison with conventional arthrography. *Arthroscopy* 1998;14:2-8.

Burstein D, Gray M: New MRI techniques for imaging cartilage. *J Bone Joint Surg Am* 2003;85-A(suppl 2):70-77.

Chapter 11

Form and Function of Tendon and Ligament

Cyril B. Frank, MD, FRCSC
Nigel G. Shrive, MA, DPhil
Ian K.Y. Lo, MD, FRCSC
David A. Hart, PhD

Introduction

Despite the fact that tendons and ligaments look similar, simple, homogeneous, and biologically inert, they are, in fact, actually surprisingly different, complex, heterogeneous, and dynamic. To successfully replace or restore tendon or ligament, their complex functions must be duplicated (or at least substituted) and to do that it is likely essential that key elements of their anatomic structures be reproduced and highly likely that at least some of their composition and microscopic substructures will also need to be recreated. These characteristics of both tendons and ligaments need to be appreciated by anyone proposing to either restore or fully "replace" these structures.

Quite simply, from a gross anatomic perspective, tendons connect muscles to bones, whereas ligaments connect bones to bones. Tendons carry the loads that are generated by their respective muscles. Thus tendons both support joints and also cause the joints that they cross to move. Tendons thus transmit forces to bones to power joints in all activities. Ligaments, on the other hand, are much more "passive structures" in the sense that they have no muscular attachments and they must simply serve to guide joint motions and to add stability to their respective joints under various conditions.

Both tendons and ligaments are composed of surprisingly similar-looking dense fibrous connective tissue, which has often caused them to be confused as being "identical." This is not the case, however, from many different perspectives—beginning with their gross anatomy and functions as previously noted, but also at more microscopic levels of organization. Several reviews have provided detailed comparisons of tendon and ligament structure and function. This chapter focuses more on the clinically relevant details of ligament structures and functions. Both tendons and ligaments have some fairly easily characterized mechanical properties that must be duplicated if they are to be replaced. Each anatomic structure has load-deformation behaviors that are structure-specific; both ligaments and tendons are very strong compared with other soft connective tissues such as skin. Different structures range in strength as a function of their sizes and thus can range in structural tensile strength from hundreds to thousands of newtons. They are also very stiff structurally (again with increasing stiffness as a function of size). In addition to these important nonlinear structural and material properties, both tendons and ligaments exhibit nonlinear viscoelastic behaviors that occur in response to deformations or stresses, respectively, but must contribute somehow to the rather amazing resistance to fatigue damage that tendons and ligaments display. This factor is particularly important as both tendons and ligaments are likely loaded cyclically in various degrees of tension more than almost any other structures in the body and after maturity, they must either resist (or repair) tensile fatigue damage over a lifetime. Each also must have quite specific lengths—to allow specific but minimal tensile displacement before their fibers are recruited to distribute the loads that they carry. This load-carrying ability of tendons and ligaments, resulting from their unique structural organization, is a hallmark requirement of these normal structures.

It is of great significance that analogous to bones, both tendons and ligaments adjust their mechanical properties in response to their load history. Several studies have shown that with joint immobility (load deprivation), ligament properties deteriorate quickly and exponentially (they become less stiff and strong within a few weeks of immobility). These studies and others have shown that with exercise-related loading, tendons and ligaments can improve their properties from their normal state and/or recover their properties after a period of immobility. However, the rate of recovery is much slower than the rate of the deterioration that occurs during immobility, taking many months to recover after much shorter periods of immobility. Many of the cellular mechanisms of these changes have been documented recently, generally demonstrating that the balance between synthesis and degradation of key matrix molecules is definitely linked to the loading state and loading history of the tissue.

Tendons

Classification and Anatomy

Tendons may be classified in several different manners including shape, location, and anatomy. Round tendons (such as flexor digitorum profundus) and flat tendons (such as rotator cuff tendon, bicipital aponeurosis) can be seen throughout the body and have subtle differences in structure and function. Although round tendons are generally subjected to tensile loads and exhibit a typical arrangement of parallel bundles of collagen fibers, flat tendons such as the rotator cuff may undergo more complex loading including compression and shear and have a more complex microanatomy consisting of longitudinal, oblique and transverse collagen fibers. Tendons may also be extra-articular (such as Achilles tendon) or in rare instances intra-articular (such as long head of the biceps tendon, popliteus tendon). Although most tendons are extra-articular, an intra-articular location may inhibit the healing process of tendons following injury similar to that of an intra-articular ligament (for example, anterior cruciate ligament).

Frequently, tendons are classified as sheathed or synovial-covered tendons (such as the long flexors of the fingers) and unsheathed or paratenon-covered tendons (such as the Achilles tendon). These two tendon types have differences in their soft-tissue envelope and vascularity. Extensive research has focused on the healing process and potential of these two tendons.

Gross Morphology, Histology, Microanatomy, and Cell Biology

Tendons attach muscles to bones and their primary function is to transmit load generated from muscles to bones. Because tendons are a part of a larger integrated muscle-tendon-bone unit, the entire structure must be considered to understand tendon anatomy and function. For example, not all muscles have tendons. Those muscles that shorten by significantly angulating bones at a joint have tendons. The flexor carpi radialis muscle has a tendon attachment to the bones of the wrist and when contracted flexes the wrist volarly. Conversely, the quadratus femoris

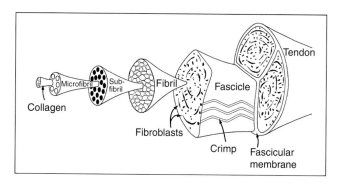

Figure 1 Schematic representation of the microarchitecture of a tendon. *(Reproduced with permission from Kastelic J, Baer E: Deformation in tendon collagen, in Vincent JFV, Currey JD (eds): The Mechanical Properties of Biologic Materials. Cambridge, England, Cambridge University Press, 1980, pp 397-435.)*

has no tendon and simply acts by pulling the femur toward the ischial tuberosity with minimal change in the joint angle. The presence of a tendon also allows a muscle to be at a distance away from its point of action, and in general muscles with long tendons (such as flexor digitorum superficialis) traverse regions where space is limited (such as the wrist). Restricted spaces such as the carpal tunnel, which contains several tendons and nerves, could not accommodate a similar number of muscle bellies. Tendons such as the Achilles tendon may also serve to centralize forces and loads from several muscles (for example, the gastrocnemius or soleus). Alternatively, tendons such as the tibialis posterior may distribute a single muscle load to several different bones by virtue of multiple tendon attachments. Generally, however, tendons attach immediately distal to the joint on which they predominantly act, which maximizes the speed of muscle action but decreases its mechanical advantage.

The shapes of tendons vary greatly throughout the human body. Tendons may appear as long, rounded or rope-like cords (such as the Achilles tendon) or as short, flattened bands of tissue (such as the bicipital aponeurosis). As rounded tendons, their cross-sectional area is generally proportional to the maximal isometric force the corresponding muscle can produce. Although most tendons attach muscles to bones, some tendons may act as origins for muscles (the lumbrical muscles arise from the flexor digitorum profundus) or connect two muscle bellies together (omohyoid, digastric muscle). In addition, a large portion of the tendon may form within the muscle belly itself (such as with the soleus and gastrocnemius). For example, in pennate muscles, tendons extend far into the muscle belly and the muscle attaches to the tendon at an angle. This action allows a larger number of muscle fibers to attach to the tendon, and thus increases the strength of the muscle-tendon unit but decreases its range of motion.

The general structure of tendons is shown in **Figure 1**. Tendons are formed primarily of collagen fibrils, which are evident ultrastructurally. These molecules form fibers that

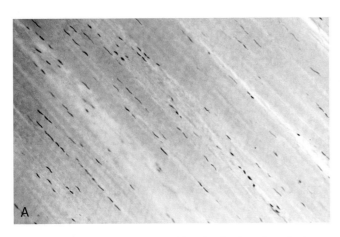
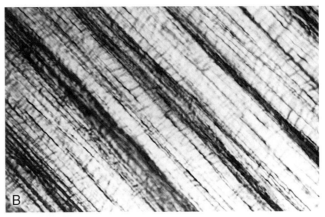

Figure 2   **A,** Photomicrograph of longitudinal section of a human flexor tendon. Note the parallel rows of fibroblasts lying between collagen bundles. **B,** Photomicrograph of the same section under polarized light microscopy, illustrating the parallel, longitudinally arranged collagen bundles (hematoxylin and eosin, X100). *(Reproduced from Woo SL-Y, An K-N, Frank CB, et al: Anatomy, biology, and biomechanics of tendon and ligament, in Buckwalter JA, Einhorn TA, Simon SR (eds): Orthopaedic Basic Science: Biology and Biomechanics of the Musculoskeletal System, ed 2. Rosemont, IL, American Academy of Orthopaedic Surgeons, 2000, pp 581-616.)*

are visible on light microscopy (**Figure 2**). A collection of fibers forms a fiber bundle, a group of fiber bundles forms a fascicle, and a group of fascicles forms the tendon. Fiber bundles and fascicles are surrounded by a loose connective tissue network called the endotenon and the entire tendon is enveloped by a similar and contiguous (with the endotenon) structure called the epitenon. In addition to binding the tendon subunits together, both the epitenon and endotenon support blood vessels, lymphatics, and nerves. Most tendons such as the Achilles tendon, patellar tendon, and flexor tendons of the finger contain multiple fascicles that spiral along the length of the tendon. This permits adjacent fascicles and fiber bundles to slide relative to one another along the longitudinal length of the tendon.

Although collagen is the primary component of tendon, representing 70% to 80% of the dry weight of tendon, it should be remembered that this represents only the dry weight of tendon, and water is still the primary constituent of tendons. Water accounts for 50% to 60% of the wet weight of a tendon and this component may be critical during normal and pathologic tendon function. Changes in water content, whether experimentally or as seen clinically (such as following injury and inflammation) can affect the viscoelastic properties of tendon, particularly at low load stress states.

The general structure of a collagen molecule consists primarily of a triple chain (α chains) helix that may have one or more nonhelical domains interrupting this chain (**Figure 3**). Each chain possesses a characteristic tripeptide sequence (glycine-x-y), where every third residue is glycine and x is frequently proline and y is frequently hydroxyproline. Three separate α chains of collagen form a right-handed superhelix with a rod-like conformation with a diameter of approximately 1.5 nm. Each α chain is composed of amino acids numbering some 1,050 residues

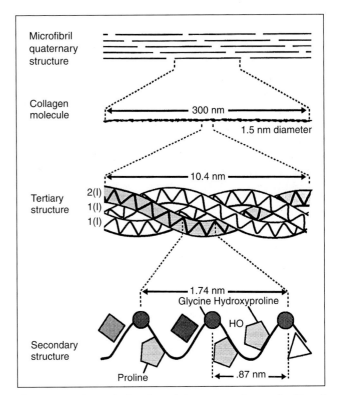

Figure 3   Schematic drawing of the structural organization of collagen into the microfibril. *(Reproduced from Woo SL-Y, An K-N, Frank CB, et al: Anatomy, biology, and biomechanics of tendon and ligament, in Buckwalter JA, Einhorn TA, Simon SR (eds): Orthopaedic Basic Science: Biology and Biomechanics of the Musculoskeletal System, ed 2. Rosemont, IL, American Academy of Orthopaedic Surgeons, 2000, pp 581-616.)*

per chain and giving a total chain length of approximately 300 nm.

The biosynthesis of collagen occurs in cellular organelles known as the rough endoplasmic reticulum. The

Table 1	Types of Collagen	
Type	**Tissue**	**Polymeric Form**
Class 1 (300-nm triple-helix)		
Type I	Skin, bone, etc.	Banded fibril
Type II	Cartilage, disk	Banded fibril
Type III	Skin, blood vessels	Banded fibril
Type V	With type I	Banded fibril
Type XI (Iα, 2α, 3α)	With type II	Banded fibril
Class 2 (basement membranes)		
Type IV	Basal lamina	Three-dimensional network
Type VII	Epithelial basement membrane	Anchoring fibril
Type VII	Endothelial basement membrane	Unknown
Class 3 (short chain)		
Type VI	Widespread	Microfilaments, 110-nm banded aggregates
Type IX	Cartilage (with type II)	Cross-linked to type II
Type X	Hypotrophic cartilage	Unknown
Type XII	Tendon, other?	Unknown
Type XIII	Endothelial cells	Unknown

(Reproduced from Mankin HJ, Mow VC, Buckwalter JA, Iannotti JP, Ratcliffe A: Articular cartilage structure, composition, and function, in Buckwalter JA, Einhorn TA, Simon SR (eds): Orthopaedic Basic Science, ed 2. Rosemont, IL, American Academy of Orthopaedic Surgeons, 2000, p 447.)

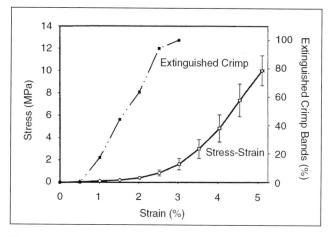

Figure 4   Illustration of the average stress-strain curve for all tendon fascicles tested (mean ± SEM, N = 8 fascicles) and percent of crimp bands extinguished as a function of applied tensile strain. Note that crimp patterns always disappeared completely in the toe region of the stress-strain curve before 3% axial strain was reached. SEM = standard error of the mean. *(Reproduced with permission from Hansen KA, Weiss JA, Barton JK: Recruitment of tendon crimp with applied tensile strain. J Biomech Eng 2002;124:72-77.)*

first product of synthesis is the procollagen α chain, which is subsequently modified by posttranslational events such as hydroxylation of proline and lysine residues, proteolytic processing to mature forms, and glycosylation with oligosaccharide side chains. These and other modifications are required before its triple helical structures can associate normally in the extracellular matrix. Various types and families of collagen have been identified and categorized on the basis of common physicochemical properties (**Table 1**).

Tendons consist mainly of type I collagen (95%) with a small amount of type III collagen (< 5%) normally present. There are also minor quantities of other collagen types (type V and VI collagen). One conspicuous feature seen histologically in both tendons and ligaments is a longitudinal wavy pattern or "crimp" seen in the collagen fibers when viewed under polarized light microscopy and sectioned along the longitudinal length of the ligament (**Figure 2, B**). This pattern or crimp has been characterized and its wavelength and angle varies depending on several factors, including sampling location, animal age, strain

state of the tissue during fixation, type of fixative, and the time of fixation. Although the exact functional implications of crimp remain to be determined, many authors have suggested that crimp may in part be responsible for the low load, nonlinear behavior of tendons. This factor likely corresponds to the toe region of the stress-strain curve of tendons under load (**Figure 4**). That is, under low loads, the initial compliance of tendons is in part secondary to recruitment of "crimped fibers" and the stretching out of crimped collagen.

In addition to collagen, proteoglycans account for approximately 1% to 5% of the dry weight of tendons. Proteoglycans are a diverse group of macromolecules defined by a protein core with at least one or more specialized carbohydrate side chains, known as glycosaminoglycans, attached to it. Glycosaminoglycans are essentially linear chains consisting of repeating disaccharide units. One of the important characteristics of proteoglycans is that their glycosaminoglycan side chains are highly negatively charged and capable of becoming extremely hydrated. This characteristic helps maintain the hydration of healthy tendon, which is important to maintaining normal viscoelastic behavior. The proteoglycan superfamily contains more than 30 full or part-time molecules with a broad range of functions including interactions with other members of the extracellular matrix. For example, decorin is probably the most common proteoglycan in tendon and has been demonstrated to bind to the surface of collagen and delay collagen fibril formation in vitro and significantly affect collagen fibrillogenesis in vivo. Another important component of the tendon extracellular matrix is tenascin-C, a glycoprotein that contributes to

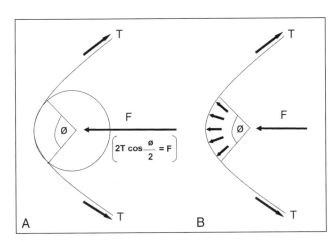

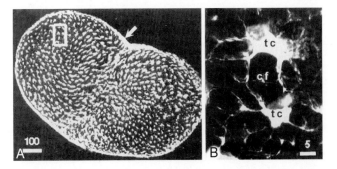

Figure 5   In **A**, equilibrium requires F = 2T cos ø/2 whereas in **B**, assuming no friction, the distribution of F as lateral compression on the tendon around the contact zone is shown. T = tension, F = force.

Figure 6   Confocal microscope images of DiI-stained cryosections and whole mounts of rat digital flexor tendons. Scale bars are labeled in µm. **A**, Low magnification of transverse cryosection of whole tendon. Cells are brightly fluorescent; close examination reveals a fine network of fluorescent cell processes between cells (boxed area enlarged in **B**). The whole tendon is enclosed by two to three layers of flattened cells, the epitenon (*arrow*). **B**, High-magnification three-dimensional projection (look-through reconstruction) of boxed region in **A**. Tendon cells (tc) extend broad flattened lateral cell processes, meeting up with those from adjacent cells. The processes wrap up collagen fiber bundles, occupying the dark tunnels (cf). (*Reproduced with permission from McNeilly CM, Banes AJ, Benjamin M, Ralphs JR: Tendon cells in vivo form a three dimensional network of cell processes linked by gap junctions. J Anat 1996;189(Pt 3):593-600.*)

matrix structure and influences the behavior of cells in contact with the extracellular matrix. It is abundant in the tendon body and at the osteotendinous and myotendinous junctions. Following stress-induced unfolding of its fibronectin type III domains, it also likely functions as an elastic protein in tendons that are known to be subjected to heavy tensile loading. Tenascin-C expression appears to be regulated by mechanical strain and it is known to be upregulated in tendinopathy where it might play a role in collagen fiber alignment and orientation.

In areas where tendons are subject to nontensile loads (compressive loads), the composition of tendons may change. For example, as a tendon travels toward its insertion site it may change directions before inserting into bone by wrapping around a bony prominence (such as malleoli) or underneath a fibrous band (such as extensor retinaculum of ankle). These changes in direction can improve a tendon's angle of approach and potentially increase its mechanical advantage. However, as a tendon curves around a pulley, it is also subjected to more complex forces including compression. Theoretically, this force is approximately twice the tension generated in the tendon multiplied by the cosine of half the angle through which it changes its direction (**Figure 5**). In these areas, tendons may contain type II collagen with an increased glycosaminoglycan content. In addition, the large proteoglycan aggrecan, characteristic of cartilaginous tissue, may also be expressed.

Because most of the mechanical behavior of tendons is related to its extracellular matrix and there are relatively few cells within tendon, the cells within tendons have largely been ignored. Less information is known about their organization and biology than in other tissues. Although mast cells, endothelial cells, and axons are known to be present, the predominant cell type in mature tendon is a tenocyte. In a newborn, the tendon cells are called

tenoblasts. All the morphologic characteristics of tenoblasts support the theory of the high metabolic activity of these cells and point to intense synthesis of the matrix components. With aging, the tenoblasts transform to tenocytes that are metabolically less active than tenoblasts. Tendon cells have the enzyme chains for all three main pathways of energy metabolism—aerobic Krebs cycle, anaerobic glycolysis, and pentose phosphate shunt. In young tendons with high growth rates, all three pathways are extremely active. With aging, Krebs cycle and pentose phosphate shunt decrease whereas the anaerobic glycolysis remains more constant. Therefore, the metabolic pathways for energy production change from aerobic to more anaerobic. The low metabolic rate of mature tenocytes is suited to the main purpose of tendons, which is to carry loads and remain in tension for periods of time without the risk of ischemia and necrosis. Classically, the cells within tendons have been described as spindle- or rod-shaped, arranged in parallel rows between bundles of collagen fibers. More recently, however, the complex shape and organization of cells has been elucidated. Tendon cells exhibit prominent sheet-like cytoplasmic processes that extend for long distances through the extracellular matrix and connect to cytoplasmic processes from adjacent cells and cell bodies (**Figure 6**). At points of contact between cell processes and cell bodies, gap junctions are detected, forming the basis for potential cell-to-cell communication and suggesting that the cells form an elaborate three-dimensional network extending throughout the tendon. Although the functional significance of this arrangement remains to be determined, some authors have suggested that this cellular network may form the basis of a load-sensing system. This scenario potentially allows a coordinated response by tendon cells to respond to changes in load or other stimuli. Recent studies at the molecular level have indicated that the gene expression patterns of cells in different parts of a complex tendon, such as the flexor tendon, reflect the biochemical heterogeneity of the tendon.

In addition to the biochemical changes noted in tendons wrapping around pulleys and under compressive loads, tendon cells and organization are also distinctly different and appear more fibrocartilaginous in nature. For example, in the peroneus longus tendon, as the tendon grooves the plantar surface of the cuboid, tendon cells appear large and round surrounded by collagen fibers arranged in a "basket-weave" fashion. This basket-weave arrangement presumably prevents tendons from delaminating or splaying apart under compressive force. These matrix and cellular changes are dynamic in nature so that when tendons are experimentally removed from their pulleys, tendons respond to their new mechanical environment by modulating their structure. These areas are also hypovascular and are prone to many clinical conditions including posterior tibial tendinosis and de Quervain's disease. Although the role of hypovascularity in the etiology of tendon degeneration remains controversial, once injured the ability to repair a tendon with a poor blood supply may be compromised.

The junction between tendon and bone may take two forms—fibrous or fibrocartilaginous. Fibrous insertions or indirect insertions (such as pes anserinus) are found in the metaphysis and diaphysis of long bones whereas fibrocartilaginous insertions or direct insertions (such as rotator cuff) are typical of tendon insertions into the epiphyses and apophyses of bone. In a fibrous insertion, the collagen fibers of the tendon insert into the periosteum during growth and development and directly into bone at maturation. Conversely, in a fibrocartilaginous insertion, there is a gradual transition from tendon to bone that is characteristically composed of four zones: tendon, uncalcified fibrocartilage, calcified fibrocartilage, and bone. This gradual transition dissipates load at the insertion site and ensures that the collagen fibers in the tendon bend gradually with joint motions.

Blood Supply and Innervation

When compared with other musculoskeletal tissues such as muscle, synovium, or bone, mature tendons are considered to have a poor blood supply. Blood flow has been estimated to be approximately 0.27 ml/g/min in rabbit muscle, but only 0.10 ml/g/min in comparable rabbit tendons. Despite the relative paucity of blood flow, blood supply is important for both normal function and during healing of injuries.

The blood supply to tendons arises principally from arteries derived from the muscle through its myotendinous junction, the paratenon or synovial sheath along the length of the tendon, or from the bone at its insertion site. These vessels form a network in the epitenon. From this network, longitudinal vessels arise and run in the endotenon between and around the collagen bundles. Because there is a layer of cartilage at the insertion site between bone and tendons, the blood supply from the bone-tendon junction does not pass directly from the bone into the tendon. Instead vessels anastomose with those of the periosteum, forming an indirect connection to the osseous circulation.

Tendons, such as the Achilles tendon, have a paratenon that allows vessels from the surrounding connective tissue to penetrate into the tendon at any point along the length of the tendon. Other tendons (for example, those of the hands and feet), however, are surrounded by a true synovial sheath. These sheaths resemble the synovium of joints and are organized in a manner similar to the peritoneum of the abdomen. The tendon is enveloped by a visceral synovial sheath (similar to the visceral peritoneum), which is linked to the outer parietal sheath (similar to the parietal peritoneum) by a mesotenon. Through the mesotenon, the tendon receives its blood, lymph, and nerve supply. In tendons around the ankle, there is a continuous mesotenon connecting the parietal and visceral synovial sheaths. In contrast, the mesotenon of the long flexors of the fingers and toes is isolated to only a few triangular bands or threads called vincula. Vincula limit the potential blood supply provided by the mesotenon. Alternatively, these tendons are dependent on the diffusion of nutrients from surrounding synovial fluid. For example, the digital flexor tendons receive up to 90% of their nutrient supply from the synovial fluid, whereas the corresponding extensor tendon receives only 58% of its nutrients from the synovial fluid. In addition to providing a source of nutrition, synovial sheaths are responsible for producing the necessary lubrication for smooth excursion of tendons (by boundary lubrication), and are a source of healing following injury as well as being involved in adhesion formation following injury or repair.

Tendons are considered to have a rich nerve supply and are typically innervated by the nerve(s) in its associated muscle(s) in addition to local cutaneous and other nerves. Nerve end-organs including Golgi organs, pacinian corpuscles, and Ruffini endings generally lie adjacent to the myotendinous junction whereas free nerve endings are typically adjacent to the bone-tendon junction.

The Golgi organs are large corpuscles and are stimulated only by large changes in mechanical deformation by pressure or compression. However, the function of the Golgi organ is dependent on its location. For example, Golgi organs found in joints relay joint angle information whereas Golgi organs found in tendons relay force information generated from its muscle. Golgi organs continue to relay information for a relatively prolonged period of time following stimulus at its new steady state environment. Pacinian corpuscles are nerve endings with an encapsulated tip. This specialized tip is highly sensitive to deformation and relays information during application or removal of a stimulus. Pacinian corpuscles are considered fast-adapting mechanoreceptors because they are stimulated by dynamic changes in deformation and are insensitive to constant, steady state events. Ruffini endings consist of multiple thinly encapsulated tips that emerge from a single axon. Ruffini endings are slow-adapting mechanoreceptors because they are stimulated during changes in deformation but also continue to relay information for an extended period of time at the new steady state level. Free nerve endings normally respond to nonphysiologic stimuli in that they relay nociceptive or pain information. In addition to their proposed role in proprioception (see below), nerves may play a role in vasoregulation.

Tendon Functions
Mechanical
The primary and most obvious function of tendons is to transmit force generated from muscle to bone. As described previously, tendons can center the action of several muscles (such as the Achilles tendon) into a single line of pull, they can distribute the contractile force of one muscle to several bones (such as with the posterior tibialis tendon), they allow muscles to be at a distance to their insertion, they allow muscle pull to travel through narrow areas of the body (such as the wrist or ankle), and they allow the direction of pull to be changed in conjunction with a pulley (for example, the posterior tibialis tendon around the medial malleolus).

In addition, tendons may have other less obvious functions. Some tendons can store elastic energy during locomotion by cyclically lengthening and shortening. Tendons appear to be efficient at this and can store 400 to 1,800 times more elastic strain energy/unit mass than muscle. For example, the percentage of elastic energy stored in the Achilles tendon during squat jumping and hopping is estimated to be 23% and 34%, respectively, of the total calf muscle work, clearly improving the efficiency of the musculoskeletal system. Because of their viscoelastic properties, tendons may also serve to prevent or reduce muscle injury, particularly during high-speed injuries or the sudden application of force. Other tendons can replace ligaments in reinforcing the capsule of synovial joints and may serve as an articulating surface (such as the extensor tendon of the proximal interphalangeal joint in the flexed position).

Tendons also act to stabilize joints. In addition to their neurosensory or proprioceptive function, tendons may also act as static or dynamic stabilizers of joints. Tendons in conjunction with muscle-generated force can act as passive viscoelastic stabilizers to the joint when not active

(passive tone) or can apply dynamic viscoelastic activation of tendons across joints as a result of voluntary or reflexive muscle contraction. This concept is an important component of joint stability and can lead to or prevent injury. For example, an unopposed contraction of the quadriceps muscle will cause the tibia to translate anteriorly and laterally, and rotate internally with a corresponding increase in the force of the anterior cruciate ligament (ACL). However, a corresponding co-contraction of the hamstring muscles can reduce these abnormal translations as well as reduce the in situ forces of the ACL, thus minimizing the risk of injury. Furthermore, load across joints (whether applied by muscle co-contraction or weight bearing) can enhance the stability of joints by physically pressing the joint together, enhancing the congruency of articulating surfaces (such as the menisci of the knee). Importantly, tendons in conjunction with muscles can contribute to joint stability (in response to external load, pain, etc) at any joint position while performing the task set by the individual (such as joint motion).

In contrast to other tissues (liver, spleen, kidney), connective tissues such as tendon and ligament must perform specific biomechanical functions for normal function of joints. Thus, these tissues generally have a large volume excess of extracellular matrix to cells. This arrangement is typical of force-transmitting (tendon) or force-dissipating and restraining structures (articular cartilage, ligaments, meniscus). The extracellular matrix, therefore, in part accounts for many of the fundamental biomechanical properties of tendons. Because tendons are primarily water, collagen, and ground substance, the biomechanical properties of tendons are therefore largely based on these components.

When evaluating the mechanical properties of tendon, both structural and material properties should be considered. Material properties are characteristics of the tendon itself whereas structural properties are characteristics of the muscle-tendon-bone complex and thus also include the properties of the muscle, muscle-tendon junction, the bone-tendon junction, and bone.

Of particular importance to tendons is their nonlinear anisotropic biomechanical behavior (Figure 7). Under low loading conditions, tendons are relatively compliant. With increasing tensile loads, tendons become increasingly stiff until they reach a range where they exhibit nearly linear stiffness. At this point, elastic elongation is occurring as a result of slippage of the fibers; tearing then occurs through molecular slippage (increased gap between adjacent molecules). Beyond that range, tendons then continue to absorb energy up to the point of their tensile failure. This initial low-load, nonlinear behavior called the toe region is caused, in part, by the recruitment of "crimped" collagen fibers, as well as the viscoelastic behaviors and interactions of collagen and other matrix materials. When compared with ligaments, tendons have smaller toe regions because most fibers in tendon are oriented along the longitudinal

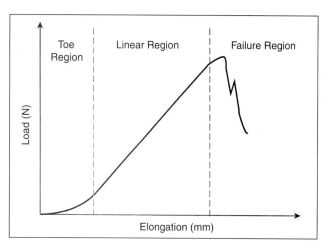

Figure 7   A schematic load-elongation curve for tendon, indicating three distinct regions of response to tensile loading. *(Reproduced from Woo SL-Y, An K-N, Frank CB, et al: Anatomy, biology, and biomechanics of tendon and ligament, in Buckwalter JA, Einhorn TA, Simon SR (eds): Orthopaedic Basic Science: Biology and Biomechanics of the Musculoskeletal System, ed 2. Rosemont, IL, American Academy of Orthopaedic Surgeons, 2000, pp 581-616.)*

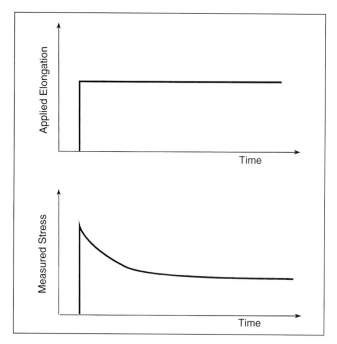

Figure 8   Typical curves demonstrating the stress-relaxation behavior of soft tissue. *(Reproduced from Woo SL-Y, An K-N, Frank CB, et al: Anatomy, biology, and biomechanics of tendon and ligament, in Buckwalter JA, Einhorn TA, Simon SR (eds): Orthopaedic Basic Science: Biology and Biomechanics of the Musculoskeletal System, ed 2. Rosemont, IL, American Academy of Orthopaedic Surgeons, 2000, pp 581-616.)*

length of the ligament requiring less realignment during loading. In the linear region, slippage initially occurs within collagen fibrils, then between collagen fibrils, and finally tearing of the fibrils or fibers until tissue failure. From this load-elongation curve, the stiffness (slope of the curve), the ultimate load (load at failure), and the energy absorbed to failure (area under the curve) can be calculated.

Not all parts of a tendon are under the same conditions of strain at any point in time and loads may be distributed across or along the structure, depending on the conditions under which it is loaded. Failures may therefore occur in various ways across the width of a tendon, along its length, or in combined configurations—all dependent on the boundary conditions of how loads were applied to the joint in question. However, oblique applied loads during eccentric contractions pose the high risk of tendon ruptures. The structural properties of tendon have been studied, however, and vary considerably according to the structure tested and the loading conditions. In general, the ultimate load of tendon is greater than that of muscle or its insertion and thus muscle ruptures or tendon avulsions are more common than rupture of the tendon itself.

Material properties are represented by a stress-strain curve and are biomechanical characteristics of the tendon substance itself. These properties are therefore normalized to the cross-sectional area of the tendon and its original length. Stress is defined as force per unit area (usually N/mm^2 in soft-tissue testing) whereas strain is defined as the change in length divided by its original length. A stress-strain curve will look similar to a load elongation

curve except that its values have been normalized to the dimensions of the tendon being tested. From the stress-strain curve the elastic modulus (slope of the curve), the tensile strength (stress at failure), the ultimate strain (strain at failure), and the strain energy density (area under the curve) can be calculated. In human tendons, the elastic modulus has been measured from 1,200 to 1,800 MPa, the ultimate tensile strength from 50 to 105 MPa, and the ultimate strain from 9% to 35%.

Tendons are viscoelastic, meaning they possess time-dependent and history-dependent properties. Therefore their mechanical behaviors depend on the manner in which they have been loaded (loading rate, loading limits, loading history) and on their environments (such as temperature and water content). This behavior can be represented by several properties including load relaxation, creep, and hysteresis. To determine load relaxation, a constant elongation is applied to the tendon and a time-dependent nonlinear decrease in load is observed (**Figure 8**). Load relaxation may also be observed in a cyclic fashion by repetitively applying a set elongation to a tendon (**Figure 9**). With an increasing number of cycles under similar conditions of displacement, tendons reach progressively lower peak loads. Ultimately, tendons appear to reach an optimum or at least a repeatable peak load, suggesting that they adapt structurally when being cycled to achieve a new biomechanical equilibrium (**Figure 9**).

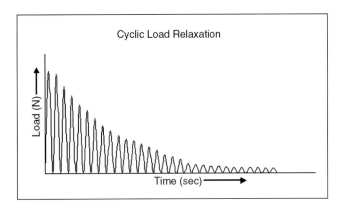

Figure 9 Cyclic load relaxation behavior of a tendon showing a decreasing peak load with repeated similar deformations over time. Note the nonlinear pattern and tendency for tendon to reach a new equilibrium as the number of cycles increases.

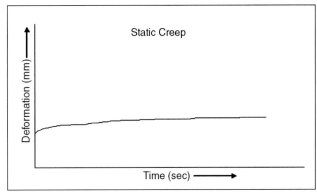

Figure 10 Static creep behavior of normal tendon. A sustained stress causes a nonlinear creep (deformation) through the tendon complex over time.

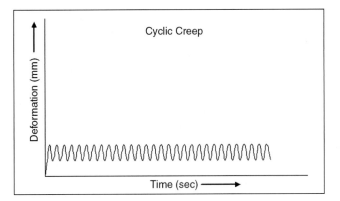

Figure 11 Cyclic creep behavior of normal control tendon, showing increasing deformation with repeated similar stresses over time. Note the nonlinear pattern and the tendency for tendon to reach a new equilibrium as the number of cycles increases.

Although these two low-load behaviors have previously been evaluated in detail, recent evidence suggests that tendons and also ligaments may function in normal daily activity not just under the action of repeated displacements or elongations, but also under the action of sustained low loads (static creep) (**Figure 10**) or of repeated low loads (cyclic creep) (**Figure 11**). For example, the same step repeated in walking requires the same acceleration and deceleration of the limbs and thus the same loads at the joint. Therefore, tendons under this environment would respond through creep rather than relaxation. Creep is defined as the deformation (or elongation) under a constant or cyclically repetitive load. This type of behavior is particularly relevant clinically, because such creep must be recoverable in normal situations but pathologic creep could result in laxity of a joint following joint injury, repair, or reconstructive surgery.

Interestingly, creep results cannot be predicted from stress relaxation tests, suggesting that a fundamental difference exists in the way soft tissues respond to creep versus relaxation conditions. Under conditions of stress relaxation, the viscoelastic response of tendon or ligament likely results from an unchanging subset of fibers within a tendon or ligament, whereas under conditions of creep, the viscoelastic properties are a result of a progressive recruitment of fibers. With progressive fiber recruitment, there is an increase in the load-bearing area of the tendon or ligament over time. Thus, the initial stress is redistributed, reducing stress on the fibers initially loaded. Therefore, tendons and ligaments seem to be uniquely designed to resist creep and excessive elongation through fiber recruitment. As with cyclic relaxation, the ability of tendons and ligaments to adjust their load-carrying capabilities to suit a particular set of environmental circumstance indicates that these tissues are adaptable, and likely represent one of the "fine-tuning" mechanisms of joint loading that may help to control tissue behaviors.

During cyclic stress relaxation testing (**Figure 12**), in addition to observing a nonlinear decrease in peak loads, the load elongation curves of a tendon during its loading and unloading phase within a single cycle will follow different paths. During one cycle, the difference between the loading and unloading curves forms a hysteresis loop and the area between the curves (area of hysteresis) represents energy loss within the tendon. This difference in these two pathways is a result of the history-dependent behavior of tendons.

The final viscoelastic behavior of tendons is that of strain rate sensitivity. In vitro failure tests have shown that tendons themselves are relatively strain rate-insensitive when compared with bone. At higher strain rates, tendons become slightly stiffer and can absorb slightly more energy than when strained slowly. Bones, on the other hand, such as the bone at the insertion of tendons, are more strain rate-dependent, exhibiting even more strength and stiffness when strained more quickly. The implications of these responses are that bone-tendon complexes can adapt, to some extent, to high strain rates in a way that would help to minimize their injury.

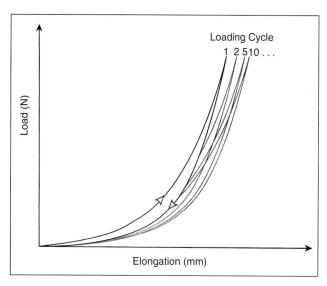

Figure 12 Typical loading (top) and unloading (bottom) curves from cyclic tensile testing of soft tissue. The area between the curves, called the area of hysteresis, represents the energy losses within the tissue. *(Reproduced from Woo SL-Y, An K-N, Frank CB, et al: Anatomy, biology, and biomechanics of tendon and ligament, in Buckwalter JA, Einhorn TA, Simon SR (eds): Orthopaedic Basic Science: Biology and Biomechanics of the Musculoskeletal System, ed 2. Rosemont, IL, American Academy of Orthopaedic Surgeons, 2000, pp 581-616.)*

Proprioceptive

In addition to these mechanical functions, tendons may also serve a role in joint proprioception. Proprioception is now generally referred to as the conscious perception of limb position in space. The central nervous system receives input from several sources of stimuli, which ultimately define the perception and sensation of joint movement and position. These stimuli—visual, auditory, vestibular, cutaneous, joint, and muscle—provide proprioceptive information to three distinct levels of motor control: the spine; the brain stem; and the cerebellum, basal ganglia, and motor cortex.

Although the visual, auditory, and vestibular systems aid in keeping body balance, providing visual cues, and providing reference points for orientation, in joints such as the knee, proprioception is provided primarily by joint, muscle, and cutaneous receptors.

Muscle spindles, although not strictly within tendon, can also contribute to proprioception. In essence this innervation, although relatively sparse, may be critical to joint physiology and may have supplied the impetus for an explosion of investigations. However, the significance of these connections and a feedback system of proprioceptors and nociceptors in tendons to potentially "protect joints" remains controversial. It does appear, however, that proprioception and neuromuscular control can be affected by several factors including training, fatigue, injury, surgery, and rehabilitation. Although a comprehensive review of proprioception is beyond the scope of this chap-

ter, its relationship to ligament injury and reconstruction are described in the ligament section

Clinically Relevant Injuries

Tendon disruptions may occur as a result of direct trauma or by indirect trauma. Direct trauma commonly occurs during sharp lacerations and is frequently seen in the hand and wrist region. These injuries usually occur in tendons with no preexisting disease and the healing of such injuries is in part dependent on whether the tendon is paratenon-covered or sheathed.

Tendon disruptions may also occur indirectly by tensile overload of the muscle-tendon-bone complex and failure then occurs at the weakest link of this complex; however, disruptions are also dependent on the anatomic location, vascularity, skeletal maturity of the patient, and magnitude of the force applied. Most normal tendons can withstand the physiologic forces applied by muscles better than can be withstood by bone. Thus, failure through bone or the musculotendinous junction is more common than midsubstance failure of a normal tendon. For example, indirect disruptions of the flexor digitorum profundus of the hand commonly occur by avulsion of the bony insertion and particularly those in the ring finger.

In contrast, midsubstance disruptions of a tendon occur in a tendon with preexisting disease before tensile overload. This statement is largely based on multiple studies of different tendon disruptions that have universally demonstrated a pathologic ongoing degenerative process. Histologic changes observed during tendinosis may include absence of inflammatory cells, collagen degeneration, fiber disorientation, hypercellularity, vascular ingrowth, and increased interfibrillar glycosaminoglycans. For example, acute Achilles tendon disruptions commonly occur in the middle-aged athlete involved in some physical activity. In patients with no premorbid symptoms and a history of sudden snapping or popping sensation in the calf with pain and disability, pathologic study of these tendons have demonstrated "angiofibroblastic hyperplasia" a characteristic of degenerative disease or preexisting tendinosis.

In tendons, such as the supraspinatus tendon of the rotator cuff, these degenerative histologic changes have been characterized and have included loss of cellularity, thinning and disorganization of tendon fibers, the presence of granulation tissue, glycosaminoglycan infiltration, fibrocartilaginous changes, calcification, abnormalities of the tidemark, loss of staining, and incomplete tears. Although the etiology of tendon degeneration is unclear, there is an emerging consensus that tendon degeneration is multifactorial. Factors that may be implicated can include mechanical compression, impingement, and tensile overload. Some of the potential mechanisms likely involved in tendon degeneration are ischemia, oxygen-free radicals, hypoxia, pathologic alignment, tenocyte apopto-

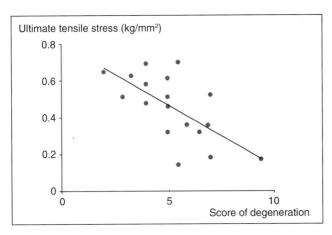

Figure 13   Correlation between the score of degeneration and the ultimate tensile stress. Degeneration at the supraspinatus tendon insertion shows a negative correlation with the ultimate tensile stress ($r = -0.60$; $P = 0.013$). *(Reproduced with permission from Sano H, Ishii H, Yeadon A, Backman DS, Brunet JA, Uhthoff HK: Degeneration at the insertion weakens the tensile strength of the supraspinatus tendon: A comparative mechanical and histologic study of the bone-tendon complex. J Orthop Res 1997; 15: 719-726.)*

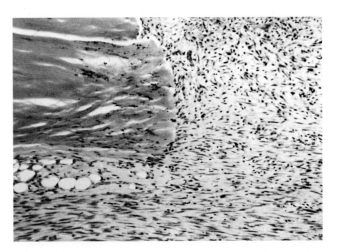

Figure 14   Longitudinal section of a rabbit tendon 1 week after surgical transection and suture reapposition. Note the increase of fibroblasts from the paratenon migrating into the wound. *(hematoxylin and eosin, X100; courtesy of Dr Larry Stein, University of Illinois.)*

sis, and fluoroquinolone. The presence of these changes not only precede but also predispose patients to rotator cuff disruptions and have been correlated to weakening of the tendon in vitro (**Figure 13**). That is, when subjected to tensile overload, muscle-tendon-bone complexes with degenerative tendons are more likely to fail in midsubstance because of preexisting weakening of the tendon substance.

The current status of tendon-to-tendon or tendon-to-bone repair suggests that the mechanical constructs of repair have been relatively optimized. In contrast, enhancement of healing through biologic intervention remains in its infancy. Identifying key factors remains the roadblock to rational and substantive augmentation of tendon repair. In the future, techniques including gene therapy, tissue engineering, and cytokine modulation may provide avenues for enhanced repair.

Tendon Repair
Healing Processes and Principles and Healing Deficiencies
The healing of most dense connective tissues (ligament, tendon, meniscus) follows the same generalized healing process (with minor modifications) and results in the production of scar tissue. Although this tissue is clearly both biologically and biomechanically inferior to normal tendon tissue, in many instances healing by the production of scar tissue can lead to functional healing. In other situations, however, the endogenous healing process may be inadequate.

Tendon healing has been classically divided into tendons that are paratenon-covered and those that are sheathed. The Achilles tendon (calcaneal tendon) of the

rabbit and rat has been extensively studied as an example of healing of a paratenon-covered tendon. Although this information has been important regarding the general healing process of tendons, it should be remembered that these models are examples of healing of a normal, paratenon-covered tendon following direct injury (such as laceration). Healing of a degenerative paratenon-covered tendon, which is more common clinically, has rarely been studied.

Paratenon-Covered Tendon
The general healing process of tendons undergoes three distinct but overlapping phases: inflammatory, fibroblastic or proliferative, and remodeling. In the inflammatory phase, following laceration, the gap between the tendon ends is filled with a hematoma and contains a mixture of inflammatory cells and products, blood cells, fibrin, and debris. This initial blood clot is resorbed and both degradative processes (to remove damaged material) and reparative processes (to replace material) are initiated by both cellular and vascular factors. During this phase proliferating tissue from the adjacent paratenon invades the gap and is replaced by a milieu of disorganized and undifferentiated fibroblasts and adjacent capillary buds. This tissue has limited structural integrity or tensile strength.

The proliferative phase of tendon healing involves the production of what grossly appears as "scar tissue." Hypertrophic fibroblastic cells produce a dense, cellular, collagenous connective tissue matrix that bridges torn tendon ends. Collagen synthesis can be detected as early as 3 days following injury. This matrix is initially disorganized and has quite a different histologic appearance than the organization of normal tendon matrix (**Figure 14**). By 2 weeks, the tendons appear grossly contiguous by a fibrous bridging scar; however, histologically the matrix is

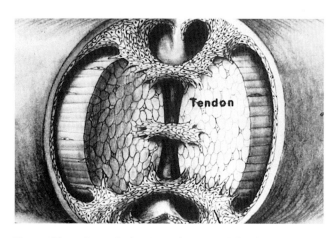

Figure 15   Schematic drawing of an immobilized tendon illustrating extrinsic and intrinsic repair. *(Courtesy of Richard H. Gelberman, MD, Boston, MA.)*

still disorganized with collagen fiber deposition and migration occurring perpendicular to the longitudinal axis of the tendon.

As collagen production and deposition continue, the gap is eventually filled histologically with bridging collagen fibers and fibroblasts. The fibrovascular proliferative tissue from the adjacent tissue regresses and becomes contiguous with the epitenon forming a tendon callus.

By 3 to 4 weeks, realignment of the scar tissue begins as both the fibroblasts and collagen fibers begin to reorient themselves along the longitudinal axis of the tendon presumably in response to tensile stress at the repair site. This remodeling process continues for many months with an accompanying improvement in the mechanical properties of the scar tissue and decrease in the mass of scar tissue (improvement in material properties). As the remodeling phase progresses there is a gradual decrease in the cellularity, vascularity, and improvement in the collagen fiber alignment and cross-linking with accompanying increase in biomechanical properties. Although at 20 weeks this tissue can demonstrate minimal histologic differences when compared with normal tendon, closer investigation has demonstrated differences in tendon biochemistry (collagen content, collagen composition), tendon ultrastructure (collagen fibril organization, collagen fibril diameters), and tendon biomechanics during early tendon remodeling. Although some tendon properties may return to normal levels, it is likely that despite months or even years of healing, some tendon characteristics will likely never reach completely normal levels.

Sheath-Covered Tendons

The presence of a synovial sheath covering a tendon such as in zone II of the long flexors of the fingers can significantly affect the healing of a tendon following direct injury. A similar process initially occurs with the formation of scar tissue resulting in physical continuity between the disrupted ends. However, an overexuberant response, particularly between the tendon and adjacent tissues, can lead to adhesion formation and restrict tendon gliding, critically important for normal function of tendons of the hand.

Similar to healing of paratenon-covered tendons, flexor tendon healing follows three sequential phases—an inflammatory phase, a fibroblastic phase, and a remodeling phase. The inflammatory phase is characterized by migration of inflammatory cells from the surrounding tissues, which phagocytose necrotic tissue and clot. The fibroblastic phase is characterized by fibroblast proliferation and extracellular matrix synthesis, and the remodeling phase is characterized by the production of newly synthesized collagen, organized and oriented along the longitudinal axis of the tendon.

The source of healing of sheathed tendons has long been a subject of controversy (**Figure 15**). Both intrinsic and extrinsic mechanisms of healing have been proposed. The extrinsic mechanism was initially proposed when early investigations suggested that flexor tendon healing occurred primarily by granulation tissue from the tendon sheath. This mechanism of healing relies on inflammatory and fibroblast cell invasion from the periphery to the site of healing with no actual tendon cells participating in the healing response. More recently, however, several investigations have demonstrated an intrinsic capacity of a sheathed tendon to heal and authors have proposed an alternative mechanism of healing via the intrinsic mechanism. The intrinsic mechanism relies on cell invasion from the tendon and epitenon healing site. Although it is likely that both of these processes are occurring clinically, the extrinsic mechanism appears to predominate early in the healing process whereas the intrinsic mechanism is more delayed. When the extrinsic mechanism predominates, it is believed that this results in a reduction in collagen organization, a decrease in material properties, and the production of adhesions between the tendon and surrounding structures. For this reason, methods of suppressing the extrinsic healing mechanism while enhancing the intrinsic healing mechanism may lead to improved functional outcomes following tendon repair.

Degenerative Tendons

The healing of tendons following indirect trauma has rarely been studied experimentally. This has largely been hindered by the fact that clinically these tendon disruptions occur in degenerative tendons and that no universally acceptable model has been developed to study healing of a naturally-occurring degenerative tendon or following experimental degeneration. Although a moot point, clinically the healing of degenerative tendon disruptions such as rotator cuff tears is distinctly different. For example, in patients with chronic rotator cuff tears follow-up imaging studies have demonstrated that up to 80% of tears may recur. This suggests, in addition to other factors (such as a biomechanical environment), that degenerative tears may have a diminished capacity to heal.

Clinically Relevant Variables Affecting Tendon Repair

Successful tendon repair requires a delicate balance between stability of the repair construct and mobility. It seems inherent that for a successful tendon repair, stability of the construct should be optimized. However, those factors that enhance stability (such as immobilization) also restrict mobility and can lead to scarring and stiffness. In contrast, enhancing mobility (for example, by early postoperative motion) can minimize adhesion formation and increase the strength of the repair. However, early postoperative motion risks early disruption and gap formation at the repair site. Early postoperative motion is particularly relevant during repair of the flexor tendon of the hand. An ideal flexor tendon repair would be easy to perform, create minimal bulk and low friction, allow adequate tendon nutrition, maximize tendon-to-tendon healing while minimizing tendon-to-surrounding-tissue healing, and be strong enough to resist disruption while allowing adequate force across the repair site to enhancing remodeling and motion.

Numerous studies have been performed evaluating the strength of different repair constructs that have varied the core suture configuration, the configuration and placement of the epitendinous suture, the number of sutures traversing the repair site, and suture caliber and materials. These studies are based on the principle that a stronger repair construct will require less postoperative protection, allowing for early aggressive postoperative motion. This in turn should minimize adhesion formation and enhance the strength of the repair construct.

Although a review of these studies is beyond the scope of this chapter, these studies have collectively established several important principles for flexor tendon repair. First, a combined core suture and epitendinous suture technique provides the most stable construct that minimizes gap formation at the repair site. Second, the strength of the repair construct is proportional to the size and number of sutures traversing the repair site. Third, nonabsorbable braided sutures (3-0, 4-0) are likely optimal for core suture placement. Fourth, equal tension should be applied to all suture strands. Fifth, although placement of the core suture dorsally (as opposed to volarly) enhances the mechanical strength of the repair it may impede the dorsally located nutrient vessels. Sixth, stress at the repair site increases collagen deposition, improves matrix organization, and improves repair strength.

Although much of the focus on flexor tendon repair has concentrated on surgical technique, rehabilitation following flexor tendon repair has similarly evolved. Early flexor tendon repair, in particular of zone II injuries, often resulted in poor outcomes and led to this region being called "no-man's land." Adhesion formation, proximal interphalangeal joint contractures, and repair dehiscence were major complications facing early hand surgeons. Eventually, the advantages of controlled early motion were

determined and the concept of passive motion was introduced using elastic band traction. Excellent results were reported using this rehabilitation protocol that included an extension block splint, active digital extension, and passive digital flexion using rubber bands attached at the wrist and to the fingernail of the injured digit. These results were a striking improvement over previous reports and heralded the beginning of modern flexor tendon repair and rehabilitation.

More recently, the addition of a palmar pulley has been reported to improve flexion of the both the proximal and distal interphalangeal joints, and a splint with a mobile wrist has been developed to further enhance tendon excursion by the synergistic effect of wrist position on finger flexion. In conjunction with specialized splinting programs, a rehabilitation program has proved useful in improving results. Three to 5 mm of excursion was necessary to prevent adhesion formation and this was achieved through a passive digital motion protocol. Subsequently, various rehabilitation protocols have been developed with variable success and reported rerupture rates. In general, however, most splinting and rehabilitation programs position the distal and proximal interphalangeal joints at rest in extension, position the wrist and metacarpophalangeal joints at rest in flexion, and include frequent application of motion (active or passive).

Many authors have observed the difficulties in repairing chronic tendon disruptions in different tendons and have developed heroic measures to reconstitute tendon continuity (for example, local soft-tissue flaps/turndowns, free tendon autograft, allograft, xenografts). Although much of the attention of tendon repair has focused on the tendon only, it is important to remember that the tendon is only one part of a muscle-tendon-bone complex. In particular, changes in the muscle following disruption may significantly affect functional outcome even in the presence of an optimized tendon repair. Furthermore, surgical tenotomy is often performed (for example, long head of biceps tenotomy, correction of deformity in cerebral palsy) with little regard for the subsequent changes in the muscle-tendon-bone complex. Many studies have evaluated the muscle response following tenotomy and have noted significant structural, molecular, and functional changes (**Table 2**).

Clinically, this has been particularly relevant in chronic tears of the rotator cuff where some authors have described "fatty degeneration" and atrophy of the rotator cuff muscles on imaging studies such as CT and MRI. In some instances, fatty degeneration and atrophy of the rotator cuff muscles correlated with functional deficits both preoperatively and postoperatively and did not improve following "successful" rotator cuff repair. Furthermore, the surgical technique of tendon repair may affect tendon healing. For example, during rotator cuff repair, maintenance of the subacromial bursa and decortication of the cortical bone on the humeral head may provide a source

Table 2   Structural, Molecular, and Functional Changes Following Tenotomy
Structural
Myofiber disorganization
Central core necrosis
Z-line streaming
Fibrosis of fibers
Fibrosis of Golgi tendon organs
Changes in sarcomere number
Alterations in number of membrane particles
Molecular
Changes in myosin heavy chain composition
Changes in expression of neural cell adhesion molecule
Functional
Decreased maximum tetanic and twitch tension

of blood supply for healing of tendon to bone. Furthermore, the area of healing during repair may be an important factor in maintaining the structural integrity of the repair. In the rotator cuff this corresponds to reconstructing the entire three-dimensional architecture of the rotator cuff footprint.

Ligaments
Classification and Anatomy

Most ligaments in the human body are discrete anatomic structures that are classified according to a variety of features including their bony attachments (for example, coracoacromial), their relationships to a joint (for example, collateral), their relationships to each other (for example, cruciate), or their gross anatomic shape (for example, deltoid). There are several hundred such ligaments in the body that all serve unique local functions in guiding joint kinematics and helping to prevent abnormal displacements of bones relative to each other during function. They have been likened to "slightly stretchy ropes" that link bones in specific anatomic locations to serve these mechanical functions. In addition, it is appreciated that, like tendons, ligaments also display subtle "viscoelastic behaviors" that contribute to minor readjustments of lengths, loads, and load distributions within each structure, and thus within the joint as a whole.

There is a second family of ligamentous structures that are much more poorly defined, known as capsular ligaments. These ligaments are much less discrete anatomically, actually blending into each other in the periarticular dense capsule of a diarthrodial joint. With effort, discrete bands of some of these ligaments have been delineated, with a few being capsular expansions of tendinous attachments (for example, the posterior oblique ligament of the knee extends from the insertion of semimem-

branosus), but most have no proximity to tendon attachments. In addition to their obvious encapsulating role (being lined with synovium on their intra-articular side), as their names would imply, these structures likely have important roles similar to those of their more discrete neighbors in helping guide bony movements during joint function.

The attachment sites of the ligaments onto the bones at either end are in unique and critical locations on the bone and often involve unusual shapes on the bone. Very few ligament insertion sites are what would be considered "simple" in shape and these shapes are likely critical to how the fibers within that ligament are recruited as its joint moves. The specific (average) shapes of only a few ligaments have thus far been well defined, generally those requiring surgical reconstruction.

Gross Morphology, Histology, Microanatomy, and Cell Biology

Like tendons, ligaments are dense bands of collagenous connective tissue that appear white and relatively avascular. Most ligaments have a thin surface layer known as an "epiligament" (analogous to the tendon epitenon) that appears more vascular than the actual body of the underlying ligament itself. This epiligament is often indistinguishable from and merges into the periosteum of the bone around the attachment sites of the ligament. It obscures the surface of the ligament and can make the ligament appear smooth rather than fibrous.

Ligaments are (somewhat) parallel-fibered, dense, collagenous tissues that are more difficult to dissect than tendons because they are generally less distinct. Ligaments also appear to have more fiber-fiber interactions than tendons, with more "intertwining" of functional subunits. Compared with tendons, ligaments also generally contain slightly plumper but still elongated fibroblasts or fibrocytes between their fibers, with these cells running parallel to the ligament fibers. In addition, there are some potentially important differences in cell shapes and cellular behaviors between different ligaments. Midsubstance cells from normal ACLs are more chondroid in appearance; they grow and migrate more slowly in vitro than cells derived from medial collateral ligaments (MCLs) (**Figure 16**). There appear to be subtle differences in the matrix produced by these fibroblasts of ACL versus MCL. These characteristics are collectively believed to have relevance to the rates and ability of ACL to heal.

Compared with tendons, ligaments have a similarly complex morphology at their bone insertions, also involving transition zones from soft midsubstance, through zones of stress-distributing fibrocartilage and calcified fibrocartilage, before merging into bone. Sharpey's fibers are the calcified collagenous anchors within bone that (as with tendons) attach the ligament to bone so firmly in the adult state. Intrinsic collagen fibers actually appear to run

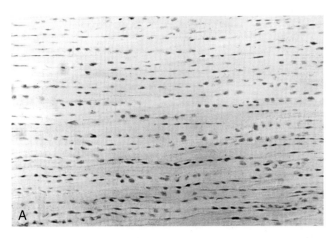
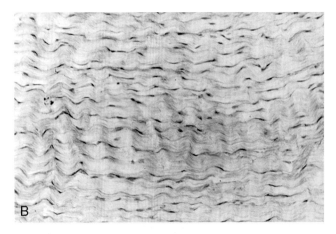

Figure 16   Differing appearances of cells in the ACL of the New Zealand White rabbit (**A**) and the MCL of the New Zealand White rabbit (**B**). Note the more rounded appearance of the ACL nuclei in contrast to the elongated MCL nuclei. *(Reproduced with permission from Frank CB: Ligament injuries: Pathophysiology and healing, in Zachazewski JE, Magee DJ, Quillen WS (eds): Athletic Injuries and Rehabilitation. Philadelphia, PA, WB Saunders, 1996, p 14.)*

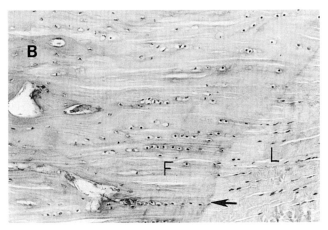
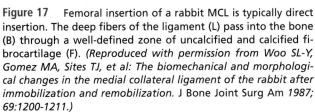

Figure 17   Femoral insertion of a rabbit MCL is typically direct insertion. The deep fibers of the ligament (L) pass into the bone (B) through a well-defined zone of uncalcified and calcified fibrocartilage (F). *(Reproduced with permission from Woo SL-Y, Gomez MA, Sites TJ, et al: The biomechanical and morphological changes in the medial collateral ligament of the rabbit after immobilization and remobilization. J Bone Joint Surg Am 1987; 69:1200-1211.)*

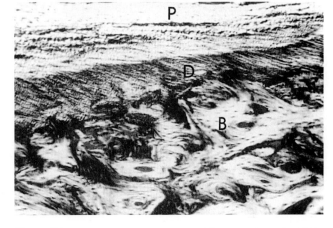

Figure 18   Indirect insertion of a rabbit MCL into the tibia showing superficial fibers (P) inserting into periosteum, and the deep fibers (D) inserting obliquely into bone (B). (hematoxylin and eosin staining, x50). *(Reproduced with permission from Woo SL-Y, Gomez MA, Sites TJ, et al: The biomechanical and morphological changes in the medial collateral ligament of the rabbit after immobilization and remobilization. J Bone Joint Surg Am 1987;69:1200-1211.)*

from the substance of each structure directly into the bone where they are literally cemented into place. Developmental studies have shown that these direct ligament insertions, which are by far the most common ligament insertion type in the body, are actually formed by bone growing in and around preexisting ligament collagen fibers, anchoring them into place (**Figure 17**). There are a few examples of indirect ligament insertions (ligaments that insert by merging with adjacent periosteum into bone) during growth and development—for example, the tibial insertion of the MCL in the immature state (**Figure 18**). These periosteal attachments in growing ligaments likely contribute somewhat to the strength of the ligament

at that time (as well as to injury patterns, including epiphyseal avulsions).

Ligament composition is similar to that of tendons with some subtle but potentially important differences that likely make ligaments slightly more viscous and slightly less strong and stiff than tendons (**Figure 19**). Water and collagen contents of ligaments are similar to those of tendons (60% to 70% water) with most of their dry weight (> 80%) being collagen. Ligaments likely have slightly higher water contents and slightly lower collagen contents than tendons (by a few percent), but these amounts probably vary between structures and between individuals.

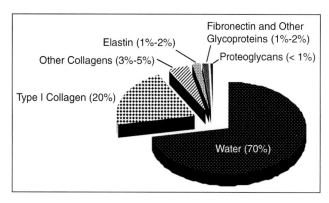

Figure 19   Pie chart illustrating the biochemical constituents of a typical ligament. Note the predominance of water. *(Reproduced with permission from Frank CB: Ligament injuries: Pathophysiology and healing, in Zachazewski JE, Magee DJ, Quillen WS (eds): Athletic Injuries and Rehabilitation. Philadelphia, PA, WB Saunders, 1996, p 15.)*

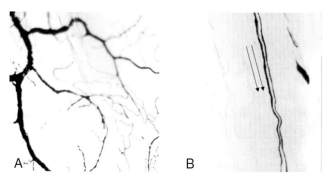

Figure 20   Vascular perfusion of the New Zealand White rabbit lateral collateral ligament with an ink/gelatin solution. Collagen and matrix are unstained and therefore not visible. Bar = 100 μm. **A,** Blood vessel plexuses and random vessel orientation in epiligament. **B,** Longitudinal orientation of ligament midsubstance vessels. Double arrows indicate long axis of ligament. *(Courtesy of Dr. Robert C. Bray of the University of Calgary, Department of Surgery, Calgary, Alberta, Canada.)*

Collagen type I is the main collagen type in ligaments (> 90% of the collagen present), but there are smaller proportions of type III and type VI, as well as some types V, XI, and XIV (the latter nearer insertions). Ligament proteoglycans, which represent about 1% of the dry weight of the ligament but which are likely critical for binding of water and growth factors and for determining fiber spacing and fiber sliding interactions, are primarily decorin and biglycan. The latter seems to be found more in ligaments than tendons, but this has not yet been characterized in a large enough sample of ligaments to be confirmed. Other small proteoglycans are also found (lumican, fibromodulin) in ligaments, as well as very small quantities of larger aggregating proteoglycans, as seen in compressive areas of tendons, perhaps because ligaments also interact with bones. The distributions of these larger proteoglycans and their relationships to local characteristics of that ligament have not yet been demonstrated.

Blood Supply and Innervation

Ligament blood supply is relatively sparse compared with that of skin and is again similar to that of tendons. However, vascular injection studies demonstrate that ligaments are more vascular than their white appearance suggests (**Figure 20**). Perigeniculate arteries supply penetrating superficial arterioles that enter the ligaments from their surfaces (not through bone insertion sites), branch in those surface "epiligament" layers, and then enter the underlying ligament substance in several locations. The blood supply of the ACL in the knee is derived from the middle geniculate artery, which enters the joint and ramifies through the surface synovium on the ACL to enter its substance between its fascicles. These vessels are more abundant at the surfaces nearer to the ligament insertions but they are variable. Although sparse, they likely play critical roles in supply of nutrients and distribution of water within the ligament.

There are some nerves on and within ligaments and, as with blood vessels, there appear to be more of these nerves nearer to the ligament attachments to bone (**Figure 21**). Both nociceptive pain sensors and some proprioceptive nerve elements occur within ligament substance, suggesting that ligaments do have roles in sensation, position sense, and likely in neuromuscular feedback to the muscles of the joint that it serves. Although proprioceptive nerves are present in ligaments and are known to play some role in joint position sense along with tendons and other periarticular tissues, a quantitative analysis of the physiologic role(s) of ligament proprioceptors has proven to be difficult. There is considerable ongoing work in this area and more information is needed to define just how important nerves in ligaments are to their functions.

Ligament Functions
Mechanical
The main functions of ligaments are known to be mechanical, working as passive restraints of bones in diarthrodial joints. They connect bone to bone across a joint space, passively helping to guide the motion of the joint that they serve. Individual ligaments have "dominant functions," resisting certain abnormal displacements of bones more than others, thus making it easier to determine when that ligament is deficient on a physical examination. Importantly, however, there is some redundancy between ligament functions; they share load-carrying functions to a small extent. For example, the posterolateral structures in the knee (the arcuate complex) serve a complementary role to that of the ACL in resisting anterior translation of the lateral side of the tibia, explaining why that corner of the knee can "stretch out" chronically after an ACL injury.

In addition to long-standing evidence that ligaments are not as totally functionally unique and "isolated" as

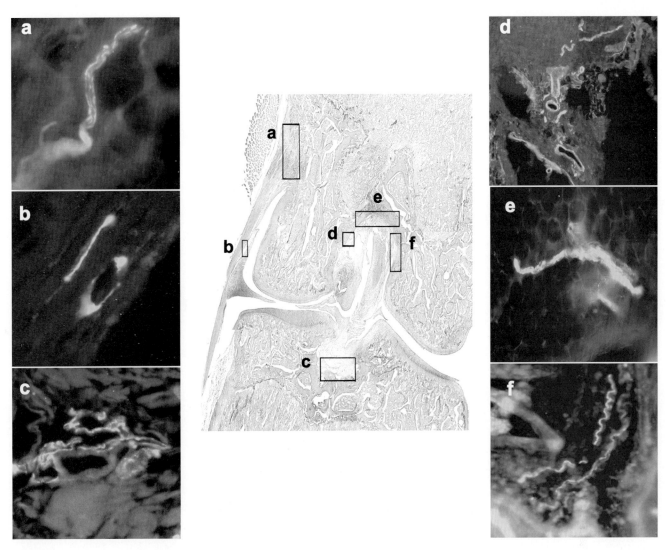

Figure 21   Coronal section of a rat knee joint showing the femoral and tibial attachments of the cruciate ligaments, and the femoral attachment of the lateral collateral ligament (LCL) (x25). Side images (**a** through **f**) show typical fluorescent-labeled protein gene product profiles. Fluorescent images are: **a,** femoral attachment of LCL; **b,** meniscal attachment of LCL; **c,** tibial attachments of cruciates; **d,e,** and **f,** cruciate attachment points in femoral groove. (The section is stained with hematoxylin, safranin O, and fast green, x400, found within the corresponding outlined areas shown above.) *(Courtesy of Dr. Paul Salo, University of Calgary.)*

may be assumed is the second fact, based on considerable evidence, that during normal joint movements the ligaments carry only small loads (a small fraction of their failure load capabilities). The neuromuscular system powers the joints and with extrinsic loads being added to the body loads, the loads on individual ligaments likely increase. However, collectively these pieces of evidence demonstrate that each joint clearly has some redundancy in terms of shared load-carrying functions; loads on individual structures are likely kept a bit lower than might be expected. At lower loads, ligaments are more viscous-dominated and at higher loads they are more elastic-dominated; however, in reality they are considered viscoelastic. Within any given ligament there are many strong and stiff collagen fibers, which can be recruited into action as loads are applied. Tensile forces are thus distrib-

uted over an increasing number of fibers as required (as bones tend to displace under increasing unbalanced forces), causing the nonlinear tensile mechanical behavior that is seen for each ligament. In so doing, fiber stresses within that ligament stay low and within their failure and fatigue limits.

Compared with any other connective tissues in the body, ligaments, like tendons, in skeletally mature individuals are known to be very strong and very stiff at higher loads. Because ligaments are connected to bone at both ends, their bony attachment sites are very important to their structural strength. Forces directed perpendicular to these insertions have been shown to cause "shear failure" of the ligament at that bony interface at relatively low loads. As Woo and associates have shown, when forces are aligned with the ligament fibers and with the direction of insertion into bone,

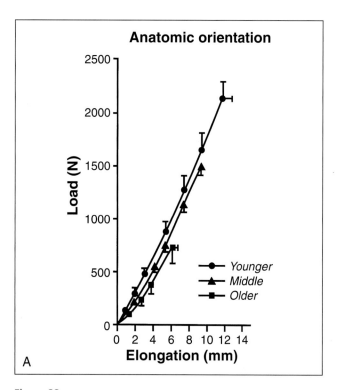

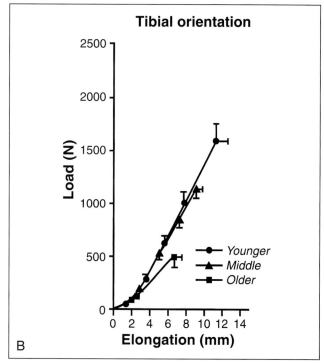

Figure 22   The structural properties (load-elongation curves) for femur-ACL-tibia complexes tested at 30° of flexion in the **(A)** anatomic orientation and **(B)** tibial orientation for younger, middle-aged, and older human donors. *(Reproduced with permission from Woo SL-Y, Hollis JM, Adams DJ, Lyon RM, Takai S: Tensile properties of the human femur-anterior cruciate ligament-tibia complex: The effects of specimen age and orientation.* Am J Sports Med *1991;19:217-225.)*

the ligaments reach their maximum strength (up to three times as strong as when they fail in shear at bony interfaces) (**Figure 22**). This fact has important implications to both clinical injury patterns, but also to experimental mechanical testing protocols of ligament properties, in which ligament orientations relative to loads are critical to the apparent maximum strength of ligaments. Ligament stiffness and strength has also been shown to be a function of age, partly because of weakness of insertions during growth and development, and partly because of postnatal maturation of the matrix in the ligament (**Figure 23**).

Ligament insertion sites with their specific locations and insertion shapes on the bone are absolutely crucial to the function of each ligament. Insertion sites often have unusual shapes in particular locations on the surface of the connected bones and these shapes, along with internal characteristics of the fiber microarchitecture, determine how fibers running between insertion sites are recruited. In general, there are different subparts of a ligament recruited into tension as the joint passes through its normal range of motion, creating functional bands within each otherwise independently identified ligament. For example, within the ACL there are anteromedial and posterolateral bands that tighten in flexion and extension of the knee, respectively.

This principle of functional bands within ligaments has several clinically important implications and is likely true of all ligaments (**Figure 24**). First, it implies that individual ligaments really do not function as homogeneous units. Tensile loads are distributed between different parts of each structure internally, depending on the three-dimensional position of the bones and that different parts of a ligament are responsible for restraining abnormal displacements of the bones in different positions of the joint. Distribution of tensile loads has implications to both physical examination for ligament functions and to ligament injury in that only the tight, or recruited part of the ligament will be damaged if bones are forcibly (and abnormally) displaced. The three-dimensional position of the joint will determine which part of each ligament guiding it will be tight in that position and therefore potentially damageable. The magnitude and direction of loads (intrinsic muscle loads and extrinsic forces; contact versus momentum-related extrinsic forces on that joint) will then determine which fibers then get recruited and the order in which they will be damaged. Fibers are slightly slack, then recruited into increasing tension, and ultimately they reach their tensile limit and fail.

To fully test the function of all parts of a ligament on physical examination, therefore, the joint must be tested throughout its range of motion. For example, the ACL, which limits AP displacements of the knee, should actually be tested as a passive restraint to anterior tibial displacement throughout the range of motion of the knee and not

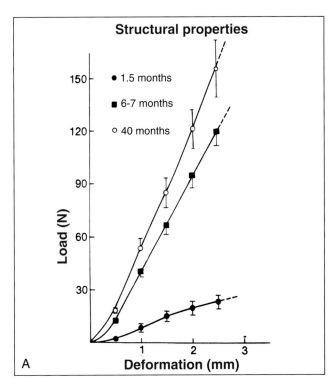

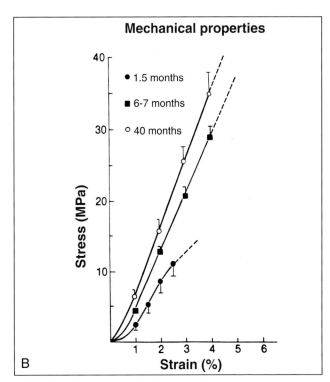

Figure 23   A, The structural properties (load deformation curves) of the femur-MCL-tibia complex and **B,** the mechanical properties of the ligament substance (stress-strain curves) for three age groups: 1.5 months (open epiphysis), 6 to 7 months (closed epiphysis), and 40 months (closed epiphysis). *(Reproduced with permission from Woo SL-Y, Young EP, Kwan MK: Fundamental studies in knee ligament mechanics, in Daniel D, Akeson WH, O'Connor JJ (eds):* Knee Ligaments: Structure, Function, Injury and Repair. *New York, NY, Raven Press, 1990, pp 115-134.)*

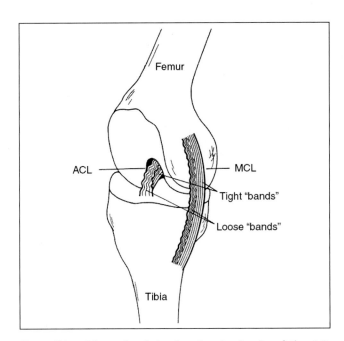

Figure 24   Schematic of the functional subunits of the ACL and the MCL. At approximately 15° of flexion, the anterior portion of both the ACL and the MCL is relatively "loose" in comparison with the "tight" posterior parts. *(Reproduced with permission from Frank CB: Ligament injuries: Pathophysiology and healing, in Zachazewski JE, Magee DJ, Quillen WS (eds):* Athletic Injuries and Rehabilitation. *Philadelphia, PA, WB Saunders, 1996, p 10.)*

just at convenient positions of 30° and 90° of flexion. Unique parts of the ACL should be tight in each of those positions but other subdivisions should be tight in other positions in the remaining arc of knee motion. For the knee, the posterolateral band of the ACL should be tight as the knee approaches extension (the Lachman position) whereas the anteromedial portion should be tighter as the knee is flexed to the anterior drawer position. Positive tests are interpreted as a knee flexion angle-specific increase in anterior tibial displacement of the injured knee versus the normal knee, indicating the functional loss of that part of that ligament (a positive Lachman test is indicated by a disrupted posterolateral band of the ACL). If abnormal displacements occur with examination at all joint angles (positive Lachman and anterior drawer tests), it suggests a probable complete disruption of that structure.

Ligament "sprains" are classified clinically and experimentally according to what proportion of a ligament is torn. A grade I sprain is a partial tear in which one part of a functional band is disrupted. There should be minimal (or no) abnormal displacements of bones—assuming forces are applied at the right joint angle and in the correct direction(s) to reveal such laxity. A grade II injury indicates enough tearing of enough fibers within a structure for clinically detectable laxity. Some part(s) of the structure, however, must remain intact (otherwise it is a grade III or complete injury of that structure).

Material and Viscoelastic Properties

Like tendons, ligament properties can also be expressed on a material basis; that is, corrected for size. Force per unit area describes tensile stress within a structure and again like tendons, on this stress-strain basis, ligaments are relatively stiff and strong. Along with tendons, they are among the strongest tensile tissues in the body (> 80 MPa failure stresses).

Key viscoelastic properties of ligaments are also like those of tendons; they "load relax" (loads/stresses decrease within the structure if they are pulled to constant deformations) and/or they creep (increasing deformation over time if they are held under constant loads/stresses) (**Figures 7 through 12**). These microadjustments of ligament loads/stresses and lengths are likely important to their ability to distribute loads internally and to balance loads among structures in a joint. Although not studied in as much detail as failure properties, they may have important roles in controlling local stresses and thus influencing cellular homeostasis in the variable loading environments experienced by these tissues.

Proprioceptive

As noted previously, ligaments have been shown to have some proprioceptive role in joint functioning. Ligament strains invoke neurologic feedback signals and appear to play a role in joint position sense. The magnitude and physiologic/clinical impact of this role under different loading circumstances, with aging and with injury, has proved difficult to quantify and requires ongoing analysis.

Clinically Relevant Injuries

Ligaments are most often torn in traumatic joint injuries, which are collectively known as sprains. The injury can be modest, in which fibers are stretched but none are actually torn, or the fibers can be partially disrupted (some fibers torn), or completely disrupted (all fibers torn). As noted previously, based on progressive fiber recruitment, it is easy to imagine that only the tight parts of a ligament will be torn when the bones are forcibly displaced. The more severe the force, the more fibers that are progressively torn and the more severe the resulting objective instability or laxity of the damaged joint. Assuming no other compensation, such injuries would be more likely to become symptomatic. Combined ligament injuries—that is, to multiple ligaments around any given joint—render the joint the most unstable and less likely for spontaneous healing.

As might be expected because of the increasing instability with damage to an increasing number of compensatory structures, the functional outcomes of combined injuries are poorer than isolated ligament injuries and are thus more likely to require either acute or chronic surgical repair. Replacement of injured cruciate ligaments in the knee, especially the ACL, is frequently required because of functional instabilities that occur in combination with collateral ligament injuries. These types of combined injuries are particularly common in athletic populations at high risk for injury (young, aggressive, athletic males). In these situations collateral ligament healing is also functionally impaired, leading to chronic combined laxity and symptomatic instabilities that can require surgery. Improvement of the natural healing ability of both cruciate and collateral ligaments of the knee is a common challenge. Similarly, inadequate healing or subsequent reinjury and failure of damaged ligaments is also common in and around other joints (such as the shoulder, some finger and intercarpal ligaments, wrist ligaments, and ankle ligaments).

Factors That Influence Healing Outcomes

The healing response may be influenced by several factors, including the age of the patient, genetic contributions, gender, hormonal effects, presence of comorbidities, quality of the tissue before injury from a mechanical and biologic perspective, and changes in neurovascular regulation.

Like most connective tissues, ligaments change as a function of age. Generally, ligaments achieve their peak performance, in a mechanical sense, at the time of skeletal maturity, because of an optimization of their cellular and matrix behaviors. Prior to skeletal maturity, ligaments are more viscous (have higher water content) and have smaller cross-sectional areas, making them relatively compliant (low stiffness). Upon clinical evaluation, these joints appear relatively loose, and at higher loads the ligament insertions are common sites of injury (particularly in children) because the ligaments have not yet firmly cemented into the bones. After skeletal maturity, ligament cells begin to slow down their metabolic functions, maintaining the matrix as opposed to adding to it as was the case during growth. They reach their maximum size and structural stiffness and are less viscous (more elastic) than their immature counterparts. During middle age, both ligament and ligament insertions begin to weaken, resulting in progressive loss of structural strength. Viscosity decreases further and ligament collagen becomes more highly cross-linked. Ligaments become less compliant and the joints appear to tighten over time. With old age, bones are usually more fragile than ligaments and become clinically significant sites of weakness in joint injuries. Ligaments lose mass, stiffness, strength, and viscosity in elderly people. Because elderly people generally are less active, the changes in the ligaments are usually not part of any obvious clinical problem. If the joints deform as the result of changes in bone shapes causing ligaments to experience excessive loads as a result, ligaments may experience excessive creep and contribute to pathologic joint laxities.

Studies from many areas and organ systems clearly point to an age-related loss of neuroregulation. Whether these changes are intrinsic to the systems studied or secondary effects of alterations in other physiologic systems remains unclear. Animal model studies of the knee joint have shown a definite correlation between loss of neuronal elements and the onset of osteoarthritic changes in such joints, although isolation of the contribution of age-related neuronal loss in specific ligaments is difficult and requires further study.

Gender-specific and hormone-related variables impact both the risk for ligament injuries as well as the potential response to such injuries. Several reports have indicated that female athletes experience a much higher rate of noncontact-initiated ACL injuries than do males participating in the same sports at the same level. Although some of the knee ligament injuries may be caused by anatomic considerations, and running and cutting maneuvers that are correctible, the fact that changes in hormonal levels have been implicated indicates that such fluctuations contribute to the risk environment. Females tend to have a more vigorous inflammatory response than males and because the inflammatory response to injury is a central initial step in the healing process, this is a consistent pattern of observation. Healing responses in postmenopausal women decline separately from the decline associated with aging.

At present, it is not clear what role genetic factors play in knee ligament injury and wound healing. Genetic factors do play a role in some pathologic scarring or wound healing such as keloid formation, which is more common in some races than others. Recent animal studies examining skin healing in two genetically distinct pig types point to a genetic component in skin wound healing, but whether these findings are skin-specific or can be extrapolated to wound healing in other tissues following overt injury remains an area of investigation.

The quality of the tissue before overt injury may play a role in the wound healing process and the final outcome, and therefore should be considered. Some animal studies have demonstrated that depriving healing ligaments of mechanical loading has a detrimental effect on healing outcome. Similar studies have shown that reinjury of an acutely healing MCL leads to alterations in gene expression of the healing tissue with reexpression of proinflammatory molecules. Tissue history is an area of study plagued by a paucity of information so that discussions are speculative and the relative importance of this variable on outcome is largely unknown.

The presence of comorbidities such as diabetes can impact the healing outcome. Diabetic patients have a compromised wound healing response, caused in part by an impaired inflammatory response and elaboration of growth factors. Comorbidities could also impact the healing process indirectly through the treatment interventions designed to control the comorbidities. As an example, rheumatoid arthritis patients are being treated with biologics such as those designed to neutralize inflammatory components. Patients with certain inflammatory diseases are treated with glucocorticoids that are known to have profound effects on inflammatory processes.

The neural and vascular components also likely play important roles in influencing healing outcomes. The difference in healing capacities between different knee ligaments has recently been associated with the superior potential of some ligaments to increase their blood supply through angiogenesis, and because increased flow is essential for ligament healing to occur, this factor may be the major difference in healing potential between different knee ligaments. Knee joints possess abundant nerve supplies that relay sensory and motor information on such aspects as proprioception, nociception, and vasoregulation. Studies of injured knee ligaments in animal models show higher than normal levels of immunoreactivity in and adjacent to the healing zone; however, the nerve fibers appear to be tangled and truncated and do not look like those in the ligaments from normal animals. Studies such as these have established that knee ligaments contain an abundant nerve and vascular supply and that these elements likely play a major role in healing outcomes.

Ligament Repair
Healing Processes, Principles, and Healing Deficiencies
Evidence has accumulated over many years showing that the natural healing ability of ligaments is variable, with some structures either having adequate compensatory mechanisms when injured or truly healing adequately (functionally), and some not. Physical, anatomic, and biologic reasons can be invoked to explain these differences. Generally speaking, in the most severe complete injuries of either tendons or ligaments, retraction of torn ends leaves a gap that must be bridged. Some gaps are insurmountable, with many centimeters of space between retracted muscle and tendon insertion sites onto bone (for example, biceps tendon ruptures in the upper arm). Other gaps are likely minimal, offering the potential for successful bridging by local repair responses. These physical, anatomic barriers can be compounded by local biologic deficiencies that still remain ill-defined in many instances, but include inadequate cellular division within these hypocellular tissues, lack of local blood supply, potential interference with local nerve supply, and perhaps interference with the formation of local repair responses by local inhibitors of healing (for example, in the synovial space). For a combination of these reasons, certain structures therefore have notoriously poor healing potential and require attempts at repair or restoration. It should be noted, however, that these same complications (such as inadequate blood supply) will be the same for any bioengineered replacement, a fact that must be taken into account for any approaches. Because of local deficiencies (in anatomy, load, or lubrication) the functional and biologic

demands on any graft replacement will be somewhat unique—and one approach may therefore not work in all circumstances.

As noted in the tendon section, despite significant healing challenges, there is considerable experimental evidence from animal models suggesting that many ligaments and tendons do have the potential to heal naturally by virtue of what should be called scar formation. Scar is a unique connective tissue that forms in the adult, apparently as a consequence of bleeding and inflammation surrounding the damaged connective tissue in the area of injury. Like skin wounds, ligament scars are collagenous matrices built on fibrin clots with early cellular (fibroblastic) division and progressive deposition of increasingly dense fibrous matrix that then remodels slowly to align along the main tensile axis of the structure. There are several morphologic, ultrastructural, biochemical, and biomechanical changes that occur within the scar as it forms and remodels, with progressive but ultimately limited improvement over months to years of healing.

Some of the specific reasons for scar weakness have been identified and include flaws within the matrix (**Figure 25**), abnormal collagen types, inadequate collagen cross-linking, and abnormally small collagen fibril sizes (**Figure 26**) (the latter perhaps related to abnormal cellular production of proteoglycans). As previously noted, scars of tendons and ligaments apparently stop improving after reaching 30% to 50% of normal tissue quality; that is, at roughly 25 to 40 MPa of ultimate tensile strength. Viscoelastic behaviors of ligament scars (creep and load-relaxation behaviors) are also abnormal. Scars creep considerably more than normal ligaments under low load stresses, thereby affecting joint stability and kinematics during normal daily activities. Scars improve slowly, but their recovery is apparently slightly better than that of high load properties, at least in extra-articular healing environments. Clinically, it is important to keep loads low on healing ligaments during the initial healing period to minimize stretching out of the ligaments and thus the potential for reinjury. The fatigue behaviors of these scars are not yet known.

Clinically Relevant Variables Affecting Ligament Repair

There is considerable evidence to suggest that scar tissue has definite potential to be improved. It is hypermetabolic and hypercellular and is responsive to many variables. Joint motion and tissue loading are particularly important factors. Animal model research over the past 50 years has strongly suggested that although immobility may lead to a slightly "tighter" healing joint with less ligament and joint laxity when tested at low loads, some joint motion, if appropriately controlled to stay within subfailure and subdamage loads, can improve the structural strength of most healing ligaments (**Figure 27**). Canine models by Woo and associates as well as other authors, have clearly

shown that immobilization compromises ligament scar strength, whereas some motion increases scar strength (**Figure 28**). This fact has supported empirical clinical observations that short periods of immobility (if any) are required to lead to optimal clinical results (stability with least recurrent instability) secondary to serious ligament injuries.

Some authors have argued that continuous passive motion leads to optimal results for healing extra-articular ligaments, whereas others have suggested that active motion, where kinematics can presumably be controlled if neuromuscular function is not abnormal, can be equally effective. Optimal loads/stresses are not known and may be scar- or structure-specific, but some amount of tensile loading appears to be good for the endogenous repair of all ligaments, with the possible exception of the ACL.

Biochemical methods of improving scar quality and composition have also been examined with evidence that scar can, in fact, also be modified by several other extrinsic factors (anti-inflammatory agents, growth factors, cytokines). Platelet-derived growth factor appears to be an early stimulator of ligament scar formation, whereas transforming growth factor-β1 and insulin-like growth factor-1 have also been shown to have some slightly later stimulatory effects on collagen synthesis and remodeling. Hyaluronic acid may stimulate scar formation and type III collagen synthesis in ACLs. Interestingly, scar has some pluripotential capabilities, with compressive forces on it apparently being able to upregulate some cartilage-like molecules in vitro. This factor has important implications to scar remodeling in vivo but raises the interesting and only minimally investigated possibility of scar harvesting, expansion, and modification ex vivo for possible reimplantation purposes.

As previously noted, another clinically relevant variable is the effect of gap size on ligament repair. Experimental studies have suggested that increasing gap sizes between disrupted ends leads to a structurally weaker scar, likely caused by an increased number or size of fatal flaws. Based on their similarity to tendons, where surgical repair was clearly seen to restore some function to muscle-tendon units, suture apposition of torn ends of ligamentous structures became fashionable for most acute ligament ruptures. The supporting concept was that such suture reapposition of torn ligament ends should lead to better quality repair (presumably tighter and stronger repairs) than nonsurgical approaches. This concept was based on the general notion that the natural history of untreated healing of ruptured ligaments would not be as strong or as tight as sutured repairs, a concept that was tested scientifically only within the past 25 years.

It has become more obvious over time that the subjective and objective clinical natural history of healing of many ligament injuries, when treated with appropriate physiotherapy, is not detectably different from suture repairs. Although there is some evidence that acute suture

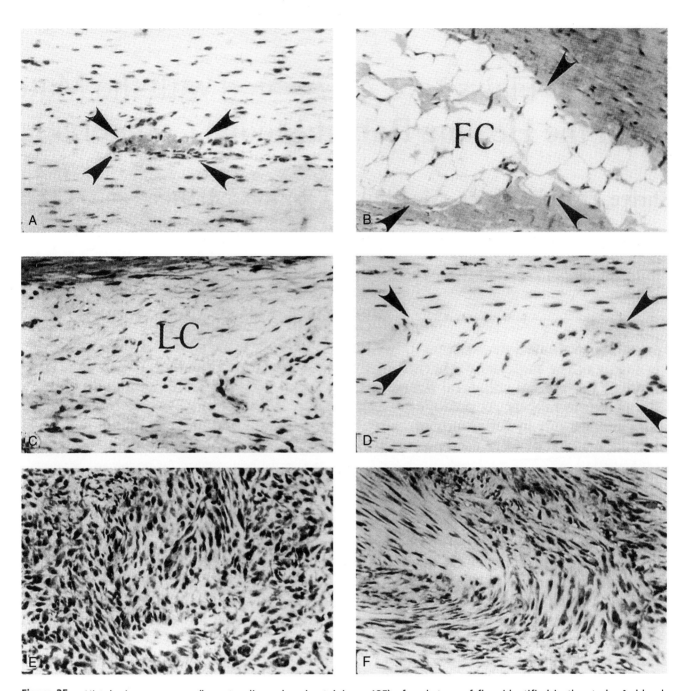

Figure 25   Histologic appearance (hematoxylin and eosin staining; x125) of each type of flaw identified in the study: **A,** blood vessels, **B,** fat cells (FC), **C,** loose collagen (LC), **D,** disorganized collagen, **E,** cellular infiltrates, and **F,** a combination of any or all of these flaws. The longitudinal axis of the MCL runs right to left. *(Reproduced with permission from Shrive N, Chimich D, Marchuk L, Wilson J, Brant R, Frank C: Soft-tissue "flaws" are associated with the material properties of the healing rabbit medial collateral ligament. J Orthop Res 1995;13:923-929.)*

repairs of certain ligaments, including the ACL in the knee, can result in improved proportions of functional results, most data still suggest that for whatever reasons, acute ligament suturing often does not meaningfully change the natural history of joint stability (tightness or stiffness) or reinjury of that ligament (its strength).

Based on this failure to demonstrate improved outcomes definitively, and while still being debated by some,

acute suture repair of most ligament injuries (except those in serious combined injuries and dislocations) has more recently been abandoned in favor of nonsurgical rehabilitation. Although it cannot be stated that nonsurgical approaches achieve success by virtue of improving healing of damaged structures themselves, as opposed to compensatory changes in complementary elements around each joint (other musculotendinous structures, remodeling of

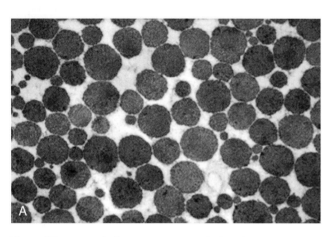
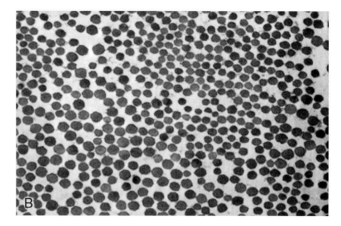

Figure 26   A, Typical transverse transmission electron microscope sections of control MCL and **B,** 14-week MCL scar. Note the distribution of large and small fibril diameters in the control MCL in contrast with only small fibril diameters in the scar MCL (x30,000).

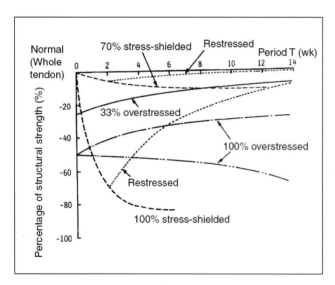

Figure 27   Summary of experimental results on the effects of stress shielding, restressing after stress shielding, and stress increase on the structural properties of rabbit patellar tendons. *(Reproduced with permission from Hayashi K: Biomechanical studies of the remodeling of knee joint tendons and ligaments.* J Biomechanics *1996;29:707-716.)*

Tendon and Ligament Grafting and Replacement
Using Normal Tissues as Grafts

Based on a long history of clinical and basic investigation that dates back over 100 years, grafting of dense connective tissues from other sources, either within the same individual (autografting) or postmortem tissue harvested from another individual of the same species (allografting), has become the gold standard for tendon and ligament replacement. Grafting of animal tissues (xenografting) has received less attention, with the possibility of immunologic rejection being a major barrier—with most clinicians and investigators focusing for the past several decades on the other two options. Tendons and fascia have become the two major sources of harvestable tissues because it has been shown that some of these structures are potentially "expendable" without a huge clinical cost. Unlike tendon and fascial tissues, which can be harvested with what is perceived to be relatively little morbidity from an individual, there have not been any spare ligaments identified within an individual that can be transplanted to another site without significant potential loss of function at the donor site. Again, based on a long series of empirical and subsequent semiquantitative clinical studies dating back over 50 years, for autografting purposes, hamstring tendon grafts and partial patellar tendon grafts have become the two gold standard tendon grafts in the lower extremity, with palmaris longus tendons, if present, being a graft source of low functional risk. Similarly, fascial strips from the lower extremity (fascia lata) also have been harvested as tendon and ligament graft materials. Given the lack of concern for donor site morbidity in allografting, there are many additional tendon and even potential ligament graft options (Achilles, tibialis anterior, ACL). There has been considerable work done on all of these grafts, clinically and experimentally, over the past 25 years to determine their efficacy and shortcomings (if any) in a variety of sit-

other tissues), they are known to achieve equal and often at least adequate clinical success in relatively safe ways.

Also as previously noted, some ligament injuries have continued to have relatively poor functional clinical outcomes with both natural healing plus aggressive and appropriate therapy, as well as with attempted suture repairs plus therapy, particularly in certain categories of patients (high-risk young aggressive athletic males with ACL injuries). This factor has suggested that in certain injuries in certain subsets of individuals, some other surgical or biologic approaches were required. Various types of reconstructive surgery have evolved to treat these lesions.

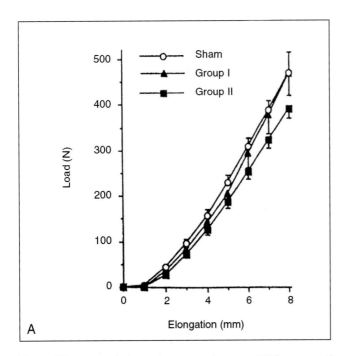
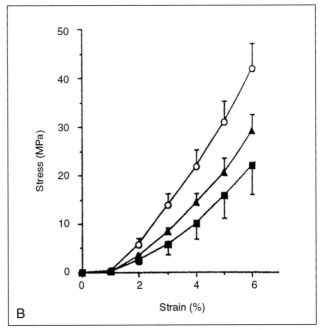

Figure 28   **A,** Load-elongation curves (mean ± SEM) representing the structural properties of the FMTC (femur-MCL-tibia complex) for group 1 (not repaired, no immobilization) and group II (repair, 6 weeks of immobilization) at 48 weeks postoperatively. Experimental samples from group II were the furthest from the controls at all time periods. **B,** Stress-strain curves representing the mechanical properties of the MCL substance of group I (not repaired, no immobilization) and group II (repair, 6 weeks of immobilization) at 48 weeks postoperatively. Note that these properties did not recover to the level of control as did the structural properties. SEM = standard error of the mean. *(Reproduced with permission from Inoue M, Woo SL-Y, Gomez MA, Amiel D, Ohland KJ, Kitabayashi LR: Effects of surgical treatment and immobilization on the healing of the medial collateral ligament: A long-term multidisciplinary study.* Connect Tis Res *1990; 25:13-26.)*

uations. In the context of this chapter, on attempting to bioengineer ideal tendon and ligament replacements, it is helpful to review these grafts as the current gold standards for comparison. In the pursuit of optimizing any bioengineered tendon and ligament, it is also helpful to review what is known about the healing processes, successes and failures of these so-called perfectly engineered tissue grafts, which can potentially start out nearly identical to the adult tissues that they are being used to replace. Knowledge about autograft and allograft successes and failures clinically, and more importantly, knowledge concerning their healing processes over time, experimentally, will be reviewed.

There is a long clinical history of use of autograft and allograft tendons and ligaments to reconstruct their damaged counterparts. They have become the gold standards for replacing some damaged structures, such as the ACL in the knee. Both patellar tendon grafts and multiply looped hamstring grafts have become nearly equal in terms of current use based on similar successes and relatively modest morbidities. Some morbidity and potential risks exists with the harvesting of either type of tendon graft in an autograft situation, including pain, swelling, numbness caused by local nerve damage, scarring, stiffness, potential weakness, atrophy, tendinitis, and infection. They involve significant surgical procedures and they

recover slowly over many months; however, their ultimate clinical outcomes are quite good. Recent evidence suggests an 80% success rate of grafts in restoring knee stability, at least over the short term. Although only a small proportion of these chronic reconstructions create abnormal knees from a symptomatic point of view, many do restore functional stability for a significant period of time. Longer term clinical outcomes may show decreased success rates because of stretching out or increased creep of the graft over time; however, this postulate requires further study, likely in more controlled animal studies.

Although both autograft and allograft tendons appear to have reasonable clinical success in terms of functional stability, there is considerable clinical and experimental evidence that their structures and functions are altered over time. The cellularity and collagen matrix architecture of tendon grafts is likely altered shortly after transplantation. Cells and vessels grow onto and into grafts, penetrating their dense matrix and contributing to local and generalized remodeling. Normally large collagen microfibrils are either replaced by new small scar-like fibrils, or the normal fibrils become eroded to the smaller size. Either way, the normal tendon tissue apparently becomes less stiff, weaker, and more prone to damage than at the time of transplantation. Grafts may also be softened by increased water and proteoglycan contents, potentially con-

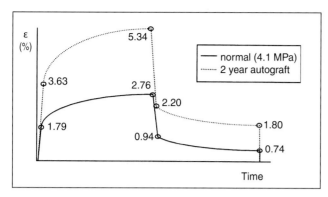

Figure 29   Creep and creep recovery of 2-year MCL autografts and normal MCLs. "ε" indicates strain and mean strains are shown. *(Reproduced with permission from Thornton GM, Boorman RS, Shrive NG, Frank CB: Medial collateral ligament autografts have increased creep response for at least 2 years and early immobilization makes this worse.* J Orthop Res *2002; 20: 346-352.)*

tributing to altered viscoelastic properties. Although not yet proven to be the case, there is some experimental evidence in an animal model of collateral ligament grafting that even a supportive healing environment in the extra-articular space can cause fresh ligament grafts to change quite significantly. Both autograft and allograft ligament grafts have shown increased potential to stress-relax under fixed deformations and increased potential to creep under fixed loading conditions (**Figure 29**), both possibly contributing to altered load-carrying ability of grafts at low functional loads and increases in relative laxity in vivo. These subtle changes could have important implications to joint laxity at low loads—potentially not being large enough to cause symptoms from instability but potentially contributing to altered joint mechanics, remodeling, and degradation of cartilage. This theory is currently being investigated in animal models.

Summary

Tendons and ligaments are normally very complex structures that are anatomically and biologically diverse and dynamic. Injured tendons and ligaments do have some intrinsic healing capacity (some more than others), generally via scar formation and remodeling. Scarring is a ubiquitous process that can vary in quality and quantity in and around the damaged structures, being improved by appropriate rehabilitation (presumably some aspect of force application to the healing complex). Scarring, however, even in its most optimal circumstances, does have some discrete structural and biologic limitations that prevent its ability to restore normal tendon and ligament.

When scarring is inadequate or when it fails to restore functional tendon or ligament tissue (such as in the ACL), graft replacement is a viable clinical option. Clinical and experimental evidence suggests that grafting of tendons

and ligaments by dense connective tissue autografts and allografts is quite successful. However, even these optimized grafts are often not normal and sometimes fail. These scenarios collectively suggest that despite progress in this area, further understanding of both biologic and biomechanical aspects of normal healing and transplanted ligaments and tendons is still required.

Selected Bibliography

General

Amis AA, Dawkins GP: Functional anatomy of the anterior cruciate ligament: Fibre bundle actions related to ligament replacements and injuries. *J Bone Joint Surg Br* 1991;73:260-267.

Benjamin M, Ralphs JR: The cell and developmental biology of tendons and ligaments. *Int Rev Cytol* 2000; 196:85-130.

Butler DL: Anterior cruciate ligament: Its normal response and replacement. *J Orthop Res* 1989;7:910-921.

Frank CB: The pathophysiology of ligaments, in Arendt EA (ed): *OKU: Sports Medicine*, ed 2. Rosemont, IL, American Academy of Orthopaedic Surgeons, 1999, pp 11-17.

Frank CB, Hart DA, Shrive NG: Molecular biology and biomechanics of normal and healing ligaments: A review. *Osteoarthritis Cartilage* 1999;7:130-140.

Jackson DW, Arnoczky SP, Woo SL-Y, Frank CB, Simon TM (eds): *The Anterior Cruciate Ligament: Current and Future Concepts*. New York, NY, Raven Press, 1993.

Lo IK, Randle JA, Majima T, et al: New directions in understanding and optimizing ligament and tendon healing. *Curr Opin Orthop* 2000;11:421-428.

Sharma P, Mafulli N: Tendon injury and tendinopathy: Healing and repair. *J Bone Joint Surg Am* 2005;87:187-202.

Woo SL-Y, An K-N, Frank CB, et al: Anatomy, biology, and biomechanics of tendon and ligament, in Buckwalter TA, Einhorn TA, Simon SR (ed): *Orthopaedic Basic Science: Biology and Biomechanics of the Musculoskeletal System*, ed 2. Rosemont, IL, American Academy of Orthopaedic Surgeons, 2000, pp 581-616.

Tendons

Ahmed IM, Lagopoulos M, McConnell P, Soames RW, Sefton GK: Blood supply of the Achilles tendon. *J Orthop Res* 1998;16:591-596.

Amiel D, Chu CR, Lee J: Effect of loading on metabolism and repair of tendons and ligaments, in Gordon SL, Blair SJ, Fine LJ (eds): *Repetitive Motion Disorders of the Upper Extremity*. Rosemont, IL, American Academy of Orthopaedic Surgeons, 1995, pp 217-230.

Benjamin M, Qin S, Ralphs JR: Fibrocartilage associated with human tendons and their pulleys. *J Anat* 1995;187:625-633.

Berglund M, Wiig M, Torstensson M, Reno C, Hart DA: Assessment of mRNA levels for matrix molecules and TGF-β1 in rabbit flexor and peroneus tendons reveals regional differences in steady-state expression. *J Hand Surg [Br]* 2004;29:165-169.

Blevins FT, Djurasovic M, Flatow EL, Vogel KG: Biology of the rotator cuff tendon. *Orthop Clin North Am* 1997;28:1-16.

Butler DL, Malaviya P, Awad H: A multidisciplinary approach to analyzing tendon fibrocartilage mechanics, structure and chemistry. *Abstracts of the Third World Congress of Biomechanics*. Sapporo, Japan, 1998, p 213.

Chansky HA, Iannotti JP: The vascularity of the rotator cuff. *Clin Sports Med* 1991;10:807-822.

Chiquet-Ehrismann R, Tucker RP: Connective tissues: Signaling by tenascins. *Int J Biochem Cell Biol* 2004;36:1085-1089.

Clark JM, Harryman DT II: Tendons, ligaments, and capsule of the rotator cuff: Gross and microscopic anatomy. *J Bone Joint Surg Am* 1992;74:713-725.

Cook CS, McDonagh MJN: Measurement of muscle and tendon stiffness in man. *Eur J Appl Physiol Occup Physiol* 1996;72:380-382.

Danielson KG, Baribault H, Holmes DF, Graham H, Kadler KE, Iozzo RV: Targeted disruption of decorin leads to abnormal collagen fibril morphology and skin fragility. *J Cell Biol* 1997;136:729-743.

Fuchs B, Weishaupt D, Zanetti M, Hodler J, Gerber C: Fatty degeneration of the muscles of the rotator cuff: Assessment by computed tomography versus magnetic resonance imaging. *J Shoulder Elbow Surg* 1999;8:599-605.

Fukashiro S, Komi PV, Jarvinen M, Miyashita M: In vivo Achilles tendon loading during jumping in humans. *Eur J Appl Physiol Occup Physiol* 1995;71:453-458.

Goutallier D, Postel JB, Bernageau J, Lavau L, Voisin MC: Fatty muscle degeneration in cuff ruptures: Pre- and postoperative evaluation by CT scan. *Clin Orthop Relat Res* 1994;304:78-83.

Holden JP, Grood ES: Korvick DL, Cummings JF, Butler DL, Bylski-Austrow DI: In vivo forces in the anterior cruciate ligament: Direct measurements during walking and trotting in a quadruped. *J Biomech* 1994;27:517-526.

Jozsa L, Kannus P, Jarvinen TA, Balint J, Jarvinen M: Number and morphology of mechanoreceptors in the myotendinous junction of paralysed human muscle. *J Pathol* 1996;178:195-200.

Khan U, Kakar S, Akali A, Bentley G, McGrouther DA: Modulation of the formation of adhesions during the healing of injured tendons. *J Bone Joint Surg Br* 2000;82:1054-1058.

Khan U, Occleston NL, Khaw PT, McGrouther DA: Differences in proliferative rate and collagen lattice contraction between endotenon and synovial fibroblasts. *J Hand Surg [Am]* 1998;23:266-273.

Lephart SM, Fu FH: Proprioception and neuromuscular control, in Lephart SM, Fu FH (eds): *Joint Stability*. Champaign, IL, Human Kinetics, 2000.

Lephart SM, Fu FH: The role of proprioception in the treatment of sports injuries. *Sports Exerc Inj* 1995;1:96-102.

Lephart SM, Henry TJ: Functional rehabilitation for the upper and lower extremity. *Orthop Clin North Am* 1995;26:579-592.

Lephart SM, Henry TJ: The physiological basis for open and closed kinetic chain rehabilitation for the upper extremity. *J Sports Rehab* 1992;1:188-196.

Li G, Rudy TW, Sakane M, Kanamori A, Ma CB, Woo SL: The importance of quadriceps and hamstring muscle loading on knee kinematics and in-situ forces in the ACL. *J Biomech* 1999;32:395-400.

McNeilly CM, Banes AJ, Benjamin M, Ralphs JR: Tendon cells in vivo form a three dimensional network of cell processes linked by gap junctions. *J Anat* 1996;189(Pt 3):593-600.

Ramachandran GN, Reddi AH (eds): *Biochemistry of Collagen*. New York, NY, Plenum, 1976.

Reddy GK, Stehno-Bittel L, Enwemeka CS: Matrix remodeling in healing rabbit Achilles tendon. *Wound Repair Regen* 1999;7:518-527.

Sano H, Ishii H, Yeadon A, Backman DS, Brunet JA, Uhthoff HK: Degeneration at the insertion weakens the tensile strength of the supraspinatus tendon: A comparative mechanical and histologic study of the bone-tendon complex. *J Orthop Res* 1997;15:719-726.

Sano H, Uhthoff HK, Backman DS, et al: Structural disorders at the insertion of the supraspinatus tendon: Relation to tensile strength. *J Bone Joint Surg Br* 1998;80:720-725.

Sarkar K, Uhthoff HK: Pathophysiology of rotator cuff degeneration, calcification, and repair, in Burkhead WZ (ed): *Rotator Cuff Disorders*. Baltimore, MD, Williams & Wilkins, 1996, pp 36-44.

Thornton GM, Frank CB, Shrive NG: Ligament creep behavior can be predicted from stress relaxation by incorporating fiber recruitment. *J Orthop Res* 2002;20:967-974.

Thornton GM, Frank CB, Shrive NG: The effect of fibre recruitment during creep of ligaments, in Middleton J, Jones ML, Shrive NG, Pande GM (eds): *Computer Methods in Biomechanics and Biomedical Engineering*, ed 3. (Proceedings of the International Symposium, Lisbon, Portugal, 1999). London, United Kingdom, Gordon and Breach Publishers, 2001, pp 343-348.

Thornton GM, Oliynyk A, Frank CB, Shrive NG: Ligament creep cannot be predicted from stress relaxation at low stress: A biomechanical study of the rabbit medial collateral ligament. *J Orthop Res* 1997;15:652-656.

Uhthoff HK, Sano H: Pathology of failure of the rotator cuff tendon. *Orthop Clin North Am* 1997;28:31-41.

Uhthoff HK, Sarkar K: Pathology of rotator cuff tendons, in Watson MS (ed): *Surgical Disorders of the Shoulder*. London, England, Churchill Livingstone, 1991, pp 258-270.

Uhthoff HK, Sarkar K: The effect of aging on the soft tissues of the shoulder, in Matsen FA III, Fu FH, Hawkins RJ (eds): *The Shoulder: A Balance of Mobility and Stability*. Rosemont, IL, American Academy of Orthopaedic Surgeons, 1993, pp 269-278.

Vogel KG: Fibrocartilage in tendon: A response to compressive load, in Gordon SL, Blair SJ, Fine LJ. (eds): *Repetitive Motion Disorders of the Upper Extremity*. Rosemont, IL, American Academy of Orthopaedic Surgeons, 1995, pp 205-215.

Williams PL, Bannister LH, Berry MH, et al (eds): *Gray's Anatomy*, ed 38. Edinburgh, Scotland, Churchill Livingstone, 1995.

Yamamoto N, Takauchi M: In vivo measurement of patellar tendon force in rat during running on a treadmill. *Abstracts of the Third World Congress of Biomechanics*. Sapporo, Japan, 1998, p 461.

Ligaments

Ahmed AM, Burke DL, Duncan NA, Chan KH: Ligament tension pattern in the flexed knee in combined passive anterior translation and axial rotations. *J Orthop Res* 1992;10:854-867.

Altman GH, Horan RL, Martin I, et al: Cell differentiation by mechanical stress. *FASEB J* 2002;16:270-272.

Anderson AF: Rating scales, in Fu FH, Harner CD, Vince KG (eds): *Knee Surgery*. Baltimore, MD, Williams & Wilkins, 1994, pp 275-296.

Awad HA, Butler DL, Boivin GP, et al: Autologous mesenchymal stem cell-mediated repair of tendon. *Tissue Eng* 1999;5:267-277.

Awad HA, Butler DL, Harris MT, et al: In vitro characteristics of mesenchymal stem cell-seeded collagen scaffolds for tendon repair: Effects of initial seeding density on contraction kinetics. *J Biomed Mater Res* 2000;51:233-240.

Batten ML, Hansen JC, Dahners L: Influence of dosage and timing of application of platelet-derived-growth factor on the early healing of the rat medial collateral ligament. *J Orthop Res* 1996;14:736-741.

Beynnon BD, Fleming BC, Johnson RJ, Nichols CE, Renmstrom PA, Pope MH: Anterior cruciate ligament strain behaviour during rehabilitation exercises in vivo. *Am J Sports Med* 1995;23:24-34.

Bosch U, Krettek C: Tissue engineering of tendons and ligaments: A new challenge. *Unfallchirurg* 2002;105:88-94.

Buckley SL, Barrack RL, Alexander AH: The natural history of conservatively treated partial anterior cruciate ligament tears. *Am J Sports Med* 1989;17:221-225.

Butler DL, Awad HA: Perspectives on cell and collagen composites for tendon repair. *Clin Orthop* 1999;367(suppl):S324-S332.

Butler DL, Goldstein SA, Guilak F: Functional tissue engineering: The role of biomechanics. *J Biomech Eng* 2000;122:570-575.

Cartmell JS, Dunn MG: Effect of chemical treatments on tendon cellularity and mechanical properties. *J Biomed Mater Res* 2000;49:134-140.

Casteleyn PP, Handelberg F: Non-operative management of anterior cruciate ligament injuries in the general population. *J Bone Joint Surg Br* 1996;78:446-451.

Cunningham KD, Musani F, Hart DA, Shrive NG, Frank CB: Collagenase degradation decreases collagen fibril diameters: An in vitro study of the rabbit medial collateral ligament. *Connect Tissue Res* 1999;40:67-74.

Daniel DM: Selecting patients for ACL surgery, in Jackson DW, Arnoczky, SP, Woo SL-Y, Frank CB, Simon TM (eds): *The Anterior Cruciate Ligament: Current and Future Concepts*. New York, NY, Raven Press, 1993, pp 251-258.

DesRosiers EA, Yahia L, Rivard CH: Proliferative and matrix synthesis response of canine cruciate ligament fibroblasts submitted to combined growth factors. *J Orthop Res* 1996;14:200-208.

Donnelly NI, Hart DA, Frank CB: Matrix mRNA levels in ligament tissue versus cells. *In Vitro Cell Dev Biol Anim* 1998;34:617-618.

Frank CB, McDonald DB, Wilson JE, Eyre DR, Shrive NG: Rabbit medial collateral ligament scar weakness is associated with decreased collagen pyridinoline crosslink density. *J Orthop Res* 1995;13:157-165.

Frank C, McDonald D, Shrive N: Collagen fibril diameters in the rabbit medial collateral ligament scar: A longer term assessment. *Connect Tissue Res* 1997;36:261-269.

Frank C, Shrive N, Hiraoka H, Nakamura N, Kaneda Y, Hart D: Optimisation of the biology of soft tissue repair. *J Sci Med Sport* 1999;2:190-210.

Germain L, Goulet F, Muolin V, Berthod F, Auger FA: Engineering human tissues for in vivo applications. *Ann N Y Acad Sci* 2002;961:268-270.

Hart DA, Nakamura N, Marchuk L, et al: Complexity of determining cause and effect in vivo after antisense gene therapy. *Clin Orthop Relat Res* 2000;379(suppl):S242-S251.

Hildebrand KA, Frank CB: Scar formation and ligament healing. *Can J Surg* 1998;41:425-429.

Hildebrand KA, Jia F, Woo SL-Y: Response of donor and recipient cells after transplantation of cells to the ligament and tendon. *Microsc Res Tech* 2002;58:34-38.

Hidebrand KA, Woo SL-Y, Smith DW, et al: The effects of platelet-derived growth factor-BB on healing of the rabbit medial collateral ligament: An in vivo study. *Am J Sports Med* 1998;26:549-554.

Hodde J: Naturally occurring scaffolds for soft tissue repair and regeneration. *Tissue Eng* 2002;8:295-308.

Jackson DW, Simon TM: Tissue engineering principles in orthopaedic surgery. *Clin Orthop Relat Res* 1999;(367 suppl):S31-S45.

Krauspe R, Schmidt M, Schaible HG: Sensory innervation of the anterior cruciate ligament: An electrophysiological study of the response properties of single identified mechanoreceptors in the cat. *J Bone Joint Surg Am* 1992;74:390-397.

Laurencin CT, Ambrosio AM, Borden MD, Cooper JA Jr: Tissue engineering: Orthopaedic applications. *Annu Rev Biomed Eng* 1999;1:19-46.

Letson AK, Dahners LE: The effect of combinations of growth factors on ligament healing. *Clin Orthop Relat Res* 1994;308:207-212.

Li WJ, Laurencin CT, Caterson EJ, Tuan RS, Ko FK: Electrospun nanofibrous structure: A novel scaffold for tissue engineering. *J Biomed Mater Res* 2002;60:613-621.

Lin VS, Lee MC, O'Neal S, McKean J, Sung KL: Ligament tissue engineering using biodegradable fiber scaffolds. *Tissue Eng* 1999;5:443-452.

Lo IK, Chi S, Ivie T, Frank CB, Rattner JB: The cellular matrix: A feature of tensile bearing dense soft connective tissues. *Histol Histopathol* 2002;17:523-537.

Lo IK, Marchuk L, Hart DA, Frank CB: Messenger ribonucleic acid levels in disrupted human anterior cruciate ligaments. *Clin Orthop Relat Res* 2003;407:249-258.

Majima T, Marchuk LL, Sciore P, Shrive NG, Frank CB, Hart DA: Compressive compared with tensile loading of medial collateral ligament scar in vitro uniquely influences mRNA levels for aggrecan, collagen type II and collagenase. *J Orthop Res* 2000;18:524-531.

Menetrey J, Kasemkijwattana C, Day CS, et al: Direct-, fibroblast- and myoblast-mediated gene transfer to the anterior cruciate ligament. *Tissue Eng* 1999;5:435-442.

Müller W, Biedert R, Hefti F, Jakob RP, Munzinger U, Stäubli HU: OAK knee evaulation: A new way to assess knee ligament injuries. *Clin Orthop Relat Res* 1988;232:37-50.

Murray MM, Spector M: The migration of cells from the ruptured anterior crucaite ligament into collagen-glycosaminoglycan regeneration templates in vitro. *Biomaterials* 2001;22:2393-2402.

Nakamura N, Hart DA, Boorman RS, et al: Decorin antisense gene therapy improves functional healing of early rabbit ligament scar with enhanced collagen fibrillogenesis in vivo. *J Orthop Res* 2000;18:517-523.

Nakamura N, Timmermann SA, Hart DA, et al: A comparison of in vivo gene delivery methods for antisense therapy in ligament healing. *Gene Ther* 1998;5:1455-1461.

Rodeo SA, Arnoczky SP, Torzilli PA, Hidaka C, Warren R: Tendon-healing in a bone tunnel. A biomechanical and histological study in the dog. *J Bone Joint Surg Am* 1993;75:1795-1803.

Ross SM, Joshi R, Frank CB: Establishment and comparison of fibroblast cell lines from the medial collateral and anterior cruciate ligaments of the rabbit. *In Vitro Cell Dev Biol* 1990;26:579-584.

Shrive NG, Chimich D, Marchuk L, Wilson J, Brant R, Frank C: Soft tissue "flaws" are associated with the material properties of the healing rabbit medial collateral ligament. *J Orthop Res* 1995;13:923-929.

Thornton GM, Shrive NG, Frank CB: Altering ligament water content affects ligament pre-stress and creep behaviour. *J Orthop Res* 2001;19:845-851.

Thornton GM, Shrive NG, Frank CB: Ligament creep recruits fibres at low stresses and can lead to modulus-reducing fibre damage at higher creep stresses: A study in a rabbit medial collateral ligament model. *J Orthop Res* 2002;20:967-974.

Tomasek JJ, Gabbiani G, Hinz B, Chaponnier C, Brown RA: Myofibroblasts and mechano-regulation of connective tissue remodeling. *Nat Rev Mol Cell Biol* 2002;3:349-363.

Wiig ME, Amiel D, VandeBerg J, Kitbayashi L, Harwood FL, Arfors KE: The early effect of high molecular weight hyaluronan (hyaluronic acid) on anterior cruciate ligament healing: An experimental study in rabbits. *J Orthop Res* 1990;8:425-434.

Winters SC, Seiler JG, Woo SL-Y, Gelberman RH: Suture methods for flexor tendon repair: A biomechanical analysis during the first six weeks following repair. *Ann Chir Main Memb Super* 1997;16:229-234.

Woo SL-Y, Smith DW, Hildebrand KA, Zeminski JA, Johnson LA: Engineering the healing of the rabbit medial collateral ligament. *Med Biol Eng Comput* 1998;36:359-364.

Yoshida M, Fujii K: Differences in cell properties and responses to growth factors between human ACL and MCL cells. *J Orthop Sci* 1999;4:293-298.

Zhang F, Lineaweaver WC: Growth factors and gene transfer with DNA strand technique in tendon healing. *J Long Term Eff Med Implants* 2002;12:105-112.

Tendon and Ligament Grafting and Replacement

Aglietti P, Buzzi R, D'Andria S, Zaccherotti G: Long-term study of anterior cruciate ligament reconstruction for chronic instability using the central one-third patellar tendon and a lateral extraarticular tenodesis. *Am J Sports Med* 1992;20:38-45.

Aglietti: Buzzi R, Zaccherotti G, DeBiase P: Patellar tendon versus doubled semitendinosus and gracilis tendons for anterior cruciate ligament reconstruction. *Am J Sports Med* 1994;22:211-217.

Altman GH, Horan RL, Lu HH, et al: Silk matrix for tissue engineered anterior cruciate ligaments. *Biomaterials* 2002;23:4131-4141.

Amiel D, Billings E Jr, Akeson WH: Ligament structure, chemistry and physiology, in Daniel DM, Akeson WH, O'Connor JJ (eds): *Knee Ligaments: Structure, Function, Injury and Repair.* New York, NY, Raven Press, 1990, pp 77-91.

Anderson AF, Snyder RB, Lipscomb AB Sr: Anterior cruciate ligament reconstruction using the semitendinosus and gracilis tendons augmented by the Losee iliotibial band tenodesis: A long-term study. *Am J Sports Med* 1994;22:620-626.

Bellincampi LD, Closkey RF, Prasad R, Zawadsky JP, Dunn MG: Viability of fibroblast-seeded ligament analogs after autogenous implantation. *J Orthop Res* 1998; 16:414-420.

Beynnon BD, Johnson RJ, Fleming BC: The mechanics of anterior cruciate ligament reconstruction, in Jackson DW, Arnoczky SP, Woo SL-Y, Frank CB, Simon TM (eds): *The Anterior Cruciate Ligament: Current and Future Concepts.* New York, NY, Raven Press, 1993, pp 259-272.

Blatter G, Tissi R: Is suture of the ruptured anterior cruciate ligament without augmentation sensible? *Unfallchirurgie* 1991;17:232-235.

Dunn MG, Avasarala PN, Zawadsky JP: Optimisation of extruded collagen fibers for ACL reconstruction. *J Biomed Mater Res* 1993;27:1545-1552.

Dunn MG, Liesch JB, Tiku ML, Zawadsky JP: Development of fibroblast-seeded ligament analogs for ACL reconstruction. *J Biomed Mater Res* 1995;29:1363-1371.

Dunn MG, Tria AJ, Kato YP, et al: Anterior cruciate ligament reconstruction using a composite collagenous prosthesis: A biomechanical and histologic study in rabbits. *Am J Sports Med* 1992;20:507-515.

Engebretsen L: The acute repair of anterior cruciate ligament tears, in Jackson DW, Arnoczky SP, Woo SL-Y, Frank CB, Simon TM (eds): *The Anterior Cruciate Ligament: Current and Future Concepts.* New York, NY, Raven Press, 1993, pp. 273-279.

Engebretsen L, Benum P, Fasting O, Molster A, Strand T: A prospective, randomized study of three surgical techniques for treatment of acute ruptures of the anterior cruciate ligament. *Am J Sports Med* 1990;18:585-590.

Gisselfalt K, Edberg B, Flodin P: Synthesis and properties of degradable poly (urethane urea)s to be used for ligament reconstructions. *Biomacromolecules* 2002;3: 951-958.

Goodship AE, Wilcock SA: Shah JS: The development of tissue around prosthetic implants used as replacements for ligaments and tendons. *Clin Orthop Relat Res* 1985;196:61-68.

Goulet F: Tissue-engineered ligament, in Lanza R, Langer R, Chick WL (eds): *Principles of Tissue Engineering.* San Diego, CA, Academic Press Ltd, 1997, pp 633-644.

Graf BK, Vanderby R Jr: Autograft reconstruction of the anterior cruciate ligament: Placement, tensioning, and preconditioning, in Jackson DW, Arnoczky SP, Woo SL-Y, Frank CB, Simon TM (eds*): The Anterior Cruciate Ligament: Current and Future Concepts.* New York, NY, Raven Press, 1993, pp 281-289.

Jackson DW, Lemos MJ: Autograft reconstruction of the anterior cruciate ligament: Bone-patellar tendon-bone, in Jackson DW, Arnoczky SP, Woo SL-Y, Frank CB, Simon TM (eds*): The Anterior Cruciate Ligament: Current and Future Concepts.* New York, NY, Raven Press, 1993, pp 291-303.

Jackson DW, Simon TM, Kurzweil PR, Rosen MA: Survival of cells after intra-articular transplantation of fresh allografts of the patellar and anterior cruciate ligaments: DNA-probe analysis in a goat model. *J Bone Joint Surg Am* 1992;74:112-118.

Kato YP, Dunn MG, Zawadsky JP, Tria AJ, Silver FH: Regeneration of Achilles tendon with a collagen tendon prosthesis: Results of a one-year implantation study. *J Bone Joint Surg Am* 1991;73:561-574.

Kaplan N, Wickiewicz TL, Warren RF: Primary surgical treatment of anterior cruciate ligament ruptures: A long-term follow-up study. *Am J Sports Med* 1990;18: 354-358.

King GJ, Edwards P, Brant RF, Shrive NG, Frank C: Intraoperative graft tensioning alters viscoelastic but no failure behaviours of rabbit medial collateral ligament autografts. *J Orthop Res* 1995;13:915-922.

Koski JA, Ibarra C, Rodeo SA: Tissue-engineered ligament: Cells, matrix and growth factors. *Orthop Clin North Am* 2000;31:437-452.

Majima T, Marchuk LL, Shrive NG, Frank CB, Hart DA: In vitro cyclic tensile loading of an immobilized and mobilized ligament autograft selectively inhibits mRNA levels for collagenase MMP-1. *J Orthop Sci* 2000;5:503-510.

Milthorpe BK: Xenografts for tendon and ligament repair. *Biomaterials* 1994;15:745-752.

Mohtadi NG: Quality of life assessment as an outcome in anterior cruciate ligament reconstructive surgery, in Jackson DW, Arnoczky SP, Woo SL-Y, Frank CB, Simon TM (eds)*: The Anterior Cruciate Ligament. Current and Future Concepts.* New York, NY, Raven Press, 1993, pp 439-444.

Ng GY, Oakes BW, Deacon OW, McLean ID, Lampard D: Biomechanics of patellar tendon autograft for reconstruction of the anterior cruciate ligament in the goat: Three-year study. *J Orthop Res* 1995;13:602-608.

Ng GY, Oakes BW, Deacon OW, McLean ID, Lampard D: The long-term biomechanical and viscoelastic performance of repairing anterior cruciate ligament after hemitransection injury in a goat model. *Am J Sports Med* 1996;24:109-117.

Noyes FR, Barber-Westin SD: Reconstruction of the anterior cruciate ligament with human allograft: Comparison of early and later results. *J Bone Joint Surg Am* 1996;78:524-537.

Rodeo SA, Arnoczky SP, Torzilli PA, Hidaka C, Warren RF: Tendon-healing in a bone tunnel. A biomechanical and histological study in the dog. *J Bone Joint Surg Am* 1993;75:1795-1803.

Sabiston P, Frank C, Lam T, Shrive N: Allograft ligament transplantation: A morphological and biochemical evaluation of a medial collateral ligament complex in a rabbit model. *Am J Sports Med* 1990;18:160-168.

Sabiston P, Frank C, Lam T, Shrive N: Transplantation of the rabbit medial collateral ligament: I. Biomechanical evaluation of fresh autografts. *J Orthop Res* 1990;8: 35-45.

Shelbourne KD, Nitz P: Accelerated rehabilitation after anterior cruciate ligament reconstruction. *Am J Sports Med* 1990;18:292-299.

Shino K, Inoue M, Nakamura H, Hamada M, Ono K: Arthroscopic follow-up of anterior cruciate ligament reconstruction using allogeneic tendon. *Arthroscopy* 1989;5:165-171.

Shino K, Oakes BW, Horibe S, Nakata K, Nakamura N: Collagen fibril populations in human anterior cruciate ligament allografts: Electron microscopic analysis. *Am J Sports Med* 1995;23:203-208.

Sun ZY, Zhao L: Feasibility of calcium pyrophosphate fiber as scaffold material for tendon tissue engineering in vitro. *Zhongguo Xiu Fu Chong Jian Wai Ke Za Zhi* 2002;16:426-428.

Tan W, Krishnaraj R, Desai TA: Evaluation of nanostructured composite collagen-chitosan matrices for tissue engineering. *Tissue Eng* 2001;7:203-210.

Thornton GM, Boorman RS, Shrive NG, Frank CB: Medial collateral ligament autografts have increased creep response for at least two years and early immobilization makes this worse. *J Orthop Res* 2002; 20:346-352.

Chapter 12

Form and Function of Skeletal Muscle

Richard L. Lieber, PhD

Introduction

An understanding of skeletal muscle structure and function is important to the orthopaedic surgeon. Tendon transfers are performed to restore lost motor function, flexor tendon repairs restore digital motion, joint arthroplasty requires the movement and reorientation of skeletal muscles, and muscles are often removed during spine surgery or fracture repair. Because muscle is required for movement, the orthopaedic surgeon must make judicious choices when it comes to transferring or transecting skeletal muscles. In this chapter, skeletal muscle microanatomy and macroanatomy will be discussed with emphasis on those physiologic and mechanical properties that have clinical significance.

Skeletal Muscle Anatomy

Skeletal Muscle Cell Microstructure

Skeletal muscle fibers are cells that, in many ways, are like any other body cell. However, because muscle cell function is highly specialized to produce force and movement, the cellular components are also highly specialized (**Figure 1**). Muscle cells or fibers are cylindrical, with a diameter ranging from approximately 10 μm to about 100 μm—less than the diameter of a human hair. Muscle fiber diameter is profoundly important for at least two reasons. First, a muscle fiber's diameter determines its strength, and second, when altered fiber diameters are observed in mature muscle, this suggests that the level of muscle use has changed. Muscle fiber length is also highly variable, depending on the muscle's architecture. Fiber length has a profound influence on fiber contraction velocity and the distance over which the fiber can shorten (for example, muscle fiber excursion).

The scaffolding that surrounds the muscle cell is known as the basal lamina. The normal physiologic role of the basal lamina is poorly understood; however, it is clear that the basal lamina plays an important role in muscle fiber recovery from injury. When the basal lamina remains intact after injury (such as a crush injury), recovery is relatively complete, similar to nerve crush as opposed to nerve injury that includes axotomy. Conversely, when the basal lamina is destroyed (such as in a traumatic cut), fiber regeneration first requires the laying down of a new scaffold. If a muscle fiber is destroyed and denervated, but the basal lamina remains intact, when the motor nerve reinnervates the fiber it will do so at the original site dictated by the basal lamina, even though no muscle fiber is present. Thus the basal lamina, which demarcated functional myotubes during development, retains a good deal of identity later in cellular life. It is likely that the basal lamina expresses a variety of extracellular matrix proteins that create a "molecular fingerprint" that remains even if the muscle fiber itself is destroyed.

A mesh-like sheath of collagenous tissue, called the endomysium, surrounds the muscle fiber. The role of the endomysium in the passive mechanical properties of the fiber has not been clearly quantified. Electron micrographs of the muscle endomysium show a complex structure with intimate interaction between the endomysium and the muscle fiber (**Figure 2**). Bundles of fibers, each surrounded by endomysial tissue, are organized into muscle fascicles, each surrounded by a more stout perimysium. Bundles of fascicles are organized into muscles, surrounded by epimysium connective tissue.

Myofibrils: The Muscle Contractile Apparatus

Perhaps the most distinctive feature of a muscle cell is its ordered array of contractile filaments (**Figure 3**). There is a well-defined hierarchy of filament organization that proceeds from a large scale (10^{-6} m) to a small scale (10^{-10} m). The largest functional unit of contractile filaments is the myofibril. Myofibrils are simply a string of sarcomeres arranged in series. Myofibrillar diameter is approximately 1 μm, which means that thousands of myofibrils are typically packed into a single muscle fiber. One way in which a muscle fiber grows is to increase the number of myofibrils that it contains. Myofibrils are arranged in parallel to make up the muscle fiber. However, their arrangement might not simply resemble a bundle of spa-

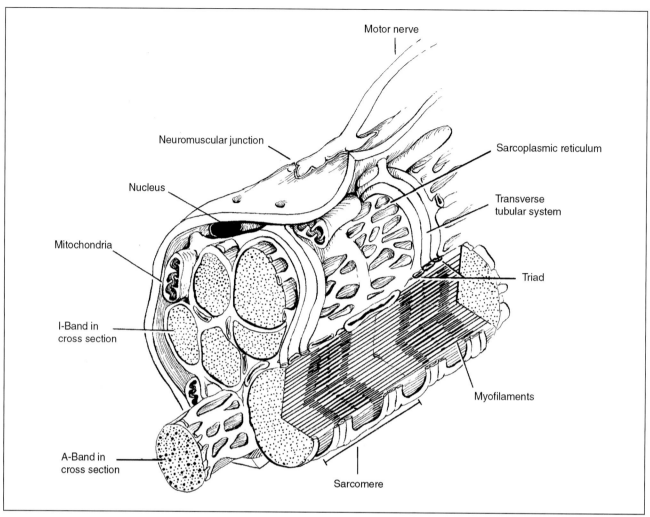

Figure 1   Schematic representation of the muscle cell. The muscle cell, which is specialized for the production of force and movement, contains an array of filamentous proteins as well as other subcellular organelles such as mitochondria, nuclei, satellite cells, sarcoplasmic reticulum, and transverse tubular system. Note the formation of "triads," which represent the T-tubules flanked by the terminal cisternae of the sarcoplasmic reticulum. Also note that when the myofilaments are sectioned longitudinally, the stereotypic striated appearance is seen. When myofilaments are sectioned transversely at the level of the A- or I-bands, the hexagonal array of the appropriate filaments is seen. *(Reproduced with permission from Lieber R (ed): Skeletal Muscle Structure, Function, and Plasticity. Philadelphia, PA, Lippincott Williams & Wilkins, 2002, p 15.)*

ghetti; there is some evidence that myofibrils within the fiber are arranged similar to the weave in a rope.

Myofibrils are interconnected with one another by a set of specialized proteins known as intermediate filaments. In mature skeletal muscle, the major intermediate filament is desmin, which provides a cytoskeletal support system that permits efficient mechanical coupling of the force generated by one myofibril to the adjacent myofibril. The intermediate filament network can dynamically remodel in response to intense exercise and may be profoundly important to a muscle's ability to grow in response to mechanical stress.

Sarcomeres

Myofibrils can also be subdivided into subunits called sarcomeres, the functional unit of muscle contraction. A my-

ofibril is several sarcomeres (or muscle segments) arranged in series. The total number of sarcomeres within a fiber depends on the muscle fiber length and diameter and is the most important determinant of muscle fiber function. Because of the series arrangement of sarcomeres within a myofibril, the total distance of myofibrillar shortening is equal to the sum of the shortening distances of the individual sarcomeres. This is why a whole muscle may shorten several centimeters even though each sarcomere can only shorten about 1 µm. The number of sarcomeres in a mature muscle can change given the appropriate stimulus, which means that muscle fibers have a great capacity for adaptation.

Sarcomeres are composed of contractile filaments called myofilaments. Two major sets of contractile filaments, one thick and the other relatively thin, exist in the

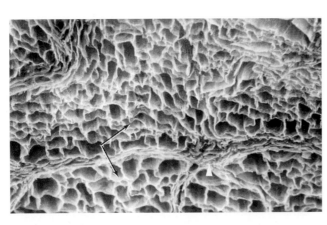

Figure 2   Scanning electron micrograph of the endomysial connective tissue within skeletal muscle. This image was generated by scanning electron microscopy of a muscle whose fibers were removed by acid digestion. The arrowhead points to perimysial connective tissue. The arrows point to individual endomysial tubes. *(Reproduced with permission from Trotter JA, Purslow PP: Functional morphology of the endomysium in series fibered muscles.* J Morphol *1992;212:109-122.)*

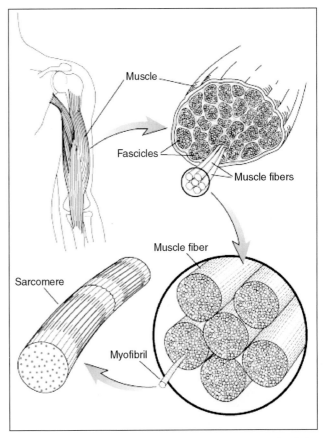

Figure 3   Structural hierarchy of skeletal muscle. Whole skeletal muscles are composed of numerous fascicles of muscle fibers. Muscle fibers are composed of myofibrils arranged in parallel. Myofibrils are composed of sarcomeres arranged in series. Sarcomeres are composed of interdigitating actin and myosin filaments. *(Reproduced with permission from Lieber R (ed):* Skeletal Muscle Structure, Function, and Plasticity. *Philadelphia, PA, Lippincott Williams & Wilkins, 2002, p 18.)*

sarcomere. These thick and thin filaments represent large polymers of the proteins myosin and actin, respectively. The myosin-containing filaments (thick filaments) and the actin-containing filaments (thin filaments) interdigitate to form a hexagonal lattice. It is the active interdigitation of these microscopic filaments that produces muscle shortening. It is also this interdigitated, repetitive dark and light banding pattern that gives the muscle its striated or striped appearance that is observable on light microscopy (**Figure 4**).

Various regions of the sarcomere are named based on their appearance (**Figure 5**). For example, the sarcomere region containing the myosin filaments is known as the A-band (anisotropic, an optical term describing what this band does to incoming light). The region containing the actin filament is known as the I-band (isotropic). The region of the A-band where there is no actin-myosin overlap is called the H-zone (helle, a German word for "light"). The dark narrow line that bisects the I-band is the Z-band (zwitter, a German word for "between"). The relatively dense zone in the center of the A-band is known as the M-band. Most investigators who quantify sarcomere dimensions use the distance from one Z-band to the next as the definition of the sarcomere length, which is an important variable relative to force generation.

Muscle Cell Membrane Systems

In addition to the well-defined arrangement of force-generating components present in muscle cells, an intricate system exists for activating these force generators. The membrane system present is actually a specially designed version of the endoplasmic reticulum within normal cells. Although longitudinal micrographs of muscle provide a dramatic representation of the contractile fila-

ments, the membrane system that activates them is less obvious. The two main components of this system are the transverse tubular system (T-system) and the sarcoplasmic reticulum (SR). The T-system begins as invaginations of the surface membrane and is therefore physically contiguous with the sarcolemma. If a surface "scan" of a muscle fiber is observed at very high magnification, periodic invaginations of the surface membrane will appear as holes that actually extend deep into the muscle fiber. These invaginations extend transversely across the long axis of the muscle fiber. The function of the T-system is to convey the activation signal received from the motoneuron to the myofibrils, which are themselves not in direct contact with the motoneuron. The SR is much more complex than the T-system. It is directly involved in the storage of calcium that activates muscle and the removal of calcium from the myofilaments that causes muscle relaxation. Embedded in the SR membrane are specific calcium channels and calcium pumps that accomplish the functions of calcium release and uptake, respectively. The

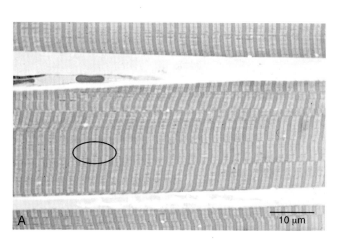
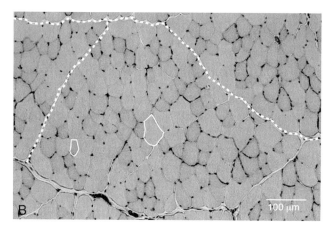

Figure 4 **A,** Longitudinal section of a tibialis anterior muscle biopsy specimen that was chemically fixed, embedded in plastic, sectioned at 1 µm thickness, and stained with toluidine blue. The alternating light and dark regions correspond to the sarcomere A- and I-bands. The circled area is shown under electron microscopy in Figure 5. Several fibers are shown in this section. **B,** Cross section of a vastus lateralis muscle biopsy specimen that was frozen, sectioned at 8-µm thickness, and stained with hematoxylin and eosin for inspection of normal fiber morphology. Note that, in cross section, muscle appears to be a collection of densely packed polygonal fibers. Each muscle fiber is surrounded by a sheath of endomysial connective tissue (shown for one fiber as a solid line), and collections of muscle fibers (fascicles) are surrounded by more dense perimysial connective tissue (shown for one region as a dashed line). Calibration bars correspond to a distance of 100 µm. *(Reproduced with permission from Lieber R (ed):* Skeletal Muscle Structure, Function, and Plasticity. *Philadelphia, PA, Lippincott Williams & Wilkins, 2002.)*

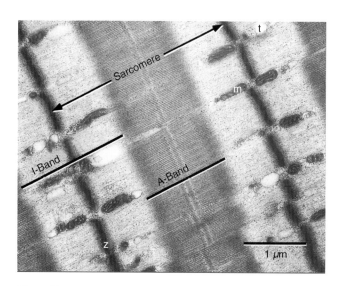

Figure 5 Longitudinal electron micrograph of a rabbit tibialis anterior muscle that was fixed in glutaraldehyde, embedded in plastic, sectioned at an approximate thickness of 60 nm, and stained with heavy metal. This more severe processing is necessary to view the tissue with an electron microscope. Note the much greater magnification of the A- and I-bands in this electron micrograph compared with the longitudinal light micrograph shown in Figure 4. The region in this micrograph corresponds roughly to the circled region of Figure 4. Calibration bar corresponds to a distance of 1 µm. (m = mitochondrion, z = Z-band, and t = transverse tubular system.) *(Reproduced with permission from Lieber R (ed):* Skeletal Muscle Structure, Function, and Plasticity. *Philadelphia, PA, Lippincott Williams & Wilkins, 2002, p 23.)*

SR envelops each myofibril to permit intimate contact between the activation and force-generation systems. The SR is also in contact with the T-system and therefore acts as the "middleman" in skeletal muscle activation and relaxation.

Whole Skeletal Muscle Structure
Skeletal Muscle Architecture

Skeletal muscle is not only highly organized at the microscopic level, the arrangement of muscle fibers at the macroscopic level also demonstrates a striking degree of organization. In making comparisons among various muscles, certain factors such as fiber type distribution are important, but there is no question that an important factor in determining a whole muscle's contractile properties is the muscle's architecture.

Skeletal muscle architecture can be defined as the arrangement of muscle fibers relative to the axis of force generation. Although muscle fibers have a relatively consistent fiber diameter among muscles of different sizes, the arrangement of these fibers can be quite different. Thus, it would be impossible to estimate the force a muscle would generate if fiber diameter from a muscle biopsy were measured because there would be no estimate of the number of muscle fibers generating the force. Similarly, even if the total muscle volume were estimated, the myriad ways to arrange fibers within that volume would preclude producing a valid force estimate. In fact, the various types of muscle fiber arrangement within whole muscles are as numerous as the muscles themselves, but for convenience three general types of fiber architecture are presented here.

Muscles with fibers that extend parallel to the muscle force-generating axis are termed parallel or longitudinally arranged muscles (**Figure 6, A**). Although the fibers extend

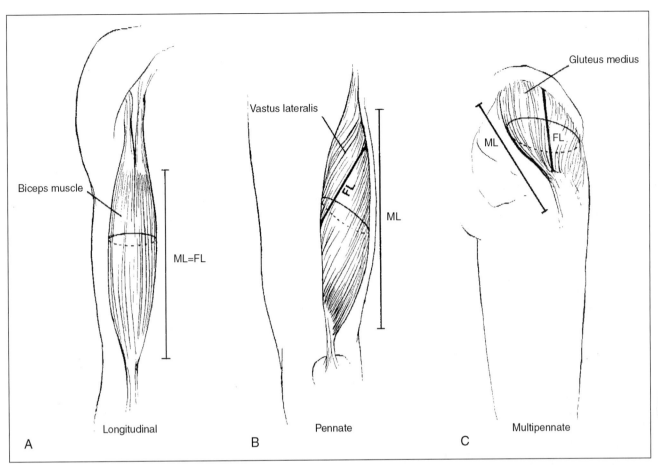

Figure 6   Muscle architectural types. Skeletal muscle fibers may be oriented parallel to the muscle's force-generating axis **(A)**, at a fixed angle relative to the force-generating axis **(B)**, or at multiple angles relative to the force-generating axis **(C)**. Each of these drawings represents an idealized view of muscle architecture and probably does not adequately describe any single muscle. (ML = muscle length, FL = fiber length.) *(Reproduced with permission from Lieber R (ed):* Skeletal Muscle Structure, Function, and Plasticity. *Philadelphia, PA, Lippincott Williams & Wilkins, 2002, p 28.)*

parallel to the force-generating axis, they never extend the entire muscle length. Muscles with fibers that are oriented at a single angle relative to the force-generating axis are called unipennate muscles (**Figure 6,** *B*). The angle between the fiber and the force-generating axis generally varies from 0° to 30°. It is obvious when preparing muscle dissections that most muscles fall into the final and most general category, multipennate muscles—muscles composed of fibers that are oriented at several angles relative to the axis of force generation (**Figure 6,** *C*). An understanding of muscle architecture is critical to understanding the functional properties of different muscles.

Physiologic Cross-Sectional Area
After measurement of a muscle's architectural properties, the so-called physiologic cross-sectional area (PCSA) can be calculated. PCSA is directly proportional to the maximum tetanic tension that can be generated by the muscle. This value is almost never the cross-sectional area of the muscle in any of the traditional anatomic planes, as would be obtained, for example, using a noninvasive imaging

method such as MRI, CT, or ultrasound. Theoretically, PCSA represents the sum of the cross-sectional areas of all of the muscle fibers within the muscle. It is calculated using the equation below. This equation is important to understand normal muscle and to make valid estimates of PCSA in human studies where the attempt is to evaluate patient performance in a physiologic context. In the equation, ρ represents muscle density (1.056 g/cm^3 for mammalian muscle) and θ represents surface pennation angle.

$$\text{PCSA (cm}^2) = \frac{\text{Muscle Mass (g)} \times \text{cosine } \theta}{\rho \text{ (g/cm}^3) \times \text{Fiber Length (cm)}}$$

The usefulness of this equation was highlighted by Powell and associates in an experimental comparison between the estimated maximum muscle tetanic tension (based on PCSA calculations) and measured maximum tetanic tension (measured using traditional physiologic testing techniques). These investigators found that the estimations and predictions agreed within experimental error. The only exception to that conclusion was the soleus muscle. Interestingly, this was the only muscle tested that contained a large proportion of slow muscle fibers. These data may suggest that slow fibers generate less tension per unit area compared with fast fibers, but the evidence is not conclusive in this regard.

It is important to emphasize that PCSA (and therefore maximum muscle tension) is not simply proportional to muscle mass (as is clear from the equation). In other words, given information on muscle mass or on muscle mass change (say, due to immobilization or spinal cord injury), no statement can be made with respect to muscle force. Although mass is proportional to the amount of contractile material in the muscle, the arrangement of that material is of critical importance. In some pathologic conditions, mass may change because of noncontractile proteins (increased connective tissue or inflammatory cells). In such instances, even calculated PCSA will not accurately predict tetanic tension.

Muscle Fiber Length

Unfortunately, even though it is often stated that muscle fiber length is proportional to fiber excursion (or velocity), there has not been a comprehensive study in mammalian muscle, analogous to the study just described for PCSA that confirms this relationship quantitatively. However, experimental evidence exists in the literature to suggest that this relationship is valid. First, in mechanical studies of isolated frog single muscle fibers, in which fiber length and thus, the number of sarcomeres in series, is easily measured, maximum contraction velocity is directly proportional to fiber length as is the width of the isometric length-tension relationship. This is the reason that muscle contraction velocities are often normalized and expressed in fiber length/s or sarcomere length/s. Second, in a mechanical and anatomic study of the cat semitendinosus muscle, which represents a unique model in that it is composed of distinct proximal and distal heads separated by a tendinous inscription and has distinct innervation to each head, the maximum contraction velocity of the two heads stimulated simultaneously was the same as the sum of the maximum contraction velocity of the two heads stimulated individually.

Architecture of Human Skeletal Muscles

Several architectural investigations have been performed in human upper and lower limbs. The relevant architectural characteristics are presented in **Tables 1 and 2**. Pennation angles normally range from about 0° to 30°. Thus, pennation probably has a relatively small influence on muscle PCSA calculations and function. In addition, the ratio of muscle fiber length to muscle length typically ranges from approximately 0.2 to 0.6. In other words, even the most longitudinally oriented muscles have fibers that

extend only about 60% of the muscle length. Finally, there is a very poor correlation between muscle mass and muscle PCSA. Again, mass gives little information that is relevant to function.

Muscles of the Lower Limb

Although each muscle is unique in terms of its architecture, taken as functional groups (for example, hamstrings, quadriceps, dorsiflexors, plantar flexors) several generalizations can be made (**Figure 7**). In terms of architecture, the typical properties of the various groups can be articulated. Quadriceps femoris muscles are characterized by their relatively high pennation angles, large PCSAs, and short fibers. In terms of design, these muscles appear suited for the generation of large forces (because force is proportional to PCSA). The hamstrings, on the other hand, by virtue of their relatively long fibers and intermediate PCSAs, appear to be designed for large excursions (because excursions are proportional to fiber length). A similar generalization can be made for the plantar flexors and dorsiflexors—plantar flexors appear to be designed for high force production whereas dorsiflexors appear to be designed for moderate forces, but high excursions. A very general (and a bit dangerous) conclusion might be that the antigravity extensors are more designed toward force production, whereas the flexors are more designed for high excursions. This generalization will break down upon close scrutiny but might provide a useful memory tool.

The two most important muscle architectural parameters are muscle PCSA (which is proportional to maximum muscle force) and muscle fiber length (which is proportional to maximum muscle excursion). These two parameters can be used to make general comparisons between muscles in terms of design. For example, the sartorius, semitendinosus, and gracilis muscles have extremely high fiber lengths and low PCSAs, which permit high excursions at low forces (**Figure 7**). At the other end of the spectrum is the soleus muscle, with its high PCSA and short fiber length, suitable for generating high forces with small excursions.

Muscles of the Upper Limb

Because of the specialization observed in the lower limb and the growing interest in upper extremity surgical procedures, it is important to understand the architectural features of muscles in the human arm and forearm. Although no such clear-cut generalizations regarding functional group design could be made for upper extremity muscles as were made for the lower limb, a high degree of architectural specialization is present in many upper limb muscles. The details of these results are presented in **Table 2**. Again, each of these muscles has a high degree of specialization by virtue of design. For example, the superficial and deep digital flexors to each digit are similar to one another but quite different from the digital extensors (**Figure**

Table 1	Architectural Properties of Human Lower Limb*					
Muscle	**Muscle Mass (g)**	**Muscle Length (mm)**	**Fiber Length (mm)**	**Pennation Angle (°)**	**Cross-Sectional Area (cm²)**	**FL/ML Ratio**
RF (n=3)	84.3 ± 14	316 ± 5.7	66.0 ± 1.5	5.0 ± 0.0	12.7 ± 1.9	.209±.002
VL (n=3)	220 ± 56	324 ± 14	65.7 ± 0.88	5.0 ± 0.0	30.6 ± 6.5	.203±.007
VM (n=3)	175 ± 41	335 ± 15	70.3 ± 3.3	5.0 ± 0.0	21.1 ± 4.3	.210±.005
VI (n=3)	160 ± 59	329 ± 15	68.3 ± 4.8	3.3 ± 1.7	22.3 ± 8.7	.208±.007
SM (n=3)	108 ± 13	262 ± 1.5	62.7 ± 4.7	15 ± 2.9	16.9 ± 1.5	.239±.017
BF$_l$ (n=3)	128 ± 28	342 ± 14	85.3 ± 5.0	0.0 ± 0.0	12.8 ± 2.8	.251±.022
BF$_s$ (n=3)	—	271 ± 11	139 ± 3.5	23 ± 0.9	—	.517±.032
ST (n=2)	76.9 ± 7.7	317 ± 4	158 ± 2.0	5.0 ± 0.0	5.4 ± 1.0	.498 ± 0.0
SOL (n=2)	215 (n=1)	310 ± 1.5	19.5 ± 0.5	25 ± 5.0	58.0 (n=1)	.063±.002
MG (n=3)	150 ± 14	248 ± 9.9	35.3 ± 2.0	16.7 ± 4.4	32.4 ± 3.1	.143±.010
LG (n=3)	—	217 ± 11	50.7 ± 5.6	8.3 ± 1.7	—	.233±.016
PLT (n=3)	5.30 ± 1.9	85.0 ± 15	39.3 ± 6.7	3.3 ± 1.7	1.2 ± 0.4	.467±.031
FHL (n=3)	21.5 ± 3.3	222 ± 5.0	34.0 ± 1.5	10.0 ± 2.9	5.3 ± 0.6	.154±.010
FDL (n=3)	16.3 ± 2.8	260 ± 15	27.0 ± 0.58	6.7 ± 1.7	5.1 ± 0.7	.104±.004
PL (n=3)	41.5 ± 8.5	286 ± 17	38.7 ± 3.2	10.0 ± 0.0	12.3 ± 2.9	.136±.010
PB (n=3)	17.3 ± 2.5	230 ± 13	39.3 ± 3.5	5.0 ± 0.0	5.7 ± 1.0	.170±.006
TP (n=3)	53.5 ± 7.3	254 ± 26	24.0 ± 4.0	11.7 ± 1.7	20.8 ± 3	.095±.015
TA (n=3)	65.7 ± 10	298 ± 12	77.3 ± 7.8	5.0 ± 0.0	9.9 ± 1.5	.258±.015
EDL (n=3)	35.2 ± 3.6	355 ± 13	80.3 ± 8.4	8.3 ± 1.7	5.6 ± 0.6	.226±.024
EHL (n=3)	12.9 ± 1.6	273 ± 2.4	87.0 ± 8.0	6.0 ± 1.0	1.8 ± 0.2	.319±.030
SAR (n=3)	61.7 ± 14	503 ± 27	455 ± 19	0.0 ± 0.0	1.7 ± 0.3	.906±.017
GR (n=3)	35.3 ± 7.4	335 ± 20	277 ± 12	3.3 ± 1.7	1.8 ± 0.3	.828±.017
AM (n=3)	229 ± 32	305 ± 12	115 ± 7.9	0.0 ± 0.0	18.2 ± 2.3	.378±.013
AL (n=3)	63.5 ± 16	229 ± 12	108 ± 2.0	6.0 ± 1.0	6.8 ± 1.9	.475±.023
AB (n=3)	43.8 ± 8.4	156 ± 12	103 ± 6.4	0.0 ± 0.0	4.7 ± 1.0	.663±.036
PEC (n=3)	26.4 ± 6.0	123 ± 4.5	104 ± 1.2	0.0 ± 0.0	2.9 ± 0.6	.851±.040
POP (n=2)	20.1 ± 2.4	108 ± 7.0	29.0 ± 7.0	0.0 ± 0.0	7.9 ± 1.4	.265±.048

*AB = adductor brevis; AL = adductor longus; AM = adductor magnus; BF$_l$ = biceps femoris, long head; BF$_s$ = biceps femoris, short head; EDL = extensor digitorum longus; EHL = extensor hallucis longus; FDL = flexor digitorum longus; GR = gracilis; FHL = flexor hallucis longus; FL/ML = fiber length/muscle length; LG = lateral gastrocnemius; MG = medial gastrocnemius; PEC = pectineus; PB = peroneus brevis; PL = peroneus longus; PLT = plantaris; POP = popliteus; RF = rectus femoris; SAR = sartorius; SM = semimembranosus; SOL = soleus; ST = semitendinosus; TA = tibialis anterior; TP = tibialis posterior; VI = vastus intermedius; VL = vastus lateralis; VM = vastus medialis.
(Reproduced with permission from Wickiewicz TL, Roy RR, Powell PL, Edgerton VR: Muscle architecture of the human lower limb. Clin Orthop Relat Res 1983;179:275-283.)

8). As with the lower extremity, this type of scatter plot can be used to compare functional properties between muscles of the forearm. Clearly, such differences could be considered in surgical and rehabilitative procedures involving the upper limb or in designing artificial muscles that might restore lost function. It could be expected that when a muscle is surgically transferred to perform the function of another muscle whose function has been lost, matching of architectural properties may prove beneficial. This is a popular area of study that has been discussed at length.

Clinical Significance of Skeletal Muscle Architecture

In addition to improving understanding of muscle anatomy and function, elucidation of muscle architecture provides information useful for selection of muscles used in tendon transfers. To substitute lost muscle function, the distal tendons of muscles are often transferred from one position to another (tendon transfer). It would seem reasonable to select a donor muscle with architectural properties that are similar to the original muscle to perform the original muscle's function. Several factors influence

Table 2   Architectural Properties of the Human Arm and Forearm[*][†]

Muscle	Muscle Mass (g)	Muscle Length (mm)	Fiber Length (mm)	Pennation Angle (°)	Cross-Sectional Area (cm²)	FL/ML Ratio
BR (n=8)	16.6±2.8	175±8.3	121±8.3	2.4±.6	1.33±.22	.69±.062
PT (n=8)	15.9±1.7	130±4.7	36.4±1.3	9.6±.8	4.13±.52	.28±.012
PQ (n=8)	5.21±1.0	39.3±2.3	23.3±2.0	9.9±.3	2.07±.33	.58±.021
EDC I (n=8)	3.05±.45	114±3.4	56.9±3.6	3.1±.5	.52±.08	.49±.024
EDC M (n=5)	6.13±1.2	112±4.7	58.8±3.5	3.2±1.0	1.02±.20	.50±.014
EDC R (n=7)	4.70±.75	125±10.7	51.2±1.8	3.2±.54	.86±.13	.42±.023
EDC S (n=6)	2.23±.32	121±8.0	52.9±5.2	2.4±.7	.40±.06	.43±.029
EDQ (n=7)	3.81±.70	152±9.2	55.3±3.7	2.6±.6	.64±.10	.36±.012
EIP (n=6)	2.86±.61	105±6.6	48.4±2.3	6.3±.8	.56±.11	.46±.023
EPL (n=7)	4.54±.68	138±7.2	43.6±2.6	5.6±1.3	.98±.13	.31±.020
PL (n=6)	3.78±.82	134±11.5	52.3±3.1	3.5±1.2	.69±.17	.40±.032
FDS I(P) (n=6)	6.0±1.1	92.5±8.4	31.6±3.0	5.1±0.2	1.81±.83	.34±.022
FDS I(D) (n=9)	6.6±0.8	119±6.1	37.9±3.0	6.7±0.3	1.63±.22	.32±.013
FDS I(C) (n=6)	12.4±2.1	207±10.7	67.6±2.8	5.7±0.2	1.71±.28	.33±.025
FDS M (n=9)	16.3±2.2	183±11.5	60.8±3.9	6.9±0.7	2.53±.34	.34±.014
FDS R (n=9)	10.2±1.1	155±7.7	60.1±2.7	4.3±0.6	1.61±.18	.39±.023
FDS S (n=9)	1.8±0.3	103±6.3	42.4±2.2	4.9±0.7	0.40±.05	.42±.014
FDP I (n=9)	11.7±1.2	149±3.8	61.4±2.4	7.2±0.7	1.77±.16	.41±.018
FDP M (n=9)	16.3±1.7	200±8.2	68.4±2.7	5.7±0.3	2.23±.22	.34±.011
FDP R (n=9)	11.9±1.4	194±7.0	64.6±2.6	6.8±0.5	1.72±.18	.33±.009
FDP S (n=9)	13.7±1.5	150±4.7	60.7±3.9	7.8±0.9	2.20±.30	.40±.015
FPL (n=9)	10.0±1.1	168±10.0	45.1±2.1	6.9±0.2	2.08±.22	.24±.010

*Data from: Lieber RL, Fazeli BM, Botte MJ: Architecture of selected wrist flexor and extensor muscles. J Hand Surg [Am] 1990;15:244-250, and Lieber RL, Jacobson MD, Fazeli BM, Abrams RA, Botte MJ: Architecture of selected muscles of the arm and forearm: Anatomy and implications for tendon transfer. J Hand Surg [Am] 1992;17A:787-798.
† BR = brachioradialis; EDC I, EDC M, EDC R, and EDC S = extensor digitorum communis to the index, middle, ring and small fingers, respectively; EDQ = extensor digiti quinti; EIP = extensor indicis proprius; EPL = extensor pollicis longus; FDP I, FDP M, FDP R, and FDP S = flexor digitorum profundus muscles; FDS I, FDS M, FDS R, and FDS S = flexor digitorum superficialis muscles; FDS I (P) and FDS I (D) = proximal and distal bellies of the FDS I; FDS I (C) = the combined properties of the two bellies as if they were a single muscle; FL/ML = fiber length/muscle length; FPL = flexor pollicis longus; PL = palmaris longus; PQ = pronator quadratus; PT = pronator teres.

donor selection, including donor muscle availability, donor muscle morbidity, preoperative strength, integrity, expendability, synergism, transfer route and direction, and surgeon experience and preference.

Surgical Restoration of Digital Extension

As an example of the way in which architectural differences might be useful in tendon transfer, consider the case of surgical restoration of digital extension after high radial nerve palsy. Potential donor muscles, that are transferred into the extensor digitorum communis (EDC) include the flexor carpi radialis (FCR), the flexor carpi ulnaris (FCU), the flexor digitorum superficialis to the middle finger (FDS (M)), and the FDS to the ring finger (FDS (R)). From the standpoint of architecture alone, the FDS (M) most closely resembles the EDC in terms of force generation (cross-sectional area) and excursion (fiber length). This can be appreciated by the relatively close position in "architectural space" of the FDS (M) to the EDC (**Figure 8**). If individual architectural properties are

compared, it is clear that the FDS (M) has more than enough excursion in comparison with the EDC, whereas the FCU has excessive force-generating potential but may lack sufficient excursion. Thus, if the concern were sufficient force, the FCU might be chosen, and if the concern were excursion, the FDS (M) might be chosen. A knowledge of muscle architecture is necessary so that an informed decision can be made.

Skeletal Muscle Physiology
Excitation-Contraction Coupling

The process by which neural activation culminates in muscle contraction is known as excitation-contraction coupling, or EC coupling (**Figure 9**). EC coupling is a sequence of microscopic events, each of which is necessary for contraction to occur. If any single step of EC coupling is impaired, muscle contraction does not occur normally. This impairment might be interpreted as muscle paralysis or fatigue. However, such a general classification is not

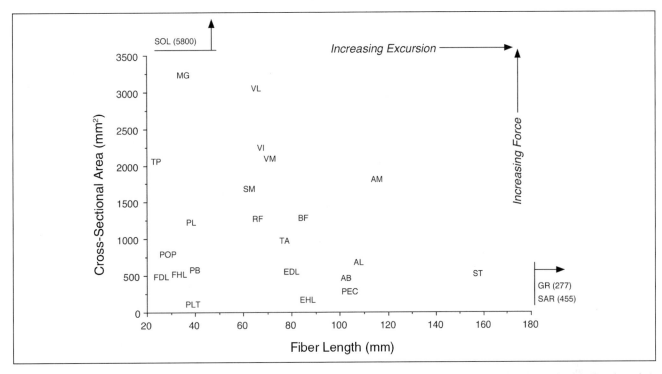

Figure 7   Scatter graph of fiber length and physiologic cross-sectional areas of muscles in the human lower limb. Fiber length is proportional to muscle excursion whereas physiologic cross-sectional area is proportional to maximum muscle force. This graph can be used to compare the relative forces and excursions of leg muscles. See Table 1 for abbreviations. Muscles placed at extremes of graph (SOL, GR, and SAR) would be plotted off this scale at the position shown. *(Reproduced with permission from Lieber R (ed): Skeletal Muscle Structure, Function, and Plasticity. Philadelphia, PA, Lippincott Williams & Wilkins, 2002, p 38.)*

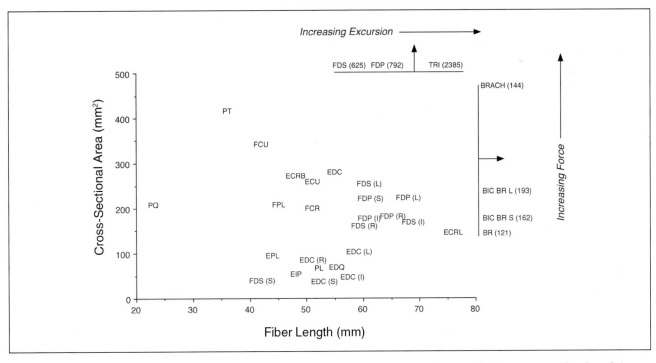

Figure 8   Scatter graph of the fiber length and physiologic cross-sectional areas of muscles in the human arm. Fiber length is proportional to muscle excursion whereas physiologic cross-sectional area is proportional to maximum muscle force. Thus, this graph can be used to compare the relative forces and excursions of arm and forearm muscles. Muscles placed at extremes of the graph (FDS, FDP, TRI, BRACH, BR, and BIC BR) would be plotted off this scale at the position shown. BIC = biceps; BRACH = brachialis; ECRB = extensor carpi radialis brevis; ECRL = extensor carpi radialis longus; ECU = extensor carpi ulnaris; FCR = flexor carpi radialis; FCU = flexor carpi ulnaris, TRI = triceps brachii. See Table 2 for additional abbreviations. *(Reproduced with permission from Lieber R (ed): Skeletal Muscle Structure, Function, and Plasticity. Philadelphia, PA, Lippincott Williams & Wilkins, 2002, p 39.)*

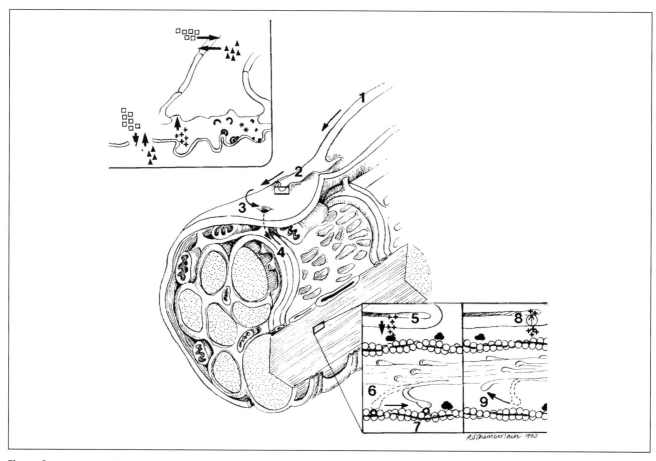

Figure 9   Sequence of events involved in EC coupling of a nervous impulse to muscle contraction. 1, Action potential conducted by nerve to muscle (inset, squares represent Na^+ ions entering nerve, and triangles represent K^+ ions leaving the nerve to conduct the action potential). 2, Nervous impulse transmitted across neuromuscular junction to muscle fiber (inset, crosses represent Ca^{2+} ions entering nerve end, half-moons represent the neurotransmitter ACh, and asterisks represent the enzyme acetylcholinesterase degrading ACh). 3, Action potential conducted along fiber surface (inset, squares represent Na^+ ions entering fiber, and triangles represent K^+ ions leaving the fiber to conduct the action potential). 4, Action potential conducted deep into fiber via the T-system. 5, Ca^{2+} released from SR to bind troponin and thus activate the actin filament. 6 and 7, Cross-bridge produces force and filament sliding. 8, Ca^{2+} is pumped back into SR when electrical impulses cease. 9, Cross-bridges relax because of lack of Ca^{2+} filament activation. *(Reproduced with permission from Lieber R (ed): Skeletal Muscle Structure, Function, and Plasticity. Philadelphia, PA, Lippincott Williams & Wilkins, 2002, p 46.)*

useful unless the underlying cause is known.

Nerve Action Potential

The first step in the EC coupling chain is the generation of the peripheral nerve action potential. An action potential results from activation of the peripheral nerve axon that innervates the muscle. The "normal" way to activate an axon is by generation of a signal from the central nervous system to initiate movement. However, the axon may be depolarized in several additional ways, including trauma to the peripheral nerve or application of an external electrical stimulating device. An electrical stimulating device can be used clinically to substitute lost function in patients with paralysis, muscle weakness after surgery, or in those whose motor system is unable to activate a muscle after surgery. Regardless of the manner of initiation, the resulting action potentials that propagate down the

peripheral nerve are identical. The action potential arrives at the neuromuscular junction, the interface between muscle and nerve. The indentation on the muscle fiber surface in which the motor nerve rests is known as the synaptic cleft.

Acetylcholine Release

The end of the peripheral nerve contains packets of the neurotransmitter acetylcholine (ACh), which causes muscle fiber excitation. ACh is synthesized by the cell body of the motor nerve and is transported down the axon where it is stored at nerve endings for later use. Following nerve depolarization, a quantum or unit of ACh is released into the synaptic cleft where it diffuses across the synaptic cleft and binds to the ACh receptor. ACh binding results in depolarization of the muscle fiber sarcolemma and an action potential that propagates from the neuromuscular junction outwardly in all directions. Communication between the nerve and muscle therefore occurs via a standard synapse in which the neurotransmitter is ACh. This type of synapse is referred to as cholinergic.

The storage and release of ACh to cause muscle activation is accomplished by the interaction of numerous active enzymes. The function of these enzymes has been studied in isolation and a therapy for "overactive" or "spastic" muscles was developed based on discoveries made. One method for blocking neuromuscular transmission is injection of botulinum toxin into the muscle, near the motor point (the anatomic location where the motor nerve enters the muscle and is near the neuromuscular junction). This toxin acts by entering the presynaptic nerve terminal and blocking ACh release by interrupting the activity of one of the enzymes involved in the release process. Such chemical "blocks" typically act for 3 to 6 months before they are no longer needed or before another dose is required.

Calcium Release and Uptake Regulates Muscle Contraction

After the T-system signals the SR that the fiber has been activated, the SR releases calcium ions in the region of the myofilaments. This release process is extremely fast—much faster than the resulting contraction/relaxation cycle. The calcium ions bind to troponin, the actin filament regulatory protein, which in turn releases the inhibition on the actin filament, permitting interaction between the myosin and actin filaments and resulting in cross-bridge cycling and, therefore, force generation and movement. As long as neural impulses arrive at the neuromuscular junction and, therefore, calcium concentrations remain high in the region of the myofilaments, force generation continues. However, when the impulses cease, calcium levels drop and force decreases as calcium is pumped back into the SR by the calcium-activated adenosine triphosphatase (ATPase) enzyme. The calcium-activated ATPase enzyme is an integral protein that is embedded within the SR membrane. The mechanism of action of this enzyme has been thoroughly studied and is one of the best understood of the ion transport enzymes. The calcium pumping process is energy dependent and requires ATP. When calcium levels in the region of the myofilaments drop below a critical level, thin filament inhibition again resumes, and actin-myosin interaction is prevented. Muscle fiber relaxation parallels the drop in calcium levels. Muscles with high SR/calcium pumping ability can thus relax faster compared with muscles with less SR/calcium pumping ability. This ultrastructural difference among muscles allows some muscles to function at extremely high contraction/relaxation rates.

Temporal Summation

A well-known muscle contractile property follows directly from an understanding of the EC coupling sequence. First, it should be obvious that the time required for activation, contraction, and then relaxation to occur is finite. Excitation (with accompanying calcium release) is relatively rapid (on the order of approximately 5 msec), whereas contraction and relaxation are relatively slow (on the order of about 100 msec). The mechanical consequence of the activation process (the muscle twitch) lags far behind the activation process itself. Because contraction and relaxation are relatively slow processes, if multiple impulses activate muscle, a higher force results compared with activation by a single impulse alone. If a "train" of such pulses (say, 50 pulses in a row) is delivered to the muscle, separated in time by different amounts, this results in a tetanic contraction, and the force generated is quite different from a twitch. Higher forces result when stimuli are delivered at higher frequencies because there is less time for relaxation (frequency = 1/interpulse interval; low intervals correspond to high frequencies). At relatively low frequencies (10 Hz), the contractile record almost completely relaxes between successive pulses. This is referred to as an unfused tetanic contraction, because it is still possible to distinguish individual contractile events within the force record. However, as stimulation frequency increases, the tetanic record becomes more fused, until at very high frequencies (100 Hz), the contractile record becomes a fused contraction. A fused tetanic contraction appears as such because calcium is released onto the myofilaments much faster than the rate at which the myofilaments can relax.

Skeletal Muscle Mechanics
The Active Length-Tension Relationship

Since the late 1800s, it has been known that the force developed by a muscle during isometric contraction (when the muscle is not allowed to shorten) varies with its starting length. The isometric length-tension curve is generated by maximally stimulating a skeletal muscle at a variety of discrete lengths and measuring the tension generated at each length. When maximum tetanic tension at each length is plotted against length, a relationship such as that shown in **Figure 10** is obtained. Although a general description of this relationship was established early in the history of biologic science, the precise structural basis for the length-tension relationship in skeletal muscle was not elucidated until the sophisticated mechanical experiments of the early 1960s were performed. It was these experiments that defined the precise relationship between myofilament overlap and tension generation, which is currently referred to as the length-tension relationship. In its most basic form, the length-tension relationship reflects the fact that tension generation in skeletal muscle is a direct function of the magnitude of overlap between the ac-

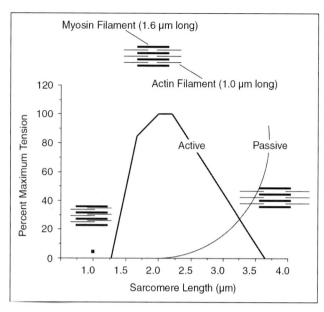

Figure 10 The sarcomere length-tension curve for frog skeletal muscle obtained using sequential isometric contractions in single muscle fibers. Insets show schematic arrangement of myofilaments in different regions of the length-tension curve. Curved line represents passive muscle tension. *(Reproduced with permission from Lieber R (ed): Skeletal Muscle Structure, Function, and Plasticity. Philadelphia, PA, Lippincott Williams & Wilkins, 2002, p 52.)*

tin and myosin filaments. The shape and amplitude of this curve has significant implications for surgical reconstruction. Briefly, because muscles can be stretched in the operating room to lengths well beyond those at which they generate any tension at all, surgeons must be aware of the fact that, when suturing a muscle into a distal tendon or into the periosteum, the chosen length will have a profound functional effect. If the length is too long and the sarcomeres generate little or no active tension (**Figure 10, right side**), the patient will experience a poor functional recovery unless the muscle adapts dramatically. Experimental evidence has been provided that demonstrates, on average, that transferred muscles are overstretched during normal surgical procedures to the point where they are predicted to generate less than 30% of maximum force. Perhaps this is why it is often stated in the literature that a muscle will lose one "strength grade" after transfer. Muscle force is, in effect, "wasted" because myofilament overlap at these long lengths is so unfavorable. If the functional consequences of muscle length are carefully considered during the surgical procedure, there is no apparent reason why muscle strength should decrease dramatically after tendon transfer surgery.

The Passive Length-Tension Relationship
The solid line in **Figure 10** represents the tension generated if a muscle is stretched to various lengths without stimulation. Note that near the optimal length, passive

tension is almost zero. However, as the muscle is stretched to longer lengths, passive tension increases dramatically. These relatively long lengths can be attained physiologically, and therefore, passive tension can play a role in providing resistive force even in the absence of muscle activation. What is the origin of passive tension? Obviously, the structure(s) responsible for passive tension are outside of the cross-bridge itself because muscle activation is not required. Several recent studies have shed light on what has turned out to be a fascinating and huge protein with skeletal muscle, aptly named titin. Magid and Law measured passive tension in whole muscle, single fibers, and single fibers with membranes removed and showed that each relationship scaled to the size of the specimen. The source for passive force-bearing in muscle was within the normal myofibrillar structure, not extracellular as had previously been supposed. In parallel with these studies, it has been demonstrated that the size of the protein responsible for passive force-bearing in muscle was in the megadalton range (relatively large). Because most proteins are in the tens to hundreds of kilodaltons, this was a startling observation.

The discovery of titin has tremendous clinical significance because during the traditional physical examination, it is the passive properties of skeletal muscles that are the most readily appreciated and quantified and that are used to make clinical decisions. Because passive properties are dominated by titin, it is probably the titin molecule that most strongly influences such an examination. Although it is certainly premature to make definitive statements, it is possible that the titin molecule will become as important for clinicians as the myosin molecule has become for physiologists. The passive tension properties of muscle are clinically relevant in that they determine the "feel" of a muscle intraoperatively. However, this "feel" is not a good predictor of function because sarcomere length (which determines force generated) and passive tension are only loosely related.

Force-Velocity Relationship Describes Isotonic Muscle Contraction
The length-tension relationship describes a muscle's behavior at constant length (under isometric conditions). However, much of muscle use involves movement that is better described by the force-velocity relationship. Unlike the length-tension relationship, the force-velocity relationship does not have a precise, anatomically identifiable basis. The force-velocity relationship describes the force generated by a muscle as a function of velocity under conditions of constant load (isotonic conditions). It can also be stated in the reverse, such that the velocity of muscle contraction is dependent on the force resisting the muscle. Historically, the force-velocity relationship was investigated to a much greater degree than the length-tension

relationship because such mechanical studies were used to define the kinetic properties of the cross-bridges.

Experimentally, the force-velocity relationship, like the length-tension relationship, is a curve that actually represents the results of many experiments plotted on the same graph. Experimentally, a muscle is stimulated maximally and allowed to shorten (or lengthen) against a constant load. The muscle velocity during shortening (or lengthening) is measured and plotted against the resistive force. The general form of this relationship is plotted in **Figure 11.** On the horizontal axis, muscle velocity relative to maximum velocity (V_{max}) is plotted, while on the vertical axis muscle force is plotted relative to maximum force (P_o).

Concentric Contractions

When a muscle is activated and required to lift a load that is less than the maximum tetanic tension it can generate, the muscle begins to shorten. Contractions that permit the muscle to shorten are known as concentric contractions. The word "concentric" in this context traditionally describes shortening contractions of muscle. In concentric contractions, the force generated by the muscle is always less than the muscle's maximum force (P_o). As the load the muscle is required to lift decreases, contraction velocity increases. This occurs until the muscle finally reaches its maximum contraction velocity, V_{max}. V_{max} is a parameter that can be used to characterize muscle, which is related to both fiber type distribution and architecture.

The force-velocity relationship is a very steep rectangular hyperbola; force drops off rapidly as velocity increases. For example, in a muscle that is shortening at only 1% of its maximum contraction velocity (extremely slow), tension drops by 5% relative to maximum isometric tension. Similarly, as contraction velocity increases to only 10% maximum (easily attainable physiologically), muscle force drops by 35%. Even when muscle force is 50% maximum, muscle velocity is only 17% V_{max}.

Eccentric Contractions

As the load on the muscle increases, it finally reaches a point where the external force on the muscle is greater than the force that the muscle can generate. Even though the muscle may be fully activated, it is forced to lengthen because of the high external load. There are two main characteristics regarding eccentric contractions. First, the absolute tensions achieved are very high relative to the muscle's maximum tetanic tension-generating capacity; second, the absolute tension is relatively independent of lengthening velocity. These characteristics suggest that skeletal muscles are very resistant to lengthening, a property necessary for many normal movement patterns. The basic mechanics of eccentric contractions are still a source of debate because the cross-bridge theory that so nicely describes concentric contractions does not adequately describe eccentric contractions.

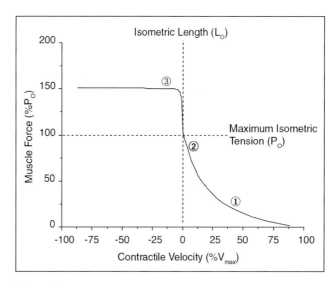

Figure 11   The muscle force-velocity curve for skeletal muscle obtained using sequential isotonic contractions. Note that force increases dramatically upon forced muscle lengthening and drops precipitously upon muscle shortening. *(Reproduced with permission from Lieber R (ed):* Skeletal Muscle Structure, Function, and Plasticity. *Philadelphia, PA, Lippincott Williams & Wilkins, 2002, p 62.)*

Clinical Implications of the Force-Velocity Relationship

There are clinical implications of the force-velocity relationship for both lengthening (eccentric) and shortening (concentric) contractions. With regard to exercise and strengthening, it is believed that muscles are strengthened as a result of the high forces they experience during the exercise itself—higher forces producing greater strengthening. Therefore, exercises performed with muscle activated in a way that allows them to shorten at high velocities necessarily implies that the muscles are producing relatively low forces. This is intuitively obvious as a light load is compared with a heavy load—the light load can be moved much more quickly. However, these rapid movements would have very small strengthening effects because the muscle forces are so low. With regard to exercise including muscle lengthening, it can be seen from **Figure 11** that very high muscle forces would be involved. Indeed, lengthening contractions are often invoked in power training, with the goal being to cause increases in muscle mass and strength. In human studies, muscle injury and soreness are selectively associated with eccentric contraction. This concept may be the reason why many strength trainers use the phrase, "no pain, no gain" or "break it down to build it up." Although this association appears to be true in terms of phenomenology, there is little evidence at the cellular level that muscle cell injury is required for muscle cell strengthening.

Table 3 Fiber Type Classification Schemes*				
Basis for Scheme		**Fiber Type Spectrum**		**Authors**
Metabolic	SO	FOG	FG	Peter et al 1972
Morphology and physiology	Slow red	Fast white	Fast white	Ranvier 1873
Z-line width	Red	Intermediate	White	Gauthier 1969
Histochemistry	III	II	I	Romanul 1964
Histochemistry	Type 1	Type 2A	Type 2B	Brooke and Kaiser 1972
Immunohistochemistry	Type 1	Types 2A and 2X	Type 2B	Schiaffino et al 1989

*SO = slow oxidative; FOG = fast oxidative glycolytic; FG = fast glycolytic.

Muscle Fiber Types

To this point, it may have been implied (by omission) that all muscle fibers are created equal. Although this statement is true in terms of value, it is clearly not true in terms of properties. By understanding the anatomic differences between fiber types, insight is gained into the rationale for the anatomic features themselves. The idea that all muscle fibers are the same is an oversimplification based on the overwhelming evidence that skeletal muscle fibers are heterogeneous. In the early 1800s it was observed that the gross appearance of different skeletal muscles ranged in color from pale white to deep red. One of the earliest classification schemes for muscle was based on color, and thus muscles were classified as "red" or "white" (**Table 3**). However, as experimental methods became more sophisticated, it became clear that numerous other differences existed between muscles. For example, certain muscles contracted very rapidly, whereas others contracted more slowly. Certain muscles could maintain force for a long period of time, whereas others fatigued very rapidly. Certain muscles generated large forces, and others generated very small forces. Thus, muscles were also classified as fast or slow, and fatigable or nonfatigable. In addition, with the advent of light microscopy and histochemistry, it became possible to classify individual fibers based on their appearance after a particular staining protocol. Many of these schemes did not correlate with muscle color, and many of them did not correlate with one another. **Table 3** presents a few of the classification schemes used historically and the bases for them. The main drawback associated with fiber type classification schemes was that the classification only worked for one property but had no relationship to others. For example, anatomists identified type 1 and type 2 fibers, and physiologists spoke of fast twitch and slow twitch muscles. In addition, it was not clear whether muscle fibers were mutable over their life span.

The current view of muscle fiber types is that skeletal muscle fibers possess a wide and nearly continuous spectrum of morphologic, contractile, and metabolic properties. The appropriate view of any classification scheme, therefore, is that it is an artificial system superimposed on a continuum for convenience. The most useful scheme is one that can be related to other types of measurements (physiologic and biochemical) to understand more fully muscle's normal and adaptive properties. Fortunately, most modern muscle fiber type classification schemes are based on some type of measurement of the myosin molecule.

Common Methods Used for Typing Muscle Fibers
The Metabolic Classification Scheme

To date, many agree that the so-called metabolic classification scheme is the most useful in terms of making a connection between fiber type and function. That is, the metabolic scheme allows switching back and forth between anatomic and physiologic studies and permits understanding one type of study based on the other. (Unfortunately, this scheme is not the one most widely used for study of human muscle). In the metabolic method, three muscle fiber properties are identified using histochemical methods. These methods rely on the fact that enzymes located in thin (6 to 8 μm) frozen sections of muscle fibers can be chemically reacted with certain products to visualize the activity of the enzyme. The most modern histochemical methods are actually able to quantify the activity of the enzymes in standard units (similar to in vitro biochemical studies) based only on measurements of optical density in frozen tissue sections. A 6-μm section is still two to four sarcomeres thick, so many proteins are available that can participate in chemical reactions.

The basic requirement for a histochemical assay is similar, at least in principle, to the requirement for any biochemical assay. First, a substrate (fuel) is provided for the enzyme to be studied. Second, an energy source is provided that allows the enzyme to use the substrate. Third, a reaction product is linked to another product that can be visualized microscopically. Of course, the entire reaction takes place in the tissue itself, not in a test tube. The three histochemical assays typically used to determine muscle fiber types are the myofibrillar ATPase (MATPase) assay, the succinate dehydrogenase (SDH) assay, and the α-glycerophosphate dehydrogenase (αGP) assay.

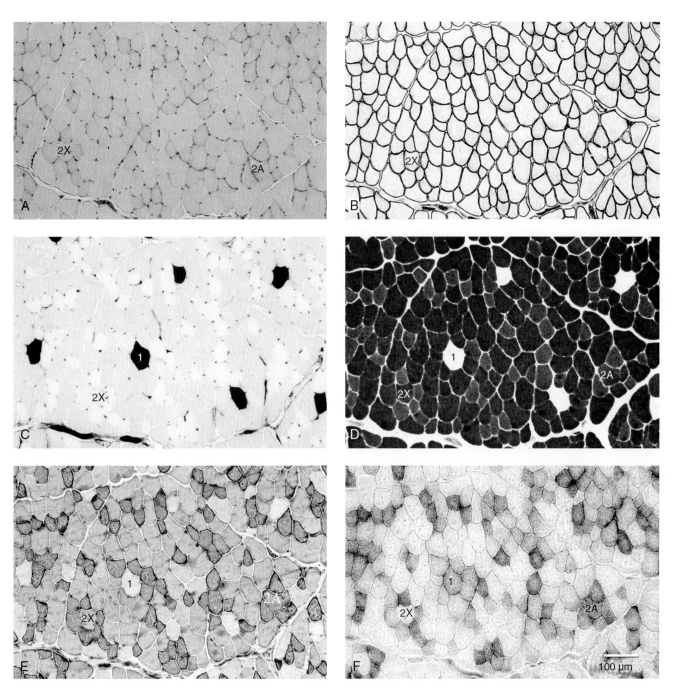

Figure 12   Serial cross sections of rabbit tibialis anterior skeletal muscles under various staining conditions. **A,** Hematoxylin and eosin, demonstrating general muscle fiber morphology. **B,** Dystrophin immunohistochemistry showing the subsarcolemmal nature of this protein. **C,** Myofibrillar ATPase under acid preincubation conditions. Under these conditions, slow fibers stain darkly as do the extracellular capillaries whereas fast fibers stain lightly. **D,** Myofibrillar ATPase under alkaline preincubation conditions. Under these conditions, slow fibers stain lightly whereas fast fibers stain darkly. Note that in both panels C and D, fast fiber staining intensity occurs at two levels. **E,** Immunohistochemical reaction for fast myosin heavy chain antibody. In rat skeletal muscle, this antibody labels type 2A fibers darkly and type 2X fibers more lightly and is negative for types 2B and 1 fibers. **F,** SDH used to demonstrate muscle fiber oxidative capacity. Note that the slow fibers (sample fiber labeled with a "1") as well as the type 2A fast fibers (sample fiber labeled with a "2A") have higher oxidative capacity compared with the type 2X fibers (sample fiber labeled with a "2X"). *(Reproduced with permission from Lieber R (ed): Skeletal Muscle Structure, Function, and Plasticity. Philadelphia, PA, Lippincott Williams & Wilkins, 2002.)*

Myofibrillar ATPase

In a classic example of combined physiologic and biochemical experimentation, V_{max} was measured in several skeletal muscles and shown to be proportional to myofibrillar ATPase activity. Thus, the histochemical assay for myofibrillar ATPase activity is used to distinguish between fast- and slow-contracting muscle fibers (although, strictly speaking, a fiber should not be histochemically typed and called fast or slow because the classification method does not actually measure speed but histochemical appearance) (**Figure 12**).

Succinate Dehydrogenase

The histochemical assay for SDH is used to distinguish between oxidative and nonoxidative (less oxidative) fibers. Fibers with a high oxidative capacity generate ATP via oxidative phosphorylation. This sequence of reactions occurs in the mitochondria, which is one reason that highly oxidative fibers have a high volume fraction of mitochondria. Fibers rich in SDH (and thus rich in mitochondria) stain with a speckled pattern of the mitochondria, proportional to the number of mitochondria and the SDH activity within them (**Figure 12**). Oxidative fibers have a relatively dense, purple speckled appearance, whereas nonoxidative fibers have only scattered purple speckles. Therefore, this histochemical assay reflects the relative oxidative potential of muscle fibers.

α-Glycerophosphate Dehydrogenase

The αGP enzyme is used to distinguish fibers based on their relative glycolytic potential. Glycolysis is used to generate ATP in the absence of oxygen (anaerobically). The chemical reactions involved in glycolysis take place in the muscle cell cytoplasm (myoplasm). As such, the αGP stain is not confined to a specific cellular organelle as is the SDH stain, and the appearance is much more continuous across the cell. αGP is not actually involved with direct steps in glycolysis. Rather, the αGP enzyme is responsible for shuttling the nicotinic acid dehydrogenase produced by glycolysis into the mitochondria where ATP can be produced. This assay can thus distinguish between glycolytic and nonglycolytic fibers.

Fiber Type Classifications Using Histochemical Methods

In their most basic form, the three histochemical methods just described can classify muscle fibers into fast or slow, oxidative or nonoxidative, and glycolytic or nonglycolytic. Potentially, if a given muscle fiber is stained for all three properties, any of the eight (2^3) fiber types could be obtained. In reality, however, more than 95% of normal muscle fibers can be classified into one of only three categories. These three categories represent the three major fiber types which are called FG (fast contracting, glycolytic), FOG (fast contracting, and oxidative and glycolytic), and SO (slow contracting, oxidative). This scheme can classify most muscle fibers, and it can be related to physiologic, biochemical, and morphologic measurements. Although classification schemes are, by definition, artificial, this one is less so in that it interleaves well with many different experimental methodologies.

Classification by Immunohistochemistry

Although histochemical fiber type identification can yield valuable insights into muscle function, it is limited in its ability to identify specific cellular proteins. Can it be concluded that the fast fibers from one muscle contain the identical protein to fast fibers in the other muscle? Of course not. For this purpose, specific identification methods must be used to identify proteins with the same specificity as a human fingerprint.

Muscle fibers are fairly easily classified using immunohistochemistry because different forms of the myosin heavy chain molecule (different isoforms) are expressed within the different fiber types. The most complete set of myosin heavy chain isoforms were developed on rat skeletal muscle and these sets have been applied to other mammalian systems.

Regarding these antibodies used on human muscle, in a subsequent study it was shown, using in situ hybridization, that the muscle fibers that had been identified as type 2B were actually expressing messenger RNA transcripts of the type 2X isoform. This type of study demonstrates that, just because a fiber type is "named," for example, type 2B, this is merely a placeholder name until definitive identification of the protein product is made using modern molecular methods.

Classification by ATPase Stability

A scheme used often in human muscle pathology and even in animal experiments is the so-called ATPase-based classification scheme. In this classification scheme, several repetitions of the ATPase assay mentioned previously are performed on serial sections of muscle (serial sections are consecutive 6- to 8-μm sections in which the same fiber can be identified on one section and then the next, etc.). However, although the routine ATPase assay is performed under alkaline conditions (pH, 9.4), in the ATPase-based classification scheme, several other assays are performed under increasingly acidic conditions (pH, 4), and optical density is measured. Thus the assay determines the sensitivity of the ATPase enzyme to the pH of the medium. For reasons that are not clear, fast muscle myosin has a different pH sensitivity than slow muscle myosin. At acid pH, slow fibers stain more darkly than fast fibers, whereas at alkaline pH the opposite is true. In fact, the scheme takes this differential pH sensitivity a step further. Fast fibers themselves can be subdivided based on differential pH sensitivity over the range of pH 4.3 to 4.6. This classification scheme can thus differentiate between fast fibers (type 2) and slow fibers (type 1), and between (at least) two fast fiber subtypes (type 2A and type 2B). **Table 4** presents the definitions of type 1, 2A, and 2B fibers based on the ATPase scheme. Note that this technique must be fine tuned to accurately and repeatedly obtain valid results on various tissues. The values presented are those obtained in the study by Brooke and Kaiser for human muscle.

It has been indirectly concluded that type 2A fibers have a greater oxidative capacity than type 2B fibers, and therefore many equate them (incorrectly) with type FOG fibers. Several studies have directly demonstrated that the metabolic scheme does not correlate well with the ATPase-based scheme. This realization should not be surprising based on an understanding of what the two schemes measure. Why should the pH sensitivity of the ATPase molecule be related to the oxidative or glycolytic capacity of the cell? A relationship may exist in general, as most cellular metabolic processes are complementary. However, the relationships may not hold following a perturbation of the cellular environment and, therefore, fiber type determination with this method must be used with great caution. It seems most prudent to measure directly the property of interest (for example, oxidative capacity) rather than relying on an indirect measure associated with the property of interest.

Physiologic Properties of Muscle Fiber Types

It is difficult to obtain a precise measurement of the properties of a single fiber type population. It is not technically possible to perform all of the interesting physiologic measurements on intact mammalian single muscle fibers. The best information comes either from physiologic experiments on muscles composed mainly of one fiber type, or on single "skinned" muscle fibers whose type is determined immunohistochemically. The drawback associated with the whole muscle approach is that it assumes that a muscle's properties are simply the sum of all the available fibers in the muscle and that each fiber exerts the same relative influence.

Maximum Contraction Velocity of Different Muscle Fiber Types

The force-velocity relationship described previously provides a convenient tool for muscle fiber type-specific characterization of speed (how quickly the muscle contracts). The parameter V_{max} can be compared between muscles that have large differences in fiber type distribution to measure fiber type-specific values for V_{max}. Muscle architecture has a profound influence on absolute contraction velocity, and therefore, all absolute velocities measured experimentally must be expressed in terms of a normalized velocity such as fiber lengths per second or sarcomere lengths per second to determine the intrinsic value of V_{max} for a fiber.

Assuming that the correct type of experiment is performed, fast-contracting muscle fibers shorten two to three times faster than slow-contracting fibers at V_{max}. Despite the popular discussion of fiber type distribution, this factor probably has very little to do with performance.

Table 4   Fiber Type Definition Using the ATPase Assay

Preincubation pH	Type 1	Type 2A	Type 2B
9.4	Light	Dark	Dark
4.6	Dark	Light	Medium
4.3	Dark	Light	Medium

Maximum Tension Generated by Different Muscle Fiber Types

In a manner similar to that used for measurement of V_{max}, maximum tetanic tension (P_o) can be measured in muscles of different fiber type distributions. Again, differences in architecture must be accounted for to attribute differences in force to fiber type differences and not to architectural differences (PCSA). This value is then normalized to the PCSA of the muscle studied, to yield the value known as specific tension, or force of contraction per unit area of muscle.

In measuring the specific tension of whole skeletal muscle, most investigators find that muscles composed mainly of fast fibers have a greater specific tension than muscles composed mainly of slow fibers. The typical value for specific tension of fast muscle is approximately 22 N/cm^2 (250 kPa in SI units) whereas that for slow muscle is 10 to 15 N/cm^2 (approximately 125 kPa in SI units). The common interpretation of these whole muscle experiments has been that fast muscle fibers have a greater specific tension than slow muscle fibers. Of course the problem with this interpretation is that it assumes that a muscle fiber from a mixed muscle has the same properties as a muscle fiber of the same type that is in a homogeneous muscle. This assumption may not be true.

The best estimates of specific tension come from isometric contractile experiments of single motor units. Muscle fibers within a motor unit can be classified and are generally the same fiber type. Thus, if the force generated by a motor unit is measured, and the motor unit PCSA is determined, specific tension of different motor unit types (and therefore muscle fiber types) can be calculated. The advantage of this method is that the contractile properties are all measured from the same fiber type. The difficulty with this scenario is that measurement of motor unit PCSA is extremely technically difficult. Generally, methods used for motor unit PCSA determination are extremely indirect, relying on a series of questionable assumptions as previously discussed in the motor unit section of this chapter. In only one experiment have all of the fibers belonging to a motor unit been identified and summed to yield PCSA. These experiments showed that fast muscle fibers develop just slightly more tension than slow muscle fibers. This is the best information available to date on this subject.

Endurance of Different Muscle Fiber Types

The endurance (or its opposite, fatigue) of muscle fibers is even more difficult to precisely define than speed or strength. Endurance depends on the type of work the muscle is required to perform. For example, if the workload is extremely light, there is almost no difference between fiber types. If the workload is extremely heavy, the muscle fibers themselves do not fatigue; rather, the neuromuscular junction fatigues, and again, there is no difference between types. Because EC coupling involves a chain of events, it is possible to produce fatigue by interrupting any point in the chain. Thus, a danger exists in simply ascribing a drop in force to muscle fiber fatigue without understanding the reason for the drop. The currently used method for fatigue measurement was developed for classification of single motor units and will thus be deferred until the motor unit presentation. The endurance of the various motor units (and muscle fiber types) differs considerably. However, it is difficult to give a quantitative difference unless the work conditions are known. Generally, SO fibers have the greatest endurance, followed by FOG fibers, and FG fibers. This is not surprising in that FG fibers have a very low oxidative capacity.

Morphologic Properties of Different Muscle Fiber Types

If the histochemical and physiologic differences between muscle fiber types are understood, structural differences between the various fiber types generally follow logically.

Contractile Protein Differences Between Fiber Types

Although myosin isoform differences are profound, there is really not a large structural difference between the different myosins as determined by electron microscopy and x-ray diffraction. In terms of sarcomere force-generating components, whereas the proteins have very different functional properties, structurally they are quite similar. Fast and slow myosin have approximately the same mass and shape. Muscles composed of either fast or slow sarcomeres have approximately the same filament spacing and cross-bridge density.

Metabolic Differences Between Fiber Types

Clearly, the large difference in oxidative and glycolytic capacity is represented in the cell as large differences in the concentration of the metabolic enzymes. For example, in the fast fibers, the cytoplasm has a much higher concentration of all of the glycolytic intermediates. Similarly, all of the oxidative fibers (FOG and SO) have a much higher concentration of oxidative enzymes. Because oxidative phosphorylation occurs in the mitochondria, oxidative fibers have a higher mitochondrial density than nonoxidative fibers. In a detailed quantitative study of the ultrastructure of the various fiber types, it was demonstrated that highly oxidative fibers have a high concentration of mitochondria (up to 25%) and may contain twice the volume fraction of lipid. This finding alone is one reason why it is difficult to compare the specific tension of the various fiber types even if intact single fibers could be isolated. Not all of the space within the fiber is contractile material, and the difference between the fibers in the amount that is contractile material is type-specific.

Membrane Differences Between Fiber Types

Recall that the T-system and SR are involved in the excitation portion of EC coupling. It makes sense that muscles that are required to respond rapidly (fast fibers) would have a well-developed membranous activation system. This is exactly what has been demonstrated in quantitative studies. The SR and T-system of fast fibers may occupy two to three times more volume in fast fibers than slow fibers. Thus, differences in speed between fast and slow fibers result from differences in cross-bridge cycling rates and differences in activation speed.

Z-Disk Structural Differences Between Fiber Types

A final interesting structural difference between fiber types that is very useful but poorly understood is the difference between muscle fiber type Z-disk thickness. It has been shown that FG fibers have the most narrow Z-disks (60 nm) whereas SO fibers have the widest Z-disks (150 nm). The thickness of the Z-disk in FOG fibers is intermediate (80 nm). As stated, the reason for this difference is not clear, but in eccentric contraction-induced muscle injury, the Z-disk appears to be the weak link that is most susceptible to injury.

Plasticity of Muscle Fiber Type

Despite classification of fiber types into specific categories, it must be emphasized that muscle fiber type is extremely plastic given the right conditions. The classic studies of the 1960s and 1970s revealed that chronic electrical stimulation of skeletal muscle can progressively transform fast skeletal muscle cells into slow muscle cells. Although there are subtle differences among muscles in terms of the nature, extent, and time course of the transformation, the results are surprisingly consistent. There is general agreement that chronic electrical stimulation produces increased capillary density, increased percentage of type 1 muscle fibers, decreased fiber size (if the stimulation duration is long enough), increased endurance, and decreased strength. This serves as a template that describes the changes that occur in skeletal muscle with increased use. Voluntary exercise, especially when performed for long durations, results in many of the same muscular changes. Spasticity is often believed to result in changes typically seen in increased-use models.

The opposite model, chronic decreased use of skeletal muscle, which can be studied using models of simulated weightlessness, tenotomy, immobilization in a shortened position, or spinal cord isolation, causes muscle fibers to decrease their size and transform in the direction of the faster phenotype. One of the most extreme examples of such a transformation was reported in a rat spinal cord injury model in which the rats lived about half their life span with upper motor neuron lesions and, as a result, converted almost all of their muscle fibers to the fastest phenotype, even in the very slow soleus muscle. Similar results have been reported in humans after traumatic spinal cord injury. With this knowledge, it becomes clear that an analysis of skeletal muscle fiber type distribution can be a useful indicator of the amount and type of activity that a muscle has received over an extended period of time. In addition to fiber type distribution, muscle fiber size provides insights into the extent of fiber use. Obviously, increased use of skeletal muscle at high loads produces muscle fiber hypertrophy, whereas decreased use yields muscle cellular atrophy. Both responses appear to be load dependent. Thus, fiber size is typically interpreted as an indirect indicator of the amount of force imposed on a muscle.

Muscle fiber type distribution and muscle fiber size distribution are parameters that provide insight into the overall type and amount of muscle use. Therefore, these parameters are often studied in spastic muscle in an attempt to determine its use pattern. However, despite the ease of measuring these parameters, they are not extremely specific and probably only provide a general indicator of muscle use.

Summary

Skeletal muscle is highly organized at the microscopic and macroscopic levels. It is clear that skeletal muscles, arranged using different architectural strategies, are able to produce the high forces or high excursions required for human movement and postural control. The mechanical properties of muscle and the length-tension and force-velocity relationships provide muscle with the length and load sensitivity needed to move with great coordination or power. Finally, the diversity among fiber types permits different muscles to perform functions requiring high loads for brief periods or low continuous loads for extended periods. These properties should all be understood and put to use by the orthopaedic surgeon when planning and performing procedures that affect human movement.

Selected Bibliography

General

Aidley DJ: *The Physiology of Excitable Cells.* New York, NY, Cambridge University Press, 1989.

Engel AG, Banker AQ (eds): *Myology.* New York, NY, McGraw-Hill Book Company, 1986.

Enoka R (ed): *Neuromechanical Basis of Kinesiology.* Champaign, IL, Human Kinetics, 1994.

Lieber R (ed): *Skeletal Muscle Structure, Function, and Plasticity.* Philadelphia, PA, Lippincott Williams & Wilkins, 2002.

Pette D (ed): *The Dynamic State of Muscle Fibers.* Berlin, Germany, Walter de Gruyter, 1990.

Skeletal Muscle Anatomy

Belcastro A: Skeletal muscle calcium-activated neutral protease (Calpain) with exercise. *J Appl Physiol* 1993; 74:1381-1386.

Lazarides E: Intermediate filaments as mechanical integrators of cellular space. *Nature* 1980;283:249-256.

Lieber RL, Thornell L-E, Fridén J: Muscle cytoskeletal disruption occurs within the first 15 minutes of cyclic eccentric contraction. *J Appl Physiol* 1996;80:278-284.

Peachey LD, Eisenberg BR: Helicoids in the T system and striations of frog skeletal muscle fibers seen by high voltage electron microscopy. *Biophys J* 1978;22: 145-154.

Whole Skeletal Muscle Structure

Bodine SC, Roy RR, Meadows DA, et al: Architectural, histochemical, and contractile characteristics of a unique biarticular muscle: The cat semitendinosus. *J Neurophysiol* 1982;48:192-201.

Burkholder TJ, Fingado B, Baron S, Lieber RL: Relationship between muscle fiber types and sizes and muscle architectural properties in the mouse hindlimb. *J Morphol* 1994;221:177-190.

Gans C, Bock WJ: The functional significance of muscle architecture: A theoretical analysis. *Ergeb Anat Entwicklungsgesch* 1965;38:115-142.

Lieber RL, Friden J: Functional and clinical significance of skeletal muscle architecture. *Muscle Nerve* 2000;23:1647-1666.

Powell PL, Roy RR, Kanim P, Bello M, Edgerton VR: Predictability of skeletal muscle tension from architectural determinations in guinea pig hindlimbs. *J Appl Physiol* 1984;57:1715-1721.

Sacks RD, Roy RR: Architecture of the hindlimb muscles of cats: Functional significance. *J Morphol* 1982; 173:185-195.

Architecture of Human Skeletal Muscle
Friden J, Albrecht D, Lieber RL: Biomechanical analysis of the brachioradialis as a donor in tendon transfer. *Clin Orthop Relat Res* 2001;383:152-161.

Friden J, Lieber RL: Mechanical considerations in the design of surgical reconstructive procedures. *J Biomech* 2002;35:1039-1045.

Friden J, Lieber RL: Tendon transfer surgery: Clinical implications of experimental studies. *Clin Orthop Relat Res* 2002;(suppl 403):S163-S170.

Jacobson MD, Raab R, Fazeli BM, Abrams RA, Botte MJ, Lieber RL: Architectural design of the human intrinsic hand muscles. *J Hand Surg [Am]* 1992;17:804-809.

Lieber RL, Fazeli BM, Botte MJ: Architecture of selected wrist flexor and extensor muscles. *J Hand Surg [Am]* 1990;15:244-250.

Lieber RL, Jacobson MD, Fazeli BM, Abrams RA, Botte MJ: Architecture of selected muscles of the arm and forearm: Anatomy and implications for tendon transfer. *J Hand Surg [Am]* 1992;17:787-798.

Skeletal Muscle Physiology
Dykstra DD: Botulinum toxin in the management of bowel and bladder function in spinal cord injury and other neurologic disorders. *Phys Med Rehabil Clin N Am* 2003;14:793-804.

Ebashi S, Maruyama K, Endo M (eds): *Muscle Contraction: Its Regulatory Mechanisms*. New York, NY, Springer Verlag, 1980.

Entman ML, van Winkle WB (eds): *Sarcoplasmic Reticulum in Muscle Physiology*. Boca Raton, FL, CRC Press, 1986.

Hambrecht FT, Reswick JB (eds): *Functional Electrical Stimulation: Applications in Neural Prostheses*. New York, NY, Marcel Dekker, 1977.

Skeletal Muscle Mechanics
Freehafer AA, Peckham PH, Keith MW: Determination of muscle-tendon unit properties during tendon transfer. *J Hand Surg [Am]* 1979;4:331-339.

Friden J, Lieber RL: Evidence for muscle attachment at relatively long lengths in tendon transfer surgery. *J Hand Surg [Am]* 1998;23:105-110.

Horowits R, Kempner ES, Bisher ME, Podolsky RJ: A physiological role for titin and nebulin in skeletal muscle. *Nature* 1986;323:160-164.

Labeit S, Kolmerer B: Titins: Giant proteins in charge of muscle ultrastructure and elasticity. *Science* 1995; 270:293-296.

Lieber RL, Murray W, Clark DL, Hentz VR, Fridén J: Biomechanical properties of the brachioradialis muscle: Implications for surgical tendon transfer. *J Hand Surg [Am]* 2005;30:273-282.

Magid A, Law DJ: Myofibrils bear most of the resting tension in frog skeletal muscle. *Science* 1985;230:1280-1282.

Podolsky RJ, Shoenberg M: Force generation and shortening in skeletal muscle, in *Handbook of Physiology*. Baltimore, MD, American Physiological Society, 1983, pp 173-187.

Force-Velocity Relationship Describes Isotonic Muscle Contraction
Harry JD, Ward AW, Heglund NC, Morgan DL, McMahon TA: Cross-bridge cycling theories cannot explain high-speed lengthening behavior in frog muscle. *Biophys J* 1990;57:201-208.

Morgan DL: New insights into the behavior of muscle during active lengthening. *Biophys J* 1990;57:209-221.

Common Methods Used for Typing Muscle Fibers
Barany M: ATPase activity of myosin correlated with speed of muscle shortening. *J Gen Physiol* 1967;50:197-218.

Brooke MH, Kaiser KK: Muscle fiber types: How many and what kind? *Arch Neurol* 1970;23:369-379.

Dubowitz V, Brooke MH (eds): *Muscle Biopsy: A Modern Approach*. Philadelphia, PA, WB Saunders, 1973.

Eisenberg BR: Quantitative ultrastructure of mammalian skeletal muscle, in Peachey LD, Adrian RH, Geiger SR (eds): *Skeletal Muscle*. Baltimore, MD, American Physiological Society, 1983, pp 73-112.

Smerdu V, Karsch-Mizrachi I, Campione M, Leinwand L, Schiaffino S: Type IIx myosin heavy chain transcripts are expressed in type IIb fibers of human skeletal muscle. *Am J Physiol* 1994;267:C1723-C1728.

Physiologic Properties of Muscle Fiber Types
Bodine SC, Roy RR, Eldred E, Edgerton VR: Maximal force as a function of anatomical features of motor units in the cat tibialis anterior. *J Neurophysiol* 1987; 57:1730-1745.

Close RI: Dynamic properties of mammalian skeletal muscles. *Physiol Rev* 1972;52:129-197.

Morphologic Properties of Different Muscle Fiber Types
Gonzalez-Serratos H: Inward spread of activation in vertebrate muscle fibers. *J Physiol* 1971;212:777-799.

Haselgrove JC: Structure of vertebrate striated muscle as determined by x-ray-diffraction studies, in *Handbook of Physiology*. Bethesda, MD, American Physiological Society, 1983, pp 143-171.

Zappe HA, Maeda Y: X-ray diffraction study of fast and slow mammalian skeletal muscle in the live relaxed state. *J Mol Biol* 1985;185:211-214.

Plasticity of Muscle Fiber Type
Booth FW, Kelso JR: Effect of hind-limb immobilization on contractile and histochemical properties of skeletal muscle. *Pflugers Arch* 1973;342:231-238.

Buller AJ, Lewis DM: Some observations on the effects of tenotomy in the rabbit. *J Physiol* 1965;178:326-342.

Eisenberg BR, Salmons S: The reorganization of subcellular structure in muscle undergoing fast-to-slow type transformation: A stereological study. *Cell Tissue Res* 1981;220:449-471.

Grimby G, Broberg C, Krotkiewska I, Krotkiewski M: Muscle fiber composition in patients with traumatic cord lesion. *Scand J Rehabil Med* 1976;8:37-42.

Lieber RL, Friden JO, Hargens AR, Feringa ER: Long-term effects of spinal cord transection of fast and slow rat skeletal muscle: II. Morphometric properties. *Exp Neurol* 1986;91:435-448.

Lieber RL, Johansson CB, Vahlsing HL, Hargens AR, Feringa ER: Long-term effects of spinal cord transection on fast and slow rat skeletal muscle: I. Contractile properties. *Exp Neurol* 1986;91:423-434.

Maier A, Cocket JL, Simpson DR, Saubert CI, Edgerton VR: Properties of immobilized guinea pig hind limb muscles. *Am J Physiol* 1976;231:1520-1526.

Pette D (ed): *Plasticity of Muscle*. New York, NY, Walter de Gruyter, 1980.

Pette D, Smith M, Staudte H, Vrbova G: Effects of long-term electrical stimulation on some contractile and metabolic characteristics of fast rabbit muscles. *Pflugers Arch* 1973;338:257-272.

Roy R, Bello M, Bouissou P, Edgerton R: Size and metabolic properties of fibers in rat fast-twitch muscles after hindlimb suspension. *J Appl Physiol* 1987;62: 2348-2357.

Roy RR, Pierotti DJ, Flores V, Rudolph W, Edgerton VR: Fibre size and type adaptations to spinal isolation and cyclical passive stretch in cat hindlimb. *J Anat* 1992;180:491-499.

Roy RR, Sacks RD, Baldwin KM, Short M, Edgerton VR: Interrelationships of contraction time, Vmax, and myosin ATPase after spinal transection. *J Appl Physiol* 1984;56:1594-1601.

Salmons S, Henriksson J: The adaptive response of skeletal muscle to increased use. *Muscle Nerve* 1981;4: 94-105.

Salmons S, Streter FA: Significance of impulse activity in the transformation of skeletal muscle type. *Nature* 1976;263:30-34.

Salmons S, Vrbova G: The influence of activity on some contractile characteristics of mammalian fast and slow muscles. *J Physiol* 1969;201:535-549.

Saltin B, Gollnick PD (eds): Skeletal muscle adaptability: Significance for metabolism and performance, in *Handbook of Physiology*. Baltimore, MD, American Physiological Society, 1983, pp 539-554.

Chapter 13

Form and Function of the Peripheral Nerves and Spinal Cord

Ranjan Gupta, MD
Tahseen Mozaffar, MD

Introduction

At the beginning of the 20th century, Spanish anatomist Cajal wrote that "each nerve cell, whatever its functional category, appears to be constructed according to the same model and to possess the same texture and chemical composition." The human nervous system defines the very nature of humanity. Through this complex and intricate system, effective communication and response is possible within the body and to the environment. Over the course of thousands of years, this system has evolved to allow complex, coordinated movements (such as playing a Beethoven piano concerto) while retaining basic reflexes (such as withdrawal from pain). These capabilities are facilitated by a variety of cells that make up the central nervous system (CNS) (brain and spinal cord) and the peripheral nervous system (PNS). The PNS provides the mechanism for relaying information between the CNS and the environment. Although the complexity and detail of this system still remain beyond the understanding of modern neuroscientists, the system has an innate simplicity as indicated by Cajal. The nervous system is composed of relatively few different cell types including neurons and glial cells. Neurons are composed of a cell body, dendrite, axon, and presynaptic terminal. Nerves are bundles of axons enclosed in specialized connective sheaths. Within the nerve, there are several different satellite cells known as glial cells. This basic framework organizes the nervous system.

Anatomy and Physiology of Peripheral Nerves

The primary cell of the nervous system is the neuron. This polarized cell, with dendrites to receive information and axons to send information, is responsible for relaying and storing information. The transfer of information is effectively performed as the axon of one neuron relays infor-mation to the dendrite of another neuron at a region known as the synapse. Each neuron usually has several dendrites that meet at the cell body, also known as the perikaryon or the soma. The axon hillock is a specialized region of the perikaryon that functions to generate an action potential for signal propagation. It is from this region of the perikaryon that the axon originates. The axon is responsible for the propagation of the action potential from one neuron to the next. The axon will terminate at either a synapse to relay information to an adjacent dendrite or at the motor end plate (neuromuscular junction) to relay information to a muscle cell. Both axons and dendrites contain not only mitochondria, but also cytoskeletal elements such as microtubules and neurofilaments. At the ultrastructural level, axons differ from dendrites; axons typically lack ribosomes and extend for substantial distances before branching or terminating. Axons require several intracellular transport systems that are dependent on adenosine 5'-triphosphate (ATP), calcium, and microtubules. The transport of molecules from the perikaryon toward the terminus is known as anterograde transport and may occur by either slow or fast anterograde transport mechanisms. Fast anterograde transport occurs at speeds up to 400 mm/day and relies on the carrier protein kinesin. Although fast anterograde transport uses this ATPase to transport macromolecules and mitochondria, slow anterograde transport is responsible for the movement of neuronal structural components. Retrograde transport allows the neuron to recycle proteins (empty neurotransmitter vesicles) and occurs at one half to one third the rate of fast anterograde transport. This transport mechanism relies on the carrier protein dynenin, and picks up signals from the environment (such as chromatolysis after axonotomy). Retrograde axonal transport plays a critical role in many clinical conditions including herpes simplex virus, polio, rabies, and tetanus because they are all transported by this mechanism. Axonal transport mechanisms are altered with both diabetes and amyotrophic lateral sclerosis.

Although possessing an electrical charge is not a unique characteristic of neurons, the ability of neurons to control their own charge and that of surrounding cells is unique. This electrical charge allows information to be transferred between the nervous system and the environment through a series of electrical and chemical signals. The interior of a cell has a resting potential because of the unequal distribution of monovalent ions that cannot cross the plasma membrane (Na^+, K^+, Cl^-, A^-). Ion channels, formed by proteins with a hydrophilic core, exist within the plasma membrane to control the flow of ions based on the specificity of the channel. At rest, the channels are relatively permeable to K^+ and Cl^- ions, but not to Na^+ ions and the proteins within the neuron that are aggregately negatively charged. Based on the concentration differences across the plasma membrane, each ion has a diffusion potential that dictates the equilibrium potential for each ion. For ion A, the equilibrium potential for that ion is calculated with the Nernst equation:

$$E = \frac{RT}{FZ} \ln \frac{[A] \text{ outside}}{[A] \text{ inside}}$$

Where E is the membrane potential, R is the universal gas constant, T is the temperature in absolute degrees Kelvin, F is the Faraday constant, and Z is the ion valence. At 25°C, RT/FZ= 26 mV.

In addition to the unequal distribution of ions, an ATP pump transports three Na^+ ions out of the cell while transporting two K^+ ions into the cell. Each ion creates a voltage difference across the membrane based on its equilibrium potential and its own internal resistance as related to the membrane permeability. Without a sodium-potassium pump, there would be a net flow of ions that would equalize the equilibrium potentials. The resting potential is maintained with the sodium-potassium pump between 50 and 80 mV. The inside of the neuronal cell is negatively charged relative to the outside of the cell. At the resting state, the resistances of Na^+ and Cl^- batteries are relatively high compared with K^+. As such, the resting transmembrane potential of the neuron is closest to the K^+ equilibrium potential and can be determined by the Goldman-Hodgkin-Katz equation (V = voltage; g = conductance; K = potassium; E = membrane potential):

$$V_{membrane} = \frac{g_K E_K + g_{Na} E_{Na} + g_{Cl} E_{Cl}}{g_K + g_{Na} + g_{Cl}}$$

Neurons may develop a graded potential, either a hyperpolarizing or depolarizing local change in membrane potential that is related to the intensity of the stimuli and varies continuously in amplitude. Different types of graded potentials include the receptor potential, the pace-maker potential (cardiac versus gastrointestinal), and the synaptic potential. These potentials depend on the passive properties of the cell membrane including the internal resistance (Ri; longitudinal) of the axon, the transverse/membrane resistance (Rm; across the axon), and the capacitance (Cm). The neuron is a leaky capacitor governed by the following laws of physics: V = IR and τ = RC (V = voltage/potential difference; I = current; R = resistance; C = capacitance). τ is the time constant and is used to express the rate of change of the capacitance as related to the resistance. When a current pulse is applied across a membrane, the voltage pulse spreads down the membrane and declines as it progresses. This rate of decline is defined by the length constant or space constant λ. Because unmyelinated axons and dendrites have a λ of 10 to 100 μ, graded potentials such as receptor or synaptic potentials do not travel far before degrading. A decrease in the intracellular longitudinal resistance or an increase in transmembrane resistance will serve to increase λ. A decrease in membrane capacitance will decrease the time constant (τ). These three natural strategies are used to propagate the voltage pulse more rapidly while preventing the decline in amplitude over distance.

An action potential is used to transmit messages rapidly over long distances. This depolarization occurs when the graded potentials summate beyond a threshold level. When initiated, the membrane no longer follows the equation V = IR. The neuron becomes more permeable as the conductance to Na^+ increases and the Na^+ voltage-gated channels open. At the point where Na^+ permeability exceeds K^+ permeability, the potential reverses and now approaches the Na^+ equilibrium potential. At the peak of the action potential, the inward Na^+ current will briefly equal the outward K^+ current. The inactivation of the Na^+ gates and increased activation of the K^+ gates bring the membrane potential back to the resting potential as the ion permeabilities return to normal levels. During the rising phase and the early falling phase of the action potential, the membrane will not respond to additional stimuli during the absolute refractory period (all or none phenomenon). As the falling phase continues, a relative refractory phase occurs during which a smaller action potential may be generated with a stronger depolarization trigger. The rate of action potential conductance is related to passive membrane properties including the internal resistance of the axoplasm. The internal resistance of the axon decreases as the square of the axonal diameter increases. When the axonal diameter becomes greater than 1 μm, only mild increases in conduction velocity occur. In vertebrates, this adaptation is unreasonable secondary to the large number of axons. As such, the increase in conduction velocity is created with the formation of myelin to increase membrane resistance and decrease capacitance; thus, the rate of passive current flow increases as τ decreases. The net result is that current from an active node will jump to the next node to produce saltatory conduction and will avoid the high resistance of myelinated regions of the axons. At the nodes of Ranvier, there is a high concentration of voltage-gated sodium channels.

Myelin is a complex structure that is formed by oligodendrocytes and Schwann cells to increase the speed of conduction of the action potential. Myelin is 70% lipid and 30% protein. Although the lipids such as cholesterol, phospholipids, and galactolipids are not unique to myelin, the myelin proteins are unique. The primary myelin proteins of the CNS include proteolipid and myelin basic proteins. The myelin proteins of the PNS are P0 glycoprotein, myelin-associated glycoprotein, and plasma membrane protein-22. Larger diameter axons have an increased ability to propagate an action potential because these axons have a thicker myelin sheath, which increases the rate of action potential conduction. Although Schwann cells and oligodendrocytes belong to the family of glial cells known as macroglia, they differ in that oligodendrocytes are present in the CNS and can insulate several axons, whereas Schwann cells are present in the PNS and myelinate only a region of one axon. The CNS nodes are exposed to the extracellular environment, whereas the nodes of the PNS are covered by a basal lamina. Each PNS axon may be myelinated by as many as 500 Schwann cells. Whereas Schwann cells are usually present at an interval of 0.1 to 1.0 mm along the axon with intervening nodes of Ranvier, oligodendrocytes are usually present at intervals of 0.2 mm. The nodes of Ranvier are regions of the nerve where the myelinated sheath is discontinuous at regular intervals to allow salutatory conduction of the action potential.

Other glial cells exist within the nervous system. The astrocyte, which provides both support and structure to the brain and spinal cord, is a CNS cell and member of the macroglia family. Astrocytes terminate in cellular processes that are known as end-feet, and line the external surfaces of the CNS (glia limitans) or the CNS blood vessels (blood-brain barrier). Astrocytes located in the gray matter of the spinal cord are known as protoplasmic astrocytes, whereas those in the white matter are known as fibrous astrocytes, secondary to the increased content of intermediate filaments. Astrocytes may be identified immunohistochemically by the presence of glial fibrillary acidic protein, which is found in the intermediate filaments. These cells maintain the extracellular ionic environment, secrete a variety of growth factors and cytokines, and provide a framework for neuronal migration during development. Whereas macroglial cells are derived from the neuroectoderm, the second family of glial cells (known as the microglia) is derived from the mesoderm. Microglial cells are made up of macrophages or phagocytes that are mobilized after injury, infection, or disease and are the predominant cells involved with CNS inflammation. Although these cells are vital for the removal of cellular debris through the activation of interleukin-1β and tumor necrosis factor-α, these cells are also believed to be responsible for secondary injury after trauma such as spinal cord injury.

Neurons communicate with each other at specialized regions known as synapses, which may be electrical or chemical. Electrical synapses are ion channels on two different neurons that appose one another and form connexons to create a low resistance bridge between the neurons. Electrical synapses are rare in mammals. Chemical synaptic transmission follows a fairly well-characterized pathway. Neurotransmitters are synthesized and stored in membrane-bound vesicles within the presynaptic area. When an action potential depolarizes this area, Ca^{2+} influx occurs through voltage-gated Ca^{2+} channels that enable the vesicles to bind to the neuronal membrane. Through exocytosis, the neurotransmitters enter the synaptic cleft and diffuse across the cleft to bind to the receptor on the postsynaptic neuron. The binding of the neurotransmitter-receptor complex induces ion-channel opening, which results in the depolarization or hyperpolarization of the postsynaptic membrane. This process may occur through direct conformational change of the ion channel or through secondary messenger synapses. These later synapses activate a guanosine nucleotide-binding protein that may be coupled to cyclic adenosine monophosphate (cAMP), phospholipase C, or phospholipase A. Unlike single message synapses that remain active only for the length of time that the neurotransmitter-receptor complex exists, the guanosine nucleotide-binding protein-linked synapses persist as the signal is amplified in strength and duration. Neurotransmitters can be classified as either a small-molecule messenger (less than 10 carbons) or as larger neuropeptides. Although small-molecule neurotransmitters including amino acids (gamma-aminobutyric acid, glycine, aspartate, and glutamate), biogenic amines (acetylcholine, dopamine, histamine, and serotonin), and nucleotides (adenosine triphosphate) are located diffusely throughout the nervous system, the neuropeptides including endorphins, cholecystokinin, and oxytocin are located primarily within the CNS.

Classification of Nerve Fibers

Nerve fibers can be classified based on diameter and conduction velocity or neuronal function. Afferent fibers are nerve fibers that carry sensory information from the peripheral receptors to the dorsal ganglion and on to the spinal cord and higher levels. Afferent fibers from the viscera are termed visceral afferents and those from receptors in muscles, skin, and sensory organs of the head are called somatic afferents. Motor information from the CNS is carried to motor effector organs (skeletal muscles) by nerve fibers called efferent fibers; the nerves carrying these efferent fibers to the skin, skeletal muscles, and the joints are called somatic nerves. Efferent nerve fibers that carry information to the visceral organs, and that are in-

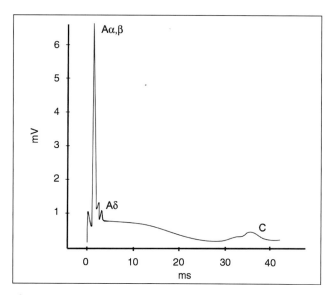

Figure 1   Nerve fiber type. Conduction velocities of peripheral nerves are measured clinically from compound action potentials. Aα and Aβ fibers, being the largest, have large early potentials that occur almost immediately. Aδ nerve fibers fire next and C fibers, which are unmyelinated, have action potentials that fire much later than other nerve fibers. mV = millivolt, ms = millisecond.

Table 1 Afferent Fiber Groups in Peripheral Nerves				
	Muscle Nerve*	Cutaneous Nerves*	Fiber Diameter (μm)	Conduction Velocity (m/s)
Myelinated				
Large	I	Aα	12-20	72-120
Medium	II	Aβ	6-12	36-72
Small	III	Aδ	1-6	4-36
Unmyelinated	IV	C	0.2-1.5	0.4-2.0

* Sensory nerves in muscle are classified according to their fiber diameters. Sensory afferents in cutaneous nerves are classified by conduction velocities.

volved with the function of these organs, are called autonomic efferents; the nerves are called autonomic nerves.

Nerve fibers were originally classified on the basis of axon diameter and conduction velocity (**Figure 1**). Nerve fibers are currently classified into types A, B, and C, with subcategories for A fibers; each has distinct histologic and electrophysiologic characteristics (**Table 1**). The A fibers are myelinated somatic axons, either afferent or efferent. The B fibers are myelinated efferent axons that constitute the preganglionic axons of the autonomic nerves. The unmyelinated C fibers consist of the efferent postganglionic axons of autonomic nerves and the small afferent axons of the dorsal root and peripheral nerves. These C fibers, unlike the large A and B fibers, are unmyelinated; several C fibers share a single Schwann cell. These characteristics and the absence of myelin sheath allow histologic identification of the C fibers.

Peripheral Nerve Development, Structure, and Biomechanics
Development
The origin of the PNS is ectodermal; most of the cells are derived from the neural crest. These cells arise from the lateral edge of the neural plate and migrate laterally to the neural tube. The extracellular matrix in a limb provides path guidance and promotes growth. The matrix proteins responsible for this specificity and guidance include N-cadherin, neural cell adhesion molecules (expressed on neural ectoderm and axons of differentiated neurons),

laminin (most effective in promoting neurite growth), fibronectin, collagen, and tenacin. Schwann cells also are derived from the neural crest and migrate in a segmental manner following the outgrowing developing fibers.

Myelin is a multilamellar, membranous sheath with a high lipid-to-protein ratio that surrounds the axons of CNS and PNS nerves to improve the conduction of action potentials through saltatory conduction. After the first half of the gestational period, before the nervous system becomes fully functional, oligodendrocytes form CNS myelin and Schwann cells form PNS myelin. This process is usually complete by 2 years of age. Myelination in the CNS proceeds along the neuroaxis (spinal cord, brainstem, and forebrain) and continues until the third decade of life. The interaction between axons and glia is critical for development and for nerve regeneration. One of the critical axonally derived Schwann cell survival signals is the β-neuregulins that bind to the erb B4 receptors of Schwann cells. Data from studies on mice lacking either neuregulin or its receptor provide confirmation that these factors are important for survival and maturation of Schwann cell precursors. Although it is known that the presence of an axonal signal is necessary for the initiation of myelination, the actual signal for this process has not been identified. It is known that axon-Schwann cell contact is critical and that a diffusible molecule is probably produced by axons with a diameter greater than 0.7 μm. When Schwann cells receive this signal, gene expression patterns change as the Schwann cells transition from nonmyelinating to myelinating cells and synthesize a variety of myelin components. Transcription factors are believed to regulate this Schwann cell gene expression. The gene nuclear factor kappa B is one of the earliest transcription factors that must be activated along the progression from nonmyelinating to myelinating Schwann cells. This activation is followed by activation of Oct-6 (a POU domain transcription factor), also known as cAMP-inducible POU (SCIP), which is expressed in late Schwann cell progenitors and promyelinating Schwann cells, but is not expressed in the terminal differentiation phase of mature

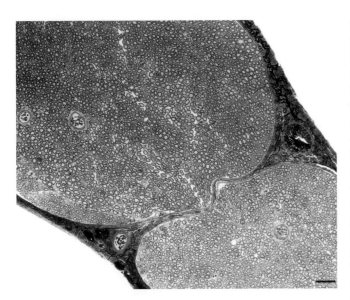

Figure 2   Histologic appearance of normal nerve with two distinct group fascicles (toluidine blue stained). Scale bar 80 μm.

myelinating Schwann cells. After Oct-6 expression is downregulated, the *Krox-20* gene encodes a zinc finger transcription factor that is necessary for myelination. *Krox-20* regulates not only myelin-specific genes, but also cell adhesion molecules and growth factors. Its absence blocks Schwann cell differentiation and prevents myelin formation. Prior to myelination, Schwann cells express nerve growth factor receptor and several adhesion molecules, which are downregulated after contact with axons. After Schwann cells receive the axonally derived signal to initiate myelination, upregulation occurs in several myelin-specific proteins including myelin-associated glycoprotein, myelin basic protein, and P0 glycoprotein. P0 glycoprotein is an integral membrane adhesion molecule because it promotes the compaction of myelin through homophilic interactions. Myelin basic protein works with P0 glycoprotein to maintain the major dense line of the myelin. Data collected from multiple studies with transgenic null, mutant mice have clearly shown that the formation of myelin is relatively insensitive to molecular changes, whereas the maintenance of myelin is far more labile.

Nerve Architecture

Peripheral nerves are organized by several different layers of connective tissue, including a blood-nerve barrier (**Figure 2**). The external epineurium is the outermost layer of the peripheral nerve that provides a supportive and protective framework. The internal epineurium surrounds individual fascicles, cushions against external pressure, and allows longitudinal excursion. It has a well-developed vascular plexus with channels feeding endoneurial plexuses. Along the nerve path, larger amounts of this layer occur at the level of joints. The next layer, the perineurium, is a

thin, dense sheath that surrounds each fascicle and acts as the blood-nerve barrier (an extension of the blood-brain barrier). It is composed of up to 10 layers and has flattened mesothelial cells with tight junctions that act as a bidirectional barrier to diffusion. It provides high tensile strength that resists up to 750 mm Hg. The deepest layer and smallest unit of the perineurium is the endoneurium, the loose collagenous matrix that surrounds individual nerve fibers. Neural tissue is organized into fascicles, with groups of axons packed with endoneurial connective tissue. The fascicle is also the smallest unit of the nerve that can be surgically manipulated. It forms plexuses that are not simply parallel, and that possess a high degree of variability. This structure changes rapidly; along the length of a major nerve the maximal unaltered segment will be 15 to 20 mm. The blood supply of the peripheral nerve is composed of well-developed intraneural microvascular plexuses. Both intrinsic and extrinsic segmental longitudinal vessels run in loose connective tissue surrounding the nerve and communicate with the intraneural microvascular plexuses.

Nerve Biomechanics

It is important to understand the biomechanical properties of nerves to better appreciate the effects of injury and the repair and regenerative processes. Nerves are complex, heterogeneous composite structures that are composed of neurons, Schwann cells, fibroblasts, and collagen. Nerves exhibit nonlinear stress-strain viscoelastic behavior with both creep and stress relaxation properties. Early studies have detailed the time-dependent nature of nerves. A rapid decrease in nerve tension occurs after acute fixed lengthening. This change suggests that a nerve repair with gradual apposition of nerve fibers would lower the peak tension at the time of repair and would reduce the potential stretch-induced injury. Greater stress relaxation also occurs at the lower strain rates. With increased time after transection of the peripheral nerve, the stress relaxation properties of the nerve significantly decrease and may subsequently increase the tension at the suture line with a delayed neurorrhaphy. Under tension, rabbit nerves exhibit a low modulus that increases gradually with increasing strain. When the nerve fails under tension, the perineurium ruptures, whereas the epineurium remains intact. In situ, the resting nerve is under minimal stress, but is under significant strain that varies with changes in limb position.

Several cadaveric studies have provided knowledge concerning changes in nerve tension and strain resulting from changes in limb position. In one study, the excursion and strain of the median nerve was measured with the limb in several different positions. Shoulder motion created median nerve excursion at the elbow of 9.1 mm and a change in strain of 13.3%. Although elbow motion induced 12.3 mm of median nerve excursion at the elbow, no significant change in nerve strain occurred. Although wrist motion caused 5.6 mm of excursion and 14.8% strain of the median nerve at the wrist, digital motion only resulted in 3.4 mm of excursion and 10.3% change in strain. Factors limiting this motion are believed to alter normal nerve function. Similar cadaveric studies performed on the ulnar nerve at the elbow confirmed that significant motion of the ulnar nerve normally occurs with a potential for 21.9 mm of excursion at the elbow and 23.2 mm of excursion at the wrist. Other studies of the ulnar nerve have detailed the changes in intraneural pressure that occur with changes in elbow posture. With increasing elbow flexion, the mean intraneural pressure increased relative to the extraneural pressure as the ulnar nerve also decreased in mean cross-sectional area. These changes are not limited to the cubital tunnel, but include the medial epicondyle and the region deep to the flexor carpi ulnaris. The fact that the ulnar nerve has at least a 10% increase in strain levels at the medial epicondyle with maximum elbow flexion provides evidence that cubital tunnel syndrome occurs secondary to both compression and traction forces. In another study, normal ulnar nerve strain at the elbow measured 5.3% and decreased to 4.3% after decompression, and −0.54% after decompression and medial epicondylectomy. Other surgical procedures for cubital tunnel syndrome involve ulnar nerve mobilization and transposition anterior to the medial epicondyle. These anterior transposition procedures have been shown to cause significant changes in neural excursion, ultimate strain, ultimate strength, and modulus; the procedures may lead to improved function.

Many early studies have attempted to evaluate the biomechanical properties of nerves by focusing on stress-strain curves in a manner similar to that used to evaluate ligaments and tendons. Other studies have focused on the relationship between increased tension and blood flow. A study by Lundborg and Rydevik showed that nerve elongation of more than 8% to 10% of resting length caused impairment of intraneural blood flow. A 15% increase in nerve elongation caused complete occlusion of intraneural blood flow. Other studies have shown that 8% nerve elongation decreased neural blood flow by 50%; however, the flow level recovered after the increase in tension. A 16% nerve elongation decreased blood flow by 80% and the nerve did not recover after stretch. Recent studies have evaluated how changes in the biomechanical properties of the nerve affect the neural physiology. Sustained increases in nerve tension alter the neural electrophysiology; an in situ strain of 8% prevents compound muscle action-potential generation and propagation. Because changes in the biomechanical parameters that alter nerve conduction velocity and latency values have not been shown to correlate with blood flow changes, it is suggested that ischemia alone is not responsible for the electrophysiologic changes. Limited understanding currently exists regarding the cellular, biochemical, and molecular changes of the neurons and surrounding glia in response to altered me-

chanical loading. Less information is known about how altered mechanical loading of nerves may detrimentally affect neural regeneration and promote gliosis. Answers to these important clinical questions will help improve the functional outcomes of patients after neural injury.

Anatomy of the Spinal Cord

The spinal cord is a vital part of the CNS that relays sensory input from the environment to higher levels of the neuroaxis, directs motor activity through somatic and visceral motor neurons, possesses intrinsic reflex properties, and influences the activity of spinal neurons through descending tracts. The spinal cord is derived from a specialized portion of the ectoderm that is posterior to the notochord, the neural plate. The caudal portion of the neural plate develops into the cervical, thoracic, and lumbar regions of the spinal cord. The sacral and coccygeal regions of the spinal cord are derived from the caudal eminence. The neural plate begins to fold (moving in a rostral to caudal direction) and meets at the midline (starting at day 21 of gestation) to form the neural tube. If the neural folds do not meet and undifferentiated neuroectoderm remains, the embryo will have severe defects such as rachischisis or anencephaly. If the neural tube is formed, but the overlying vertebrae fail to develop, the resulting range of defects include spina bifida occulta and meningocele.

The spinal cord spans the distance from the foramen magnum to the second lumbar vertebrae. Axons enter and exit the spinal cord via the spinal nerves, each of which consists of a ventral or efferent root and a dorsal or afferent root. The ventral roots carry output to the striated muscles from the myelinated nerve fibers of the alpha and gamma motor neurons in the gray matter of the ventral horn. The dorsal roots carry sensory input from myelinated and unmyelinated nerve fibers that originate from somatic sensory receptors. The cell bodies of the afferent fibers are located in the dorsal root ganglia. The spinal cord has 8 cervical, 12 thoracic, 5 lumbar, 5 sacral, and 1 coccygeal levels that produce spinal nerves that exit through the corresponding intervertebral foramina (Figure 3). At both the C4 to T1 region and the L1 to S2 region, the spinal cord is enlarged and forms the basis for the brachial and lumbar plexuses, respectively. The nomenclature of the spinal nerves is such that the C1 through C7 nerve roots exit rostral to their corresponding vertebral body; the C8 nerve root exits caudal to the C7 vertebral body. All subsequent nerve roots exit caudal to their corresponding vertebral bodies. The spinal cord is further subdivided into white and gray matter. The descending tracts from the cortex and subcortical parts of the brain and the ascending fiber tracts are organized into well-demarcated and somatotopically arranged columns. These columns contain both myelinated and unmyelinated nerve axons. The central portion of the spinal cord contains the gray matter; it is an x-shaped structure, which contains longitu-

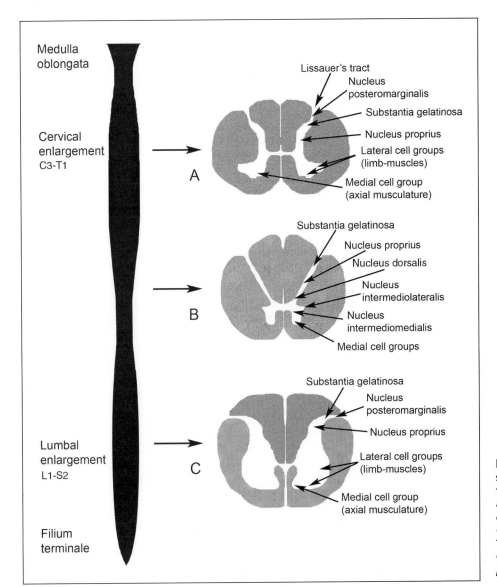

Figure 3   Illustrations of cross sections of the spinal cord at the cervical **(A)**, thoracic **(B)**, and lumbar **(C)** regions. *(Reproduced with permission from Gluhbegovic N, Williams TH: The Human Brain and Spinal Cord. Philadelphia, PA, JB Lippincott, 1980.)*

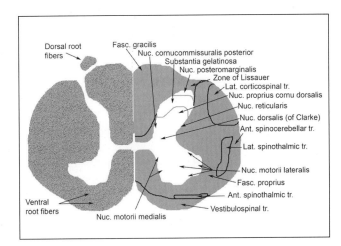

Figure 4   Illustration of the cellular organization of the spinal cord. Fasc = fasciculus, Nuc = nucleus, Lat = lateral, Ant = anterior, tr = tract. *(Reproduced with permission from Carpenter MB: Human Neuroanatomy. Baltimore, MD, Williams & Wilkins, 1976.)*

dinally arranged neuronal cell bodies and supporting structures such as glial cells, dendrites, and myelinated and unmyelinated axons. The gray matter is divided into the dorsal horn (predominately sensory), the intermediate zone, and the ventral horn (purely motor). The ventral horn is populated by motor efferent neurons that project their axons out of the CNS via the ventral roots: the alpha and gamma motoneurons. The dorsal horns contain the first order neurons that receive afferent input from the sensory dorsal root ganglion neurons, and in turn project their axons centrally along the various sensory tracts. The intermediate zone contains neurons with projections that remain within the spinal cord and end on another neuron. These are the interneurons that play an important role in generating spinal reflexes. The spinal cord is histologically divided into nine lamellae (starting posteriorly and continuing anteriorly); each lamella contains a specific neuron and receives axonal projections from specific sensory axons and descending pathways (**Figure 4**). Laminae X is the region around the central canal. The laminae include the posteromarginal nucleus (I), substantia gelatinosa (II), nucleus proprius (III and IV), and the dorsal nucleus of Clarke within the thoracic zone (VII).

The ascending and descending tracts link the spinal cord to the neuroaxis and the propriospinal fibers project from one spinal level to another and form the basis of intraspinal reflexes. The spinal cord has several superficial landmarks that help to delineate different functional units. The anterior median fissure divides the spinal cord into two halves and contains both pia mater and sulcal branches of the anterior spinal artery. The pia mater within the posterior median sulcus is known as the posterior median septum. The posterior root or sensory fibers enter the spinal cord at the posterolateral sulcus. The posterior intermediate sulcus is located between the posterior median sulcus and the posterolateral sulcus and serves to divide the regions between the medial gracile fasciculus and lateral cuneate fasciculus. These tracts or fasciculi are also known as the dorsal columns within the white matter of the spinal cord. These fibers convey tactile, proprioceptive, and vibratory information from the ipsilateral side of the body. Whereas the gracile fasciculus fibers originate from sacral, lumbar, and lower thoracic regions, the cuneate fasciculus fibers originate from the upper thoracic and cervical regions. The lateral funiculus is located between the posterolateral and anterolateral sulci and includes the lateral corticospinal tract and the anterolateral system (ALS). The posterior and anterior spinocerebellar tracts are located on the lateral side of the cord with fibers originating from the thoracic nucleus of Clarke for the posterior tracts and the spinal border cells at the lumbosacral levels for the anterior tracts. The ALS contains the spinothalamic, the spinomesencephalic, and spinoreticular fibers. These fibers primarily arise from posterior horn cells and convey pain, temperature, and crude touch across the contralateral side of the body. The fibers are somatotopically arranged so that the lower portions of the body are posterolateral and the upper portions are anteromedial within the ALS. The lateral funiculus also contains the descending lateral corticospinal and rubrospinal tracts. Corticospinal fibers that cross the midline at the junction of the medulla and spinal cord form the lateral corticospinal tract, whereas the fibers on the ipsilateral side descend within the anterior corticospinal tract. These fibers also are somatotopically arranged with lower extremity fibers located laterally and upper extremity fibers located medially. The rubrospinal fibers serve to excite flexor motor neurons and inhibit the extensor motor neurons. The anterior funiculus includes the reticulospinal, the vestibulospinal, portions of the ALS, the anterior corticospinal tract, and the medial longitudinal fasciculus. Reticulospinal and vestibulospinal fibers function to excite extensor motor neurons and inhibit flexor motor neurons. The medial longitudinal fasciculus includes the medial vestibulospinal, the tectospinal, the interstitiospi-

nal, and the reticulospinal fibers and directs axial and neck motor neurons.

The pia mater, the deepest of the three meninges, intimately surrounds the spinal cord. The pia mater is bathed in cerebrospinal fluid within the subarachnoid space. Lumbar punctures aspirate fluid from this region. The arachnoid mater is relatively adherent to the most superficial meningeal layer, the dura mater. The dura extends from the foramen magnum and continues caudally to the filum terminale internum and externum. The dura is separated from the vertebrae by the epidural space. The anterior and posterior spinal arteries and branches of segmental arteries provide the blood supply to the spinal cord. The segmental arteries that supply the spinal nerve roots and the dorsal root ganglia are known as radicular arteries, whereas the segmental arteries that supply the cord directly are known as the spinal medullary arteries. One of the largest spinal medullary arteries is located at the L2 level on the left side of the body and is known as the artery of Adamkiewicz. The posterior spinal artery supplies the posterior, lateral, and anterior funiculi, whereas the central branches of the anterior spinal artery supply the gray matter and the adjacent white matter.

The spinal cord has distinct regional characteristics. Within the cervical region, there is significantly more white matter because of the presence of an increased number of ascending/descending tracts. Although the anterior and posterior horns of the gray matter are relatively small from C1 to C3, these regions are relatively large from C4 to C8 because these levels provide the sensory and motor innervation for the upper extremities. The anterior and posterior horns are relatively small within the thoracic region and make the white matter appear proportionately large. The dorsal nucleus of Clarke is located within this region and contains axons that project to the cerebellum. At the lumbar level, the spinal cord is round with relatively large anterior and posterior horns and less white matter. At the sacral levels, the cord consists primarily of gray matter with relatively little white matter; the substantia gelatinosa is quite obvious. The sacral levels also include the preganglionic parasympathetic cell bodies.

Sensory Systems

Sensory information is required for three main functions: sensation, control of movement, and maintaining arousal. Although sensation is a conscious experience, much of the sensory information used to control movement is not perceived. Similarly, many other somatic sensibilities controlling autonomic functions never reach consciousness. Somatic sensibility arises from information provided by a variety of receptors distributed throughout the body. The four major categories of these sensibilities are discriminative touch, proprioception, nociception, and thermal thresholds. Touch is mediated by mechanoreceptors in the skin. Mechanoreceptors differ in morphology and skin lo-

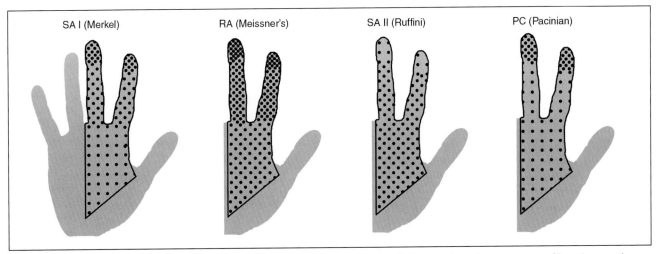

Figure 5   The distribution of the various mechanoreceptors in the human hand. The number of sensory nerve fibers innervating an area is indicated by stippling density, with the highest density of receptors shown by the heaviest stippling. (RA= rapidly adapting, SA = slowly adapting, PC = pacinian corpuscle.)

Table 2   Receptor Types

Receptor Type	Fiber Type	Modality
Nociceptors		
Mechanical	Aδ	Sharp, pricking pain
Thermal and mechanothermal	Aγ	Sharp, pricking pain
Thermal and mechanothermal	C	Slow, burning pain
Polymodal	C	Slow, burning pain
Cutaneous and subcutaneous mechanoreceptors		
Meissner's corpuscle	Aα,β	Touch (stroking)
Pacinian corpuscle	Aα,β	Vibration
Merkel disk receptor	Aα,β	Pressure, texture
Ruffini endings	Aα,β	Skin stretch
Thermal receptors		
Cool receptors	Aδ	Skin cooling (25° C)
Warm receptors	C	Skin warming (41° C)
Heat nociceptors	Aδ	Hot temperatures (> 45° C)
Cool nociceptors	C	Cold temperatures (< 5° C)
Muscle and skeletal mechanoreceptors		
Muscle spindle primary	Aα	Muscle length and speed
Muscle spindle secondary	Aβ	Muscle stretch
Golgi tendon organ	Aα	Muscle contraction
Joint capsule mechanoreceptor	Aβ	Joint angle

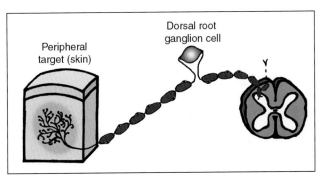

Figure 6   Illustration of the anatomy of the dorsal root ganglion. The cell body lies in a ganglion on the dorsal root of a spinal nerve. The axon has two branches, one projecting to the periphery and one projecting to the CNS. Sensory information regarding touch and limb proprioception is carried by the medial lemniscal tract and information concerning pain and temperature is carried by the anterolateral tract.

endings are located in the deeper subcutaneous tissues. These receptors are much larger than the Meissner corpuscles or the Merkel disk receptors. The pacinian corpuscle is physiologically similar to Meissner corpuscle. Ruffini endings are slowly adapting receptors. **Table 2** describes types of receptors and their individual functions.

This distinct system of receptors and pathways is responsible for receiving and mediating these specific modalities of sensory information from an external stimulus to the central structures where processing occurs. The sensory information goes through a common class of sensory neurons: the dorsal root ganglion neuron. The dorsal root ganglion neuron performs the functions of sensory transduction and transmission of encoded stimulus information. The morphology of the dorsal root ganglion neuron is shown in **Figure 6**.

These sensory tracts relay information to a layer of receptor neurons. The first layer of neurons is called the first

cation (**Figure 5**). The two principal mechanoreceptors in the superficial skin are the Meissner corpuscle and the Merkel disk receptor. Meissner corpuscles are rapidly adapting receptors, whereas Merkel disk receptors are slowly adapting receptors. Pacinian corpuscles and Ruffini

Table 3 Types of Muscle Fibers			
Nomenclature			
Myosin heavy chain	Type I	Type II A	Type II B/X
Twitch and fatigue characteristics	Slow	Fast resistant	Fast fatigue
Twitch and enzymatic characteristics	Slow oxidative	Fast oxidative-glycolytic	Fast glycolytic
Metabolic Characteristics			
Glycogen	Low	High	High
Glycolytic enzymes	Low	High	High
Oxidative enzymes	High	High	Low
Cytochrome c	High	High	Low
Capillary supply	Very rich	Rich	Sparse
ATP	Low	High	High
Twitch and Fatigue Characteristics			
Twitch speed	Low	High	High
Twitch tension	Low	High	High
Resistance to fatigue	High	High	Low
Characteristics of Motor Neurons			
Size of cell body	Small	Large	Large
Size of motor unit	Small	Large	Large
Diameter of axons	Small	Large	Large
Conduction velocity	Low	High	High
Threshold for recruitment	Low	High	High
Firing frequency	Low	High	High

order neuron or the primary afferent. This neurite is the efferent output of the dorsal root ganglion neurons. With the peripheral nerves, or the individual ganglia of the cranial nerves, this neurite projects to the spinal cord or the brainstem, where they synapse with the second order neurons. The neurons in subcortical regions are referred to as lower order neurons. The information from the lower order neurons is passed through relay nuclei to higher order neurons in the cerebral cortex. In the sensory system, the thalamus serves an important role as a relay nucleus. Sensory information from the thalamus is relayed to specific sensory regions of the cortex where it is perceived.

Motor Systems

Motor movements in mammals are initiated in the spinal cord. These movements are regulated by input from other levels including the brainstem (and its reticular formulation), the motor cortex, and the subcortical structures such as the basal ganglia and the cerebellum. At each of these levels, individual neural circuits are interconnected to the neural circuits from the other division. The end result is well-planned, well-coordinated, and well-executed motor movement.

The spinal cord has the circuitry responsible for the reciprocal activation of flexor and extensor muscles during locomotion. Spinal cord neurons are the primary recipient

of the afferent information from the peripheral neurons; they also receive input from the various neurons in the spinal cord and from descending pathways from the cortical and subcortical motor regions. These descending pathways are further subclassified into pyramidal pathways (those arising from the cerebral cortex) and extrapyramidal pathways (those arising from the basal ganglia, the red nucleus of the brainstem, the reticular activating system, and the efferent nucleus of the cerebellum). Striated muscle cells are innervated by ventral horn motor neurons. These lower motor neurons innervating a specific muscle are arranged in a column that extends through several spinal segments. These motor neurons are somatotopically organized within the ventral horn—the motor neurons projecting to the axial muscles are located more medially (lamella VIII), whereas those projecting to the limbs are located more laterally and in a different lamella (lamella IX). Within these distinct lamellae, further somatotopic arrangement occurs. The motor neurons projecting to the muscles around the hip are relatively more medial, whereas the motor neurons projecting to the muscles of the distal limb are placed more laterally within lamella IX. The motor neurons innervating the extensor muscles tend to be located ventral to those innervating flexor muscles.

To generate movement, the motor unit must be activated. The motor unit consists of the corresponding motor neuron, its motor axon, and all the muscle fibers innervated by this motor axon. The motor unit is the final common pathway that generates motor movement. The function of the motor unit is regulated by the descending inputs from the cortical and the subcortical system and from the sensory pathways. Interneurons also play an important role in fine tuning some of these movements.

The subdivision of the motor units depends on their histologic and physiologic profiles. Important determining factors include enzymatic properties shown by histochemical reactions; the rate of rise in twitch tension, which regulates the speed of contraction; the degree of fatigability; and the nature of motor innervation. **Table 3** summarizes the commonly used classification of muscle fibers into type I and type II according to histochemical reactions.

Spinal Cord Reflexes

Spinal cord reflexes involve the final common pathway and are an integral part of the neural circuitry believed to be involved in the maintenance of posture and the production of movement (**Figure 7**). A reflex is a stereotyped response to a specific sensory stimulus. A reflex pathway consists of the receptor (the sensory organ), the effector (the motor neuron), and the interconnecting neural elements (the interneurons). A monosynaptic reflex involves only one synapse between the receptor and the effector; a polysynaptic reflex involves more than one connection and often involves interneurons. In general, most reflexes are polysynaptic. Spinal reflex pathways can be modulated by supraspinal pathways either directly (through a mechanism known as presynaptic inhibition or indirectly (through interneurons).

Table 4 details the characteristics of these spinal reflexes. Perhaps the most important and certainly the most studied spinal reflex is the stretch reflex, a contraction of muscle that occurs when the muscle is lengthened. Clinically, the stretch reflex is most commonly elicited by tapping on a tendon to produce stretch of the extrafusal muscle fibers. The tapping is detected by the muscle spindle and transmitted to the CNS via type Ia afferent fibers. Muscle spindles sense the change of length and the afferent discharges from this spindle are carried to the spinal cord by type Ia fibers. These fibers make direct connection to

the alpha motor neurons (thus a monosynaptic reflex) and the efferent information is carried back to the muscle, causing muscle contraction. The type Ia fibers from the muscle excite not only the motor neurons innervating the muscle, but also excite innervating muscles having similar mechanical action. A reciprocal inhibition of the antagonistic muscles via the type Ia inhibitory interneurons also occurs; thus, when a muscle is stretched, the antagonist muscles relax. The stretch reflex is the strongest in the physiologic extensor muscles (muscles that oppose gravity). In humans, these muscles are the flexors of the upper extremity and the extensors of the lower extremity.

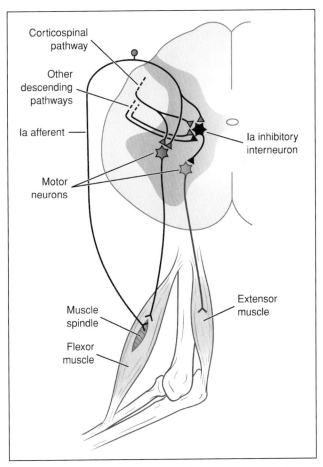

Figure 7   Pathways involved with the spinal stretch reflex, a monosynaptic reflex.

Table 4 Summary of Spinal Reflexes		
Segmental Reflex	**Receptor Organ**	**Afferent Fiber**
Phasic stretch reflex	Muscle spindle (primary endings)	Type Ia (large myelinated)
Tonic stretch reflex	Muscle spindle (secondary endings)	Type II (intermediate myelinated)
Clasp-knife response	Muscle spindle (secondary endings)	Type II (intermediate myelinated)
Flexion-withdrawal reflex	Nociceptors (free nerve endings), touch and pressure receptors	Flexor-reflex afferents: small unmyelinated cutaneous afferents (A-delta, C and muscle afferents, group III)
Autogenic inhibition	Golgi tendon organ	Type Ib (large myelinated)

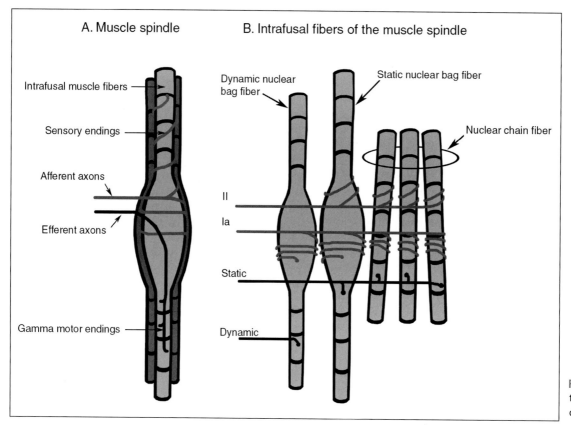

A. Muscle spindle

Intrafusal muscle fibers

Sensory endings

Afferent axons

Efferent axons

Gamma motor endings

B. Intrafusal fibers of the muscle spindle

Dynamic nuclear bag fiber

Static nuclear bag fiber

Nuclear chain fiber

II

Ia

Static

Dynamic

Figure 8 Anatomy of a muscle spindle.

Muscle spindles or Golgi tendon organs are specialized receptors distributed throughout the belly of the muscle and arranged parallel to the extrafusal muscle fibers in striated muscles (Figure 8). Each spindle consists of an encapsulated group of specialized muscle fibers called intrafusal fibers. Each intrafusal fiber within the spindle is innervated by a gamma motor neuron. Activation of the gamma motor neurons causes contraction of the ends or poles of the intrafusal fiber, resulting in stretching of the noncontractile equatorial region. When a muscle is shortened, the intrafusal fibers become slack or unloaded and are unable to monitor changes in length. The gamma motor neuron activation provides a means of controlling the length of the intrafusal fibers and the ability of the muscle spindle to detect changes in muscle length. The gamma motor neurons are generally coactivated with alpha motor neurons.

Muscle spindles have primary and secondary afferent endings. All intrafusal fibers in the spindle have a primary ending located in the center or equatorial region of the fiber, which gives rise to a large diameter, fast-conducting afferent fiber called a type Ia fiber. The primary endings are most sensitive to sudden changes in the length of the muscle and are responsible for the phasic component of the stretch reflex. The secondary endings are located primarily on the nuclear chain fibers and give rise to small diameter, slow-conducting afferent fibers called type II fibers. The secondary endings are most sensitive to steady

Table 5   Findings in Upper and Lower Motor Neuron Lesions

Findings	Upper Motor Neuron Lesion	Lower Motor Neuron Lesion
Stretch	Decreased	Decreased
Tone	Increased	Decreased
Deep tendon reflexes	Increased	Decreased
Superficial tendon reflexes	Decreased	Decreased
Babinski sign	Present	Absent
Clonus	Present	Absent
Fasciculations	Absent	Present
Atrophy	Absent	Present

changes in muscle length and are responsible for the tonic component of the stretch reflex.

Upper Motor Neuron Syndrome and Spasticity

Disruption of the descending pathways anywhere from the cerebral cortex to the spinal cord results in a clinical syndrome called the upper motor neuron syndrome. Patients with upper motor neuron syndrome have both negative (loss of function) and positive symptoms (abnormal function). Table 5 details the differences between upper and lower motor neuron syndromes. The hallmark of upper motor neuron syndrome is an increase in basal muscle tone or spasticity that results from changes in spinal proprioceptive reflexes. Spasticity is physiologically defined as a velocity-dependent increase in muscle tone, resulting in an initial burst of resistance (the spastic catch). While the muscle continues to move, the resistance ceases. Other characteristics of spasticity include increased tendon reflexes, flexor spasms associated with paraplegia, and loss of dexterity. These symptoms result in decreased strength, speed, and range of voluntary movement. Superficial (often cutaneous) reflexes are abolished in upper motor neuron syndromes. Negative symptoms include weakness and/or paresis, and fatigability. The negative symptoms usually are much more prominent when the pathologic lesion affecting the upper motor neuron is acute; with insidious onset lesions, the negative symptoms are not especially prominent except for the loss of dexterity.

Summary

A better understanding and appreciation of the PNS and spinal cord can result in improved treatment of musculoskeletal disorders. Therapeutic options are often limited for patients with neurologic deficits. Improved patient outcomes, using surgical treatment alone, have currently plateaued. Continued research into the biology of neural development and regeneration is necessary to improve functional outcomes for those patients with disorders of the musculoskeletal system.

Selected Bibliography

Anatomy and Physiology of Peripheral Nerves

Arroyo EJ, Bermingham JR Jr, Rosenfeld MG, Scherer SS: Promyelinating Schwann cells express Tst-1/SCIP/Oct-6. *J Neurosci* 1998;18:7891-7902.

Chan JR, Cosgaya JM, Wu YJ, Shooter EM: Neurotrophins are key mediators of the myelination program in the peripheral nervous system. *Proc Natl Acad Sci USA* 2001;98:14661-14668.

Cosgaya JM, Chan JR, Shooter EM: The neurotrophin receptor p75NTR as a positive modulator of myelination. *Science* 2002;298:1245-1248.

Griffin JW, Drucker N, Gold BG, et al: Schwann cell proliferation and migration during paranodal demyelination. *J Neurosci* 1987;7:682-699.

Gupta R, Gray M, Chao T, Bear D, Modafferi E, Mozaffar T: Schwann cells upregulate vascular endothelial growth factor secondary to chronic nerve compression injury. *Muscle Nerve* 2005;31:452-460.

Gupta R, Lin YM, Bui P, Chao T, Preston C, Mozaffar T: Macrophage recruitment follows the pattern of inducible nitric oxide synthase expression in a model for carpal tunnel syndrome. *J Neurotrauma* 2003;20:671-680.

Gupta R, Rowshan K, Chao T, Mozaffar T, Steward O: Chronic nerve compression induces local demyelination and remyelination in a rat model of carpal tunnel syndrome. *Exp Neurol* 2004;187:500-508.

Gupta R, Steward O: Chronic nerve compression induces concurrent apoptosis and proliferation of Schwann cells. *J Comp Neurol* 2003;461:174-186.

Kury P, Bosse F, Muller HW: Transcription factors in nerve regeneration. *Prog Brain Res* 2001;132:569-585.

Salzer JL: Nodes of Ranvier come of age. *Trends Neurosci* 2002;25:2-5.

Classification of Nerve Fibers

Gasser H: The classification of nerve fibers. *Ohio J Sci* 1941;41:145.

Steward O: *Functional Neuroscience*. New York, NY, Springer, 2000.

Peripheral Nerve Development, Structure, and Biomechanics

Byl C, Puttlitz C, Byl N, Lotz J, Topp K: Strain in the median and ulnar nerves during upper-extremity positioning. *J Hand Surg [Am]* 2002;27:1032-1040.

Clark WL, Trumble TE, Swiontkowski MF, Tencer AF: Nerve tension and blood flow in a rat model of immediate and delayed repairs. *J Hand Surg [Am]* 1992;17:677-687.

Driscoll PJ, Glasby MA, Lawson GM: An in vivo study of peripheral nerves in continuity: Biomechanical and physiological responses to elongation. *J Orthop Res* 2002;20:370-375.

Gelberman RH, Yamaguchi K, Hollstien SB, et al: Changes in interstitial pressure and cross-sectional area of the cubital tunnel and of the ulnar nerve with flexion of the elbow: An experimental study in human cadavera. *J Bone Joint Surg Am* 1998;80:492-501.

Gupta R, Truong L, Bear D, Chafik D, Modafferi E, Hung CT: Shear stress alters the expression of myelin-associated glycoprotein (MAG) and myelin basic protein (MBP) in Schwann Cells. *J Orthop Res* 2005;23:1232-1239.

Hicks D, Toby EB: Ulnar nerve strains at the elbow: The effect of in situ decompression and medial epicondylectomy. *J Hand Surg [Am]* 2002;27:1026-1031.

Kwan MK, Wall EJ, Massie J, Garfin SR: Strain, stress and stretch of peripheral nerve: Rabbit experiments in vitro and in vivo. *Acta Orthop Scand* 1992;63:267-272.

Lundborg G, Rydevik B: Effects of stretching the tibial nerve of the rabbit: A preliminary study of the intraneural circulation and the barrier function of the perineurium. *J Bone Joint Surg Br* 1973;55:390-401.

Nickols JC, Valentine W, Kanwal S, Carter BD: Activation of the transcription factor NF-kappaB in Schwann cells is required for peripheral myelin formation. *Nat Neurosci* 2003;6:161-167.

Rambukkana A, Zanazzi G, Tapinos N, Salzer JL: Contact-dependent demyelination by Mycobacterium leprae in the absence of immune cells. *Science* 2002; 296:927-931.

Rydevik B, McLean WG, Sjostrand J, Lundborg G: Blockage of axonal transport induced by acute, graded compression of the rabbit vagus nerve. *J Neurol Neurosurg Psychiatry* 1980;43:690-698.

Rydevik BL, Kwan MK, Myers RR, et al: An in vitro mechanical and histological study of acute stretching on rabbit tibial nerve. *J Orthop Res* 1990;8:694-701.

Toby EB, Hanesworth D: Ulnar nerve strains at the elbow. *J Hand Surg [Am]* 1998;23:992-997.

Toby EB, Rotramel J, Jayaraman G, Struthers A: Changes in the stress relaxation properties of peripheral nerves after transection. *J Hand Surg [Am]* 1999; 24:694-699.

Wall EJ, Kwan MK, Rydevik BL, Woo SL, Garfin SR: Stress relaxation of a peripheral nerve. *J Hand Surg [Am]* 1991;16:859-863.

Wright TW, Glowczewskie F Jr, Cowin D, Wheeler DL: Ulnar nerve excursion and strain at the elbow and wrist associated with upper extremity motion. *J Hand Surg [Am]* 2001;26:655-662.

Wright TW, Glowczewskie F, Wheeler D, Miller G, Cowin D: Excursion and strain of the median nerve. *J Bone Joint Surg Am* 1996;78:1897-1903.

Anatomy of the Spinal Cord

Haines D, Mihailoff G, Yezierski R: The spinal cord, in Huanes D (ed): *Fundamental Neuroscience*, ed 2. New York, NY, Churchill Livingstone, 2002.

Bodine S, Lieber R: Peripheral nerve physiology, anatomy, and pathology, in Buckwalter J, Einhorn T, Simon S (eds): *Orthopaedic Basic Science: Biology and Biomechanics of the Musculoskeletal System,* ed 2. Rosemont, IL, American Academy of Orthopaedic Surgeons, 2000, pp 617-682.

Chapter 14

Form and Function of the Intervertebral Disk

Andrew E. Park, MD
Scott D. Boden, MD

Introduction

The human spine is a complex structure consisting of 24 vertebrae (7 cervical, 12 thoracic, and 5 lumbar) and their intervening disks (**Figure 1**). The spine functions as the primary component of the axial skeleton, houses and protects the spinal cord and nerve roots, and allows for motion in three dimensions. The primary components of the spinal column are the vertebrae and the intervertebral disks. Their anatomic form and microstructure correlate with their functional role. The intervertebral disk plays a large role in balancing the spine's flexibility with stability. The disk also is where many pathologic processes of spinal disorders manifest clinical symptoms.

Biomechanical properties of the disk reflect its structure and function. Loading characteristics of the disk are affected by posture and aging. Spinal motion is intimately related to the mechanical properties of the intervertebral disk. Likewise, stability of the spine depends to a great extent on the integrity of the disk.

Pathologic processes occurring in the intervertebral disk are among the most common disorders encountered by spine surgeons. Disk herniations, degenerative disk disease, and degenerative spondylolisthesis represent various manifestations of altered structure and function of the disk.

Basic scientific research in the area of disk degeneration has been a promising field of investigation. Gene therapy is one of the modalities currently being studied as a possible treatment in the future.

Normal function of the axial skeleton is made possible by the intervertebral disks. They stabilize the spine and maintain its alignment by anchoring adjacent vertebral bodies onto one another. The disks allow for motion between vertebrae that gives the spine its flexibility, absorbs energy, and distributes loads applied to the body. Many of these functions are made possible by the structure of the disks, which consist of an outer ring, called the anulus fibrosus, surrounding a softer gelatinous substance, the nucleus pulposus (**Figure 2**). Although both structures are components of the intervertebral disk, each has a different composition and mechanical properties that work together to achieve the normal function of the disk. Recent investigations have advanced understanding of the unique structure-composition-function relationship of the anulus fibrosus and nucleus pulposus and thus increase the understanding of the biologic and mechanical characteristics of intervertebral disks.

Structure and Composition

The intervertebral disks increase in height and diameter from the cervical to the lumbar spine. Despite the considerable variation in size, all intervertebral disks have the same basic superstructure and composition. Like other connective tissues, they consist of a sparse population of cells in an abundant extracellular matrix. These cells synthesize the proteoglycans and collagens that make up the disk matrix. The structural integrity and mechanical properties of the nucleus pulposus depend on the macromolecules and the influx and efflux of water. Because the periphery of the normal disk is the source of the blood supply, the metabolism of disk cells is dependent on diffusion of nutrients and wastes through the permeable matrix. Movement of these nutrients and waste molecules through the matrix is related to the composition, ionic charge, and organization of the macromolecular framework, and the interstitial water content, which in turn is largely determined by the proteoglycan concentration.

The intervertebral disk is an avascular structure that includes the outer anulus fibrosus, the inner nucleus pulposus, and the cartilaginous end plates adjacent to the

American Academy of Orthopaedic Surgeons | Orthopaedic Basic Science, ed 3 **259**

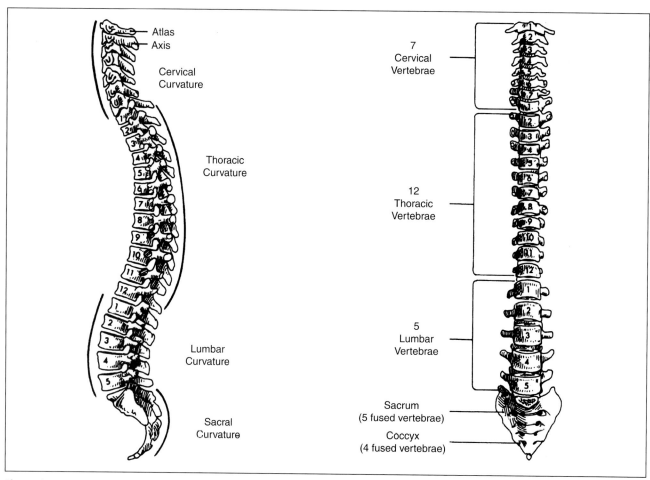

Figure 1   Drawing of the spine that shows the 24 vertebral bodies and the 23 intervertebral disks. The coronal and sagittal alignment of the spine is shown. *(Reproduced with permission from Ashton-Miller JA, Schultz AB: Biomechanics of the human spine, in Mow VC, Hayes WC (eds):* Basic Orthopaedic Biomechanics. *Philadelphia, PA, Lippincott Williams & Wilkins, 1997, pp 353-393.)*

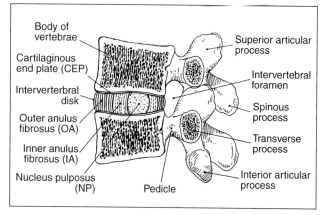

Figure 2   Sagittal section view of a motion segment comprising two vertebral bodies and an intervertebral disk forming a strong connection between the bones. The four regions of the disk are shown: cartilaginous end plate, outer anulus fibrosus, inner anulus fibrosus, and nucleus pulposus. The posterior articular and spinous processes and the articular surface of a facet joint are also shown. *(Reproduced with permission from Ashton-Miller JA, Schultz AB: Biomechanics of the human spine, in Mow VC, Hayes WC (eds):* Basic Orthopaedic Biomechanics. *Philadelphia, PA, Lippincott Williams & Wilkins, 1997, pp 353-393.)*

vertebral surfaces. The anulus fibrosus maintains the stability of the motion segment along with the interspinous ligaments, muscles, and the bony articulations. The anulus fibrosus can be divided into the outer and inner anulus layers. The nucleus pulposus is derived from the primitive notochord and its primary function is to resist compressive loads. The nucleus pulposus is clearly bordered by the anulus fibrosus in the developing infant, but the distinction between the two regions of the disk diminishes during the transition to adulthood. During the growth and development of the spine, the notochordal cells are replaced by chondrocytes. The mechanism of this transition is not understood. In spines of older adults, the nucleus pulposus becomes more difficult to distinguish from the anulus fibrosus, and eventually becomes a fibrocartilaginous mass similar to the inner zone of the anulus fibrosus. The anulus fibrosus has an outer collagenous layer of type I collagen in which the fibers are arranged in oblique layers of lamellae that insert directly into the vertebral bodies via Sharpey's fibers. The fibers of lamellae run perpendicular to one another—offering resistance to movements in all directions. The collagen fibers in the posterior portion of the disk run in a more vertical than oblique direction, which may account for the relative frequency of annular tears seen clinically in this region. Beneath the outer layer of the anulus fibrosus is the inner layer. This inner layer consists of a less dense type II collagen matrix, lacking the highly organized, crossed fibrils seen in the outer layer. The cartilaginous end plate in the immature spine is a layer of hyaline cartilage resting on the subchondral bone. This cartilage is a growth plate and is responsible for endochondral ossification during growth. The cartilaginous end plates also allow the insertion of the inner fibers of the anulus fibrosus and the diffusion of nutrients from the subchondral bone to the disk. In adulthood, the hyaline cartilage layer is replaced by calcified cartilage.

Collagens and proteoglycans are the primary structural components of the intervertebral disk. The collagens give the disk tensile strength and are the primary restraints to extension and rotational movements. Proteoglycans, through their interactions with water, provide the primary resistance to compressive forces and give the disk viscoelastic properties.

Overall, collagens account for more than 70% of the dry weight of the outer anulus fibrosus layer, but less than 20% of the dry weight of the central nucleus of the spines of younger persons. In contrast, proteoglycans account for only a small percentage (dry weight) of the outer layer of the anulus fibrosus, but as much as 50% of the dry weight of the nucleus pulposus in a child. Most of the various collagenous materials are composed of type I and type II collagens (80% of total collagen content). In the anulus fibrosus and nucleus pulposus, both type I and II collagens are highly cross-linked with pyridinoline residues. Although these mature cross-links are found in many other connective tissues, their highest concentration is in the intervertebral disk. This high concentration of cross-links helps to maintain tissue cohesiveness, an important factor for resisting high mechanical loads.

Type VI collagen is the next most common collagen type found in the disk. It does not form fibrils, but instead forms a fine filament network. There is an unusually high concentration of type VI collagen compared with other connective tissues of the body, indicating that it plays a role in the properties of the disk matrix. Other collagen types found in the disk include types III, V, IX, XI, and XII.

Composition changes that occur in the disk with aging are quite predictable and ubiquitous. In the aging disk, water content, proteoglycan content, size, and concentration are decreased, and keratan sulfate and collagen content are increased. In accordance with the changes in the microstructure, disk height loss occurs, which impacts the overall spinal alignment. The net effect of these changes is an alteration of the mechanical properties of the disk. This change in mechanical properties ultimately manifests in the different disease states of the disk seen with degeneration of the disk and with aging.

Regional variations of the disk anatomy are seen throughout the spine. These variations in structure are consistent with their functional role. Disks in the cervical spine bear the least weight and are relatively thin. The cervical disks allow some translation in the sagittal plane, but the lateral motion is limited by the uncovertebral joint anatomy. Cervical disks, as in the lumbar spine, are wedge shaped and are taller and wider anteriorly than posteriorly. This characteristic contributes to the overall sagittal contour of the spine with cervical and lumbar lordosis. Thoracic disks increase in height and width in a caudal direction, mirroring the increasing size of the vertebral bodies. However, thoracic kyphosis is primarily a result of the bony morphology, because the disks are relatively uniform in their thickness. It is the vertebral bodies in the thoracic spine that are taller posteriorly than anteriorly. In the lumbar spine the disks are taller and wider anteriorly, providing the major contribution to lumbar lordosis. The amount of normal lordosis that is attributable to the disk space increases caudally. Thus, the lower lumbar disks are more wedge-shaped and lordotic than the upper lumbar disks. Loss of lumbar lordosis is primarily a phenomenon occurring within the disk space because the vertebral bodies are fairly uniform in their height from front to back.

Nutrition, Blood Supply, and Innervation of the Disk

Despite the avascularity of the disk, nutrients are used by the disk tissue via diffusion and waste products are disposed of in a similar manner. Previously held beliefs that the disk is inert tissue have been overturned by experimental evidence of metabolic activity within the disk. Canine studies by Nachemson and others have increased the understanding of the mechanism by which the disk receives nutrients and disposes of metabolic by-products.

The peripheral vascular plexus of the anulus fibrosus and the vessels adjacent to the hyaline cartilage of the bony end plate provide the interface for the diffusion of metabolites. Through a centrifugal gradient that ranges from 80% permeability centrally to 40% permeability on the periphery, solutes between the disk and the plasma may pass down their respective concentration gradients. The partition coefficient defines the equilibrium between the solutes, and the diffusion coefficient characterizes the solute mobility.

The partition coefficient varies with the size and charge of the solute particle. Small uncharged solutes show a near-equilibrium between the plasma and disk concentrations. Charged molecules, however, are affected by the relatively negatively charged intradiskal environment. Therefore, anionic solutes have a lower intradiskal concentration with respect to the plasma. Conversely, positively charged solutes are preferentially attracted toward the intradiskal matrix. This effect is dependent primarily on the concentration of the negatively charged proteoglycans.

The solute mobility (diffusion coefficient) within the disk is slower than in the plasma because the collagen and proteoglycan matrix impedes the diffusion process. The diffusion coefficient of the disk is approximately half that of the plasma; it is greatest in the inner anulus fibrosus where the water concentration is the highest. A "pumping" phenomenon, which occurs with variations in the loading and unloading of the disk, may have a role in the transport of some of the larger solutes. This phenomenon is not likely to be a major factor for the smaller solutes, which diffuse readily.

Diffusion of metabolites is critically dependent on the fine vasculature near the cartilaginous end plates. Any process that disrupts this fine vascular system, such as aging or environmental factors such as cigarette smoking, may in turn impact disk metabolism and health. Clinically, this phenomenon is corroborated by the relatively higher incidence of degenerative disk disease among smokers.

The source of innervation of the intervertebral disk has been a topic of debate. Hirsch and associates were able to show that nerve endings exist in the posterior aspect of the anulus fibrosus. Presumably these nerve endings represent a continuum from the nerve endings in the posterior longitudinal ligament. More recent studies staining for acetylcholine have shown clear evidence for innervation of the outer layer of the anulus fibrosus. This innervation of the posterior longitudinal ligament and anulus fibrosus originates from the sinuvertebral nerve. The precise relationship between the nerve fibers innervating the disk and discogenic pain, however, is not well defined.

Function

The mechanical architecture of the intervertebral disk is basically divided between the anulus fibrosus on the outside and the inner nucleus pulposus. The two structures act in concert to withstand very large loads in a multitude of different force vectors. The nucleus is distorted by compressive loads. The result of this loading is the conversion of the compressive force to radially directed forces in the horizontal plane. The outer anulus fibrosus, with fibers oriented perpendicular to one another with a high degree of cross-linking, is perfectly designed to handle these loads. Thus, the radial forces are distributed to the high tensile strength of the anulus fibrosus.

Disk biomechanics play a stabilizing role in maintaining harmonious motion between vertebrae. Instability is defined as loss of the ability to withstand normal physiologic loads to limit motion and to prevent irritation of neurologic structures. With disk degeneration, changes in the mechanical properties of the disk are seen. Biomechanical testing on intervertebral motion segments with varying degrees of disk degeneration shows an initial in-

crease in sagittal plane motion with disk degeneration—followed by decreasing flexion and extension with more advanced degenerative disk disease. During lateral bending the flexibility of the disk decrease with increasing disk degeneration. During rotation, the flexibility of the disk increases with increasing disk degeneration—however, the load borne by the bony articulations increases with advanced disk degeneration. Although the absolute flexibility of the disk varies, depending on the plane of motion studied, the overall result of disk degeneration is that the proportion of the load dissipated by the disk decreases. As a result, the facet joints and interspinous ligaments play an increasingly important role in spinal stability.

Pressures exerted on the intervertebral disk are dependent on the posture of the spine at the time of measurement. The pressure is approximately one and a half times the compressive load divided by the cross-sectional area. Lumbar disk pressure is increased when a patient in a recumbent position stands upright. The pressures are highest for unsupported sitting. Lumbar disk pressures while sitting can be decreased with the addition of armrests, lumbar support, and inclination of the backrest. In vivo studies and experience with diskography have shown lower pressures in painful disks. This finding suggests that disk degeneration leads to abnormal mechanical properties of the disk. The pressure within the disk is believed to be relatively uniform throughout the nucleus pulposus and anulus fibrosus.

Diskography is a diagnostic technique used to identify abnormal properties in the disk. The normal anulus fibrosus resists distension and the disk will normally accept approximately 1 mL of contrast. In a degenerated disk, lower opening pressures are seen followed by the ability to infuse greater than 2 mL of contrast medium. Furthermore, the extravasation of contrast can be seen on fluoroscopy or CT following diskography. Advocates of diskography as a diagnostic procedure use the reproduction of symptoms with the procedure in conjunction with the clinical history and imaging studies to formulate treatment recommendations.

Future Treatment Considerations

Because many of the pathologic processes of the intervertebral disk are related to the degenerative changes that occur with aging, treatments directed toward addressing those changes hold great promise as a therapeutic intervention. With the degeneration of the intervertebral disk, a decrease in the synthesis of critical biologic components of the disk is seen. This issue is compounded by an increase in the degradation of the molecular components of inner disk material. Future strategies should be directed toward addressing one or both of these components to significantly impact the disease process. Along those lines several variations have been attempted in animal models to introduce the complementary DNA encoding various

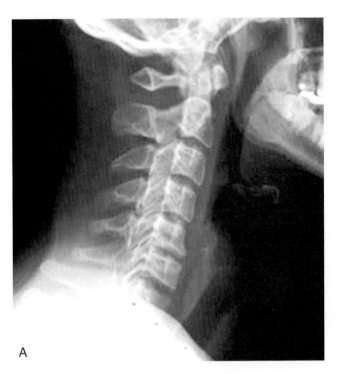
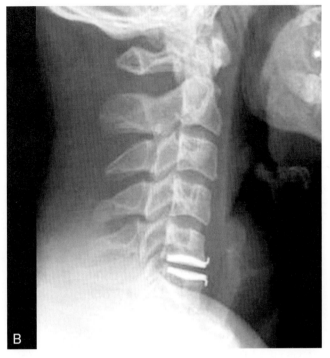

Figure 3 **A,** Preoperative lateral radiograph of a patient who underwent a Bryan cervical disk arthroplasty *(Medtronic Sofamor Danek, Memphis, TN)* for a C5/6 disk herniation. **B,** Lateral radiograph of the same patient at 1-year follow-up.

proteins for the purpose of increasing specific gene expression and to promote more favorable disk metabolic activity. Adenovirus-mediated transfer of specific genes has been successful in expressing marker proteins and growth factors within the disk of rabbits. Other laboratories have focused investigations on modifying the regulation of the proteoglycans in the extracellular matrix simulating that of the intervertebral disk. One such investigation has used osteogenic protein-1 (OP-1, Stryker Biotech, Hopkinton, MA), also known as bone morphogenetic protein-7, to stimulate the production of proteoglycans and type II collagen, both of which are primary components of the nucleus of the intervertebral disk. With an increased understanding of which growth factors are required to stimulate the production of the appropriate matrix components, the possibility of using gene therapy for this purpose may become a reality.

Currently under investigation are several forms of intervertebral disk replacement in the lumbar and cervical spine (**Figure 3**). The proposed benefit of this intervention is the elimination of the complications associated with fusion surgery and transition level disease. Degenerative disk disease and cervical disk herniations may be amenable to this form of surgical therapy. As understanding of this new treatment continues to increase, surgeons must be aware of the potential complications and adverse effects inherent to arthroplasty. Additional investigations into the consequences of wear debris and the long-term clinical results from disk arthroplasty will require careful analysis before widespread acceptance of this new technology.

Summary

The structure of the intervertebral disk illuminates the intimate relationship between anatomic structure and composition with function. With aging, predictable changes in composition and function are seen within the disk. Some of these changes ultimately manifest in a variety of clinical scenarios. Better understanding of the normal anatomy allows physicians the necessary tools to study the disk in pathologic conditions.

Currently accepted treatments are primarily directed toward decompression of neural structures and stabilization of motion segments for the different conditions resulting from disk pathology. Investigational studies of intervertebral disk replacement are ongoing. Future treatments may be directed toward either prevention of degeneration or restoration of normal disk microstructure and function.

Selected Bibliography

Structure and Composition

Herkowitz HN, Rothman RH, Simeone FA (eds): *The Spine*, ed 4. Philadelphia, PA, Elsevier Health Science, 1998.

White AA III, Panjabi MM: *Clinical Biomechanics of the Spine*, ed 2. Philadelphia, PA, JB Lippincott, 1990.

Nutrition, Blood Supply, and Innervation of the Disk

Bogduk N: The innervation of the lumbar spine. *Spine* 1983;8:286-293.

Hirsch C, Ingelmark BE, Miller M: The anatomical basis for low back pain: Studies on the presence of sensory nerve endings in ligamentous, capsular, and intervertebral disc structures in the human lumbar spine. *Acta Orthop Scand* 1963;33:1-17.

Nachemson A: Editorial comment: Lumbar discography: Where are we today? *Spine* 1989;14:555-557.

Urban JP, Smith S, Fairbank JC: Nutrition of the intervertebral disc. *Spine* 2004;29:2700-2709.

Function

Andersson BJ, Ortengren R, Nachemson AL, et al: The sitting posture: An electromyographic and discometric study. *Orthop Clin North Am* 1975;6:105-120.

Executive Committee of the North American Spine Society: Position statement on discography. *Spine* 1988;13:1343.

Panjabi MM: The stabilizing system of the spine: Part II. Neutral zone and instability hypothesis. *J Spinal Disord* 1992;5:390-397.

Future Treatment Considerations

An HS (ed): *Principles and Techniques of Spine Surgery.* Philadelphia, PA, JB Lippincott, 1998.

Kang JD, Boden SD: Orthopaedic gene therapy: Spine. *Clin Orthop Relat Res* 2000;(suppl 379):S256-S259.

Nishida K, Kang JD, Gilbertson LG, et al: Modulation of the biologic activity of the rabbit intervertebral disc by gene therapy: An in vivo study of adenovirus-mediated transfer of the human transforming growth factor beta 1 encoding gene. *Spine* 1999;24:2419-2425.

Takegami K, Thonar EJ, An HS, Kamada H, Masuda K: Osteogenic protein 1 enhances matrix replenishment by intervertebral disc cells previously exposed to interleukin 1. *Spine* 2002;27:1318-1325.

Chapter 15

Kinesiology

Kenton R. Kaufman, PhD, PE
Kai-Nan An, PhD

Introduction

Kinesiology is the study of movement of the human body. This chapter will discuss how biologic form and mechanical structure result in human functional abilities.

Kinematics is the study of the motion of rigid structures, independent of the forces that might be involved. Two types of movement, translation (linear displacement) and rotation (angular displacement), occur within three orthogonal planes; that is, movement has six degrees of freedom. Motion between skeletal segments occurs at joints. Most joint motion is minimally translational and primarily rotational. The deviation from absolute rotatory motion may be noted by the changes in the path of a joint's instantaneous center of rotation. These paths have been measured for most of the joints in the body and vary only slightly from true arcs of rotation. Kinesiology, thus, is first a study of the kinematics of the joints in the musculoskeletal system. To provide for the greatest possible function of an extremity, a joint must allow for rotatory motions in all three planes about all three axes.

The study of the forces that bring about these movements is part of the mechanical discipline called kinetics. Kinetics provides insights into the cause of the observed motion. Forces and loads are not visually observable; they must be either measured with instrumentation or calculated from kinematic data. Kinetic quantities studied include such parameters as the forces produced by muscles; reaction loads between body parts as well as their interactions with external surfaces; the load transmitted through the joints; the power transferred between body segments; and the mechanical energy of body segments. Inherent to such studies are the functional demands imposed on the body.

The structure and stability of each extremity and its joints reflect different functional demands. The functional demands on the upper extremity are quite different from those on the lower extremity. More structural strength is needed in the lower extremity. In contrast, the upper ex-

tremity is designed for more movement. These functional requirements dictate the nature of the material, size, shape, and infrastructure of the joint system. Kinesiology is thus a study of how the musculoskeletal system has adapted to the kinematic and kinetic requirements of human movement. It is the study and understanding of how motions are produced by forces at individual joints as well as the integration of requirements when a specific function is desired. This chapter will present current knowledge about the various components of the musculoskeletal system, but is not intended to be a comprehensive representation of the entire subject of kinesiology as it relates to human movement.

Structure and Function of the Shoulder Joint

The shoulder represents the group of structures connecting the arm to the thorax. The combined movements of four distinct articulations (glenohumeral, acromioclavicular [AC], sternoclavicular, and scapulothoracic) allow the arm to be positioned in space (**Figure 1**). The four articulations work together to produce mobility. Shoulder range of motion is traditionally measured in terms of flexion and extension (movement in the sagittal plane), abduction (elevation in the coronal plane), and internal/external rotation (axial rotation of the humerus). Clinical terms such as flexion, adduction, horizontal adduction, and extension are descriptive, but insufficient to describe the position of the arm with respect to the thorax. A key to understanding the kinematics of a joint is the ability to measure and describe its motion in an accurate and reproducible fashion. One method to achieve this accuracy in description is to designate various vertical planes available for elevation of the humerus similar to the longitudinal demarcations of a globe. The plane of pure abduction in the coronal plane is defined as the 0° plane and pure flexion in the anterior sagittal plane is 90° (**Figure 2**). Maximal horizontal adduction of the shoulder occurs at +124° and maximal hori-

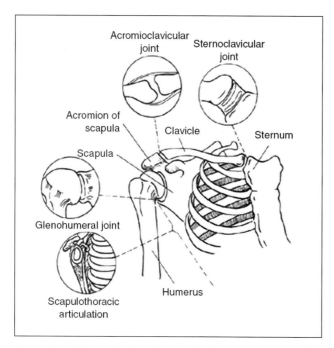

Figure 1   Schematic depiction of the bony structures of the shoulder and their four articulations. The circular insets show front views of the three synovial joints (sternoclavicular, acromioclavicular, and glenohumeral) and a lateral view of the scapulothoracic joint, a bone-muscle-bone articulation. *(Reproduced with permission from De Palma AF: Biomechanics of the shoulder, in* Surgery of the Shoulder, *ed 3. Philadelphia, PA, JB Lippincott, 1983, pp 65-85.)*

zontal abduction at -88° **(Figure 3)**. Humeral elevation within a given plane is then quantified by measuring the angle formed between the unelevated humerus and the elevated humerus. Pure abduction to 90° is described as (0, 90) whereas pure flexion to 90° is described as (+90, 90) **(Figure 2)**. The final determinant of shoulder position is the axial rotation of the humerus described by the angle formed between the forearm (elbow flexed to 90°) and a line perpendicular to the plane of elevation **(Figure 4)**. In this position, rotation is defined as 0°. External rotation from that position is designated as positive (+), and internal rotation from that position is designated as negative (-).

The wide range of motion of the shoulder (exceeding a hemisphere) is the result of synchronous, simultaneous contributions from the four distinct articulations of the shoulder complex. The most important function of the shoulder is arm elevation. Normal arm elevation has been reported as 167° in men and 171° in women. Very few activities of daily living involve movement in a single plane. The most common plane for humeral elevation in daily living is 50° to anterior of the coronal plane. This approximates the line of the scapula or the scapular plane (also called scaption), which is described as being anywhere from 30° to 50° anterior to the coronal axis **(Figure 5)**. Several investigators have attempted to relate glenohumeral and scapulothoracic motion during arm elevation in various planes **(Table 1)**. About two thirds of the motion takes

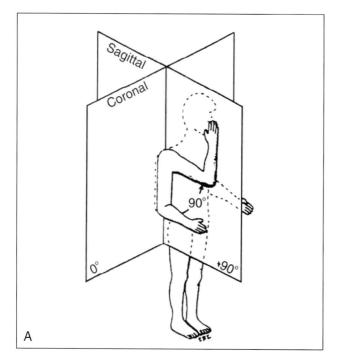

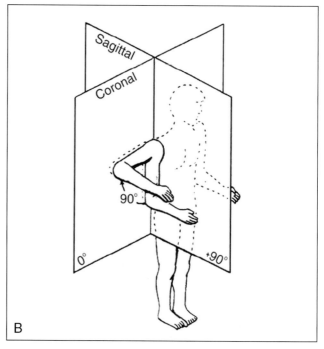

Figure 2   A, Elevation of the arm in the sagittal plane (flexion) may be defined as occurring in the +90° plane. Flexion to an angle of 90° within that plane is then described as (+90, 90). **B,** Elevation of the arm in the coronal plane (abduction) may be defined as occurring in the 0° plane. Abduction to an angle of 90° within that plane is described as (0, 90). *(Modified from Pearl ML, Harris SL, Lippitt SB, et al: A system for describing positions of the humerus relative to the thorax and its use in the presentation of several functionally important arm positions.* J Shoulder Elbow Surg *1992;1:113–115.)*

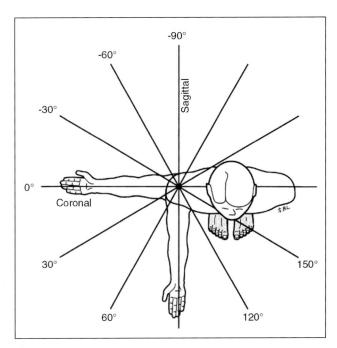

Figure 3 Planes of elevation of the arm. In normal individuals, the available planes of elevation are from -88° to +124°; therefore, there are 212 different planes of humeral elevation. *(Reproduced with permission from Pearl ML, Harris SL, Lippitt SB, et al: A system for describing positions of the humerus relative to the thorax and its use in the presentation of several functionally important arm positions. J Shoulder Elbow Surg 1992;1:113–115.)*

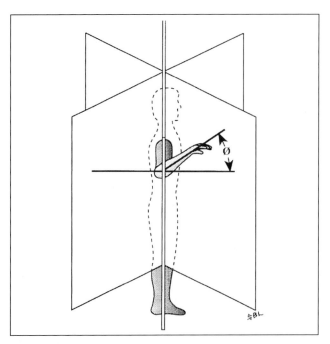

Figure 4 Rotation of the humerus is described by the angle formed by the forearm and a line perpendicular to the plane of elevation. *(Reproduced with permission from Pearl ML, Harris SL, Lippitt SB, et al: A system for describing positions of the humerus relative to the thorax and its use in the presentation of several functionally important arm positions. J Shoulder Elbow Surg 1992;1:113–115.)*

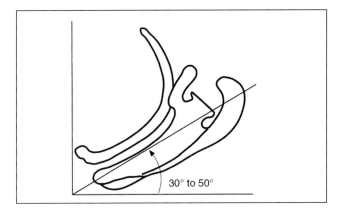

Figure 5 The plane of the scapula is approximately 30° to 50° anterior to the coronal plane of the body. *(Reproduced from Simon SR, Alaranta H, An KN, et al: Kinesiology, in Buckwalter JA, Einhorn TA, Simon SR (eds): Orthopaedic Basic Science, ed 2. Rosemont, IL, American Academy of Orthopaedic Surgeons, 2000, p 735.)*

Table 1   Arm Elevation: Glenohumeral-Scapulothoracic Rotation

Investigator(s)	Glenohumeral/Scapulothoracic Motion Ratio
Inman et al (1944)	2: 1
Freedman and Munro (1966)	1.35: 1
Doody et al (1960)	1.74: 1
Poppen and Walker (1976)	4.3: 1 (< 24° elevation)
	1.25: 1 (> 24° elevation)
Saha (1971)	2.3: 1 (30° to 135° elevation)

place in the glenohumeral joint and about one third in the scapulothoracic articulation, resulting in a 2:1 ratio.

Biomechanics of the Glenohumeral Joint

The articular surface of the humerus is approximately one third of a sphere (**Figure 6**). The articular surface is ori-

ented with an upward tilt of approximately 40° to 45° and is retroverted approximately 30° with respect to the condylar line of the distal humerus. The average radius of curvature of the humeral head in the coronal plane is 24.0 ± 2.1 mm. The radius of curvature in the anteroposterior and axillary-lateral view is similar, measuring 13.1 ± 1.3 mm and 22.9 ± 2.9 mm, respectively. The humeral articulating surface is spherical in the center. However, the peripheral radius is 2 mm less in the axial plane than in the coronal plane. Thus the peripheral contour of the articular surface is elliptical with a ratio of 0.92. The major axis is superior to inferior and the minor axis is anterior to posterior.

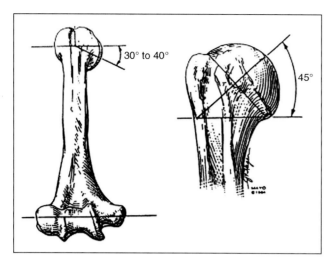

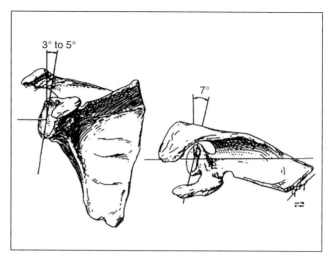

Figure 6   The two-dimensional orientation of the articular surface of the humerus with respect to the bicondylar axis. *(Reproduced with permission from Mayo Foundation.)*

Figure 7   The glenoid faces slightly superior and posterior (retroverted) with respect to the body of the scapula. *(Reproduced with permission from Mayo Foundation.)*

The glenoid fossa consists of a small, pear-shaped, cartilage-covered bony depression that measures 39.0 ± 3.5 mm in the superior/inferior direction and 29.0 ± 3.2 mm in the anterior/posterior direction. The anterior/posterior dimension of the glenoid is pear-shaped with the lower half being larger than the top half. The ratio of the lower half to the top half is 1:0.80 ± 0.01. The glenoid is more curved superior to inferior (coronal plane) and relatively fatter in an anterior to posterior direction (transverse plane). In the coronal plane, the articular surface of the glenoid comprises an arc of approximately 75° and in the transverse plane, the arc of curvature of the glenoid is about 50°. The glenoid has a slight upward tilt of about 5° with respect to the medial border of the scapula and is retroverted a mean of approximately 7° (**Figure 7**). The superior inclination of the glenoid has been shown to contribute significantly to inferior stability of the glenohumeral joint because of a cam effect resulting in tightening of the superior capsule during inferiorly directed stress on the humerus. There is more constraint to the glenoid in the coronal versus sagittal plane. These anatomic features help prevent superior-inferior translation of the humeral head but allow translation in the sagittal plane. The glenohumeral joint demonstrates laxity in every direction. A study of normal unanesthetized volunteers has demonstrated that passive humeral translation on the glenoid averaged 8 mm anteriorly, 9 mm posteriorly, and 11 mm inferiorly. Up to 2 cm of glenohumeral translation has been documented in some unanesthetized volunteers with no history of shoulder instability.

The glenohumeral contact point moves forward and inferior during internal rotation (**Figure 8**). With external rotation, the contact is posterior/inferior. With elevation, the contact area moves superiorly. The stability ratio is defined as the force necessary to translate the humeral head

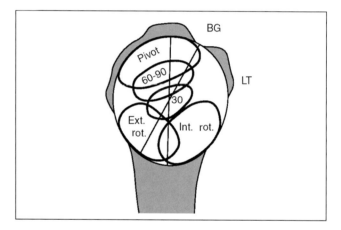

Figure 8   Humeral contact position as a function of glenohumeral motion and positions. BG = bicepetal groove; LT = lesser trochanter; Int = internal; Ext = external; rot = rotation. *(Reproduced with permission from Morrey BF, An K-N: Biomechanics of the shoulder, in Rockwood CA, Matsen FA (eds): The Shoulder. Philadelphia, PA, WB Saunders, 1990, pp 208-245.)*

from the glenoid fossa divided by the compressive load times 100. Stability ratios are in the range of 50% to 60% in the superior-inferior direction and 30% to 40% in the anterior-posterior direction. After the labrum is removed, the ratio is decreased by approximately 20%.

Surface motion at the glenohumeral joint is primarily rotational. The center of rotation has been defined as a locus of points situated within 6.0+/−1.8 mm of the geometric center of the humeral head. However, the motion is not purely rotational. The humeral head displaces with respect to the glenoid. From 0° to 30°, and often from 30° to 60°, the humeral head moves upward in the glenoid fossa by about 3 mm, indicating that rolling and/or gliding has taken place. Thereafter, the humeral head has only

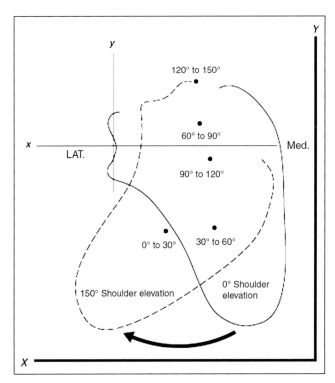

Figure 9   Rotation of the scapula on the thorax in the scapular plane. Instant centers of rotation (solid dots) are shown for each 30° interval of motion during shoulder elevation in the scapular plane from 0° to 150°. The x y axes are fixed in the scapula, whereas the X and Y axes are fixed in the thorax. From 0° to 30° the scapula rotated about its lower midportion; from 60° onward, rotation took place about the glenoid area, resulting in a medial and upward displacement of the glenoid face and a large lateral displacement of the inferior tip of the scapula. *(Reproduced with permission from Poppen NK, Walker PS: Normal and abnormal motion of the shoulder.* J Bone Joint Surg Am *1976;58:195-201.)*

about 1 mm of additional excursion.

Scapulothoracic Joint

During arm elevation in the scapular plane, the scapula moves in relation to the thorax. From 0° to 30° the scapula rotates about its lower midportion, and then from 60° onward the center of rotation shifts toward the glenoid, resulting in a large lateral displacement of the inferior tip of the scapula (**Figure 9**). The center of rotation of the scapula for arm elevation is situated at the tip of the acromion as viewed from the edge (**Figure 10**). The mean amount of scapular twisting at maximum arm elevation is 40°. The superior tip of the scapula moves away from the thorax and the inferior tip moves toward it.

Acromioclavicular Joint

The AC joint is a true diarthrodial joint that allows the articulation of the medial aspect of the acromion with the lateral aspect of the clavicle. The joint surfaces are not perfectly congruent, and a fibrocartilaginous meniscus is interposed between the clavicle and the acromion. The AC capsule is thickened superiorly, forming the AC ligament. The AC ligament and AC capsule are the initial stabilizers of the AC joint in the AP direction and for axial rotation of the clavicle. The AC capsule and ligaments are the primary stabilizers of the AC joint when this joint is subjected to relatively light loads of daily activity and recreation; however, when greater forces are applied to the AC joint, the most important stabilizing structures become the coracoclavicular ligaments composed of the trapezoid and conoid ligaments.

The scapula is essentially suspended from the clavicle by way of these two strong ligaments that span from the undersurface of the clavicle to the coracoid process of the scapula. Although the trapezoid is larger and stronger, it has been shown that during large displacements of the AC joint, the conoid resists almost four times as much force (70%) as does the trapezoid (18%). The trapezoid ligament, because of its oblique fibers, more effectively resists AC joint compression during loading of the glenohumeral joint, such as during weight lifting. This tough sling of ligamentous tissue effectively decreases the compression of the acromion against the lateral end of the clavicle.

Sternoclavicular Joint

The sternoclavicular joint forms the only true skeletal articulation or bridge between the upper extremity and the thorax. This diarthrodial joint is composed of reciprocally saddle-shaped, but incongruous, articular surfaces with an interposed fibrocartilaginous disk or meniscus. Ligamentous restraints surround the sternoclavicular joint anteriorly, posteriorly, superiorly, and inferiorly.

The clavicle moves in the AP and superoinferior directions and also rotates about its long axis both anteriorly and posteriorly during normal motion of the arm. Greater motion occurs at the sternoclavicular joint than at the AC joint. Approximately 35° of superior rotation, anterior rotation, and posterior rotation occurs in the sternoclavicular joint, and this unconstrained, saddle-shaped articulation allows 45° to 50° of axial rotation to occur. The clavicle has been shown to rotate 40° to 50° during active forward elevation of the arm. Although the clavicle rotates this amount with respect to the fixed sternum, it rotates only 5° to 8° with respect to the acromion at the AC joint because of the concomitant synchronous rotation of the scapula during forward elevation of the arm.

Structure and Function of the Elbow Joint

The bony structures of the elbow are the distal end of the humerus and the proximal ends of the radius and ulna. The elbow joint complex allows two degrees of freedom in motion: flexion/extension and pronation/supination. The elbow joint complex is three separate synovial articulations. The humeroulnar joint is the articulation between

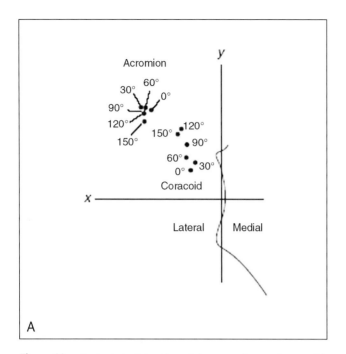

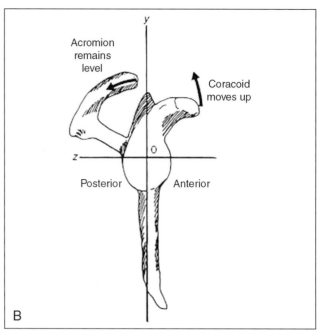

A

B

Figure 10   **A,** A plot of the tips of the acromion and coracoid process on radiograms taken at successive intervals of arm elevation in the scapular plane show upward movement of the coracoid and only a slight shift in the acromion relative to the glenoid face. This finding demonstrates twisting, or external rotation, of the scapula about the x-axis. **B,** A lateral view of the scapula during this motion would show the coracoid process moving upward while the acromion remains on the same horizontal plane as the glenoid. *(Reproduced with permission from Poppen NK, Walker PS: Normal and abnormal motion of the shoulder. J Bone Joint Surg Am 1976;58:195-201.)*

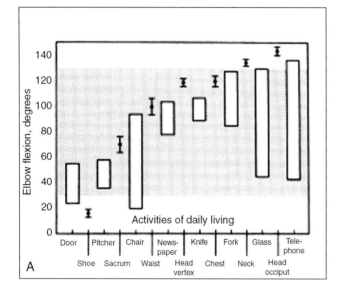

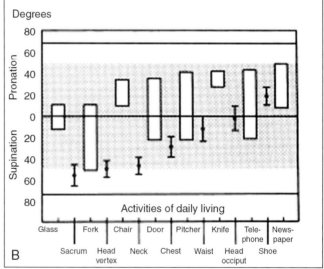

A

B

Figure 11   **A,** Functional arc of elbow motion for activities of daily living is approximately 100°, between 30° and 130°. **B,** Functional arc of forearm rotation is approximately 50° of pronation and 50° of supination for most activities of daily living. *(Reproduced with permission from Morrey BF, Askew LJ, An KN, et al: A biomechanical study of functional elbow motion. J Bone Joint Surg Am 1981; 63:872-877.)*

the trochlea of the distal humerus and the trochlear fossa of the proximal ulna. The humeroradial joint is formed by the articulation between the capitulum of the distal humerus and the head of the radius. The proximal radioulnar joint is formed by the head of the radius and the ra-

dial notch of the proximal ulna. The normal range of flexion-extension is between 0° and 140° to 160°. Forearm rotation consists of 70° to 80° of pronation and 80° to 85° of supination. The functional arc of motion for most activities of daily living is 100° from 30° to 130° of flexion-extension (**Figure 11,** *A)* with 50° of pronation and 50° of supination (**Figure 11,** *B).*

The rotational axis of flexion-extension can be approximated by a line passing through the center of the trochlea, bisecting the angle formed by the longitudinal axes of the humerus and the ulna. The instant centers of flexion and extension vary within 2 to 3 mm of this axis

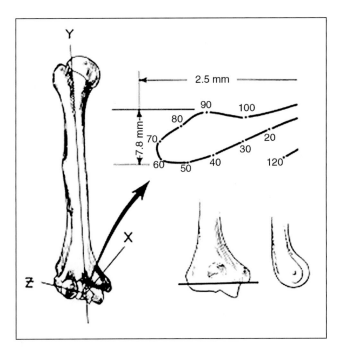

Figure 12   The very small locus of instant center of rotation for the elbow joint demonstrates that the axis may be replicated by a single line drawn from the inferior aspect of the medial epicondyle through the center of the lateral epicondyle, which is in the center of the lateral projected curvature of the trochlea and capitellum. *(Reproduced with permission from Morrey BF, Chao EY: Passive motion of the elbow joint. J Bone Joint Surg Am 1976;58:501-508.*

(**Figure 12**). With the elbow fully extended and the forearm fully supinated, the longitudinal axes of the humerus and ulna normally intersect at a valgus angle referred to as the carrying angle. In adults, the carrying angle averages 7° in men and 13° in women, varying as a function of flexion (**Figure 13**). This angle decreases with elbow flexion and there is a slight axial rotation of about 5°, first internal and then external rotation of the ulna with reference to the humerus. The optimal axis to best represent flexion-extension motion was found to be close to the line joining the centers of the capitellum and the trochlear groove.

Varus/valgus rotational motions at the elbow are restricted. Motion produced in this plane constitutes joint instability. The greatest resistance to rotational forces exists at the elbow on the medial side, where the medial collateral ligament (MCL) is the most important stabilizer, especially the anterior oblique fibers. The anterior oblique ligament is taut throughout the flexion-extension range, whereas the posterior oblique ligament is taut only during flexion. At 90° of flexion, the MCL contributes 54% of the resistance to valgus stress. The remainder is supplied by the shape of the articular surface and the anterior capsule. The articular congruity provides partial stability. The radial head provides about 30% of valgus stability and is more important in 0° to 30° of flexion and pronation. In extension, the olecranon becomes locked in its fossa. Equal contributions from the MCL, joint surface shape, and anterior capsule are important to resisting valgus stress in extension.

Stability to varus stress is provided by the lateral collateral ligament (LCL), anconeus, and joint capsule. The LCL contributes only 9% of restraint to varus stress at 90° of flexion. Approximately 78% of restraint to varus stress is provided by joint articulation and 13% by the joint capsule. In extension, the lateral ligament contributes 14% of restraint to varus stress, with 54% provided by the joint

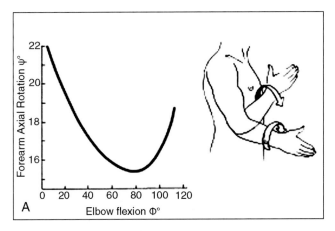

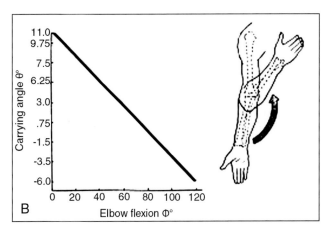

Figure 13   **A,** During elbow flexion, the ulna demonstrates a slight axial rotation referable to the humerus with an amplitude of less than 10°. **B,** During elbow flexion and extension, a linear change in the carrying angle is demonstrated, typically going from valgus in extension to varus in flexion. *(Reproduced with permission from Morrey BF, Chao EY: Passive motion of the elbow joint. J Bone Joint Surg Am 1976;58:501-508.)*

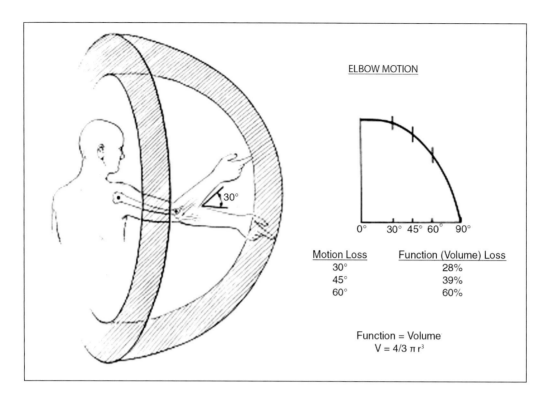

ELBOW MOTION

Motion Loss	Function (Volume) Loss
30°	28%
45°	39%
60°	60%

Function = Volume
$V = 4/3 \pi r^3$

Figure 14 Restricted elbow motion limits the sphere of influence of the hand in space. Flexion contractures of more than 30° are associated with a rapid loss of effective reach area. *(Reproduced with permission from An K-N, Morrey BF: Biomechanics, in Morrey BF, Chao EYS (eds): Joint Replacement Arthroplasty. New York, NY, Churchill Livingstone, 2003.)*

surface shape and 32% by the capsule.

Because the elbow functions as a link to position the hand in space, no single position is considered optimal for function. To understand this concept it is important to recognize that the shoulder functions as a ball joint, allowing the hand to circumscribe a portion of a spherical surface in space. With each successive change in the flexion position of the elbow, a sphere of a different radius is described. The elbow thus allows the upper extremity to operate at different distances away from the body. Loss of motion at the elbow can then be described as a loss of reach length. In actuality, the ability to reach not only is related to the diameter of the sphere but also affects the amount of the circumference of the sphere in which the hand can operate; that is, the volume of the sphere (**Figure 14**). Thus, reach capacity is not linear, but is calculated as a function of the third power of the radius. Patients can tolerate flexion contractures of approximately 30° with about a 20% functional loss; when loss is more than 30° of extension, patients readily report functional impairment. Extension contractures at the elbow also limit function, particularly if the dominant arm is involved. Inability to flex the elbow more than 100° restricts such self-care activities as dressing, feeding, and hygiene for the face and head.

Structure and Function of the Wrist

The wrist functions by allowing changes of orientation of the hand relative to the forearm. The wrist joint complex consists of multiple articulations of eight carpal bones with the distal radius, the structures of the ulnocarpal space, the metacarpals, and each other. This collection of bones and soft tissues is capable of a substantial arc of motion that augments hand and finger function.

Traditionally, the carpal bones are described as being arranged in two anatomic rows. The proximal carpal row consists of the scaphoid, lunate, and triquetrum, and the distal row is formed by the trapezium, trapezoid, capitate, and hamate. The pisiform lies within the flexor carpi ulnaris tendon and, through its articulation with the trapezium, functions as a sesamoid. Therefore, it is not included as a functional member of the proximal carpal row. The scaphoid links the proximal and distal rows. Both rows move with respect to each other in the midcarpal joint, and the proximal row moves on the radius in the radiocarpal joint.

The carpus may also be considered in terms of three functional columns (**Figure 15**). The central or flexion-extension column is formed by the distal carpal row and the lunate. This column functions as a longitudinal link between the radius and metacarpals and its integrity depends on the carpal ligaments because the muscles that produce wrist motion attach distal to the central column. The lateral or mobile column is the scaphoid. The medial or rotational column is the triquetrum.

The arrangement of the carpal bones and their ligaments is crucial to wrist stability. The two carpal rows articulate to form the midcarpal joint, which consists of three different types of articular surfaces. On the radial side, the trapezium and trapezoid (of the distal row) are concave with their articulations to the distal scaphoid and lateral capitate. The head of the capitate in the center of the midcarpal joint is convex. The ulnar-sided hamate-triquetral articulation is helicoid in nature. The proximal carpal row has a single biconvex joint surface that articulates with a more shallow, concave distal radius with two facets and a triangular fibrocartilage complex. The radiocarpal joint, therefore, appears relatively incongruent. The distal radius has an average of 14° of palmar tilt, and 22° of radial inclination. The distal radius probably contributes to the limitation of motion such that flexion is greater than extension and ulnar deviation greater than

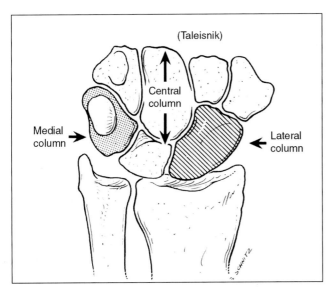

Figure 15   Three columns of the wrist with the bones in each are as follows: central, lunate, and entire distal carpal row; lateral, scaphoid; and medial, triquetrum. (*Reproduced with permission from* Regional Review of Courses in Hand Surgery, *ed 4. Aurora, CO, American Society for Surgery of the Hand, 1991.*)

radial deviation. The radial articular surface of the wrist affords no real bony stability. Stability is provided primarily by the soft-tissue envelope of the wrist.

Ligaments are the primary stabilizers of the wrist. They usually are classified into palmar and dorsal ligaments as well as extrinsic and intrinsic ligaments. The palmar ligaments, which are more numerous and substantial than the dorsal ligaments and are considered the principal stabilizers of the wrist, function mainly to resist hyperextension forces. Most of the extrinsic ligaments, which arise from the radius and ulna and attach to the carpus, insert on the proximal carpal row. The important extrinsic ligaments are the radioscaphocapitate, radiolunotriquetral, and ulnolunate. The intrinsic ligaments originate and insert on the carpus. The scapholunate ligament and the lunotriquetral ligament are important links in the proximal carpal row and provide additional stability to the wrist. The stability provided by the volar intrinsic and extrinsic ligaments may be best described by the double V configuration that they form (**Figure 16**). The arcuate ligaments, consisting of the radioscaphocapitate and ulnocapitate ligaments, converge on the capitate to form the distal V. The proximal V is formed by the radiolunotriquetral, radioscaphoid, ulnolunate, and ulnotriquetral ligaments. With ulnar deviation, the proximal V changes to an L configuration. The ulnolunate ligament assumes a more transverse orientation to essentially limit lunate displacement, and the radiolunate ligament assumes a more longitudinal configuration to limit lunate extension. The distal V ligamentous configuration similarly assumes an L configuration, but in the opposite direction. The scaphocapitate ligament becomes transverse to limit ulnar trans-

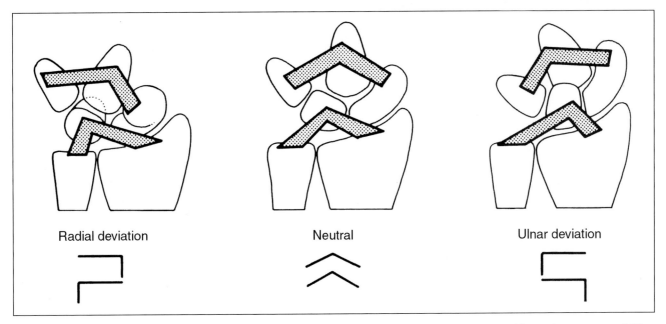

Radial deviation   Neutral   Ulnar deviation

Figure 16   Diagrammatic representation of changes in orientation of palmar radiocarpal ligaments. (*Illustration courtesy of Elizabeth Roselius, © 1985. Reproduced with permission from Taleisnik J (ed):* The Wrist. *New York, NY, Churchill Livingstone, 1985, p 26.*)

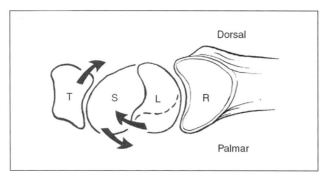

Figure 17   Schematic drawing of the trapezoid (T), scaphoid (S), lunate (L), and radius (R) in a sagittal view. The tendency of the wedge-shaped lunate (palmar pole larger than dorsal pole) to rotate into extension is counteracted by the scaphoid, which provides a palmar-flexing force induced by the trapezium and trapezoid. *(Reproduced with permission from Taleisnik J (ed): The Wrist. New York, NY, Churchill Livingstone, 1985.)*

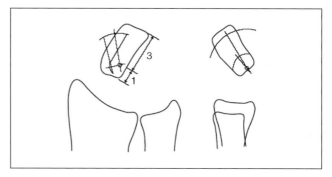

Figure 18   The location of the center of rotation during ulnar deviation (left) and extension (right), determined graphically using two metal markers embedded in the capitate. Note that during radial-ulnar deviation the center lies at a point in the capitate situated distal to the proximal end of this bone by a distance equivalent to approximately one quarter of its total longitudinal length. During flexion-extension, the center of rotation is close to the proximal cortex of the capitate. *(Reproduced with permission from McMurtry RY, Youm Y, Flatt AE, Gillespie TE: Kinematics of the wrist. II: Clinical applications. J Bone Joint Surg Am 1978;60:955-961.)*

lation of the capitate, and the triquetral capitate ligament assumes a longitudinal configuration to prevent capitate flexion. The opposite is believed to occur in radial deviation. In addition to creating movement, the extrinsic muscles of the wrist offer a dynamic component to wrist stability. There are six dedicated wrist muscles: the extensor carpi radialis brevis and longus, extensor carpi ulnaris, flexor carpi radialis, flexor carpi ulnaris, and palmaris longus muscles.

The midcarpal joints in the wrist create a double-hinged system. This bimuscular, biarticular construction is subject to collapse under compressive load. Because virtually no muscles insert on the carpus to provide dynamic stability, the compressive forces of the long flexors and extensors tend to cause the carpus to buckle at the metacarpophalangeal and midcarpal joints. Intricate ligamentous constraints and the precise opposition of multifaceted articular surfaces counteract these tendencies and afford stability. In the sagittal plane of the wrist, both the scaphoid and the lunate are wedge shaped, with the palmar aspect of both bones being wider than the dorsal aspect. Because compression tends to squeeze a wedge to its narrowest point, both the lunate and scaphoid would tend to be displaced palmarward and rotated into extension with contraction of the long flexors and extensors. As both the scaphoid and lunate tend to be forced into extension, stabilization forces must be directed primarily toward flexion. It is here that the contribution of the scaphoid spanning both the distal and proximal carpal rows can be appreciated. The natural tendency of the scaphoid to extend is stabilized at the midcarpal level. The trapezium and trapezoid articulate with the dorsal aspect of the scaphoid, pushing its distal pole down into flexion. Hence, the scaphoid counteracts the extension tendency of the lunate, lending some stability to the biarticular carpal complex (**Figure 17**). This arrangement has an advantage over a symmetric biarticular system because instability is focused

in only one direction and can be countered by a single force applied in the opposite direction or flexion.

Wrist Kinematics

The complexity of joint motion at the wrist makes it difficult to calculate the instant center of motion. However, the trajectories of the hand during radioulnar deviation and flexion/extension, when they occur in a fixed plane, are circular, and the rotation in each plane takes place about a fixed axis. These axes are located within the head of the capitate and are not altered by the position of the hand in the plane of rotation. During radioulnar deviation, the instant center of rotation lies at a point in the capitate situated distal to the proximal end of the capitate by a distance equivalent to approximately one quarter of its total length (**Figure 18**). During flexion/extension, the instant center of rotation is close to the proximal cortex of the capitate, which is somewhat more proximal than the location for the instant center of radioulnar deviation.

Normal carpal kinematics were studied in 22 cadaver specimens using a biplanar radiography method. The kinematics of the trapezium, capitate, hamate, scaphoid, lunate, and triquetrum were determined during wrist motion in the sagittal and coronal planes. The results were expressed using the concept of the screw displacement axis and converted to describe the magnitudes of rotation about and translation along three orthogonal axes. The orientation of these axes is expressed relative to the radius during sagittal plane motion of the wrist. The scaphoid exhibited the greatest magnitude of rotation and the lunate displayed the least rotation. The proximal carpal bones exhibited some ulnar deviation in 60° of wrist flexion. During coronal plane motion, the magnitude of the radioulnar deviation of the distal carpal bones were mutually similar and generally of a greater magnitude than that of the proximal carpal bones. The proximal carpal bones experience some flexion during radial deviation of the wrist and extension during ulnar deviation of the wrist.

The gross articulating surface motion of the wrist joint complex allows motion in two planes: flexion/extension (palmar flexion and dorsiflexion) in the sagittal plane and radioulnar deviation (abduction/adduction) in the frontal plane. Although small amounts of axial rotation are possible, from a practical standpoint such rotation does not occur through the carpal complex. The normal wrist range of motion is 65° to 80° of flexion and 55° to 75° of extension, but it can vary widely among individuals. Approximately 60% of flexion occurs at the midcarpal joint and 40% in the radiocarpal joint (**Figure 19**). Similarly, approximately 67% of extension takes place at the radiocarpal joint and 33% at the midcarpal joint. The total arc of radial-ulnar deviation is approximately 65° with 15° to 25° radialward and 30° to 45° ulnarward. The distal carpal row follows the finger rays during both radial and ulnar deviation, whereas the proximal carpal row glides in the direction opposite to hand movement with greater excursion during ulnar deviation. During radial deviation, the scaphoid undergoes flexion (palmarward rotation of its distal pole) as a result of its encroachment on the radial styloid process. This scaphoid motion is transmitted across the proximal row through the scapholunate ligament. Thus, in radial deviation the scaphoid flexes and so does the proximal carpal row. This conjoint movement of the scaphoid and proximal carpal row is reversed toward extension during ulnar deviation. During ulnar deviation, the triquetrum is ulnarly deviated by the proximal migration of the hamate. The motion of the triquetrum in turn causes the lunate to extend.

Structure and Function of the Hand

The hand is extremely mobile, capable of conforming to a large variety of object shapes and coordinating an infinite variety of movements in relation to each of its components. The mobility of the hand is possible because of the unique arrangement of the bones in relation to one another, the articular contours, and the action of an intricate system of muscles.

The two primary functions of the hand as an organ are touch and prehension. Prehension has been defined as the grasping or taking hold of an object between any two surfaces of the hand, or when an object is seized within the cup of the hand. Prehension may or may not include the thumb. The fundamental requirement of prehension is a firm grip. It is performed in different fashions according to the purpose of the grip, and it is described as either power grip or precision grip. Power grip is defined as forceful finger flexion used to maintain an object against the palm (**Figure 20,** *A*). The ulnar two digits, which are in-

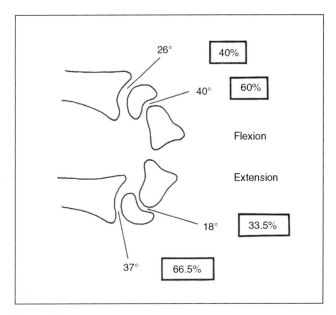

Figure 19 Approximately 60% of wrist flexion (top) occurs at the midcarpal joint, whereas approximately two thirds of wrist extension (bottom) arises at the radiocarpal joint. (*Reproduced with permission from Sarrafian, SK, Melamed JL, Goshgarian GM: Study of wrist motion in flexion and extension.* Clin Orthop Relat Res *1977;126:153-159.*)

nervated by the ulnar nerve, are more related to power grip. They provide support instead of control during power grip. Precision grip requires fine kinesthetic control and usually is associated with fine tactile sensibility at the fingertips (**Figure 20,** *B*). Precision grip is formed by clamping together the fingers and thumb, with the object held at the tips of the digits such that the palm is not involved. In this position, maximum sensation and speedy movement are available. The thumb, index, and middle fingers, which have median nerve innervation, are more related to precision grip. This radial side of the hand has been referred to as the "dynamic tridactyl" and is concerned with balance, such as in holding a coffee cup.

Three-dimensional geometric models of the articular surfaces of the hand have been constructed. The sagittal contours of the metacarpal head and proximal phalanx grossly resemble the arc of a circle. The radius of curvature of a circle fitted to the entire proximal phalanx surface ranges from 11 to 13 mm, almost twice as much as that of the metacarpal head, which ranges from 6 to 7 mm. The local centers of curvature along the sagittal contour of the metacarpal heads are not fixed. The locus of the center of curvature for the subchondral bony contour approximates the locus of the center for the acute curve of an ellipse (**Figure 21**). However, the locus of center of curvature for the articular cartilage contour approximates the locus of the obtuse curve of an ellipse.

Rolling and sliding actions of articulating surfaces exist during finger joint motion. The geometric shapes of the articular surfaces of the metacarpal head and proxi-

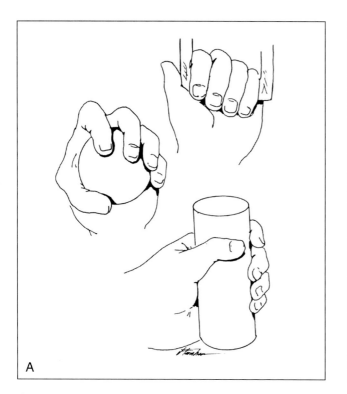

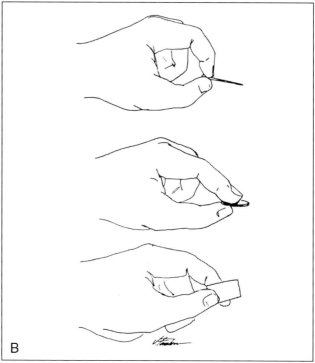

Figure 20   **A,** Power grip: hook grip (*top*), spherical grip (*center*), and cylindrical grip (*bottom*). **B,** Precision grip or handling: tip-to-tip prehension (*top*), pad-to-pad prehension (*center*), and pad-to-side prehension (*bottom*). (*Reproduced with permission from Norkin C, Le Vangie P (eds):* Joint Structure and Function: A Comprehensive Analysis. *Philadelphia, PA, FA Davis, 1990, p 243.*)

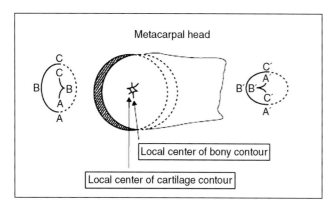

Figure 21   The loci of the local centers of curvature for sub-chondral bony contour of the metacarpal head approximates the loci of the center for the acute curve of an ellipse. The loci of the local center of curvature for articular cartilage contour of the metacarpal head approximated the loci of the bony center of the obtuse curve of an ellipse. (*Reproduced with permission from Tamai K, Ryu J, An KN, Linscheid RL, Cooney WP, Chao EY: Three-dimensional geometric analysis of the metacarpopha-langeal joint.* J Hand Surg [Am] *1988;13:521-529.*)

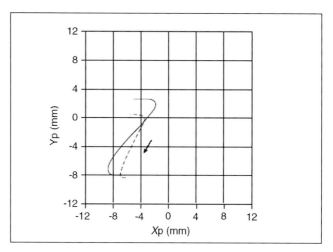

Figure 22   Intersections of the instantaneous helical angles with the metacarpal sagittal plane. They are relative to one subject tested twice in different days. The origin of the graph is coincident with the calibrated center of the metacarpal head. The arrow indicates the direction of flexion (+Xp: proximal; +Yp: dorsal). (*Reproduced with permission from Schuind F, An KN, Cooney WP III, Garcia-Elias M (eds):* Advances in the Biomechanics of the Hand and Wrist. *New York, NY, Plenum Press, 1994, pp 363-375.*)

mal phalanx, as well as the insertion location of the collateral ligaments, significantly govern the articulating kinematics, and the center of rotation is not fixed but rather moves as a function of the angle of flexion. The instant centers of rotation are within 3 mm of the center of the metacarpal head. The instantaneous helical axis of the

metacarpophalangeal joint tends to be more palmar and tends to be displaced distally as flexion increases (**Figure 22**).

The axes of rotation of the carpometacarpal joint have

been described as being polycentric. Instantaneous motion occurs reciprocally between centers of rotation within the trapezium and the metacarpal base of the normal thumb. In flexion/extension, the axis of rotation is located within the trapezium, but for abduction/adduction, the center of rotation is located distally to the trapezium and within the base of the first metacarpal. The average instantaneous center of circumduction is at approximately the center of the trapezial joint surface.

The axes of rotation of the thumb interphalangeal and metacarpophalangeal joints were located using a mechanical device. The physiologic motion of the thumb joint occurs about these axes. The interphalangeal joint axis is parallel to the flexion crease of the joint and is not perpendicular to the phalanx. The metacarpophalangeal joint has two fixed axes: a fixed flexion-extension axis just distal and volar to the epicondyles, and an abduction-adduction axis related to the proximal phalanx passing through the sesamoids. Neither axis is perpendicular to the phalanges.

The thumb is the most important digit on the hand because of its ability to oppose the fingers as a result of its moveable metacarpal. The thumb ray is believed to start with the trapezium and its articulation with the first metacarpal because there is no significant motion among the carpals with thumb motion. The flexion-extension plane of motion for the thumb is described as being approximately parallel to the palm. Flexion is motion toward the hypothenar eminence, whereas palmar abduction-adduction occurs in a plane perpendicular to the flexion-extension plane. The trapeziometacarpal joint allows approximately 45° to 70° of flexion, accompanied by some pronation. Overall thumb motion also includes approximately 0° to 30° of adduction to 40° to 70° of palmar abduction. The palmar abduction is divided between the carpometacarpal joint with an average of 42° and the metacarpophalangeal joint with a range of 0° to 20°.

Thumb opposition consists of the composite motions of abduction, which lift the thumb away from the hand, and rotation of the thumb into pronation. Thumb pronation is rotation of the thumb so that the pulp surfaces of the thumb and fingers face one another. Opposition occurs as a unit involving the interphalangeal, metacarpophalangeal, and trapeziometacarpal joints, and sequentially proceeds through abduction, flexion, and adduction accompanied by simultaneous pronation. The motion of the thumb forms a cone. The rotation is not around the axis of the first metacarpal, but is the result of an arc around a central point in the palm. It is this swinging movement in abduction that is used to draw the thumb in front of the palm and then hold an object between the thumb and finger. Full opposition proceeds through approximately 110° from full extension to complete abduction-flexion and rotation. Opposition occurs primarily at the trapeziometacarpal joint, making it the most important joint in the hand.

The trapezium is angled volarly, placing the rest of the thumb in a position palmar to the plane of the hand. In a resting position, the first metacarpal then forms an angle of approximately 45° to 60° with the second metacarpal.

The trapeziometacarpal joint is a double-saddle configuration with a ridge on the surface of the trapezium. It is concave in one plane and convex in another. This geometry permits primarily two degrees of freedom, flexion-extension and abduction-adduction. However, with distraction an average of 17° of axial rotation occurs. The prime stabilizer of the trapeziometacarpal joint is the anterior-oblique ligament, which is taut in abduction, extension, and pronation. The first intermetacarpal, ulnar-collateral, and posterior-oblique ligaments make up the secondary stabilizers. The dorsal-radial facet provides the main resistance to dorsal subluxation and becomes eroded early in degenerative arthritis.

The metacarpophalangeal joint of the thumb has a condylar configuration with two degrees of freedom. It has variable flexion-extension ranging from 0° to 90° and an average flexion of 55°. Although these motions at the metacarpophalangeal joint aid in opposition, if metacarpophalangeal joint motion is lost or the joint is fused, the adjacent joints in the thumb will compensate. Similarly, if the carpometacarpal joint is lost or fixed in an opposed position, the metacarpophalangeal joint, having good intrinsic control, can take over as the prime mobile joint. The metacarpophalangeal joint is statically stabilized by the collateral ligaments and volar plate. In addition, the thenar intrinsic muscles, by inserting onto the two sesamoids and the extensor mechanism, provide dynamic restraints to hyperextension and excessive abduction and adduction.

The interphalangeal joint is a true hinge joint with one degree of freedom. It is similarly stabilized by a volar plate and two collateral ligaments. It allows an average of 85° to 90° of flexion, which is accompanied by slight pronation. The joint also allows an average of 0° to 20° of hyperextension to increase the surface area of the thumb pad available to pinch.

Finger Kinematics

Each of the four finger rays is composed of a metacarpal, its three phalanges, and their interposed articulations. The metacarpals themselves provide a space, in length and width, to allow objects of size to be grasped. Palmar cupping allows the hand to conform to objects to increase the surface area of contact and improve application of gripping forces. This cupping is made possible by three arches of the hand. A longitudinal arch is formed by the metacarpals and flexed fingers. This arch is supplemented by two transverse arches. The first is a relatively immobile structural arch, formed by the carpals and supported by the transverse carpal ligament. The second transverse arch is distal, is formed by the metacarpal heads, and allows the hand to have greater adaptability. The progressive motion of the ulnar digits, along with the hypothenar muscles, flex and adduct the fifth metacarpal and finger to assist in cradling objects. The palm cups with metacarpal flexion and, reciprocally, the palm flattens with metacarpal extension.

Proximally, the metacarpals of each digit articulate with the wrist via the carpometacarpal joints. The primary function of these joints is to stabilize the metacarpals and, on the ulnar side, control hollowing of the palm. Joints of the index through the ring fingers are considered to be plain synovial joints with one degree of freedom, flexion and extension. The fifth carpometacarpal joint is described as a shallow saddle joint with two degrees of freedom. The carpometacarpal joints are stabilized by tough transverse intermetacarpal and longitudinal carpometacarpal ligaments. The dorsal carpometacarpal ligaments are stronger than the volar ligaments. The second carpometacarpal joint is relatively immobile, but progressively more mobility is seen in the fourth and fifth metacarpals. The fourth carpometacarpal joint exhibits 8° to 10° of motion, whereas the fifth carpometacarpal joint exhibits 15° to 20° of flexion with supination.

The metacarpophalangeal joints are considered the key element in the kinematic chain of the fingers as they position the interphalangeal joints in space. Their surfaces are described as being condyloid, with predominantly two degrees of rotational freedom. Motion is primarily in the flexion-extension axis, followed by abduction-adduction and accompanied by slight rotation. The metacarpal head has an eccentric articular surface that is broader on the palmar surface. This structure, combined with the eccentric insertion of its collateral ligaments, permits more abduction and adduction with the joint in extension than flexion. Collateral ligaments tighten with flexion, making this the most stable position. In addition to the collateral ligaments, the metacarpophalangeal joints are stabilized by the volar plate, sagittal bands of the extensor apparatus, and the deep transverse metacarpal ligament. The deep transverse metacarpal ligament or intervolar plate ligament is continuous with the volar plate and holds them together. These joints show a slight increase in the range of motion into flexion, proceeding from the radial side to the ulnar side with the index finger showing approximately 90° of flexion and the fifth metacarpophalangeal joint showing approximately 110° of flexion. The metacarpophalangeal joints have an average passive hyperextension range of 30° to 45°. Although this range is relatively constant between digits, it varies greatly between individuals and is commonly used as a measure of general flexibility. In full extension, the fingertips lie on the circumference of a circle formed in the plane of the hand, the center of which is the head of the third metacarpal. When closing the hand, the fingers flex and adduct to converge toward the base of the thenar eminence. This movement is facilitated by increased motion in the ulnar digits.

There are two separate functional positions that exist

Table 2   Joint Orientation Angles for Index Finger Function

Function	Joint Flexion Angle (°)*		
	DIP	PIP	MP
Tip pinch	25	50	48
Key pinch	20	35	20
Pulp pinch	0	50	48
Grasp	23	48	62
Baggage/hook grip	44	72	23
Holding glass	20	48	5
Opening big jar	35	55	50

*DIP = distal interphalangeal; PIP = proximal interphalangeal; MP = metacarpophalangeal

Reproduced with permission from An KN, Chao EY, Cooney WP, et al: Forces in the normal and abnormal hand. J Orthop Res 1985;3:202-211.

as the fingers flex to grasp an object. The first is the formation of the placement arc, which occurs at a position where there is full metacarpophalangeal flexion and is responsible for 77% of total finger flexion. The position during which the fingers grasp an object, known as the final encompassment, arises from motion of the proximal interphalangeal (PIP) and distal interphalangeal (DIP) joints and makes up the remaining 23% of finger flexion. The PIP joint contributes 85% and the DIP joint 15% of this motion. Thus, it can be deduced that the PIP joint is the critical joint in final encompassment, emphasizing the importance of its motion.

The interphalangeal joints, both PIP and DIP, are true hinge joints with one degree of freedom in flexion-extension. These joints are stabilized by collateral ligaments as well as by a strong volar plate that prevents hyperextension. The collateral ligaments of the interphalangeal joints are relatively taut in all positions of flexion, such that the joint is relatively stable throughout its range of motion. Consistent with the other joints of the finger rays, the interphalangeal joints show a similar pattern of increased range of motion from radial to ulnar. PIP joint flexion averages 100° to 115° at the index finger and progressively increases to approximately 135° at the little finger. Similarly, the DIP joint of the index finger has a mean flexion of 80°, which increases to 90° at the little finger. The adjacent condyles of the heads of the proximal phalanges vary such that with flexion, the middle through little fingers deviate radially at the PIP joints while the index finger's interphalangeal joint deviates ulnarly. This deviation, along with the progressive range of motion in the ulnar digits, helps to angulate these digits when flexed toward the scaphoid tubercle, thereby assisting in the opposition to the thumb as well as providing a tighter ulnar

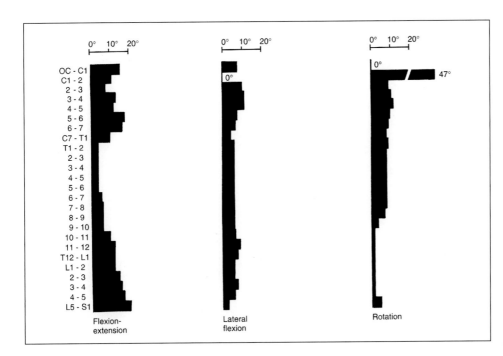

Figure 23 A composite of representative values for type and range of motion at different levels of the spine. *(Reproduced with permission from White AA III, Panjabi MN (eds): Clinical Biomechanics of the Spine. Philadelphia, PA, JB Lippincott, 1978.)*

grip. The joint orientation angles for index finger functions are presented to reinforce the overall range that is required in different joints for various functions (**Table 2**).

Structure and Function of the Spine

The human spine is a flexible column with a multicurved shape. Its principal functions are to protect the spinal cord and transfer loads from the head and trunk to the pelvis. Each of the 24 vertebrae articulates with adjacent ones to permit motion in three planes.

The vertebrae have six degrees of freedom: rotation about and translation along a transverse, sagittal, and longitudinal axis. These motions are usually coupled. Therefore, the motion produced during flexion, extension, lateral flexion, and axial rotation of the spine is a complex combined motion resulting from simultaneous rotation and translation. The relative amount of motion at different levels of the spine varies (**Figure 23**). The range of flexion and extension is approximately 4° in each of the upper thoracic motion segments, approximately 6° in the midthoracic region, and approximately 12° in the two lower thoracic segments. This range progressively increases in the lumbar motion segments, reaching a maximum of 20° at the lumbosacral level. Lateral flexion shows the greatest range in each of the lower thoracic segments, reaching 8° to 9°. In the upper thoracic segments, the range is uniformly 6°. Six degrees of lateral flexion is also found in each of all lumbar segments except the lumbosacral segment, which demonstrates only 3° of motion. Rotation is greatest in the upper segments of the thoracic spine, where the range is 9°. The range of rotation progressively decreases caudally, reaching 2° in the lower segments of

the lumbar spine. It then increases to 5° in the lumbosacral segment. The main determinant for range of motion is the orientation of the facet and intervertebral disks. The thoracic region is stabilized by the rib cage and there is generally little motion. The lumbar spine commits considerable lateral bending in the middle portion whereas flexion-extension is greatest in the lumbosacral motion segment. Rotation is remote in the lumbar region because of the orientation of the facet joints. Compared with the thoracic spine, the greater mobility in the cervical and lumbar regions corresponds with greater stresses and more clinical complaints. Motion between the surfaces of two adjacent vertebrae may be analyzed using instantaneous axes of rotation. The instantaneous center of rotation in the cervical, thoracic, and lumbar regions varies with level of the spine (**Figure 24**).

The functional motion of the spine varies with age and gender. Older people have less mobility, decreasing by approximately 30% from youth to old age. Loss of range of motion is noted in flexion and lateral bending whereas axial rotation motion is maintained with evidence of increased coupled motion. Gender differences have also been noted: men have greater mobility in flexion and extension, whereas women are more mobile in lateral flexion.

The range of motion differs at various levels of the spine and depends on the orientation of the facets of the intervertebral joints (**Figure 25**). Motion between two vertebrae is small and does not occur independently. All spinal movements involve the combined actions of several motion segments. These skeletal structures influence motion of the trunk of the rib cage, which limits thoracic mo-

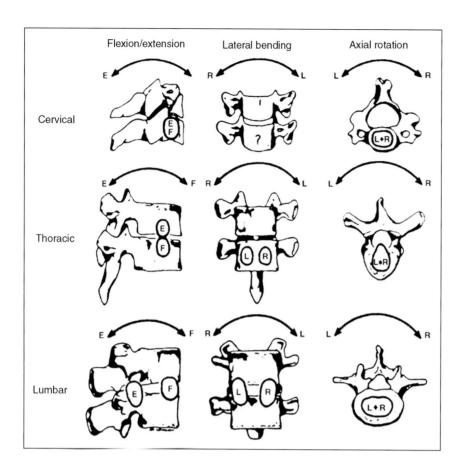

Figure 24   Approximate locations of instantaneous axes of rotation (IAR) in the three regions of the spine undergoing rotation in the three traditional planes. E = approximate location of IARs in extending from neutral position; F = IARs in flexion from neutral position; L = IARs in left lateral bending or left axial rotation. R = IARs in right lateral bending or right axial rotation. *(Reproduced with permission from White AA III, Panjabi MM (eds): Clinical Biomechanics of the Spine. Philadelphia, PA, JB Lippincott, 1978.)*

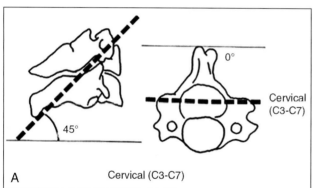

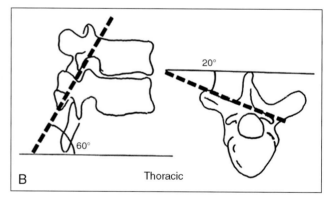

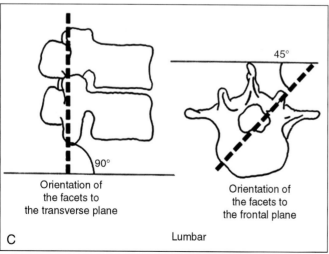

Figure 25   Orientation of the facets of the intervertebral joints (approximate values). **A,** In the lower cervical spine, the facets are oriented at a 45° angle to the transverse plane and are parallel to the frontal plane. **B,** The facets of the thoracic spine are oriented at a 60° angle to the transverse plane and at a 20° angle to the frontal plane. **C,** The facets of the lumbar spine are oriented at a 90° angle to the transverse plane and at a 45° angle to the frontal plane. *(Reproduced with permission from White AA III, Panjabi MM (eds): Clinical Biomechanics of the Spine. Philadelphia, PA, JB Lippincott, 1978.)*

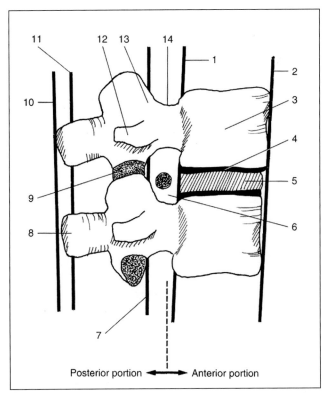

Figure 26 Schematic representation of a motion segment in the lumbar spine (sagittal view). Anterior portion: 1, posterior longitudinal ligament; 2, anterior longitudinal ligament; 3, vertebral body; 4, cartilaginous end plate; 5, intervertebral disk; 6, intervertebral foramen with nerve root. Posterior portion: 7, ligamentum flavum; 8, spinous process; 9, intervertebral joint formed by the superior and inferior facet (the capsular ligament is not shown); 10, supraspinous ligament; 11, interspinous ligament; 12, transverse process (the intertransverse ligament is not shown); 13, arch; 14, vertebral canal (the spinal cord is not depicted). *(Reproduced with permission from Nordin M, Schecter Weiner S: Biomechanics of the lumbar spine, in Nordin M, Frankel VH (eds): Basic Biomechanics of the Musculoskeletal System, ed 3. New York, NY, Lippincott Williams & Wilkins, 2001, p 257.)*

tion, and the pelvis, which augments trunk movements by tilting.

The motion segment is a basic functional unit of the spine. It consists of two adjacent vertebrae and their intervening soft tissues. It is convenient to divide the motion segment into anterior and posterior elements or columns (**Figure 26**). The dividing line is just behind the vertebral body. The anterior portion of the segment is composed of two superimposed intervertebral bodies, the intervertebral disk, and the longitudinal ligaments. The posterior portion consists of the vertebral arches, the intervertebral joints formed by the facets, the transverse and spinous processes, and various ligaments.

Anterior Portion of the Motion Segment
The vertebral bodies are designed to bear mainly compressive loads and become progressively larger caudally as

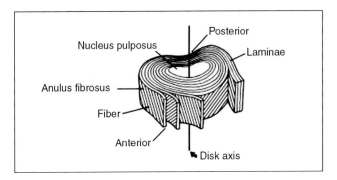

Figure 27 The intervertebral disk. *(Adapted with permission from Pope MH, Frymoyer JW, Lehmann TR (eds): Structure and function of the lumbar spine, in Occupational Low Back Pain: Assessment, Treatment, and Prevention. St. Louis, MO, CV Mosby, 1991.)*

the superimposed weight of the upper body increases. The vertebral bodies in the lumbar region are thicker and wider than those in the thoracic or cervical regions. The intervertebral disk forms the primary articulation between adjacent vertebral bodies. The disk is composed of two morphologically separate units. The outer part, the anulus fibrosus, is composed of approximately 90 collagen sheets bonded to each other. Each sheet is made of collagen fibers oriented vertically at the peripheral layer, but becoming progressively more oblique with each underlying layer (**Figure 27**). The criss-cross arrangement of the coarse collagen fiber bundles allows the anulus fibrosus to withstand high bending and torsional loads. The inner, or central, part of the disk is a gelatinous mass called the nucleus pulposus. In young individuals, the nucleus pulposus is nearly 90% water, with the remaining structure comprising collagen and proteoglycans, which bind water. The nucleus pulposus lies directly in the center of all disks except for those in the lumbar segments, where it has a slightly posterior position. In young and healthy disks, positive pressure within the nucleus pulposus increases as loads are applied to the spine. In a disk loaded in compression, the pressure is approximately 1.5 times the externally applied load per unit area. Because the nuclear material is only slightly compressible, a compressive load makes the disk bulge laterally, creating circumferential tensile stress that is sustained by the annular fibers. In the lumbar spine, the tensile stress in the posterior portion of the anulus fibrosus has been estimated to be four to five times the applied axial compressive load (**Figure 28**). The tensile stress in the anulus fibrosus in the thoracic spine is less than that in the lumbar spine because of the difference in disk geometry. The higher ratio of disk diameter to height in the thoracic disk reduces the circumferential stress.

Posterior Portion of the Motion Segment
The posterior portion of the motion segment guides its movement. The type of motion possible at any level of the

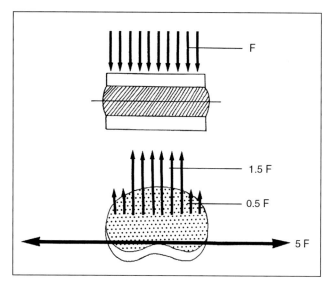

Figure 28   Distribution of stress in a cross-section of a lumbar disk under compressive loading. The compressive stress is highest in the nucleus pulposus, 1.5 times the externally applied load (F) per unit area. By contrast, the compressive stress on the anulus fibrosis is approximately 0.5 times the externally applied load. This part of the disk bears predominantly tensile stress, which is four to five times greater than the externally applied load per unit. (*Reproduced with permission from Nachemsom A: Towards a better understanding of back pain: A review of the mechanics of the lumbar disc. Rheumatol Rehabil 1975;14:129-143.*)

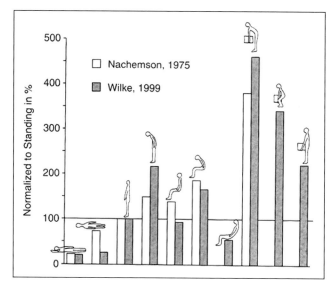

Figure 29   Data from two studies using intradiskal pressure measurements. The relative loads on the third and fourth lumbar disks measured in vivo in various body positions are compared with the load during upright standing, depicted as 100%. (*Reproduced with permission from Nachemson A: Towards a better understanding of back pain: A review of the mechanics of the lumbar disc. Rheumatol Rehabil 1975;14:129-143 and from Wilke HJ, Neef P, Caimi M, et al: New in vivo measurements of pressures in the intervertebral disc in daily life. Spine 1999;24:755-762.*)

spine is determined by the orientation of the facets of the intervertebral joints to the transverse and frontal planes. This orientation changes throughout the spine. Except for the facets of the two uppermost cervical vertebrae (C1 and C2), which are parallel to the transverse plane, the facets of the cervical intervertebral joints are oriented at a 45° angle to the transverse plane and are parallel to the frontal plane (**Figure 25,** *A*). This alignment of the joint of C3 to C7 allows flexion, extension, lateral flexion, and rotation. The facets of the thoracic joints are oriented at a 60° angle to the transverse plane and at a 20° angle to the frontal plane (**Figure 25,** *B*). This orientation allows lateral flexion, rotation, and some flexion and extension. In the lumbar region, the facets are oriented at right angles to the transverse plane and at a 45° angle to the frontal plane (**Figure 25,** *C*). This alignment allows flexion, extension, and lateral flexion, but almost no rotation. The lumbosacral joints differ from the other lumbar intervertebral joints in that the oblique orientation of the facets allows appreciable rotation.

The facets guide movement of the motion segment and have a load-bearing function. Load sharing between the facets and the disk varies with the position of the spine. The loads on the facets are greatest (approximately 30% of the total load) when the spine is hyperextended.

The ligamentous structures surrounding the spine contribute to its intrinsic stability (**Figure 26**). The liga-

ments of the spine can be divided into three systems. The nonsegmental longitudinal system includes the anterior and posterior longitudinal ligaments and the supraspinous ligaments. The segmental longitudinal system includes the intraspinous, intratransverse ligaments, and the ligamentum flavum. The articular or capsular system comprises the capsular ligaments. At the cephalad and caudal ends of the spine, specialized ligaments attach the skull and the iliac bones, respectively. Ligaments aid in the control of motion and are vital for the structural stability of the motion segment. The ligaments are also the primary tensile load-bearing structures, acting as passive elements to prevent excessive motion. The amount of strain on the various ligaments differs with the type of motion of the spine. During flexion, the intraspinous ligaments are subjected to the greatest strain, followed by the capsular ligaments and the ligamentum flavum. During extension, the anterior longitudinal ligament bears the greatest strain. During lateral flexion, the contralateral transverse ligament sustains the highest strains, followed by the ligamentum flavum and the capsular ligaments. The capsular ligaments of the facet joints bear the most strain during rotation.

Comparative Loads on the Lumbar Spine

Body position affects the magnitude of the loads on the spine (**Figure 29**). Loads on the spine are minimized when an individual assumes a supine position because the loads produced by the body's weight are eliminated. During re-

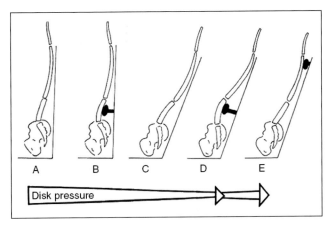

Figure 30 Influence of backrest inclination and back support on loads of the lumbar spine, in terms of pressure in the third lumbar disk, during supported sitting. **A,** Backrest inclination is 90° and disk pressure is at a maximum. **B,** Addition of a lumbar support decreases the disk pressure. **C,** Backward inclination of the backrest is 110°, but with no lumbar support it produces less disk pressure. **D,** Addition of a lumbar support with this degree of backrest inclination further decreases the pressure. **E,** Shifting the support to the thoracic region pushes the upper body forward, moving the lumbar spine toward kyphosis and increasing the disk pressure. (*Adapted with permission from Andersson BJ, Ortengren R, Nachemson, A, Elfstrom G: Lumbar disc pressure and myoelectric back muscle activity during sitting: 1. Studies on an experimental chair.* Scand J Rehabil Med *1974;6:104-114.*)

Table 3   Geometry of the Proximal Femur

Parameter	Females	Males
Femoral head diameter (mm)	45.0 ± 3.0	52.0 ± 3.3
Neck shaft angle (deg)	133 ± 6.6	129 ± 7.3
Anteversion (deg)	8 ± 10	7.0 ± 6.8

Reproduced with permission from Yoshioka Y, Siu D, Cooke TD: The anatomy and functional axes of the femur. J Bone Joint Surg Am 1987;69:873-880.

laxed upright standing, the load on the third and fourth lumbar disks is increased. Trunk flexion increases the load on the spine. The loads on the lumbar spine are lower during supported sitting than during unsupported sitting. During supported sitting, the weight of the upper body is supported by the backrest, which reduces the muscle activity, thereby relieving intradiskal pressure. Backward inclination of the backrest and use of a lumbar support further reduces the loads (**Figure 30**). The use of a support in the thoracic region, however, pushes the thoracic spine and the trunk forward and makes the lumbar spine move toward kyphosis to remain in contact with the backrest, thereby increasing the loads on the lumbar spine. Lifting activities further increase the load on the lumbar spine (**Figure 29**).

The time-dependent (viscoelastic) properties of the intervertebral disk result in diurnal changes in height. Reported diurnal height changes range from 6.3 mm to 19.3 mm, with an average of 15.7 mm. The average person is 1% shorter in the evening than in the morning. Children are 2% shorter in the evening, and the elderly are 0.5% shorter in the evening. Fifty percent of the total length change occurs during the first 2 hours in the upright posture. Thus, for most people, the first 2 hours out of bed in the morning are critical for people with degenerative disks.

Structure and Function of the Hip Joint

The hip joint is a ball-and-socket joint in which the head of the femur resides in the acetabulum of the pelvis. The hip joint is one of the most stable joints in the body. The stability is provided by the rigid ball-and-socket configuration. The constraint provided by the bony architecture minimizes the need for ligamentous and soft-tissue constraints to maintain the stability of hip articulation. The femoral head is spherical in its articular portion, which forms two thirds of its sphere. The diameter of the femoral head is smaller in females than in males (**Table 3**). In the normal hip, the center of the femoral head coincides exactly within the center of the acetabulum. The rounded part of the femoral head is spheroidal rather than spherical because the uppermost part is flattened slightly, causing the load to be distributed in a ring-like pattern around the superior pole. The head is supported by the neck of the femur, which joins the shaft. The axis of the femoral neck is obliquely set and runs superiorly, medially, and anteriorly. The angle of inclination of the femoral neck to the shaft in the frontal plane is the neck-shaft angle (**Figure 31, A**). In most adults, this angle is about 130° (**Table 3**). An angle exceeding 130° is known as coxa valga. An angle less than 130° is known as coxa vara. The femoral neck forms an acute angle with the transverse axis of the femoral condyles. This angle faces medially and anteriorly and is called the angle of anteversion (**Figure 31, B**). In the adult, this angle averages about 7.5° (**Table 3**).

The acetabulum receives the femoral head and lies on the lateral aspect of the hip. The adult acetabulum is a hemispherical socket. Together with the labrum, the acetabulum covers slightly more than 50% of the femoral head. Only the sides of the acetabulum are lined by articular cartilage, which is interrupted inferiorly by the deep acetabular notch. The articulation of the femoral head in the acetabulum permits three degrees of rotational freedom of the femur about the pelvis while essentially eliminating translation between the femoral head and the acetabulum. The rotational motion occurs around three mutually perpendicular axes that intersect at the geometric center of rotation of the spherical head. The transverse axis lies in the frontal plane and flexion and extension occur around this axis. An anterior-posterior axis lies in the

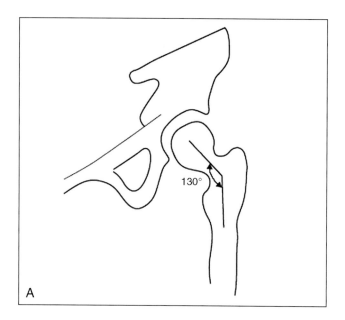

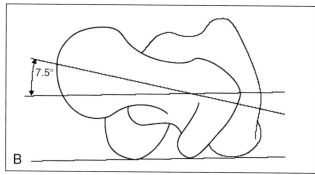

Figure 31   **A,** The hip neck-shaft angle. **B,** The normal anteversion angle formed by a line tangent to the femoral condyles and the femoral neck axis, as displayed in the superior view.

sagittal plane and adduction and abduction occur around this axis. A vertical axis coincides with the long axis of the limb when the hip joint is in the neutral position with internal and external rotation occurring around this axis. Surface motion in the hip joint can be considered a spinning of the femoral head on the acetabulum. The pivoting of the acetabulum in three planes around the center of rotation in the femoral head produces spinning of the joint surfaces.

Hip motion takes place in all three planes: sagittal (flexion-extension), frontal (abduction-adduction), and transverse (internal-external rotation). Motion is greatest in the sagittal plane, where the range of flexion is from 0° to approximately 140° and the range of extension is from 0° to 15°. The range of abduction is from 0° to 30° whereas that of adduction is somewhat less, from 0° to 25°. External rotation ranges from 0° to 90° and internal rotation from 0° to 70° when the hip joint is flexed. Less rotation occurs when the hip joint is extended because of the restricting function of the soft tissues. The range of motion of the hip joint used during activities of daily living varies (**Table 4**). Maximum motion in the sagittal plane (hip flexion) is needed for tying the shoe and bending down to pick up an object from the floor. The greatest motion in the frontal and transverse planes occurs during squatting and during shoe tying with the foot across the opposite thigh. The values obtained for these common activities indicate that hip flexion of at least 120° as well as abduction and external rotation of at least 20° are necessary for carrying out daily activities of living.

Structure and Function of the Knee

The human knee is the largest and most complex joint in the body. The knee is composed of the tibiofemoral articulation and the patellofemoral articulation. The knee is

Table 4   Mean Values for Maximum Hip Motion in Three Planes During Common Activities

Activity	Plane of Motion	Recorded Value (Degrees)
Tying shoe with foot on floor	Sagittal	124
	Frontal	19
	Transverse	15
Tying shoe with foot across opposite thigh	Sagittal	110
	Frontal	23
	Transverse	33
Sitting down on chair and rising from sitting	Sagittal	104
	Frontal	20
	Transverse	17
Stooping to obtain object from floor	Sagittal	117
	Frontal	21
	Transverse	18
Squatting	Sagittal	122
	Frontal	28
	Transverse	26
Ascending stairs	Sagittal	67
	Frontal	16
	Transverse	18
Descending stairs	Sagittal	36

Mean for 33 normal men.

Data from Johnston RC, Smidt GL: Hip motion measurement for selected activities of daily living. Clin Orthop Relat Res 1970;72:205-215.

situated between the two largest bones and longest lever arms in the body. The tibiofemoral joint is a modified hinge joint containing the articulating ends of the distal femur and the proximal tibia. The patellofemoral joint consists of the patella (the largest sesamoid bone) and the trochlea of the femur. Taken together, the knee joint's function maintains and alters given leg length, acts as a

Table 5   Range of Tibiofemoral Joint Motion in the Sagittal Plane During Common Activities

Activity	Knee Flexion (Degrees)
Walking	60[*]
Climbing stairs	94[*]
Descending stairs	87[*]
Sitting down	93[†]
Tying a shoe	106[†]
Lifting an object	117[†]

*Data from Kaufman et al (2001). Mean for 20 subjects
†Laubenthal et al (1972). Mean for 30 subjects.

shock absorber, transmits load, and provides propulsive forces for locomotion.

The shape of the articular surfaces of the proximal tibia and distal femur must fulfill the requirement that they move in contact with one another. The profile of the femoral condyles varies with the condyle examined. The lateral condyle is smaller than the medial in both the AP and proximal distal directions and contributes to the valgus and AP alignment of the knee joint. There is a slight inclination of the tibial plateau in relation to the joint line of 3° valgus and 9° posterior slope. The inclination of the tibial plateau in conjunction with the difference in condylar dimensions creates an overall valgus and slightly posterior inferior alignment of between 10° and 12° in most knees. The shape of the condyles also plays a critical role in maintaining tension in the ligamentous structures about the knee during motion. The condyles of the femur can be thought of as having two distinct circular cams of different dimensions. The central portion between these cams is flatter, that is, has a greater radius of curvature, than either the anterior or posterior portions. Tibial plateau widths are greater than the corresponding widths of the femoral condyles. However, the tibial plateau depths are less than those of the femoral condyle distances. The medial condyle of the tibia is concave superiorly whereas the lateral condyle is convex superiorly. The shape of the femoral surfaces is complementary to the shape of the tibial plateaus. In cross section, the medial and lateral tibial plateaus are roughly ovoid in shape. In the coronal plane they are nearly flat. The fibrocartilaginous medial and lateral menisci are thick peripherally and taper to thin edges centrally. The menisci deepen the tibial plateaus slightly, which provides a more congruent and constrained surface with the femoral condyles.

The anterior and posterior cruciate ligaments (ACL and PCL) function to provide joint stability. The origin of the ACL is in the posterior femoral notch and the insertion occupies about one third of the width of the tibia between the anterior and middle third. The PCL's femoral origin

lies in an AP orientation in the anterior portion of the femoral notch. The PCL inserts into the posterior sulcus of the tibia between the medial and lateral joint surfaces.

Capsule ligamentous restraints are provided by the MCL, LCL, the joint capsule, and the posterior medial and posterior lateral complexes. The supporting structures surrounding the knee can be divided into three distinct layers. On the medial side, the most superficial layer (layer one) is the deep fascia. Layer two contains the superficial MCL. Of the two components that make up the MCL (superficial and deep), the superficial MCL is clinically more important because it is the primary medial stabilizer of the knee. The superficial MCL originates on the medial epicondyle and runs approximately 10 cm to its insertion on the tibia. The posterior oblique fibers of the MCL blend posteriorly into the capsule (layer two) and, along with contributions from the semimembranosus tendon, form the oblique popliteal ligament. The lateral structure of the knee can also be divided into three layers. The most superficial layer is the lateral retinaculum, made up of the superficial oblique and deep transverse components. The middle layer (layer two) is the LCL, the fabellofibular ligament, and the arcuate ligament. The LCL originates on the lateral epicondyle of the femur and inserts on the lateral surface of the fibular head. The deepest lateral layer (layer three) is the capsule. It is a thin, weak layer anteriorly that is reinforced posteriorly by the arcuate ligament complex.

Anatomic Motion

In the tibiofemoral joint, motion takes place in all three planes but the motion is greatest in a sagittal plane. Motion in this plane is from full extension to approximately 140° of flexion. Motion in the transverse plane is influenced by the amount of knee flexion. With the knee in full extension, rotation is almost completely restricted. The range of rotation increases as the knee is flexed, reaching a maximum at 90° of flexion. In this position, external rotation ranges to approximately 45° and internal rotation ranges to approximately 30°. Motion in the frontal plane is similarly affected by the amount of joint flexion. At full extension there is little motion in the frontal plane. Frontal plane motion increases with knee flexion up to 30° and then decreases again. The functional range of tibiofemoral joint motion varies with specific activities (Table 5). During normal walking, the knee is flexed to about 60° during swing. The requirement for knee flexion increases when ascending or descending stairs. A knee range of motion of approximately 20° of flexion during stance is required for an individual to adequately perform activities of daily living.

Anterior and posterior translation of the tibia on the femur is variable and affected by the position of the knee. The AP translation on the femur is minimal in full extension and increases with flexion, reaching a maximum at

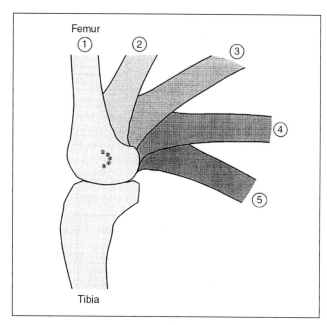

Figure 32   The instant center of rotation for the knee. (*Reproduced with permission from Frankel VH, Burstein AH, Brooks DB: Biomechanics of internal derangement of the knee: Pathomechanics as determined by analysis of the instant center of motion. J Bone Joint Surg Am 1971;53:945-961.*)

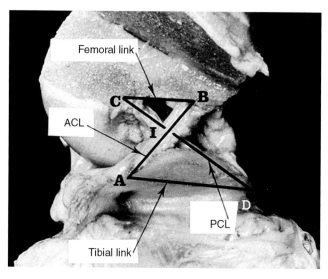

Figure 33   A human knee with the lateral femoral condyle removed, exposing the cruciate ligaments. Superimposed is a diagram of a four-bar linkage comprising the anterior cruciate ligament (ACL) AB, the posterior cruciate ligament (PCL) CD, the femoral link, CB, joining the ligament attachment points on the femur, and the tibial link, AD, joining their attachment points on the tibia. (*Reproduced with permission from O'Connor J, Shercliffe T, Fitzpatrick D, et al: Geometry of the knee, in Daniel DM, Akeson WH, O'Connor JJ (eds): Knee Ligaments: Structure, Function, Injury, and Repair. New York, NY, Raven Press, 1990, pp 163–169.*)

approximately 30° of flexion when the anterior restraints are most lax. Posterior translation is greatest at 90° of flexion. These observations support ACL laxity testing at 30° of flexion (Lachman test) and PCL testing at 90° of flexion (posterior drawer test). Tibiofemoral translation is measured in the AP plane using an instrumented laxity measurement device, such as the KT-1000 arthrometer. The manual maximum side-to-side difference has become the standard for evaluating and reporting laxity. More than 90% of normal subjects have a side-to-side difference of no more than 2 mm.

Joint Articulating Surface Motion

During normal knee motion from full extension to full flexion, the instant center pathway moves posteriorly (**Figure 32**). As the knee moves from full extension to flexion, the tibiofemoral contact point moves posteriorly on both the tibia and the femur, reflecting a combination of rolling and sliding. The ratio of rolling and sliding does not remain constant throughout the range of flexion. As the femur rolls posteriorly during flexion, the femoral condyles slide anteriorly to diminish the posterior progression of the rolling effect. Otherwise the condyles would roll off the back of the tibia. Rolling is most prominent in the initial 15° of flexion, with a rolling-sliding ratio of approximately 1:2. Sliding becomes more prominent, increasing the rolling-sliding ratio until it reaches 1:4 by the end of flexion. The unique mechanism that prevents the femur from rolling off the posterior aspect of the tibial plateau as the

knee goes into increased flexion is the four-bar linkage formed by the tibia and femoral attachment sites of the ACL and PCL and the osseous geometry of the femoral condyles (**Figure 33**). The center of rotation (or instant center) in the four-bar linkage model is where the two cruciate ligaments cross. The four-bar linkage model is useful for describing the rotation of the tibia about the femur in the sagittal plane.

The tibiofemoral joint has two degrees of freedom. The first degree of freedom allows flexion and extension in the sagittal plane. The axis of rotation lies perpendicular to the sagittal plane and intersects the femoral condyles (**Figure 34**). Both fixed axes and screw axes (instantaneous axes) have been calculated. The symmetric optimal axis is a fixed axis and is constrained in such a way that the axis is the same for both the right and left knee, whereas the screw axis is an instantaneous axis that changes with knee flexion. The screw axis may sometimes coincide with the optimal axis, but not always, depending on the motions of the knee joint. The second degree of freedom is axial rotation around the long axis of the tibia. Rotational lag around this long axis can only be found when the knee is flexed. There is also an automatic axial rotation that is involuntarily linked to flexion and extension. When the knee is flexed, the tibia internally rotates. Conversely, when the knee is extended, the tibia externally rotates. This coupled motion is called the screw-home mechanism. A clinical test, the Helfet test, is often used to determine whether ex-

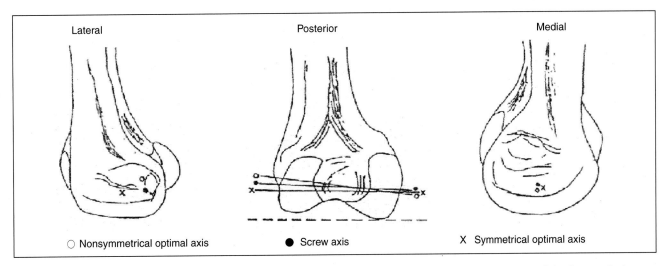

Figure 34   Approximate location of the optimal axis and the screw axis on the medial and lateral condyles of the femur of a human subject for the range of motion of 0° to 90° flexion (standing to sitting, respectively). *(Reproduced with permission from Lewis JL, Lew WD: A method for locating an optimal "fixed" axis of rotation for the human knee joint. J Biomech Eng 1978;100:187.)*

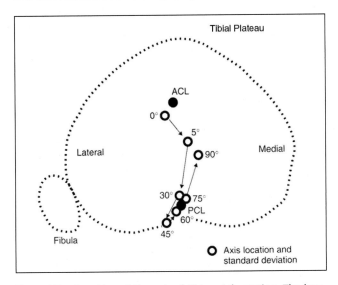

Figure 35   Location of the axis of tibia axial rotation. The location of the axis was close to the tibial insertion of the ACL at 0° of flexion and gradually moved toward that of the PCL at 45° and 90° of knee flexion. The axis then moved anterior again and was approximately at equal distance from the two insertions of the cruciate ligaments at 90° of knee flexion. ACL, insertion of the anterior cruciate ligament; PCL, tibial insertion of the posterior cruciate ligament. *(Reproduced with permission from Matsumoto H, Seedhom BB, Suda Y, et al: Axis of tibial rotation and its change with flexion angle. Clin Orthop Relat Res 2000;371:178-182.)*

ternal rotation of the tibiofemoral joint takes place during knee extension, thereby indicating whether the screw-home mechanism is intact. The location of the longitudinal rotational axis is close to the insertion of the ACL at 0° of flexion (**Figure 35**). As knee flexion continues, up to 60°, the rotational axis moves toward the insertion of the PCL. Between 60° and 90° of flexion, the rotational axis moves anteriorly again.

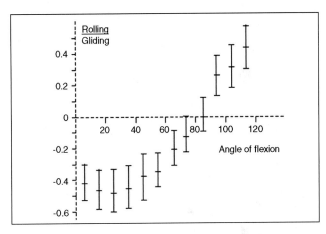

Figure 36   Calculated rolling/gliding ratio for the patellofemoral joint as a function of the knee flexion angle. *(Reproduced with permission from van Eijden TM, Kouwenhoven E, Verburg J, Weijs WA: A mathematical model of the patellofemoral joint. J Biomech 1986;19:219-229.)*

Patellofemoral Joint

The patellofemoral joint is important primarily through its role in the extensor mechanism. The patella increases the mechanical advantage of the extensor muscles by transmitting the force across the knee at a greater distance (moment arm) from the axis of rotation.

During knee flexion, the patella makes a rolling/gliding motion along the femoral articulating surface (**Figure 36**). Between 80° and 90° of knee flexion, the rolling motion of the articulating surface comes to a standstill and then changes direction. This reversal of the movement occurs at the flexion angle where the quadriceps tendon first contacts the femoral groove. Throughout the entire flexion range, the gliding motion is clockwise (**Figure 36**). In contrast, the direction of the rolling motion is counterclockwise between 0° and 90° and clockwise between 90° and 120°. The mean amount of patellar gliding for all knees is

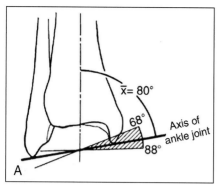

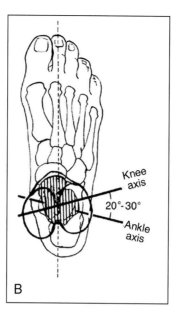

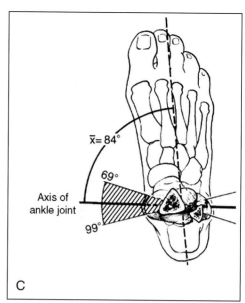

Figure 37   A, Variations in the frontal axis of the ankle joint. **B,** Relationship of the knee and ankle axes. **C,** Relationship of the ankle axis to the long axis of the foot. *(Reproduced with permission from Mann RA: Biomechanics of the foot, in Atlas of Orthotics, ed 2. St. Louis, MO, Mosby, 1985.)*

Table 6	Axis of Rotation for the Ankle	
Investigators	**Axis***	**Position**
Elftman (1945)	Fix.	67.6 ± 7.4° with respect to sagittal plane
Isman and Insman (1969)	Fix.	8 mm anterior, 3 mm inferior to the distal tip of the lateral malleolus
Inman and Mann (1979)	Fix.	79° (68° to 88°) with respect to the sagittal plane
Allard et al (1987)	Fix.	95.4 ± 6.6° with respect to the frontal plane, 77.7 ± 12.3° with respect to the sagittal plane and 17.9 ± 4.5° with respect to the transverse plane
Singh et al (1992)	Fix.	3.0 mm anterior, 2.5 mm inferior to distal tip of medial malleolus; 2.2 mm posterior, 10 mm inferior to distal tip of medial malleolus
Sammarco et al (1973)	Ins.	Inside and outside the body of the talus
D'Ambrosia et al (1976)	Ins.	No consistent patterns
Parlasca et al (1979)	Ins.	96% within 12 mm of a point 20 mm below the articular surface of the tibia along the long axis
Van Langelaan (1983)	Ins.	At an approximate right angle to the longitudinal direction of the foot; passing through the corpus tali, with a direction from the anterolaterosuperior to the posteromedioinferior
Barnett and Napier (1952)	Q-I	Dorsiflexion: down and lateral Plantar flexion: down and medial
Hicks (1953)	Q-I	Dorsiflexion: 4 mm inferior to tip of lateral malleolus to 15 mm anterior to tip of medial malleolus Plantar flexion: 5 mm superior to tip of lateral malleolus to 15 mm anterior, 10 mm inferior to tip of medial malleolus

*Fix. = fixed axis of rotation; Ins. = instantaneous axis of rotation; Q-I = quasi-instantaneous axis of rotation.

approximately 6.5 mm per 10° of flexion between 0° and 80° and 4.5 mm per 10° flexion between 80° and 120°.

Structure and Function of the Ankle

The ankle joint is composed of two joints: the talocrural (ankle) joint and the talocalcaneal (subtalar) joint. The talocrural joint is formed by the articulation of the distal tibia and fibula with the trochlea of the talus. The talocalcaneal joint is formed by the articulation of the talus with the calcaneus.

The talocrural joint forms a simple hinge consisting of the talus, medial malleolus, tibial plafond, and lateral malleolus. The tibial surface forming the superior dome of

the ankle is concave sagittally, subtly convex in the frontal plane, and oriented about 93° from the long axis of the tibia (that is, higher on the lateral than on the medial side). The shape of the cavity formed by the tibiofibular mortise, that is, the tibial plafond, matches closely the shape of the upper articulating surface of the talus. The talus is shaped like a truncated cone, or frustum, with the apex directed medially. The upper articular surface of the talus is wedge shaped, with the width 4.2 mm wider anteriorly than posteriorly. From front to back the articular surface spans an arc of about 105°.

The primary motion of the ankle joint is dorsiflexion-plantar flexion. The motion axis of the talocrural joint is obliquely oriented posterolaterally in a transverse plane and inferolaterally in the coronal plane. The general ankle axis can be estimated as passing through the inferior tips of the malleoli (Figure 37). Several authors have reported that ankle motion has more than a fixed axis of rotation, that is, a quasi-instantaneous or instantaneous axis (Table 6). A small amount of talar rotation occurs during ankle motion. During weight bearing of normal volunteers, the talus demonstrated rotational movement of 10.4° as the ankle motion varied from 30° plantar flexion to 30° dorsiflexion (Figure 38).

Stability of the talocrural joint results from congruency and the supporting ligamentous structures. The lateral ankle ligaments responsible for resistance to inversion and internal rotation are the anterior talofibular ligament, the calcaneofibular ligament, and the posterior talofibular ligament (Figure 39). Clinically, the most commonly sprained ankle ligament is the anterior talofibular ligament, followed by the calcaneofibular ligament. These two ligaments form a 105° angle between each other (Figure 39). They act synergistically to resist ankle inversion forces.

Anatomic Motion

Ankle motion occurs primarily in the sagittal plane and is described as plantar flexion and dorsiflexion (Figure 40). At heel strike, the ankle is slightly plantar flexed and continues with plantar flexion until foot-flat. This is referred to as the first rocker. At foot-flat the motion reverses to dorsiflexion during instances as the body passes over the foot. However, this movement is referred to as second rocker. The motion then returns to plantar flexion at toe-off, also called third rocker. Dorsiflexion of the ankle oc-

curs until the middle of swing phase and then ankle position returns to slight plantar flexion at heel strike. Ankle motion during normal walking averages 10° dorsiflexion

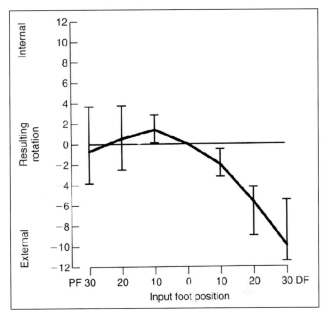

Figure 38   Horizontal rotation of the talus around the vertical axis at different positions of ankle dorsiflexion-plantar flexion. Moving from plantar flexion to dorsiflexion, the talus initially internally rotates slightly, then externally rotates markedly. (Reproduced with permission from Sammarco GJ, Hockenberry RT: Biomechanics of the foot and ankle, in Nordin M, Frankel VH (eds): Basic Biomechanics of the Musculoskeletal System. Philadelphia, PA, Lippincott Williams & Wilkins, 2001.)

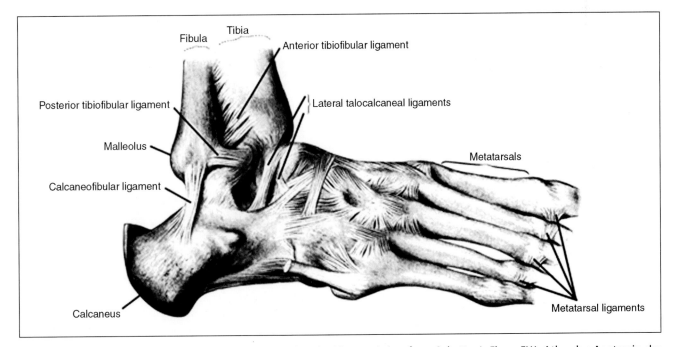

Figure 39   Ligaments of the ankle and foot. (Reproduced with permission from Sobotta J, Figge FHJ: Atlas der Anatomie des Menschen, ed 20. Munich, Germany, Urban & Schwarzenberg, 1993.)

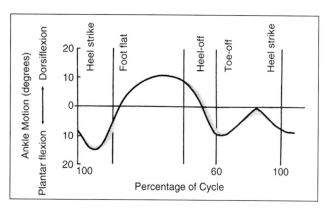

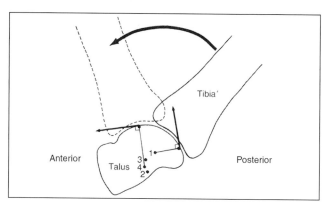

Figure 40   Range of ankle joint motion in the sagittal plane during level walking in one gait cycle. The shaded area indicates variation among 60 subjects (age 20 to 65 years). *(Reproduced with permission from Stauffer RN, Chao EY, Brewster RC: Force and motion analysis of the normal, diseased, and prosthetic ankle joint. Clin Orthop Relat Res 1977;127:189-196.)*

Figure 41   Instant center pathway for surface joint motion at the tibiotalar joint in a normal ankle from full plantar flexion to full dorsiflexion. All instant centers fall within the talus. The direction of displacement of the contact points shows distraction of the joint surfaces at the beginning of motion (points 1 and 2) and gliding thereafter (points 3 and 4). *(Reproduced with permission from Sammarco GJ, Burstein AH, Frankel VH: Biomechanics of the ankle: A kinematic study. Orthop Clin North Am 1973;4:75-96.)*

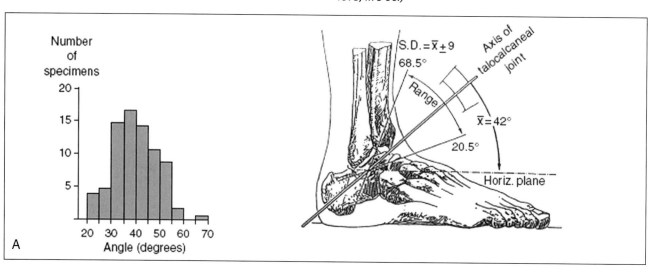

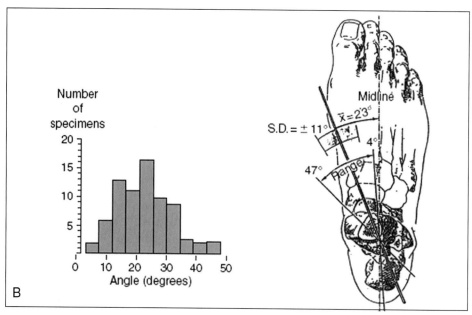

Figure 42   **A,** Variation in inclination of axis of subtalar joint as projected upon the sagittal plane. The distribution of the measurements on the individual specimens is shown in the histogram. The single observation of an angle of almost 70° was present in a markedly cavus foot. **B,** Variation in position of the subtalar axis as projected onto the transverse plane. The angle was measured between the axis and the midline of the foot. The extent of individual variation is shown on the sketch and revealed in the histogram. *(Reproduced with permission from Inman VT: The Joints of the Ankle. Baltimore, MD, Williams & Wilkins, 1976.)*

and 14° plantar flexion with the total motion of 24°. Maximum dorsiflexion occurs at 70° stance phase and maximum plantar flexion occurs at toe-off.

Extensive work has been conducted on the location of the instant center of rotation of the ankle. The instant centers of rotation fall within the tali of normal ankles but the position changes with ankle motion (**Figure 41**). This confirms that the ankle axis of rotation does not remain constant with motion. The normal ankle showed distraction tendencies in early range of plantar flexion, followed by sliding in the midportion, and compression as the close packed position is reached toward the limit of dorsiflexion.

The position of the subtalar axis (talocalcaneal joint) has been defined (**Figure 42**). The axis of motion in the talocalcaneal joint passes from the anterior medial superior aspect of the navicular bone to the posterolateral inferior aspect of the calcaneus. The motion that occurs in the talocalcaneal joint consists of inversion and eversion.

Summary

Biomechanics uses physical and engineering concepts to describe the motion of various body segments. The importance of understanding the biomechanics of the musculoskeletal system cannot be underestimated. Knowledge of the joint arthrology and arthrokinematics is essential for understanding normal and pathologic musculoskeletal conditions. Clinical treatment must take into account the various principles presented in this chapter. Knowledge of kinesiology is essential for determination of proper diagnosis and surgical treatment of joint disease; assessment of joint wear, stability, and degeneration; and design of prosthetic devices to restore function.

Acknowledgment

The authors thank Barbara Iverson for her careful preparation of this book chapter.

Selected Bibliography

General

Buckwalter JA, Einhorn TA, Simon SR (eds): *Orthopaedic Basic Science*, ed 2. Rosemont, IL, American Academy of Orthopaedic Surgeons, 2000.

Greene WB, Heckman JD: *The Clinical Measurement of Joint Motion*. Rosemont, IL, American Academy of Orthopaedic Surgeons, 1994.

Nordin M, Frankel VH: *Basic Biomechanics of the Musculoskeletal System*. Philadelphia, PA, Lea & Febiger, 1989.

Structure and Function of the Shoulder Joint

Boone DC, Azen SP: Normal range of motion of joints in male subjects. *J Bone Joint Surg Am* 1979;61:756-759.

Bowen MK, Warren RF: Ligamentous control of shoulder stability based on selective cutting and static translation experiments. *Clin Sports Med* 1991;10:757-782.

Dempster WT: Mechanisms of shoulder movement. *Arch Phys Med Rehabil* 1965;46:49-70.

DePalma AF: Biomechanics of the shoulder, in *Surgery of the Shoulder*. Philadelphia, PA, JB Lippincott, 1983, pp 65-85.

Freedman L, Munro RR: Abduction of the arm in the scapular plane: Scapular and glenohumeral movements: A roentgenographic study. *J Bone Joint Surg Am* 1966;48:1503-1510.

Fukuda K, Craig EV, An KN, Cofield RH, Chao EY: Biomechanical study of the ligamentous system of the acromioclavicular joint. *J Bone Joint Surg Am* 1986;68:434-440.

Harryman DT II, Sidles JA, Clark JM, McQuade KJ, Gibb TD, Matsen FA III: Translation of the humeral head on the glenoid with passive glenohumeral motion. *J Bone Joint Surg Am* 1990;72:1334-1343.

Inman VT, Saunders JB, Abbott LC: Observations on the function of the shoulder joint. *J Bone Joint Surg* 1944;26:1-30.

Itoi E, Motzkin NE, Morrey BF, An KN: Scapular inclination and inferior stability of the shoulder. *J Shoulder Elbow Surg* 1992;1:131-139.

Morrey BF, An KN: Biomechanics of the shoulder, in Rockwood CA, Matsen FA (eds): *The Shoulder*. Philadelphia, PA, WB Saunders, 1990.

Ovesen J, Nielsen S: Anterior and posterior shoulder instability: A cadaver study. *Acta Orthop Scand* 1986;57:324-327.

Pearl ML, Harris SL, Lippitt SB, et al: A system for describing positions of the humerus relative to the thorax and its use in the presentation of several functionally important arm positions. *J Shoulder Elbow Surg* 1992;1:113-118.

Poppen NK, Walker PS: Normal and abnormal motion of the shoulder. *J Bone Joint Surg Am* 1976;58:195-201.

Reeves B: Experiments on the tensile strength of the anterior capsular structures of the shoulder in man. *J Bone Joint Surg Br* 1968;50:858-865.

Schwartz R, O'Brien SJ, Warren RF: Capsular restraints to anterior/posterior motion of the shoulders. *Orthop Trans* 1988;12:727.

Simon SR: Kinesiology, in Simon SR (ed): *Orthopaedic Basic Science*, Rosemont, IL, American Academy of Orthopaedic Surgeons, 1994, pp 536-558.

Soslowsky LJ., Flatow EL, Bigliani LU, Mow VC: Articular geometry of the glenohumeral joint. *Clin Orthop Relat Res* 1992;285:181-190.

Turkel SJ, Panio MW, Marshall JL, Girgis FG: Stabilizing mechanisms preventing anterior dislocation of the glenohumeral joint. *J Bone Joint Surg Am* 1981;63:1208-1217.

Warren RF, Kornblatt IB, Marchand R: Static factors affecting posterior shoulder stability. *Orthop Trans* 1984;8:89.

Structure and Function of the Elbow Joint
An KN, Chao EY: Biomechanics of the elbow, in Morrey BF (ed): *The Elbow and Its Disorders*. Philadelphia, PA, Saunders, 1985.

An KN, Morrey BF: Biomechanics, in Morrey BF, Chao EY (eds): *Joint Replacement Arthroplasty*. New York, NY, Churchill Livingstone, 1991, pp 257-273.

An KN, Morrey BF: Biomechanics of the elbow, in Ratcliffe A, Woo S (eds): *Biomechanics of Diarthrodial Joints*. New York, NY, Springer-Verlag, 1990, pp 441-464.

An KN, Morrey BF, Chao EY: Carrying angle of the human elbow joint. *J Orthop Res* 1984;1:369-378.

Chao EY, Morrey BF: Three-dimensional rotation of the elbow. *J Biomech* 1978;11:57-73.

Ishizuki M.: Functional anatomy of the elbow joint and three-dimensional quantitative motion analysis of the elbow joint. *Nippon Seikeigeka Gakkai Zasshi* 1979;53:989-996.

London JT: Kinematics of the elbow. *J Bone Joint Surg Am* 1981;63:529-535.

Morrey BF, An KN: Functional evaluation of the elbow, in Morrey BF (ed): *The Elbow and Its Disorders,* ed 2. Philadelphia, PA, Saunders, 1993.

Morrey BF, Askew LJ, Chao EY: A biomechanical study of normal functional elbow motion. *J Bone Joint Surg Am* 1981;63:872-877.

Morrey BF, Chao EY: Passive motion of the elbow joint. *J Bone Joint Surg Am* 1976;58:501-508.

Ray RD, Johnson RJ, Jameson RM: Rotation of the forearm: An experimental study of pronation and supination. *J Bone Joint Surg Am* 1951;33:993-996.

Youm Y, Dryer RF, Thambyrajah K, Flatt AE, Sprague BL: Biomechanical analyses of forearm pronation-supination and elbow flexion-extension. *J Biomech* 1979;12:245-255.

Structure and Function of the Hand and Wrist
An KN: Berger RA, Cooney WP III: *Biomechanics of the Wrist Joint*. New York, NY, Springer-Verlag, 1991.

Andrews JG, Youm Y: A biomechanical investigation of wrist kinematics. *J Biomech* 1979;12:83-93.

Berger RA, Crowninshield RD, Flatt AE: The three-dimensional rotational behaviors of the carpal bones. *Clin Orthop Relat Res* 1982;167:303-310.

Brand PW, Hollister A: *Clinical Mechanics of the Hand*. St Louis, MO, Mosby, 1992.

Brumbaugh RB, Crowninshield RD, Blair WF, Andrews JG: An in-vivo study of normal wrist kinematics. *J Biomech Eng* 1982;104:176-181.

Brumfield RH, Champoux JA: A biomechanical study of normal functional wrist motion. *Clin Orthop Relat Res* 1984;187:23-25.

Cooney WP, Garcia-Elias M, Dobyns JH, et al: Anatomy and mechanics of carpal instability. *Surg Rounds Orthop* 1989;3:15-24.

De Lange A, Kauer JM, Huiskes R: Kinematic behavior of the human wrist joint: A roentgen-stereophotogrammetric analysis. *J Orthop Res* 1985;3:56-64.

Erdman AG, Al E: Kinematic and kinetic analysis of the human wrist by stereoscopic instrumentation. *J Biomech Eng* 1979;101:124.

Imaeda T, An KN, Cooney WP, Linscheid R: Anatomy of trapeziometacarpal ligaments. *J Hand Surg [Am]* 1993;18:226-231.

Kauer JM: Functional anatomy of the wrist. *Clin Orthop Relat Res* 1980;149:9-20.

Kauer JM: The mechanism of the carpal joint. *Clin Orthop Relat Res* 1986;202:16-26.

Landsmeer JMF: Anatomical and functional investigations on the articulation of the human fingers. *Acta Anat Suppl (Basel)* 1955;24:1-69.

Linscheid RL: Kinematic considerations of the wrist. *Clin Orthop Relat Res* 1986;202:27-39.

Mayfield JK, Johnson RP, Kilcoyne RF: The ligaments of the human wrist and their functional significance. *Anat Rec* 1976;186:417-428.

Minami A, An KN, Cooney WP III, Linscheid RL, Chao EY: Ligament stability of the metacarpophalangeal joint: A biomechanical study. *J Hand Surg [Am]* 1985;10:255-260.

Norkin CC, Levangie PK: *Joint Structure and Function: A Comprehensive Analysis.* Philadelphia, PA, FA Davis, 1992, pp 337-378.

Palmer AK, Werner FW: Biomechanics of the distal radioulnar joint. *Clin Orthop Relat Res* 1984;187:26-35.

Palmer AK, Werner FW: The triangular fibrocartilage complex of the wrist: Anatomy and function. *J Hand Surg [Am]* 1981;6:153-162.

Palmer AK, Werner FW, Murphy D, Glisson R: Functional wrist motion: A biomechanical study. *J Hand Surg [Am]* 1985;10:39-46.

Regional Review of Courses in Hand Surgery. Aurora, CO, American Society for Surgery of the Hand, 1991.

Ruby LK, Cooney WPI, An KN, et al: Related motion of selected carpal bones: A kinematic analysis of the normal wrist. *J Hand Surg [Am]* 1988;13:1-10.

Ryu JY, Cooney WP III, Askew LJ, An KN, Chao EY: Functional ranges of motion of the wrist joint. *J Hand Surg [Am]* 1991;16:409-419.

Sarrafian SK, Melamed JL, Goshgarian GM: Study of wrist motion in flexion and extension. *Clin Orthop Relat Res* 1977;126:153-159.

Taleisnik J: The ligaments of the wrist. *J Hand Surg [Am]* 1976;1:110-118.

Taleisnik J: *The Wrist.* New York, NY, Churchill Livingstone, 1985.

Tamai K, Ryu J, An KN, Linscheid RL, Cooney WP, Chao EY: Three-dimensional geometric analysis of the metacarpophalangeal joint. *J Hand Surg [Am]* 1988;13:521-529.

Volz RG: Lieb, M., and Benjamin, J.: Biomechanics of the wrist. *Clin Orthop Relat Res* 1980;149:112-117.

von Bonin G: A note on the kinematics of the wrist-joint. *J Anat* 1929;63:259-262.

Wright RD: A detailed study of the movement of the wrist joint. *J Anat* 1935/1936;70:137-142.

Youm Y, Flatt AE: Kinematics of the wrist. *Clin Orthop Relat Res* 1980;149:21-32.

Youm Y, McMurthy RY, Flatt AE, Gillespie TE: Kinematics of the wrist: I. An experimental study of radial-ulnar deviation and flexion-extension. *J Bone Joint Surg Am* 1978;60:423-431.

Structure and Function of the Spine

Ahmed AM, Duncan NA, Burke DL: The effect of facet geometry on the axial torque-rotation response of lumbar motion segments. *Spine* 1990;15:391-401.

Andersson BJ, Ortengren R, Nachemson A, Elfstrom G: Lumbar disc pressure and myoelectric back muscle activity during sitting: I. Studies on an experimental chair. *Scand J Rehabil Med* 1974;6:104-114.

Andersson GB, Ortengren R, Schultz A: Analysis and measurement of the loads on the lumbar spine during work at a table. *J Biomech* 1980;13:513-520.

Asmussen E, Klausen K: Form and function of the erect human spine. *Clin Orthop Relat Res* 1962;25:55-63.

Eklund JA, Corlett EN: Shrinkage as a measure of the effect of load on the spine. *Spine* 1984;9:189-194.

Frymoyer JW, Frymoyer WW, Wilder DG, Pope MH: The mechanical and kinematic analysis of the lumbar spine in normal living human subjects in vivo. *J Biomech* 1979;12:165-172.

Goode JD, Theodore BM: Voluntary and diurnal variation in height and associated surface contour changes in spinal curves. *Eng Med* 1983;12:99-101.

Gunzburg R, Hutton W, Fraser R: Axial rotation of the lumbar spine and the effect of flexion: An in vitro and in vivo biomechanical study. *Spine* 1991;16:22-28.

Horst M., Brinckmann P: Measurement of the distribution of axial stress on the end-plate of the vertebral body. *Spine* 1981; 6:217-232.

Hukins DW, Kirby MC, Sikoryn TA, Aspden RM, Cox AJ: Comparison of structure, mechanical properties, and functions of lumbar spinal ligaments. *Spine* 1990; 15:787-795.

Keller TS, Holm SH, Hansson TH, Spengler DM: The dependence of intervertebral disc mechanical properties on physiologic conditions. *Spine* 1990;15:751-761.

Kulak RF, Schultz AB, Belytschko T, Galante J: Biomechanical characteristics of vertebral motion segments and intervertebral discs. *Orthop Clin North Am* 1975;6: 121-133.

Lorenz M, Patwardhan A, Vanderby R Jr: Load-bearing characteristics of lumbar facets in normal and surgically altered spinal segments. *Spine* 1983;8:122-130.

Lumsden RM II, Morris JM: An in vivo study of axial rotation and immobilization at the lumbosacral joint. *J Bone Joint Surg Am* 1968;50:1591-1602.

Lysell E: Motion in the cervical spine: An experimental study on autopsy specimens. *Acta Orthop Scand* 1969; 123(suppl):1.

Mayer TG, Tencer AF, Kristoferson S, Mooney V: Use of noninvasive techniques for quantification of spinal range-of-motion in normal subjects and chronic low-back dysfunction patients. *Spine* 1984;9:588-595.

Miles M, Sullivan WE: Lateral bending at the lumbar and lumbosacral joints. *Anat Rec* 1961;139:387.

Moll JM, Wright V: Normal range of spinal mobility: An objective clinical study. *Ann Rheum Dis* 1971;30: 381-386.

Nachemson A: Towards a better understanding of low-back pain: A review of the mechanics of the lumbar disc. *Rheumatol Rehabil* 1975;14:129-143.

Nachemson AL, Schultz AB, Berkson MH: Mechanical properties of human lumbar spine motion segments: Influence of age, sex, disc level, and degeneration. *Spine* 1979;4:1-8.

Panjabi M, Dvorak J, Duranceau J, et al: Three-dimensional movements of the upper cervical spine. *Spine* 1988;13:726-730.

Panjabi MM, Goel VK, Takata K: Physiologic strains in the lumbar spinal ligaments: An in vitro biomechanical study. *Spine* 1982;7:192-203.

Panjabi MM, White AA III, Johnson RM: Cervical spine mechanics as a function of transection of components. *J Biomech* 1975;8:327-336.

Pearcy MJ, Bogduk N: Instantaneous axes of rotation of the lumbar intervertebral joints. *Spine* 1988;13:1033-1041.

Pope MH, Frymoyer JW, Lehmann TR: Structure and function of the lumbar spine, in Pope MH, Andersson GB, Frymoyer JW, Al E (eds): *Occupational Low Back Pain: Assessment, Treatment, and Prevention.* St Louis, MO, Mosby-Year Book, 1991, pp 3-19.

Pope MH, Wilder DG, Matteri RE, Frymoyer JW: Experimental measurements of vertebral motion under load. *Orthop Clin North Am* 1977;8:155-167.

Posner I, White AA III, Edwards WT, Hayes WC: A biomechanical analysis of the clinical stability of the lumbar and lumbosacral spine. *Spine* 1982;7:374-389.

Reichmann S: Motion of the lumbar articular processes in flexion-extension and lateral flexions of the spine. *Acta Morphol Neerl Scand* 1971;8:261-272.

Thurston AJ, Harris JD: Normal kinematics of the lumbar spine and pelvis. *Spine* 1983;8:199-205.

White AA III, Johnson RM, Panjabi MM, Southwick WO: Biomechanical analysis of clinical stability in the cervical spine. *Clin Orthop Relat Res* 1975;109:85-96.

White AA III, Panjabi MM: The basic kinematics of the human spine: A review of past and current knowledge. *Spine* 1978;3:12-20.

White AA, Panjabi M: *Clinical Biomechanics of the Spine.* Philadelphia, PA, Lippincott, 1991.

Wilke HJ, Neef P, Caimi M, Hoogland T, Claes LE: New in-vivo measurements of pressures in the intervertebral disc in daily life. *Spine* 1999;24:755-762.

Structure and Function of the Hip Joint

Crowninshield RD, Johnston RC, Andrews JG, Brand RA: A biomechanical investigation of the human hip. *J Biomech* 1978;11:75-85.

Crowninshield RD, Johnston RC, Andrews JG, Brand RA: The effects of walking velocity and age on hip kinematics and kinetics. *Clin Orthop Relat Res* 1978;132: 140-144.

Denham RA: Hip mechanics. *J Bone Joint Surg Br* 1959;41:550-557.

Johnston RC, Smidt G: Hip motion measurements for selected activities of daily living. *Clin Orthop Relat Res* 1970;72:205-215.

Johnston RC, Smidt GL: Measurement of hip-joint motion during walking: Evaluation of an electrogoniometric method. *J Bone Joint Surg Am* 1969;51:1082-1094.

Morris JM: Biomechanical aspects of the hip joint. *Orthop Clin North Am* 1971;2:33-54.

Structure and Function of the Knee

Brantigan OC, Voshell AF: The mechanics of the ligaments and menisci of the knee joint. *J Bone Joitn Surg AM* 1941;23:44-66..

Butler DL, Noyes FR, Grood ES: Ligamentous restraints to anterior-posterior drawer in the human knee: A biomechanical study. *J Bone Joint Surg Am* 1980;62:259-270..

Daniel D, Akeson WH, O'Connor J: *Knee Ligaments: Structure, Function, Injury.* New York, NY, 1990.

Frankel VH, Burstein AH, Brooks DB: Biomechanics of internal derangement of the knee: Pathomechanics as determined by analysis of the instant centers of motion. *J Bone Joint Surg Am* 1971;53:945-962.

Girgis FG, Marshall JL, Monajem A: The cruciate ligaments of the knee joint: Anatomical, functional and experimental analysis. *Clin Orthop Relat Res* 1975;106: 216-231.

Goodfellow J, Hungerford DS, Zindel M: Patello-femoral joint mechanics and pathology: 1. Functional anatomy of the patello-femoral joint. *J Bone Joint Surg Br* 1976;58:287-290.

Kaufman K, Hughes C, Morrey B, Morrey M, An K: Gait characteristics of patients with knee osteoarthritis. *J Biomech* 2001;34:907-915.

Kettelkamp DB, Johnson RJ, Smidt GL, Chao EY, Walker M: An electrogoniometric study of knee motion in normal gait. *J Bone Joint Surg Am* 1970;52:775-790.

Laubenthal KN, Smidt GL, Kettelkamp DB: A quantitative analysis of knee motion during activities of daily living. *Phys Ther* 1972;52:34-43.

Lewis JL, Lew WD: A method for locating an optimal "fixed" axis of rotation for the human knee joint. *J Biomech* 1978;100:187.

Markolf K, Mensch J, Amstutz HC: Stiffness and laxity of the knee: The contributions of the supporting structures: A quantitative in vitro study. *J Bone Joint Surg Am* 1976;58:583-594.

Matsumoto H, Seedhom BB, Suda K, Otani T Fujkawa K: Axis of tibial rotation and its change with flexion angle. *Clin Orthop Relat Res* 2000;371:178-182.

O'Connor J, Shercliff T, FitzPatrick D, et al: Geometry of the knee, in Daniel DM, Akeson WH, O'Connor JJ (eds): *Knee Ligaments: Structure, Function, Injury, and Repair.* New York, NY, Raven Press, 1990, pp 163-169.

Pope MH, Crowninshield R, Miller R, Johnson R: The static and dynamic behavior of the human knee in vivo. *J Biomech* 1976;9:449-452.

van Eijden TM, Kouwenhoven E, Verburg J, Weijs WA: A mathematical model of the patellofemoral joint. *J Biomech* 1986;19:219-229.

Structure and Function of the Ankle

Cass JR, Morrey BF, Chao EY: Three-dimensional kinematics of ankle instability following serial sectioning of lateral collateral ligaments. *Foot Ankle* 1984;5:142-149.

Close JR, Inman VT, Poor PM, Todd FN: The function of the subtalar joint. *Clin Orthop Relat Res* 1967;50:159-179.

Hicks JH: The mechanics of the foot: I. The joints. *J Anat* 1953;87:345-357.

Inman VT: *The Joints of the Ankle.* Baltimore, MD, Williams and Wilkins, 1976.

Mann RA: Biomechanics of the foot, in *American Academy of Orthopeadic Surgeons: Atlas of Orthotics.* St. Louis, MO, Mosby, 1985.

Proctor P, Paul JP: Ankle joint biomechanics. *J Biomech* 1982;15:627-634.

Rasmussen O: Stability of the ankle joint: Analysis of the function and traumatology of the ankle ligaments. *Acta Orthop Scand Suppl* 1985;211:1-75.

Sammarco GJ, Burstein AH, Frankel VH: Biomechanics of the ankle: A kinematic study. *Orthop Clin North Am* 1973;4:75-96.

Sammarco GJ, Hockenberry RT: Biomechanics of the foot and ankle, in Nordin M, Frankel H (eds): *Basic Biomechanics of the Musculoskeletal System.* Baltimore, MD, Lippincott, Williams, and Wilkins, 2001.

Sobotta J, Figge FH: *Atlas der Anatomie des Menschen.* Munich, Germany, Urban & Schwarzenberg, 1993.

Stauffer RN, Chao EY, Brewster RC: Force and motion analysis of the normal, diseased, and prosthetic ankle joint. *Clin Orthop Relat Res* 1977;127:189-196.

Wright DG, Desai SM, Henderson WH: Action of the subtalar and ankle-joint complex during the stance phase of walking. *J Bone Joint Surg Am* 1964;46:361-382.

Basic Principles and Treatment of Musculoskeletal Disease

Chapter 16

Infections in Orthopaedics

Jonathan M. Gross, MD, MPH
Edward M. Schwarz, PhD

Introduction

Although humanity has been combating infectious disease since prehistoric time, microbial pathogenesis remains one of the greatest public health issues. As testimony to its importance, the development of antibiotic drugs and prophylactic vaccines are considered among the greatest scientific achievements of the 20th century. Despite these medical advances, the current worldwide epidemic of severe acute respiratory syndrome (SARS) shows how vulnerable humanity remains to infectious disease. Musculoskeletal infections continue to be among the most difficult conditions to treat in orthopaedic surgery.

Despite the development of superior surgical techniques, newer diagnostic tools, and innovative treatments, factors such as delayed diagnosis, drug resistance, and evolving virulent pathogens present ongoing challenges. Although orthopaedic surgeons treat a spectrum of infectious processes that includes cellulitis, fasciitis, septic arthritis, and osteomyelitis, this chapter focuses on bone infections to illustrate the interplay between host and pathogen. The outcome after treatment of osteomyelitis is often unsatisfactory, with failure rates exceeding 20%. The goal of this chapter is to provide the reader with a better understanding of the mechanisms of microbial pathogenesis and the host response. The text is organized into three sections. The first section discusses modes of transmission and pathogen virulence. The second section describes host response, diagnosis and treatment. The last section reviews special infections pertinent to health care workers.

Terminology

Osteomyelitis is an infection of bone. Hematogenous osteomyelitis is an infection that seeds the bone from another location through the bloodstream. Hematogenous osteomyelitis most commonly occurs in children and occasionally in infections about indwelling prostheses, including total joints. Nonhematogenous osteomyelitis occurs when bone is directly infected and is typically associated with surgical or traumatic contamination of bone. Acute osteomyelitis is a bone infection in which there is no necrotic bone associated with the infection. By this definition the infection is diagnosed soon after the bone has been contaminated. Chronic osteomyelitis is associated with areas of bone necrosis, called a sequestrum, that are surrounded by reactive bone formation that walls off the necrotic infected area, called the involucrum. This type of biologic response requires an established infection of at least 6 weeks' duration. Thus, the accepted clinical definition of chronic osteomyelitis is clinical or radiographic evidence of infection with a duration of more than 6 weeks.

Interplay Between Host and Pathogen

Although various microbes have the ability to invade musculoskeletal tissue, among the most serious infections that require surgical attention are bacterial infections of bone (osteomyelitis). Osteomyelitis is characterized radiographically and histologically by the progressive inflammatory destruction and new apposition of bone. Clinical research on osteomyelitis is difficult because of many confounding variables that include host factors, the bone substrate within which the infection arises, the often slow pathogenesis of an infection, and the relatively low incidence of bone infections and the variety of organisms that can cause osteomyelitis. Consequently most knowledge of the pathogenesis of infection comes from animal models, which have been developed for the chicken, rat, guinea pig, rabbit, dog, and sheep. From this work it is clear that normal bone is highly resistant to infection, and that osteomyelitis most commonly results from a very large bacteria inoculum, traumatic injury to bone and the surrounding soft tissues, subsequent ischemia, and possible tissue necrosis. The process is facilitated with the presence of a foreign body. Orthopaedic surgery involves varying degrees of soft-tissue damage, possible compromised blood flow, tissue necrosis and hematoma formation, and implantation of hardware, such as plates, screws, prostheses, or cement. All of these elements increase the risk of infection.

Initiation of infection requires a pathogen to enter the host. Skin and mucous membranes are the mechanical barriers that normally protect the host from infection. To establish an infection, bacteria must break these barriers, colonize, and reproduce within the host tissue. Clinically significant infections cause damage to the host as a result of the infection. With osteomyelitis, bacteria enter the bone through two different routes: hematogenous and direct transmission. A discussion of these routes of transmission illustrates salient points concerning the interplay between the host and pathogen in the pathogenesis and bacterial diagnosis of osteomyelitis.

Hematogenous Osteomyelitis

Inoculation from the blood is known as hematogenous osteomyelitis. Hematogenously derived osteomyelitis occurs when bacteria from an infection enters into the bloodstream at a distant site and seeds the bone. This form of transmission is commonly associated with bone infections in children and in some total joint arthroplasty infections. Although fracture is known to facilitate the development of osteomyelitis from hematogenous seeding, bone damage is not a prerequisite for bacteria to invade bone. Hematogenous osteomyelitis is a good example of how intrinsic host factors can facilitate the development of acute osteomyelitis.

Skeletally immature patients have rich vascular arcades adjacent to growth plates (physes). Microorganisms can invade these metaphyseal end arterioles. Many hypotheses have been postulated as to why this region has a predilection for infection in children. One hypothesis is that the sluggish blood supply in this area of developing bone allows the bacteria to localize to these areas. Even mild bone injury can result in local inflammation and vascular congestion, which may impair the host's ability to fight infection. Further inflammation can raise the intraosseous blood pressure, further impeding the normal ability of bone to resist infection. Early intervention with antibiotics is effective and can allow the infection to be eradicated medically. Because the metaphysis is intra-articular in many joints, the acute bone infection may decompress into the joint and present as septic arthritis. In children this classically occurs in the proximal femur. The avascular nature of diarthrodial joints facilitates bacterial infection and reiterates the importance of surgical débridement once the joint has been infected. Hematogenous osteomyelitis demonstrates how host anatomy can facilitate bacterial infection. Similar opportunities are provided by indwelling prostheses and will be discussed later.

Although numerous bacteria cause bone infections, the pathogen often varies according to the patient's age, as well as according to the immune status of the patient and the circumstances of the infection. In neonates and infants, staphylococcal, streptococcal, and gram-negative species predominate. In patients 6 months up to 3 years of age, *Haemophilus influenzae* type B, streptococcal, and staphylococcal species should be considered. After 3 years of age, streptococcal and staphylococcal species predominate until the patient reaches adolescence, when *Neisseria gonorrhoeae* must also be considered.

Direct Transmission

The second mode of bacterial entry is from adjacent tissues, in which a colonized wound provides access to the host's bone. This form of bone infection is associated with ischemic ulcers in the feet of patients with diabetes or peripheral neuropathy. Polymicrobial osteomyelitis is seen when osteomyelitis arises adjacent to a colonized ulcer. Noninfectious microbes can become pathogenic when different species coexist and in concert contribute diverse factors that result in greater virulence than occurs typically with one species alone. An interesting example of this was demonstrated in an experimental model in which coinfection with *Staphylococcus epidermidis* and *Bacteroides fragilis* induced osteomyelitis. *S epidermidis* was found mainly on the foreign body and *B fragilis* was found in the marrow.

One salient feature of polymicrobial osteomyelitis is the presence of necrotic tissue and possibly the presence of a foreign body. Necrotic bone and foreign bodies provide surfaces that facilitate bacterial attachment. Once bacteria attach, certain species produce a biofilm that firmly establishes the infection. A biofilm is a protective shield that derives its protective properties from the strong bonds it forms with the glycoproteins of the host tissue. It is these bonds that have been considered the factor most responsible for the difficulty in eradicating bacteria from bone. The biofilm creates a barrier to protect the bacteria from the action of antibiotics, phagocytic cells, and antibodies, and impairs lymphocyte functions. Bacteria can produce biofilms regardless of the mode of transmission and this virulence factor is considered an important aspect of posttraumatic osteomyelitis with retained hardware as well as in osteomyelitis associated with diabetic ulcers.

Posttraumatic Osteomyelitis

The most common cause of osteomyelitis is trauma, which is usually not associated with bacteremia. Osteomyelitis is an unusual complication of closed fractures, but its incidence following an open fracture can exceed 40%. Exposure of bone does not necessarily result in osteomyelitis. Although Gustilo and Anderson found that up to 70% of surface cultures of exposed bone in open fracture were positive before the initiation of treatment, the incidence of bone infection was related to the severity of the

Table 1   Microoganisms Isolated From Patients With Bacterial Osteomyelitis

Microorganism	Most Common Clinical Association
Staphylococcus aureus (susceptible or resistant to methicillin)	Most frequent microorganism in any type of osteomyelitis
Coagulase-negative staphylococci or propionibacterium	Foreign-body-associated infection
Enterobacteriaceae or *Pseudomonas aeruginosa*	Common in nosocomial infections
Streptococci or anaerobic bacteria	Associated with bites, fist injury caused by contact with another person's mouth, diabetic foot lesions, and decubitus ulcers
Salmonella or *Streptococcus pneumoniae*	Sickle cell disease
Bartonella henselae	Human immunodeficiency virus infection
Pasteurella multocida or *Eikenella corrodens*	Human or animal bites
Aspergillus, *Mycobacterium avium* complex, or *Candida albicans*	Immunocompromised patients
Mycobacterium tuberculosis	Populations in which tuberculosis is prevalent
Brucella, Coxiella burnetii (chronic Q fever), or other fungi found in specific geographic areas	Populations in which these pathogens are endemic

cers of fistulae often identify coagulase-negative *Staphylococcus*, which represents superficial colonization without deep infection. Deep cultures taken after the establishment of infection often provide the best picture of the infective organism.

One of the rate-limiting steps in the establishment of osteomyelitis is bacterial attachment. Intact host tissue is a poor substrate for bacterial adherence, and animal models typically require some form of bone damage to reliably establish infection. In humans, the risk of subsequent infection correlates with the degree of soft-tissue injury associated with the open fracture. The injury compromises host defenses and exposes bone to bacteria. Once inside the host, pathogenic bacteria express a unique set of virulence genes and proteins that enable them to establish infection. Several of these mechanisms of pathogenesis have been elucidated for *S aureus*. One involves the bacterial expression of receptors (adhesions) to numerous host proteins, which allows effective adherence. The target of these receptors includes collagen, laminin, and bone sialoglycoprotein, all of which injury exposes, and fibronectin, which covers damaged tissue and orthopaedic implants. Greene and associates demonstrated the function of the *fnb* gene in binding fibronectin, and Fischer and associates showed the importance of the *fnb* gene for *S aureus* adhesion to titanium implants in vivo. These examples also show how a single mutation can dramatically attenuate a microbe's virulence.

Mutant strains of bacteria that have lost the ability to express functional virulence factor(s) often become nonpathogenic or attenuated, and can serve as vaccines because they express most of the antigens of the virulent strains but cannot cause disease. Although the use of attenuated pathogens has transformed health care worldwide, it is important to remember that additional mutations can suppress or complement attenuated strains, or cause them to revert to their virulent form. One such case was recently documented in a 76-year-old man who had undergone intravesical bacillus Calmette-Guérin (BCG) therapy for bladder cancer and presented with *Mycobacterium bovis* vertebral osteomyelitis 7 years later. The patient fared well with immediate antituberculous medications alone, thus highlighting the importance of appropriate consideration of the clinical setting to achieve a timely diagnosis. Common offending organisms cause osteomyelitis, but the diagnosis is made based on the clinical picture.

Virulence Factors and Host Injury

Bacteria exhibit a host of pathogenic mechanisms to establish infections in bone. These include generation of biofilms, also known as capsules, which impair antibody adhesion. This effect in turn leads to excessive release of cytokines, which can injure host tissue and provide more areas of refuge for the pathogen. Pathogens may produce adhesins, which allow bacteria to adhere to host tissues,

injury and far lower than the prevalence of positive initial cultures. Certain environmental exposures at the time of injury are associated with high risk for specific infections. *Clostridium perfringens* is associated with farm injuries, *Pseudomonas aeruginosa* and *Aeromonas hydrophila* occur after injury in fresh water, and *Vibrio* and *Erysipelothrix* infections are associated with saltwater exposures. A list of the microorganisms isolated from patients with chronic osteomyelitis is presented in Table 1.

However, in open fractures when bone is directly contaminated, chronic osteomyelitis does not generally develop. Osteomyelitis occurs as a consequence of the soft-tissue injury and the associated compromise of host defenses. Most instances of posttraumatic osteomyelitis are caused by hospital-acquired pathogens such as coagulase-positive *Staphylococcus* or enteric gram-negative bacilli such as *P aeruginosa*. Environmental exposure can be misleading, because information obtained from swabs and ul-

proteins, and other molecules. Bacteria can also produce many forms of toxins, some of which not only cause injury to the host by inappropriately stimulating the host immune system, but also actively degrade host tissues with proteolytic enzymes and disrupt host cells with pore-forming elements. *S aureus* can produce hyaluronidase to cleave proteoglycans in connective tissue and streptokinase to break down blood clots.

The Host Response to Osteomyelitis

Innate Immune Response

The immediate host response to infection is an acute inflammatory reaction. Both tissue injury and the bacteria trigger activation of the complement cascade that leads to local vasodilation, tissue edema, and migration of polymorphonuclear leukocytes (PMNs) to the inoculated area. The PMNs coat the bacteria with opsonins to facilitate phagocytosis of the bacteria. Cytokines including interleukin-1 (IL-1), IL-6, and tumor necrosis factor are released from the injured tissues and act as chemotactic factors and activators of phagocytic cells (PMNs and macrophages). Activated phagocytic cells produce free oxygen radicals (O_2^- and NO^-) that are essential for host defense. This pathway is referred to as the innate immune response and is considered the most essential aspect of the host defense against infection. Animals that are depleted of granulocytes die from sepsis only hours after inoculation and rapidly succumb to noninfectious inocula of *S aureus*. Although the effectiveness of the innate response is overwhelming under normal conditions, its power to induce host tissue damage also needs to be understood and respected. Purified bacterial components such as lipopolysaccharides from the membrane of gram-negative bacteria, or similar complex carbohydrates from gram-positive bacteria, bind to specific receptors on host cells (toll receptors), resulting in toxic shock syndrome. Florid toxic shock can result in death even faster than the infection itself.

Adaptive Immune Response

Acquired immunity functions primarily to clear low numbers of persistent bacteria and to prevent reoccurrence of the same infection. This adaptive host response involves two mechanisms, the cellular response in which cytotoxic or CD8+ T lymphocytes lyse host cells that are infected with bacteria, and the humoral response in which B lymphocytes produce antibodies against the bacteria. Central to this acquired immunity are the macrophages that phagocytose the bacteria and present their antigens to helper or CD4+ T lymphocytes, which orchestrate the cellular response by producing TH1 lymphokines (IL-12 and interferon-γ) or humoral immunity by producing TH2 lymphokines (IL-4 and IL-13). Each process takes at least 2 weeks to reach peak effectiveness. Suppressor (or regulatory) T lymphocytes downregulate this response through poorly defined mechanisms, but function to limit the extent of host tissue damage and prevent autoimmunity. Bacteria can use this downregulation to establish disease. Once bacteria are cleared, the antigenic challenge diminishes, but memory T and B lymphocytes persist to supplement the innate immune response immediately upon bacterial reactivation or reinfection.

The effectiveness of the host response is the most important determinant in the ultimate outcome of osteomyelitis. This importance is reflected in the Cierny-Mader classification of long bone osteomyelitis, which incorporates an assessment of both local and systemic host compromise into the classification algorithm. Studies using this classification system have found that the strongest predictor of treatment failure is the state of the host and not the extent of the bone involvement. It is for this reason that patients with specific defects in host defense are particularly susceptible to osteomyelitis. Patients with chronic granulomatous disease have phagocytes that are unable to produce superoxide, which is required for their bactericidal activity. Osteomyelitis has been observed in almost 33% of these patients, often with *S aureus*. Patients with abnormalities in immunoglobulin production or complement have a high risk of infection by encapsulated bacteria such as *S pneumoniae*, *H influenzae*, and *Neisseria*. These patients are also susceptible to *Mycoplasma* and *Ureaplasma* infections. Patients with defects in cell-mediated immunity are at greatest risk for infections with intracellular pathogens such as *Mycobacterium*, *Salmonella*, and *Nocardia*. General host defense abnormalities that increase the risk for osteomyelitis are found in patients with sickle cell disease or diabetes, intravenous drug users, and the elderly.

Clinical Characteristics and Diagnosis of Osteomyelitis

Patients with bone infections present with pain and swelling, and may develop sinus tract drainage from the bone to the skin surface. This is caused by the influx of host defense cells and fluid infiltrate into the infected area, which increases intraosseous pressure and impairs blood flow. The subsequent infarction of marrow fat, hematopoietic cells, and ischemic necrosis of bone results in the separation of devascularized fragments, which are called sequestra. A localized abscess, called a Brodie's abscess, may form around the necrotic sequestra, typically within the cortex of a bone. The infiltrate can also permeate through the haversian and Volkmann canal systems, lifting the periosteum off the bone, and disrupting a major blood supply to the outer cortex. This form of subperiosteal elevation is prevalent in children in whom the periosteum is thick and not as firmly attached to the bone. In an attempt to isolate the infection, the host mounts a foreign body response that encases the sequestrum in new bone in what is known as an involucrum. In florid osteomyelitis, the infection breaks through the cortex and periosteum to form soft-tissue abscesses or sinus tracts to the skin.

Osteomyelitis that develops after trauma may exhibit a slightly different pathogenesis. In skeletal trauma, such as open fractures, the periosteum may be stripped from the bone, resulting in cortical necrosis. Trauma may also devitalize the surrounding envelope of soft tissue around the bone. Soft-tissue ischemia may result in tissue necrosis and subsequent fibrosis. When the soft-tissue envelope is stripped away completely from the bone, the devitalized bone provides an ideal substrate for infection. Thus, osteomyelitis after trauma is often different from chronic osteomyelitis as necrotic bone provides an initial substrate for the development of infection.

A salient feature of established osteomyelitis is bone resorption, which can readily be detected on plain films around septic implants. This osteolysis can easily be confused with neoplasia and may require a biopsy to distinguish between the two processes. Bone resorption induced by bacterial infection occurs from the interplay of the bacterial products on the host inflammatory cascade. Bacterial products (such as lipopolysaccharides) can trigger osteolysis by inducing the synthesis of proinflammatory factors (such as prostaglandin E_2, tumor necrosis factor-α, IL-1, and IL-6). These factors act on osteoblasts to produce macrophage-colony stimulating factor and receptor activator of nuclear factor kappa (RANK) ligand, which in turn promote osteoclast differentiation and activation. They also act directly on preosteoclasts to differentiate, and mature osteoclasts to resorb bone.

Even in the presence of obvious clinical signs such as localized warmth, swelling, redness, fever, chills, loss of joint motion, and unwillingness to use an extremity, proper diagnosis requires fluid and tissue culture. The evaluation of patients with osteomyelitis should include a complete blood count with differential, erythrocyte sedimentation rate (ESR), and C-reactive protein (CRP). In acute infection, CRP concentrations rise within a few hours, reaching extremely high values (400 mg/L) within 48 hours, and can return to normal a few weeks after the infection clears; ESR may take longer to return to normal.

Because radiographic signs of osteomyelitis do not occur for at least 2 weeks, bone imaging studies are required to detect the early phase of infection. Typically, the three-phase bone scan is the first study to be performed. Technetium Tc 99m methylene diphosphonate labels bone and correlates with blood flow and osteoblast activity. The first phase of the bone scan is a flow phase consisting of 2- to 5-second images performed while the radioactive material is injected. Five minutes after the radioactive material is injected, the second phase, the blood pool phase, occurs. During the third phase, the bone is imaged approximately 3 hours after injection. Bone infection is strongly suspected when the radioactive material localizes in the bone after 3 hours. A possible fourth phase could be performed by assessing the uptake of technetium Tc 99m methylene diphosphonate that is no longer bound to the lamellar bone after 4 hours, but remains in woven bone at the site of infection up to 24 hours after the initial injection. Bone scan is sensitive for detecting acute hematogenous osteomyelitis and septic arthritis. However, these scans are less useful in neonates where false negative or "cold" scans are unacceptably high. In patients with other underlying chronic disease, bone scans can be positive for reasons other than infection. This is particularly true in patients with sickle cell disease and metastatic cancer. Bone scans are also positive in the setting of acute or healing fractures.

A similar test using gallium citrate (Ga 67) has also been used clinically, but is more time-consuming, with imaging delayed as long as 2 days after injection to detect the infection. A leukocyte-labeled nuclear imaging study (also known as a white blood cell scan) is also labor intensive. This test requires a patient to donate a sample of blood from which the white blood cells are labeled with radioisotopes. The "tagged" white blood cells are then reintroduced into the patient before a scan. The reinjected white blood cells are given up to 1 day to migrate to the site of inflammation before the scan is repeated. Technetium scans are approximately 90% sensitive, but only 50% specific. Gallium can increase the specificity to approximately 70%, and indium-labeled white blood cell scans can effect an additional increase in specificity; however, white blood cell scans are less sensitive than bone scans. Because of the cost in time, money, and labor, this test is rarely used initially for the diagnosis of osteomyelitis, but instead may have a role in clarifying results, such as when a patient's positive technetium 99 scan is believed to be falsely positive. There have recently been encouraging results with technetium antigranulocyte monoclonal antibody scans, which demonstrate better sensitivity and specificity than either tagged white cell and traditional technetium scans.

CT and MRI also are useful tools for the workup of osteomyelitis. CT provides excellent delineation of cortical bone and sequestra, which can be helpful for surgical planning. MRI may aid in the diagnosis of patients with suspected osteomyelitis and in planning their surgical treatment. MRIs are highly sensitive and specific for osteomyelitis, without exposing the patient to radioactive elements found in nuclear studies. MRI has reduced accuracy in the presence of orthopaedic implants and has been relatively expensive in the past. Both T1- and T2-weighted images provide important information. In a T1-weighted image, marrow normally produces high signal intensity; however, the low signal of the inflammatory process on T1-weighted images is indicative of infection. The T2-weighted images may produce a high signal, because the inflammatory process can cause an increase in the water content of normally fatty marrow. MRI scans are also helpful for identifying sequestra, sinus tracts, and the extent of soft-tissue edema. This information is used to map the location of infection so that the lesion can be aspirated to culture microorganisms.

Treatment

Once the diagnosis of osteomyelitis or septic arthritis is firmly established, treatment consists of the acquisition of deep and blood cultures and the surgical débridement of infected and necrotic tissue. Eradication of bone infection cannot be successfully accomplished without excision of necrotic bone. In patients with acute osteomyelitis, such as children presenting early with the signs and symptoms of osteomyelitis and positive MRI findings, medical treatment may be the only intervention necessary. In this group, prompt initiation of antibiotic therapy specific for the bacteria is the key. This treatment should begin immediately after cultures have been obtained. The typical recommended duration of antibiotic treatment is rarely more than 4 weeks. However, when longer therapy is warranted, such as in patients with diabetes, patients with metabolic or immune compromise, or those with retained hardware, patients are likely to receive 1 to 2 weeks of parenteral therapy followed by 4 to 5 weeks of oral therapy, for a total period of antibiotic administration of approximately 4 to 6 weeks. The type, duration, and route of administration of antibiotics are based on bacterial sensitivity to the antibiotic, using deep cultures (to determine the nature of the osteomyelitis—for example, infection with retained hardware). The patient's response to treatment is based on the physical findings, including temperature curves, and objective indicators to treatment in the form of serial blood work, such as ESR and CRP. If the patient has not responded, longer-term antibiotics may be continued only when it is certain that the infection has been adequately characterized and débrided, and the host does not have a correctable metabolic condition contributing to the infection. In addition to removing necrotic bone, eradication of infection typically requires removal of all contaminated hardware.

In patients with chronic infections with extensive devitalized soft tissue, soft-tissue débridement and reconstruction is required if there is any hope of eradicating the infection. The soft-tissue defect is normally covered with a rotational, free-muscle, myocutaneous or fasciocutaneous composite flap. Muscle flaps have also been used to facilitate bone healing at sites where there is little soft-tissue coverage by introducing a rich blood supply. Thus, the value of these biologic tissues is to obliterate the dead space and to provide vascularity to a previously devitalized area. Until the area of devitalized tissue has been clearly defined, the soft-tissue defects may be covered with a vacuum-assisted closure dressing after débridement or with a local antibiotic bead pouch.

The bone débridement progresses until bleeding (healthy) bone is encountered. Once the wound is clean, the bone deficit is assessed. If the bone débridement creates a critically sized bone defect, the void is eventually filled with allogeneic or autogenetic bone graft, or bone is regenerated de novo through distraction osteogenesis. Initially the "dead space" is filled with a spacer, most commonly in the form of antibiotic infused polymethylmethacrylate beads. Although polymethylmethacrylate antibiotic beads are the most commonly used vehicle for locally administered antibiotics, current antibiotic delivery systems also include implantable pumps, bioresorbable polymers, sebaceous fatty acid dimmers, and bone graft-type materials. Local antibiotics have the advantage of providing high local concentrations at the site of infection and low systemic concentrations, which accordingly have less risk of systemic complications. With the exception of local antibiotic pumps, these systems fill the empty space at the same time that they administer antibiotics. Local antibiotics can be used as an adjunct to systemic antibiotics even without mechanically unstable bone defects. Although large clinical trials evaluating the efficacy of local versus antibiotic treatments are not available, research supports their use.

Infections and Total Joint Arthroplasty

Infection following total joint arthroplasty has an incidence of less than 1% for primary surgery and up to 2% for revision surgery. Infection of total joint arthroplasty shares similarities to acute hematogenous osteomyelitis, chronic osteomyelitis, and septic arthritis. The most common clinical symptom is pain, whereas fever, chills, redness, drainage, and sinus tracts are rare. Drainage and erythema are nonspecific in the acute knee replacement. However, if any of these clinical findings are present, the physician should have a high index of suspicion for infection. The standard laboratory studies used to diagnosis infection include ESR, CRP, and a complete blood count with differential. Because these tests are not specific for microorganisms, additional invasive tests are needed to characterize the infection. These tests include aspiration of joint fluid and surgically obtained tissue samples. The aspirated fluid is examined for Gram stain, cell count, and culture results. Surgically obtained tissues are typically examined for Gram stain, culture results, and for the number of PMN white blood cells visualized per high-powered field (HPF) on frozen section. Tissue samples are taken from many sites, including granulation tissue adjacent to all components of the prosthesis. There is some debate about how many PMNs/HPF indicates infection, but typically more than five is considered indicative of infection. Selecting a criterion of one PMN/HPF lowers the threshold for infection and increases the sensitivity, but may reduce the specificity. A threshold of 10 PMNs/HPF lowers the sensitivity, but is more specific and has a higher positive predictive value. The lower sensitivity can occur from sampling errors and can produce a false-negative result. False-positive results are rare with a 10 PMNs/HPF threshold, but can occur when acutely inflamed tissue is sampled near a fracture.

One of the most powerful techniques in diagnosis and characterization of bacterial infection is the polymerase chain reaction (PCR). This assay permits the detection of as little as one molecule of DNA by generating multiple copies of the DNA target with a heat stable DNA polymerase and two oligonucleotides (primers) that flank the DNA. The key is the primer DNA. The 16S subunit of ribosomal DNA is the most conserved DNA for all phylogeny of bacteria. If a mixture of 16S DNA primers from different genus of bacteria is used, the precise genus and species of bacteria can be identified, because only a given bacterial genus' primers will amplify the DNA in question. PCR is now a standard diagnostic procedure in all microbiology laboratories. However, even with these state-of-the-art techniques, the definitive diagnostic test for periprosthetic infection remains culture of tissue obtained at the time of surgery correlated with clinical findings. In other words, a positive culture must be supported by clinical signs, symptoms, and laboratory and radiographic findings.

Plain radiographic findings often show aggressive nonfocal osteolysis, periosteal bone formation, or focal lysis adjacent to an infected prosthesis. These findings are nonspecific for infection, because aseptic loosening secondary to wear debris produces similar findings. Findings on nuclear scanning are often nonspecific and on MRI are difficult to interpret because the prosthesis may obscure the image. In these circumstances a bone scan can be combined with leukocyte scintigraphy to improve the specificity of these studies. The two most commonly used leukocyte scintigraphies are indium (In) 111 or technetium (Tc) 99m methylene diphosphonate complex to hexamethyl propyleneamine oxide. These scans together have a sensitivity of 80% to 90% and a specificity between 85% and 100%. However, leukocyte scintigraphy is expensive.

Immunoscintigraph labeling of immunoglobulins represents the newest version of nuclear imaging. Nonspecific human immunoglobulin G labeled with In 111, In 123, or Tc 99m has been studied in humans to evaluate infection and inflammation with early success. The success of these scans has been reported to be between 67% and 100% for specificity and 88% to 100% for sensitivity. Radiotracer-labeled chemotactic peptides have also been used recently, but clinical studies are not yet available.

Following a confirmed diagnosis, treatment of an infected hip or knee total joint arthroplasty follows the same basic principles for treatment of osteomyelitis. The infected site must be surgically débrided to remove all of the infected necrotic tissue. In contrast to infected fractures, in chronically infected total joint arthroplasties all foreign material including cement is removed. In frac-

tures, an infected union is preferable to an infected nonunion. Thus, in the presence of a fracture the hardware is often retained even at the risk of impairing eradication. Once the surgical débridement is completed, the tissues are sent for culture and broad-spectrum parenteral antibiotic therapy is initiated until final culture results are determined. Specific antibiotics are typically continued for 6 weeks. Repeat tissue sampling before reimplantation has been advocated. Failure to rigorously adhere to these principles will likely result in a persistent infection.

Retention of the prothesis can be considered in two special circumstances: when the diagnosis of infection is made within 3 months of the implantation of the prosthesis, or when symptoms of infection have been present for less than 1 month. However, even with these strict criteria, a 50% failure rate can be expected. The more accepted treatment involves a two-stage exchange in which the infected prosthesis is removed and replaced with an antibiotic spacer during an initial débridement and then a new prosthesis is reimplanted after a course of parenteral antibiotics. The interval between the first débridement stage and the second reimplantation stage is typically 6 weeks or longer. A single-stage débridement and prosthetic replacement can be considered, but has a lower success rate than a two-stage exchange. A three-stage program has also been described in which the initial surgical débridement is followed by an intervening stage in which a bone deficit is reconstructed with bone graft. This program is reserved for very special circumstances in which structural grafts need to be incorporated to allow for a prosthesis to be placed. More often structural bone graft material is placed at the same time as the reimplantation of the prosthesis.

Prophylactic Antibiotic Treatment of Patients With Total Joint Arthroplasties

Despite complications such as infection and aseptic loosening, total joint arthroplasty is considered one of the most successful surgical interventions in medicine. Approximately 500,000 joint arthroplasty surgeries are performed annually in the United States. More than 1.5 million procedures per year are performed worldwide. This number is expected to rise with the aging of the population and the number of people with total joint arthroplasties already is in the tens of millions. Because prevention of infection is of paramount importance for these patients, a panel of orthopaedic surgeons, infectious disease specialists, and dentists developed an advisory statement to recommend the optimal antibiotic prophylaxis in patients undergoing dental procedures. At the time the advisory statement was developed (1997), there was no evidence to support routine antimicrobial prophylaxis for patients with total joint arthroplasties before dental treatment. The task force produced three outlines identifying

Table 2   Mechanisms of Action of Common Antibiotics

Antibiotic Class	Mechanism of Action	Site of Action
β-lactams (penicillins and cephalosporins)	Inhibition of cell wall production by prevention of peptidoglycan cross linkage	Cell wall
Glycopeptides (vancomycin)	Inhibition of cell wall production by interference with addition of cell wall subunits	Cell wall
Bacitracin	Inhibition of cell wall production by interference with cell wall subunit carrier lipid	Cell wall
Aminoglycosides (gentamicin)	Inhibition of protein synthesis by binding with 30S ribosomal subunit	Protein synthesis
Macrolides (erythromycin)	Inhibition of protein synthesis by binding with 50S ribosomal subunit	Protein synthesis
Lincosamides (clindamycin)	Inhibition of protein synthesis by binding with 50S ribosomal subunit	Protein synthesis
Chloramphenicol	Inhibition of protein synthesis by binding with 50S ribosomal subunit	Protein synthesis
Tetracycline	Inhibition of protein synthesis by binding with 50S ribosomal subunit	Protein synthesis
Mupirocin	Inhibition of protein synthesis by interference with isoleucine t-RNA synthetase	Protein synthesis
Streptogramin (Synercid*)	Inhibition of early and late stages of protein synthesis at ribosomal level	Protein synthesis
Oxazolidinones (linezolid)	Inhibition of protein synthesis by binding with 50S ribosomal subunit	Protein synthesis
Novobiocin	Inhibition of DNA gyrase	DNA synthesis
Quinolones (ciprofloxacin)	Inhibition of DNA gyrase	DNA synthesis
Rifamycins (rifampin)	Inhibition of DNA-dependent RNA polymerase F	FDNA synthesis
Metronidazole	Inhibition of DNA synthesis by generation of short-lived reactive intermediates by electron transfer system	DNA synthesis
Sulfonamides and trimethoprim	Inhibition of enzymes involved in folic acid biosynthesis	Cell metabolism
Everninomicin (Ziraci†—investigational)	Unknown Unknown	

*Synercid, Monarch Pharmaceuticals, Princeton, NJ; †Ziracin, Schering-Plough Research Institute, Kenilworth, NJ.
(Reproduced with permission from the Centers for Disease Control and Prevention.)

patients with a potential increased risk for hematogenous infection: stratification for dental procedures; stratification based on the likelihood that the procedure would cause a bacteremia; and antibiotic recommendations. The advisory statement and content of the outlines are meant as guidelines only, and should not be used to replace sound clinical judgment by the dentist or orthopaedic surgeon while caring for total joint arthroplasty patients. Currently, all patients undergoing total joint arthroplasty procedures should receive antibiotic prophylaxis. Together with other clinical practice improvements, this regimen has been shown to reduce the risk of infection for primary total joint surgery from 28% to zero.

Antibiotics and Drug Resistance

Antibiotics are developed based on their ability to either inhibit the growth of (cytostatic) or kill (cytolytic) bacteria. Table 2 summarizes the mechanisms used by the most commonly used antimicrobial agents to kill or inhibit the growth of bacteria. Safe and effective antibiotics are either active against unique molecular targets within the bacteria or act more selectively against targets within the bacteria than in the human host. In general, antibiotic actions can be divided into five categories: inhibition of cell wall synthesis; alteration of cell membrane permeability; inhibition of bacterial metabolism; inhibition of protein synthe-

sis; and interference with nucleic acid synthesis. A list of common examples is summarized in Table 3. To persist within the host, the bacteria may also express phenotypic resistance to antibiotics, which also explains the high failure rate of short courses of therapy. Inadequate treatment with an antibiotic has been shown to promote resistance. Bacteroides exposed to subtherapeutic doses of tetracycline exhibit a 100-fold increase in gene transfer of tetracycline resistance transposons. Because of the extensive pathogenic mechanisms of Staphylococcus species and other bacteria associated with bone infections, osteomyelitis is difficult to eradicate and notoriously recurs, even after years of quiescence. Consequently a complete cure is an unlikely outcome.

Bacteria have derived three basic mechanisms to counter the effectiveness of an antibiotic: avoidance, decreased susceptibility, and inactivation. Bacteria may avoid an antibiotic by creating a barrier, such as a biofilm, by invading necrotic tissue, or by hiding within host cells, as can been seen with Salmonella species. Bacteria can limit exposure to an antibiotic by altering the permeability of their cell wall to an antibiotic or by producing a molecular pump that pumps out an antibiotic after it enters a cell. Bacteria may decrease their susceptibility to an antibiotic by mutating so that the molecular target upon which the antibiotic acts is no longer susceptible or the

Table 3 Mechanisms of Antibiotic Resistance

Type of Resistance and Antibiotic Class	Specific Resistance Mechanism
Altered Target	
β-lactam antibiotics	Altered penicillin binding proteins
Vancomycin	Altered peptidoglycan subunits
Aminoglycosides	Altered ribosomal proteins
Macrolides	Ribosomal RNA methylation
Quinolones	Altered DNA gyrase
Sulfonamides	Altered DNA dihydropteroate
Trimethoprim	Altered dihydrofolate reductase
Rifampin	Altered RNA polymerase
Detoxifying Enzymes	
Aminoglycosides	Phosphotransferase, acetylotransferase, nucleotidyltransferase
β-lactam antibiotics	β-lactamase
Chloramphenicol	Acetyltransferase
Decreased Uptake	
Diminished Permeability	
β-lactam antibiotics Tetracycline, quinolones, trimethoprim	Alteration in outer membrane porins
Active Efflux Pumps	
Erythromycin	Membrane transport system
Tetracycline	Membrane transport system

(Reproduced with permission from the Centers for Disease Control and Prevention.)

bacteria develops a mechanism to inactivate an antibiotic. Many strains of bacteria possess more than one of these resistance mechanisms against several classes of antibiotics.

Of all of the drug-resistant strains, *S aureus* mutants represent the most troubling to the orthopaedic surgeon because of their prevalence in wound infections, osteomyelitis, and septic joints. In the mid 1940s, when antibiotics were first used clinically, essentially all strains of *Staphylococcus* were susceptible to penicillin. Shortly afterward, resistant strains that could hydrolyze the antibiotic using β-lactamase were described. Currently, over 90% of clinical isolates are positive for β-lactamase and are resistant to first-generation penicillins.

In an effort to overcome β-lactamase, penicillinase-stable antibiotics were synthesized. The first was methicillin, which has been replaced by nafcillin and oxacillin. Predictably, methicillin-resistant *S aureus* (MRSA) strains resulted in nosocomial outbreaks shortly after the drug was in widespread use. Currently, 25% of nosocomially acquired *S aureus* isolates are resistant to methicillin. This drug resistance occurs via mutation of a gene (*mecA*), which encodes an altered penicillin-binding protein

(PBP). Because the function of PBP is to enzymatically cross-link the peptidoglycan component of the bacterial cell wall, inhibition of this enzyme causes bacterial lysis. The mutant *mecA* gene product PBPa has a very low affinity for β-lactam antibiotics and cannot be inhibited by them. Thus, MRSA is resistant to all drugs in this class, even if automated in vitro susceptibility tests indicate otherwise. An additional concern is that many MRSA strains have developed resistance to other antibiotics including aminoglycosides, tetracyclines, sulfonamides, quinolones, macrolides, and lincosamides via the mechanisms outlined in **Table 3**. This leaves vancomycin as the only available antibiotic to treat these multidrug-resistant stains of staphylococci. As intermediately susceptible isolates of *S aureus* to vancomycin are now being reported, it is likely that resistant strains will emerge that cannot be treated with antibiotics. This highlights the need to pursue the highest degree of vigilance in antibiotic use and the search for novel antibiotic drugs.

There are several investigational or recently approved drugs that may prove effective against multidrug-resistant strains, including vancomycin-resistant enterococci. These drugs include: quinupristin/dalfoprostom (a streptogramin), linezolid (an oxazolidinone), an everninomicin derivative, and glycylcyclines (tetracycline derivatives). In addition, some of the more recently introduced quinolones, including trovafloxacin and clinafloxacin, appear to have better activity versus gram-positive pathogens than their predecessors.

Although the advent of a new antibiotic arsenal to treat current and emerging pathogens is promising, it is essential to understand that new drug treatment cannot replace the surgical care of patients with orthopaedic infections. The appropriate removal of sequestra and foreign bodies will always remain an integral part of the treatment of osteomyelitis. The importance of antibiotics in conjunction with débridement is illustrated again by *S aureus*, which has been shown to exist within host osteoblasts. This phase of infection occurs under conditions of markedly reduced metabolic activity and sometimes appears as so-called small-colony variants on culture. This ability to downregulate its metabolic processes and hide within the host cell likely accounts for the bacteria's persistence despite aggressive medical and surgical management. Perhaps better antibiotics will not only combat bacteria's increasing arsenal of antibiotic resistance mechanisms, but also improve the long-term results of combined surgical and medical management of osteomyelitis.

Tuberculosis

Tuberculosis, also referred to as consumption and the white plague, has been one of the greatest threats to humanity throughout history. The disease is largely caused by *Mycobacterium tuberculosis*, but can also be caused by *Mycobacterium africanum* and *Mycobacterium bovis*. *M tu-*

Table 4   Recommendation for Treatment of Adults With Musculoskeletal Tuberculosis

Medication	Dosage
Isoniazid	300 mg/d
Rifampin	600 mg/d
Pyrazinamide	30mg/kg/d (for 2 months)
Ethambutol	Should be included in the initial regimen until the results of drug susceptibility studies are available
Pyridoxine	10 mg/d (given as prophylaxis against isoniazid-induced neuropathy)

(Reproduced with permission from the Centers for Disease Control and Prevention.)

Table 5   Tuberculosis Control Program

Control Type	Control Sections

Administrative controls	Annual risk assessment
	Written TB infection control plan
	Education program for health care workers
	Protocols for:
	  Screening patients for suspected TB
	  Diagnostic evaluation of patients with suspected TB
	  Isolation and initiation of treatment
	TST program for health care workers:
	  Routine TST at intervals established by risk assessment
	  Protocol for evaluating health care workers with positive TST
	  Protocol for identifying health care workers with possible TB
	  Protocol for investigating TST conversions in health care workers

Engineering controls	Expert evaluation of ventilation system Isolation rooms in accordance with CDC guidelines Additional air cleaning devices (HEPA, UVGI) if indicated
Respiratory protection programs	Protocol for situations requiring personal respiratory protection Education for health care workers NIOSH-certified respirators Fit testing program for health care workers

TB = tuberculosis; TST = tuberculin skin test; CDC = Centers for Disease Control and Prevention; HEPA = high efficiency particulate air; UVGI = ultraviolet; NIOSH = National Institute for Occupational Safety and Health
(Reproduced with permission from the Centers for Disease Control and Prevention.)

berculosis is an acid-fast bacillus based upon resistance to decolorization with strong mineral acids after using Ziehl-Neelsen carbolfuchsin staining methods. The bacteria grow very slowly in culture, taking 2 to 4 weeks to form a colony on agar plates.

After three decades of treating tuberculosis with antibiotics (**Table 4**), the United States declared victory over this deadly pathogen in the early 1970s. However, dramatic changes in immigration into the country, intravenous drug abuse, deterioration of public health control, and the acquired immunodeficiency syndrome (AIDS) epidemic that occurred in the 1980s produced a serious resurgence of tuberculosis throughout the nation. In addition to stressing the importance of public health surveillance, this resurgence of tuberculosis highlighted two of its unique properties, transmission and dormancy. Although most human pathogens require body fluid exchange for effective transmission, tuberculosis is readily spread from lung to lung in microscopic aerosol particles that are produced from coughing, sneezing, or even face-to-face conversation. Additionally, very few human pathogens can persist in a dormant state for decades. Tuberculosis genotyping studies have shown that most instances of the disease that occur in retirement homes are caused by reactivation of a childhood infection that occurred 60 to 80 years earlier. These remarkable features led the Centers for Disease Control and Prevention (CDC) to issues new guidelines for administrative controls, engineering controls, and respiratory protection programs (**Table 5**).

Although the CDC does not advocate vaccination for tuberculosis, it is important to know that most underdeveloped countries do use this form of prophylaxis. This consists of a vaccination with attenuated M bovis, which produces a reaction similar to that of the subcutaneous injection of tuberculin purified protein derivative used in the skin test for tuberculosis. Thus, a positive result should be expected in patients from other parts of the world and diagnosis in these individuals must be made from radiographs, cultures, and clinical signs and symptoms. In contrast, false-negative skin tests may occur in the elderly, patients infected with human immunodeficiency virus (HIV), and the chronically ill, who are immunosuppressed or malnourished and are unable to mount an immune response.

Although culture of tissue aspirates from the site of infection provides the definitive test to document the presence of tuberculosis, because of the lengthy culture period, likely presence of other microorganisms in the high-risk population, and the potential of multidrug-resistant strains, a central rule of thumb is that the diagnosis of tuberculosis is made in patients who present with a positive purified protein derivative test and radiographic findings until test cultures prove otherwise. Once appropriate specimens have been obtained, treatment tailored to the most likely type of infection should be initiated immediately. An example of this is that multidrug-resistant tuberculosis is likely to be present in HIV patients and the appropriate treatment regimen must be used in these high-risk patients.

Because of its dependence on oxygen tension, most tuberculosis infections occur in the lung. However, the CDC reported in 1991 that one in five newly diagnosed cases in the United States were extrapulmonary. These sites include the spine and extremities. Tuberculous infections of the thoracic spine were first described in the 18th century (Pott's disease); the thoracic spine remains the most common skeletal area of disease. Surgical treatment is often necessary to prevent severe spinal deformity and paraplegia, and to drain large abscesses from major joints. If the infection has destroyed the articular cartilage of a major joint, reconstruction may be possible by arthrodesis or arthroplasty. Most surgeons favor arthrodesis, but effective chemotherapeutic agents have made arthroplasty possible with promising short-term and intermediate results.

Viral Diseases

As previously discussed, vaccines have transformed medicine and eliminated the prior focus of infections in orthopaedics, most notably poliomyelitis or birth defects from maternal viral diseases. The most serious viral infections currently are caused by HIV, hepatitis B (HBV) and hepatitis C (HCV). These viruses present dangers that extend beyond the primary infection, which include postoperative complications and transmission to health care providers including the orthopaedic surgeon.

Human Immunodeficiency Virus

HIV, the virus responsible for AIDS, is a member of the *Lentivirus* subfamily of Retroviridae. After infection occurs, these enveloped RNA viruses convert their genome into DNA via a reverse transcriptase enzyme that is packaged within the viral particle. The HIV genome is packaged as a single-stranded RNA molecule with 9,300 nucleotides. This sequence encodes the regulatory elements for transcription/replication and the HIV genes including *gag, pol,* and *env.* Although there are at least nine strains of HIV, HIV-1 accounts for most infections worldwide. In comparison with other pathogens, HIV is not very hardy and can be inactivated fairly easily. Thus, transmission requires the exchange of body fluids. It is for this reason that the greatest protection and potential to eradicate HIV is to prevent this process from occurring wittingly (via unprotected sex) and unwittingly (via needle sticks).

In 1985, highly sensitive screening tests for HIV became widely available. Most screening is performed using enzyme-linked immunosorbent assay (ELISA), which determines if the patient has antibodies specific for HIV in their serum. This screening, which has a sensitivity and specificity of 98%, is performed twice and double-positives are confirmed via a more stringent immunoblot assay. Together, these tests have a false-positive rate that is less than 0.00006%. It is important to know that there is a significant lag time of up to 6 months from the initial time of infection to seroconversion using this screening test. Furthermore, some people who were exposed to HIV but failed to sustain a productive infection or have been successfully treated with chemotherapy may still have circulating antibodies specific for HIV. Thus, to determine the actual HIV viral load in an individual, a more sensitive, but less selective PCR assay is used. This test becomes positive within 1 week of infection/exposure.

Current estimates indicate that 0.5% of the US population is HIV positive. The distribution of these patients is uneven and is most highly concentrated in coastal, urban areas. Trauma centers in high endemic areas have reported that up to 10.4% of their emergency trauma patients are HIV positive. According to results from anonymous surveys conducted by the CDC, these estimates range from 0.2% to 8.9% in emergency department patients and 0.1% to 7.8% in all hospital admissions. Because of special risks to these patients and their health care providers, invasive surgeries for fractures and elective procedures are believed to be less frequently performed in HIV-positive patients compared with the general population.

HIV Pathophysiology and AIDS

Retrovirus infections are well contained by the host response and thus rarely if ever cause disease by themselves. Previously, the greatest concern with retroviral infections such as human T cell lymphoma/lymphotrophic virus type-1 (HTLV-1) was malignant transformation of the infected cell as a consequence of chromosomal mutations that occur during viral DNA integration or the transfer of potent oncogenes harbored within the viral genome. With HIV pathogenesis, clinical morbidity and mortality are the result of opportunistic infections that occur as a result of HIV-mediated immunosuppression. Thus, it is important to distinguish people infected with HIV from those with active disease, or AIDS. This distinction bears out in most clinical studies, including several on orthopaedic surgery, which found significantly poorer outcomes in AIDS patients but no differences between HIV-positive patients without AIDS and HIV-negative patients.

Although HIV can infect a broad spectrum of cells, its primary target is the CD4 lymphocyte, which is responsible for orchestrating cellular and humoral immunity. This tropism is derived from the CD4 molecule itself, which serves as the cellular receptor for gp120 on the HIV envelope. HIV also uses a family of chemokine receptors as a coreceptor for viral entry. CXCR4, which is the receptor for stromal cell-derived factor-1, is the coreceptor on T cells that is tropic for HIV. CCR5, which is the receptor for β-chemokines, is the coreceptor on monocytes and macrophages (M) that is tropic for HIV. Remarkably, a correlation between a genetic polymorphism in CCR5 and the inability to detect HIV in individuals exposed to HIV from blood transfusions has been reported. Thus, there may be some individuals who are naturally immune to HIV infection and a tremendous effort is being made to generate an intervention based on coreceptor blockade.

The acute viremia that follows the initial HIV infection in otherwise healthy people is rapidly extinguished with CD4 T cell levels returning to normal by 6 weeks.

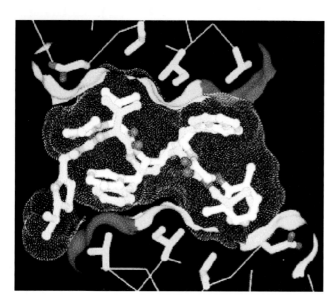

Figure 1   Active-site overlay of two inhibitors (ABT-378 and ritonavir) in contact with the HIV-1 protease. *(Reproduced with permission from Stoll V, Qin W, Stewart KD, et al: X-ray crystallographic structure of ABT-378 (lopinavir) bound to HIV-1 protease.* Bioorg Med Chem *2002;10:2803-2806.)*

However, the cellular and humoral immune responses against HIV are unable to completely eliminate the infection because of the virus' remarkable ability to mutate. It is this same characteristic that has stymied HIV vaccine development. In the next phase of the infection, termed clinical latency because patients are asymptomatic for many years, HIV replication destroys about 1% or 10^9 CD4 T cells per day. This places a high burden on the replacement system that ultimately collapses, resulting in a rapid decline in CD4 T cell level, AIDS, and death.

HIV Chemotherapy and Rational Drug Design

The first generation of anti-HIV drugs to be developed were targeted against the reverse transcriptase. Many of these (zidovudine [azidothymidine], zalcitabine [dideoxycytidine] and didanosine [dideoxyinosine]) were adopted from other antiretroviral therapies. However, the rapid drug resistance that occurs as a result of HIV mutagenesis forced a multitargeted intervention strategy. The HIV protease is a viral gene product required to process the HIV-essential Gag and Pol polypeptides into individual mature proteins. This enzyme became the next target for medical management of HIV. This effort spawned a new approach to drug development, known as rational drug design, which has emerged as a new standard in biotechnology. The pharmaceutical industry subsequently adopted this approach to produce the selective cyclooxygenase-2 inhibitors.

In contrast to traditional drug development in which large numbers of random compounds are screened for their activity against a specific target, rational drug design involves determining the atomic structure of the target

and engineering a molecule that will specifically bind to the active site, destroying its activity. With the HIV protease, this process was begun by cloning the gene into an expression vector that produced a large amount of protein in culture. The protein was then biochemically purified and concentrated to form HIV protease protein crystals. The x-ray diffraction electron density map of these crystals, which provided information about the three-dimensional structure of the protein, was then applied with the primary amino acid sequence to solve the atomic (quaternary) structure of the enzyme. From this information the desired drugs (keys) were synthesized to fit and bind to the active site (lock). As an example, **Figure 1** shows the atomic structure of ABT-378 and ritonavir bound to the HIV protease. To date the Food and Drug Administration has approved six HIV protease inhibitors: amprenavir, indinavir, lopinavir, nelfinavir, ritonavir, and saquinavir, which are commonly used in combination with the nucleoside-based drugs to effectively manage HIV infection.

Hepatitis B and C

Hepatitis viruses, which are small single-stranded RNA viruses and part of the Flaviviridae family, remain a tremendous health care concern. Although a safe and effective hepatitis B vaccine has been widely available for years, transmission of this virus remains the most common occupationally acquired bloodborne disease in the health care setting. A recent study of surgeons found that 17% were HBV positive and 14% of surgeons still susceptible to HBV had not received the vaccine. Studies have also shown that 0.5% to 5% of hospitalized patients are HBV carriers, and the CDC estimated that of the 5,100 health care workers in the United States who acquired HBV on the job in 1991, 125 will die from this infection.

HCV is primarily transmitted through the blood, and it is estimated that 90% of transfusion patients who receive HCV-positive blood will contract the disease. Approximately 4 million Americans are infected with HCV, with moderately increased prevalence in minorities: 3.2% of blacks, 2.1% of Hispanics, and 1.5% of non-Hispanic whites. Although the incidence appears to be declining since 1989, there were still 26,000 new cases in 2004. Most infections are subclinical but virtually all patients develop liver damage as detected by elevated serum aminotransferase levels. Of these patients, 85% will develop chronically elevated liver enzymes and chronic active hepatitis. At least 20% will go on to develop cirrhosis within 20 years of exposure. The risk of hepatocellular carcinoma is also elevated with HCV infection and is estimated to range from 1% to 5% within the same 20-year time frame. Persistent infection with intermittent viremia appears to occur in all infected individuals. Consequently, HCV is estimated to cause 8,000 to 10,000 deaths annually, which will likely triple over the next 10 to 20 years.

Patients are screened for HCV using an enzyme immunoassay (EIA) that detects antibodies against the virus in their serum. The current test, EIA-2, is 92% to 95% sensitive but the specificity has yet to be determined. Positive EIA-2 tests should be confirmed with a recombinant immunoblot assay. Even with a positive recombinant immunoblot assay the specificity is only 70% to 75% in low-risk donors. Seropositive patients may require PCR testing, which determines the viral load. This test should be repeated because intermittent viremia may result in a negative result. Unfortunately, the treatment of HCV is limited. Alpha-interferon has been the primary form of treatment with a response rate of only 40% to 50%, and a sustained response rate of only 15% to 20%. This therapy is recommended for patients with persistently elevated serum alanine aminotransferase levels who are at increased risk for cirrhosis.

Studies have shown that 1.7% of health care workers and 0.8% of surgeons are positive for HCV, which is similar to the reported incidence among blood donors. The percentage of surgeons testing positive correlated with age (years in practice): 30 to 39 years old were 0.4%; 40 to 49 years, 0.8%; 50 to 59 years, 1.2%; and 60 years and older, 1.4%. Parenteral transmission from patient to health care worker as well as from surgeon to patient has been reported.

Viral Transmission in the Surgical Setting

Prior reports have documented 151 instances of HIV transmission from patient to health care worker, of which 49 are described in detail. In these cases, 42 resulted from percutaneous injury, 5 from mucocutaneous exposure, 1 from both, and 1 from unknown transmission; 44 of the 49 cases involved blood. So far there have been no documented seroconversions resulting from puncture by suture needles, which is the most common cause of percutaneous exposure in surgery. Seroconversions have resulted from injuries by solid, sharp implements including scalpels, glass, and lancets. The lack of seroconversion following suture needle injury may relate to the low inoculum carried by the needle and subsequent reduction as it passes through surgical gloves.

The risk of percutaneous injury in orthopaedic procedures has been determined to be between 3% to 4%. This risk increases with the length of the procedure, amount of blood lost, and the presence of sharp objects (such as bone fragments, wires, and pins) within the surgical site. The risk of HIV seroconversion after a percutaneous injury of any type is estimated at 0.3%. The risk of HBV seroconversion to the same exposure is 30% or 100 times greater, and the risk of HCV seroconversion has been estimated to be between 2.7% and 10%.

In addition to conversions from patient to health care workers, surgeon-to-patient and patient-to-patient conversions have also been reported. For the most part, transmis-

sion in these instances appears to have resulted from breakdown in sterile technique, such as the desterilization of instruments or contamination of multidose medication vials. The American Academy of Orthopaedic Surgeons (AAOS), the CDC, and the Occupational Safety and Health Administration have published recommendations for preventing viral transmission in the health care setting with emphasis on operating room precautions. Approaches to completely prevent surface contamination of skin or conjunctiva are available and include impervious gowns, high-top shoe covers, face shields, and space suits. Cut-resistant cloth gloves can greatly reduce the risk of injury from bone spicules, wires, and pins, but cannot prevent needle punctures. Prevention of needle punctures must be accomplished by meticulous technique and may be further facilitated by the use of semisharp needles. There is also strong evidence that exposure risk following puncture is markedly reduced by using multiple layers of gloves. In the event of a significant HIV exposure (deep puncture with blood from a patient with high viral load), antiretroviral prophylaxis is recommended as outlined in **Table 6**.

Viral Transmission From Musculoskeletal Allografts

It is estimated that 150,000 musculoskeletal allografts are implanted every year in the United States. At least two cases of HIV transmission from infected donor to recipient have been reported. The first case preceded HIV antibody screening and involved transplantation of a fresh-frozen femoral head. The second case involved a donor who tested negative, but was likely to have been positive in the time frame between infection and seroconversion. In this case multiple organs were transplanted, including fresh-frozen bone and soft-tissue allografts, and processed, freeze-dried bone chips and soft tissues. All organs and three of four fresh-frozen allografts transmitted the virus. However, HIV was not transmitted from the processed freeze-dried material, which involves removal of blood and marrow elements, defatting with ethanol, and lyophilization.

In addition to HIV, transmission of HCV in fresh-frozen allografts has also been reported. Cadaver allograft screening currently includes PCR testing as well as antibody testing for HIV, HBV, and HCV. The risk of HIV transmission from musculoskeletal allografts is probably less than that for a unit of transfused blood, which is believed to be in the range of 1 in 440,000 to 600,000.

Summary

Musculoskeletal infections continue to be among the most difficult conditions to treat in orthopaedic surgery. Understanding the mechanisms of microbial pathogenesis and host response helps in the diagnosis and treatment of osteomyelitis. The age and health of the individual plays an important role in tailoring treatment. Despite advances, bacterial infection continues to hamper management, as an-

Table 6   Provisional Public Health Service Recommendations for Chemoprophylaxis After Occupational Exposure to Human Immunodeficiency Virus (HIV)

Type of Exposure	Source Material*	Antiretroviral Prophylaxis[†]	Antiretroviral Regimen[‡]
Percutaneous	Blood[§]		ZDV plus 3TC plus IDV
	Highest risk	Recommend	ZDV plus 3TC ± IDV[ǁ]
	Increased risk	Recommend	ZDV plus 3TC
	No increased risk	Offer	ZDV plus 3TC
	Fluid containing visible blood, other potentially infectious fluid, or tissue	Offer	
	Other body fluid (eg, urine)	Do not offer	
Mucous membrane	Blood	Offer	ZDV plus 3TC ± IDV[ǁ]
	Fluid containing visible blood, other potentially infectious fluid, or tissue	Offer	ZDV ± 3TC
	Other body fluid (eg, urine)	Do not offer	
Skin[¶]	Blood	Offer	ZDV plus 3TC ± IDV[ǁ]
	Fluid containing visible blood, other potentially infectious fluid, or tissue	Offer	ZDV ± 3TC
	Other body fluid (eg, urine)	Do not offer	

* Any exposure to concentrated HIV (eg, in a research laboratory or production facility) is treated as percutaneous exposure to blood with highest risk. "Other potentially infectious fluid" is defined as including semen, vaginal secretions, and cerebrospinal, synovial, pleural, peritoneal, pericardial, and amniotic fluids.

† Recommendations are defined as follows: "Recommend" indicates that postexposure prophylaxis (PEP) should be recommended to the exposed worker with counseling. "Offer" indicates that PEP should be offered to the exposed worker with counseling. "Do not offer" indicates that PEP should not be offered because these are not occupational exposures to HIV.

‡ Regimens are as follows: ZDV = zidovudine, 200 mg 3 times a day; 3TC = lamivudine, 150 mg twice daily; IDV = indinavir, 800 mg 3 times a day (if IDV is not available, saquinavir may be used, 600 mg 3 times a day). Prophylaxis is given for 4 weeks. For full prescribing information, see package inserts.

§ "Highest risk" is defined as both a larger volume of blood (eg, deep injury with large-diameter hollow needle previously in source patient's vein or artery, especially involving an injection of source patient's blood) and the presence of blood containing a high titer of HIV (eg, source patients with acute retroviral illness or end-stage AIDS; viral load measurement may be considered, but its use in relation to PEP has not been evaluated). "Increased risk" is defined as either exposure to a larger volume of blood or the presence of blood with a high titer of HIV. "No increased risk" is defined on the basis of there being neither exposure to a larger volume of blood nor the presence of blood with a high titer of HIV (eg, solid suture-needle injury from source patient with asymptomatic HIV infection).

ǁ Possible toxicity of additional drug may not be warranted.

¶ For skin, risk is increased for exposures involving high titer of HIV, prolonged contact, an extensive area, or an area in which skin integrity is visibly compromised. For skin exposures without increased risk, the risk of drug toxicity outweighs the benefit of PEP.

(Adapted from the Centers for Disease Control and Prevention: Update: Provisional Public Health Service recommendations for chemoprophylaxis after occupational exposure to HIV. MMWR Morb Mortal Wkly Rep 1996;45:458-472.)

tibiotic resistance becomes more prevalent. Tuberculosis, viral hepatitis, and HIV are of particular importance to the health care worker. Use of the advances made in the management of musculoskeletal infections will require a better understanding of the molecular mechanisms involved in infection and host response. Consequently, the management of these infections will reflect advances made not only in the management of musculoskeletal pathology, such as arthritis and fracture care, but also in the tools used to treat these recalcitrant conditions.

Selected Bibliography

General
Bloom BR: Lessons from SARS. *Science* 2003;300:701.

Haas DW, McAndrew MP: Bacterial osteomyelitis in adults: Evolving considerations in diagnosis and treatment. *Am J Med* 1996;101:550-561.

Terminology
Braun T, Lorber B: Chronic ostemyelitis, in Schlossberg D (ed): *Orthopedic Infection*. New York, NY, Springer Verlag, 1988, pp 9-20.

Interplay Between Host and Pathogen
Belmatoug N, Cremieux AC, Bleton R, et al: A new model of experimental prosthetic joint infection due to methicillin-resistant Staphylococcus aureus: A microbiologic, histopathologic, and magnetic resonance imaging characterization. *J Infect Dis* 1996;174:414-417.

Daum RS, Davis WH, Farris KB, Campeau RJ, Mulvihill DM, Shane SM: A model of Staphylococcus aureus bacteremia, septic arthritis, and osteomyelitis in chickens. *J Orthop Res* 1990;8:804-813.

Kaarsemaker S, Walenkamp GH: vd Bogaard AE: New model for chronic osteomyelitis with Staphylococcus aureus in sheep. *Clin Orthop Relat Res* 1997;339:246-252.

Lew DP, Waldvogel FA: Osteomyelitis. *N Engl J Med* 1997;336:999-1007.

Norden CW: Lessons learned from animal models of osteomyelitis. *Rev Infect Dis* 1988;10:103-110.

Passl R, Muller C, Zielinski CC, Eibl MM: A model of experimental post-traumatic osteomyelitis in guinea pigs. *J Trauma* 1984;24:323-326.

Rissing JP, Buxton TB, Weinstein RS, Shockley RK: Model of experimental chronic osteomyelitis in rats. *Infect Immun* 1985;47:581-586.

Tsukayama DT: Pathophysiology of posttraumatic osteomyelitis. *Clin Orthop Relat Res* 1999;360:22-29.

Tsukayama DT, Goldberg VM, Kyle R: Diagnosis and management of infection after total knee arthroplasty. *J Bone Joint Surg Am* 2003;85(suppl 1):S75-S80.

Varshney AC, Singh H, Gupta RS, Singh SP: Experimental model of staphylococcal osteomyelitis in dogs. *Indian J Exp Biol* 1989;27:816-819.

Worlock P, Slack R, Harvey L, Mawhinney R: An experimental model of post-traumatic osteomyelitis in rabbits. *Br J Exp Pathol* 1988;69:235-244.

Zimmerli W, Lew PD, Waldvogel FA: Pathogenesis of foreign body infection: Evidence for a local granulocyte defect. *J Clin Invest* 1984;73:1191-1200.

Hematogenous Osteomyelitis

Morrissy RT: Bone and joint infection in the neonate. *Pediatr Ann* 1989;18:33-44.

Morrissy RT, Haynes DW: Acute hematogenous osteomyelitis: A model with trauma as an etiology. *J Pediatr Orthop* 1989;9:447-456.

Direct Transmission

Caputo GM, Cavanagh PR, Ulbrecht JS, Gibbons GW, Karchmer AW: Assessment and management of foot disease in patients with diabetes. *N Engl J Med* 1994;331:854-860.

Gray ED, Peters G, Verstegen M, Regelmann WE: Effect of extracellular slime substance from Staphylococcus epidermidis on the human cellular immune response. *Lancet* 1984;1:365-367.

Gristina AG, Oga M, Webb LX, Hobgood CD: Adherent bacterial colonization in the pathogenesis of osteomyelitis. *Science* 1985;228:990-993.

Johnson GM, Lee DA, Regelmann WE, Gray ED, Peters G, Quie PG: Interference with granulocyte function by Staphylococcus epidermidis slime. *Infect Immun* 1986;54:13-20.

Mayberry-Carson KJ, Tober-Meyer B, Lambe DW Jr, Costerton JW: Osteomyelitis experimentally induced with Bacteroides thetaiotaomicron and Staphylococcus epidermidis: Influence of a foreign-body implant. *Clin Orthop Relat Res* 1992;280:289-299.

Naylor PT, Myrvik QN, Gristina A: Antibiotic resistance of biomaterial-adherent coagulase-negative and coagulase-positive staphylococci. *Clin Orthop Relat Res* 1990;261:126-133.

Rissing JP, Buxton TB, Horner JA, Shockley RK, Fisher JF, Harris R: Synergism between Bacteroides fragilis and Staphylococcus aureus in experimental tibial osteomyelitis. *J Lab Clin Med* 1987;110:433-438.

Posttraumatic Osteomyelitis

Abu-Nader R, Terrell CL: Mycobacterium bovis vertebral osteomyelitis as a complication of intravesical BCG use. *Mayo Clin Proc* 2002;77:393-397.

Buxton TB, Rissing JP, Horner JA, et al: Binding of a Staphylococcus aureus bone pathogen to type I collagen. *Microb Pathog* 1990;8:441-448.

Chuard C, Vaudaux P, Waldvogel FA, Lew DP: Susceptibility of Staphylococcus aureus growing on fibronectin-coated surfaces to bactericidal antibiotics. *Antimicrob Agents Chemother* 1993;37:625-632.

Fischer B, Vaudaux P, Magnin M, et al: Novel animal model for studying the molecular mechanisms of bacterial adhesion to bone-implanted metallic devices: Role of fibronectin in Staphylococcus aureus adhesion. *J Orthop Res* 1996;14:914-920.

Greene C, Vaudaux PE, Francois P, Proctor RA, McDevitt D, Foster TJ: A low-fibronectin-binding mutant of Staphylococcus aureus 879R4S has Tn918 inserted into its single fnb gene. *Microbiology* 1996;142:2153-2160.

Gustilo RB, Anderson JT: Prevention of infection in the treatment of one thousand and twenty-five open fractures of long bones: Retrospective and prospective analyses. *J Bone Joint Surg Am* 1976;58:453-458.

Mackowiak PA, Jones SR, Smith JW: Diagnostic value of sinus-tract cultures in chronic osteomyelitis. *JAMA* 1978;239:2772-2775.

Switalski LM, Patti JM, Butcher W, Gristina AG, Speziale P, Hook M: A collagen receptor on Staphylococcus aureus strains isolated from patients with septic arthritis mediates adhesion to cartilage. *Mol Microbiol* 1993;7:99-107.

Tsukayama DT, Gustilo RB: Antibiotic management of open fractures. *Instr Course Lect* 1990;39:487-490.

The Host Response to Osteomyelitis
Cierny G III, Mader JT: Approach to adult osteomyelitis. *Orthop Rev* 1987;16:259-270.

McGuire MH: The pathogenesis of adult osteomyelitis. *Orthop Rev* 1989;18:564-570.

Verdrengh M, Tarkowski A: Role of neutrophils in experimental septicemia and septic arthritis induced by Staphylococcus aureus. *Infect Immun* 1997;65:2517-2521.

Clinical Features and Diagnosis of Osteomyelitis
Boyle WJ, Simonet WS, Lacey DL: Osteoclast differentiation and activation. *Nature* 2003;423:337-342.

Treatment
Faber C, Stallmann HP, Lyaruu DM, et al: Release of antimicrobial peptide Dhvar-5 from polymethylmethacrylate beads. *J Antimicrob Chemother* 2003;51:1359-1364.

Klemm K: The use of antibiotic-containing bead chains in the treatment of chronic bone infections. *Clin Microbiol Infect* 2001;7:28-31.

Petri WH III: Evaluation of antibiotic-supplemented bone allograft in a rabbit model. *J Oral Maxillofac Surg* 1991;49:392-396.

Infections and Total Joint Arthroplasty
Blom AW, Taylor AH, Pattison G, Whitehouse S, Bannister GC: Infection after total hip arthroplasty: The Avon experience. *J Bone Joint Surg Br* 2003;85:956-959.

Kaim A, Ledermann HP, Bongartz G, Messmer P, Muller-Brand J, Steinbrich W: Chronic post-traumatic osteomyelitis of the lower extremity: Comparison of magnetic resonance imaging and combined bone scintigraphy/immunoscintigraphy with radiolabelled monoclonal antigranulocyte antibodies. *Skeletal Radiol* 2000;29:378-386.

Mahomed NN, Barrett JA, Katz JN, et al: Rates and outcomes of primary and revision total hip replacement in the United States medicare population. *J Bone Joint Surg Am* 2003;85:27-32.

Prophylactic Antibiotic Treatment of Patients With Total Joint Arthroplasties
Douglas P, Asimus M, Swan J, Spigelman A: Prevention of orthopaedic wound infections: A quality improvement project. *J Qual Clin Pract* 2001;21:149-153.

Antibiotics and Drug Resistance
Chuard C, Lucet JC, Rohner P: Resistance of Staphylococcus aureus recovered from infected foreign body in vivo to killing by antimicrobials. *J Infect Dis* 1991;163:1369-1373.

Hudson MC, Ramp WK, Nicholson NC, Williams AS, Nousiainen MT: Internalization of Staphylococcus aureus by cultured osteoblasts. *Microb Pathog* 1995;19:409-419.

Mader JT, Calhoun J: Long-bone osteomyelitis diagnosis and management. *Hosp Pract (Off Ed)* 1994;29:71-76.

Proctor RA, van Langevelde P, Kristjansson M, Maslow JN, Arbeit RD: Persistent and relapsing infections associated with small-colony variants of Staphylococcus aureus. *Clin Infect Dis* 1995;20:95-102.

Wilson JW, Schurr MJ, LeBlanc CL, Ramamurthy R, Buchanan KL, Nickerson CA: Mechanisms of bacterial pathogenicity. *Postgrad Med J* 2002;78:216-224.

Viral Diseases
Lam PY, Jadhav PK, Eyermann CJ, et al: Rational design of potent, bioavailable, nonpeptide cyclic ureas as HIV protease inhibitors. *Science* 1994;263:380-384.

Pomerantz RJ, Horn DL: Twenty years of therapy for HIV-1 infection. *Nat Med* 2003;9:867-873.

Stoll V, Qin W, Stewart KD, et al: X-ray crystallographic structure of ABT-378 (lopinavir) bound to HIV-1 protease. *Bioorg Med Chem* 2002;10:2803-2806.

Chapter 17

Orthopaedic Pharmacology and Therapeutics

Carol D. Morris, MD

Introduction

The list of pharmacologic agents used to treat various orthopaedic conditions is constantly expanding. Increased understanding of the molecular and cellular events responsible for many musculoskeletal diseases has led to discovery of new targets and strategies of treatment. These discoveries have led to an ever-evolving algorithm that allows many diseases to be treated using both preventive and therapeutic measures. The clinician is now challenged to make sensible choices among the growing list of pharmacologic agents. Nevertheless, it is imperative for the orthopaedic surgeon to understand the risks and benefits of drugs prescribed and to convey that information to patients when appropriate; the indications and contraindications associated with the selective cyclooxygenase-2 (COX-2) inhibitors serves as an example. This chapter discusses the pharmacologic agents used to prevent, diagnose, and treat common orthopaedic diseases.

Antibiotics

The 1928 discovery of penicillin marked the beginning of an era and laid the groundwork for modern antimicrobial therapy. Antibiotics are antibacterial compounds produced by living microorganisms that suppress the growth of other microorganisms.

Based on their spectrum of activity, antibiotics are classified as either bacteriostatic (inhibit the growth of an organism) or bactericidal (kill the organism). To make this determination, several in vitro tests are available to determine an organism's susceptibility to a given antimicrobial. The minimal inhibitory concentration (MIC) refers to the lowest concentration of an antimicrobial that prevents visible growth of an organism on antibiotic-free media after an 18- to 24-hour period. The minimal bactericidal concentration (MBC) refers to the highest dilution of an antibiotic lethal for 99% of isolate tested. Antibiot-

ics are considered to be bacteriostatic when the MIC/MBC ratio is 16 or greater for a given pathogen, and bactericidal when the MIC/MBC ratio is 4 or less. The aforementioned definition is merely a guideline and is not accepted by all clinicians because of the tremendous technical variability in performing these tests.

Five basic mechanisms by which antibiotics exert their effects have been identified: (1) inhibition of cell wall synthesis, (2) increasing cell membrane permeability, (3) ribosomal inhibition, (4) interference with DNA metabolism, and (5) antimetabolite action. These mechanisms are outlined in **Table 1**. The most commonly used antibiotics are described below.

Mechanism of Action
Inhibitors of Cell Wall Synthesis

The penicillins and cephalosporins block the transpeptidase enzyme, which is responsible for cross-linking of polysaccharide molecules in the bacterial cell wall. The natural penicillin, penicillin G, is inactivated by the enzyme β-lactamase. The synthetic penicillins (methicillin, oxacillin) are active against most β-lactamase-producing *Staphylococcus aureus*.

The cephalosporins are semisynthetic derivatives of the cephalosporin-C antibiotic isolated from the fungus *Cephalosporium acremonium*. The nucleus of the cephalosporin is a dihydrothiazine ring fused with a β-lactam ring. Cephalosporins have traditionally and somewhat arbitrarily been divided into first-, second-, and third-generation cephalosporins. The first-generation cephalosporins are primarily antistaphylococcal agents with some gram-negative coverage. The second- and third-generation cephalosporins have increased gram-negative coverage with diminished gram-positive coverage.

Vancomycin is bactericidal for gram-positive organisms. Its primary indication for usage is against methicillin-resistant *S aureus* and *Staphylococcus epidermi-*

Table 1   Mechanisms of Action for Commonly Used Antibiotics

Mechanism of Action	Antibiotic
Inhibitors of cell wall synthesis	Penicillins Cephalosporins Vancomycin Bacitracin Aztreonam Imipenem
Increase cell membrane permeability	Polymyxin Nystatin Amphotericin
Ribosomal inhibitors	Tetracycline Chloramphenicol Erythromycin Clindamycin Gentamicin Streptomycin Tobramycin Amikacin Neomycin
Interference with DNA metabolism	Quinolones Rifampin Metronidazole
Antimetabolites	Trimethoprim Sulfonamides Flucytosine

infections. Erythromycin is effective for treating *S aureus* in patients with penicillin hypersensitivity reactions. Clindamycin is active against all anaerobes and most gram-positive cocci except enterococci. The bactericidal antibiotics gentamicin, streptomycin, tobramycin, amikacin, and neomycin work by binding to the 30-S subunit, thereby causing messenger RNA to be misread, which results in the synthesis of abnormal peptides that accumulate and lead to cell death. The aminoglycosides are used primarily against gram-negative bacilli. Their toxic effects are well documented and therefore it is imperative to monitor peak and trough levels to prevent renal and auditory toxicity. Gentamicin, tobramycin, and amikacin can be administered systemically. Neomycin is used topically in wound irrigation. Streptomycin usually is used to treat tuberculosis infections by intramuscular injection.

Interference With DNA Metabolism
The quinolones inhibit the enzyme DNA gyrase. The orthopaedically useful quinolones are the fluoroquinolones that are synthetic derivatives of nalidixic acid. Nalidixic acid is unable to achieve systemic antibacterial levels after oral intake and therefore is useful only for urinary antisepsis; its fluorinated derivatives (ciprofloxacin, gatifloxacin, levofloxacin, ofloxacin) have greater antibacterial activity. Ciprofloxacin is a fluoroquinolone commonly used in managing orthopaedic infections because of its activity against both gram-positive and gram-negative microorganisms and the equivalent efficacy of both oral and intravenous preparations. Rifampin inhibits bacterial DNA-dependent RNA polymerase, thereby blocking the synthesis of RNA. It has a broad activity against gram-positive and gram-negative organisms, mycobacteria, chlamydiae, and poxviruses. Metronidazole is effective against anaerobic organisms by forming oxygen radicals that are toxic to these organisms, which lack the protective enzymes superoxide dismutase and catalase. The oxygen radicals cause loss of the helical structure of DNA and result in breakage of DNA strands.

Antimetabolites
Trimethoprim, sulfonamides, and flucytosine are analogs of naturally occurring metabolites that mimic the metabolite substrate and block the synthesis of compounds needed for replication. Trimethoprim and the sulfonamide sulfamethoxazole are most commonly prepared as a mixture. The combination blocks folic acid synthesis and has a wide spectrum of activity against aerobic gram-negative and gram-positive organisms. Flucytosine, an oral antifungal agent, blocks pyrimidine synthesis.

Clinical Applications
Antibiotics are used in orthopaedic practice for the prevention and treatment of infections. The most common clinical scenarios include surgical prophylaxis, open fractures, and osteomyelitis. Detailed knowledge of the organ-

dis, or when patients have known hypersensitivity reactions to the penicillins and cephalosporins.

Bacitracin is most active against gram-positive bacteria, including β-lactamase-producing organisms. Because of its marked toxicity when used systemically, its use is limited to local wound irrigation. Aztreonam and imipenem are structurally related to the β-lactamase resistant drugs. Aztreonam is active against gram-negative organisms only. Imipenem has perhaps the broadest antibacterial spectrum of activity of all antibiotics. As such, its use has been limited to infection with resistant organisms.

Increase Cell Membrane Permeability
Polymyxin, nystatin, and amphotericin bind to sterols in the cell membrane, thereby disrupting the functional integrity of the membrane, allowing for the passage of macromolecules and ions and resulting in cell damage or death. Nystatin and amphotericin are antifungals that are used topically and systemically, respectively. Polymyxin is active against certain gram-negative bacteria.

Ribosomal Inhibitors
The bacteriostatic agents (tetracycline, chloramphenicol, erythromycin, and clindamycin) bind to bacterial ribosomes and cause reversible inhibition of protein synthesis and prevention of bacterial multiplication. Chloramphenicol is active against gram-positive and gram-negative organisms. Tetracycline is seldom used to treat orthopaedic

isms most likely to be encountered in a given clinical setting along with a basic understanding of pharmacodynamic principles will aid in achieving the maximum desired effect. Antibiotics are most effective when directed against a single pathogen for a short period of time, and least effective and even harmful when directed against multiple pathogens for a long period of time. The development of resistant organisms as a result of routine or prolonged antibiotic use is highly debated though widely acknowledged. It is generally accepted that the administration of a narrow-range antibiotic for the shortest duration possible will best avoid the selection of resistant strains of pathogenic organisms. The drug that is least toxic, least expensive, and most effective with the narrowest spectrum of activity and best penetration should be used. As in any scenario requiring antibiotics, an unnecessarily prolonged course is associated with wound colonization with nosocomial pathogens, greater cost, and increased adverse drug reactions.

Surgical antibiotic prophylaxis refers to the administration of antibiotics to patients without clinical evidence of infection in the surgical field. The pathogens likely to cause infection during most elective musculoskeletal procedures are *S aureus*, *S epidermidis*, aerobic streptococci, and anaerobic cocci. Antibiotic prophylaxis is indicated in procedures associated with a high inherent infection rate, or procedures with a low prevalence of infection in which an infection would have catastrophic results. The latter model is best validated with prosthetic joint surgery. Clinical studies have demonstrated that antimicrobial surgical prophylaxis reduces the occurrence of infection in total joint arthroplasty to less than 1%. Similarly, administration of prophylactic antibiotics to patients who will have fracture surgery, a foreign body implanted, a bone graft procedure, or extensive dissection resulting in residual dead space or hematoma is well accepted. However, studies assessing the routine use of prophylactic antibiotics in soft-tissue procedures or diagnostic arthroscopy are inconclusive. Guidelines pertaining to the timing of perioperative antibiotic administration are well established. In general, antibiotics should be present in the tissues at the time of surgery for maximal benefit; therefore, prophylactic antimicrobials are administered within 1 hour preceding the incision.

In patients with an open fracture, antibiotics should be administered as soon as possible. The type of antibiotic administered depends on several factors, including the extent of soft-tissue injury and environmental exposures to the wound (for example, soil or fresh water). In addition, prophylaxis against tetanus is mandatory in open fracture care. A tetanus booster should be administered to patients who were immunized more than 5 years before the injury and to patients in whom immunization status is unknown.

The pharmacologic treatment of osteomyelitic and septic arthritis includes the following principles: identifying the organism, selecting the appropriate antibiotic, determining the optimum route of delivery, and planning the duration of therapy. When antibiotic therapy is first initiated in patients with bone and joint infections, the offending pathogen often has not been identified. Empiric antibacterial therapy is based on the suspected presence of the most likely organism(s). The effectiveness of systemically delivered antibiotics depends on whether adequate drug concentrations accumulate at the site of the infection to inhibit or kill the microorganism. The concentration of antibiotic in the bone interstitial fluid depends on factors such as plasma concentration, protein binding, and the ability of the antibiotic to cross the capillary membrane. Animal studies have demonstrated differences in antibiotic concentrations in normal bone versus osteomyelitic bone. The β-lactam agents, aminoglycosides, and tetracyclines are all able to achieve serum-level concentrations in bone with acute infection. In addition, certain bacteria such as *S aureus* are capable of evading the action of antimicrobials once they are ingested by macrophages. Clindamycin, the quinolones, and rifampin all have the ability to penetrate macrophages and hence treat infections that persist by this mechanism.

Effective doses of antibiotic must be balanced against systemic toxicity, which is monitored by the peak and trough concentrations. Peak concentrations are determined from blood concentration 30 minutes after intravenous administration and adjusted by changing the drug dosage. Trough concentrations are determined from blood concentration just before administration of intravenous antibiotics and adjusted by altering the time interval between doses. If the trough level is four times the MIC of the antibiotic for a specific pathogen, the pathogen is considered to be sensitive to the antibiotic.

Infections associated with orthopaedic implants create a unique biologic milieu that is particularly challenging to treat. Antibiotic therapy alone is often inadequate, and the implant must be removed to eradicate the infection. The bacteria's ability to produce a protective biofilm and the variability of different biomaterials to adhere to bacteria are factors that have generated novel treatment strategies beyond the use of routine antibiotics.

Antibiotic-impregnated polymethylmethacrylate (PMMA) has the potential advantage of delivering high local antibiotic concentrations with minimal serum concentrations. Several thermostable antibiotics, such as gentamicin, have predictable elution kinetics from PMMA. Antibiotics are eluted from PMMA in quantities that vastly exceed the MIC needed to treat most susceptible pathogens in the first 2 to 3 days, after which there is low concentration in the surrounding fluid. The mechanical strength of the cement, once it is impregnated with antibiotic powder, correlates with the amount of antibiotic added. The use of 2 g or less of antibiotic powder per 40-g pack of cement does not appear to compromise the compressive strength of bone cement, alleviating concerns about early mechanical failure resulting from antibiotic-impregnated cement.

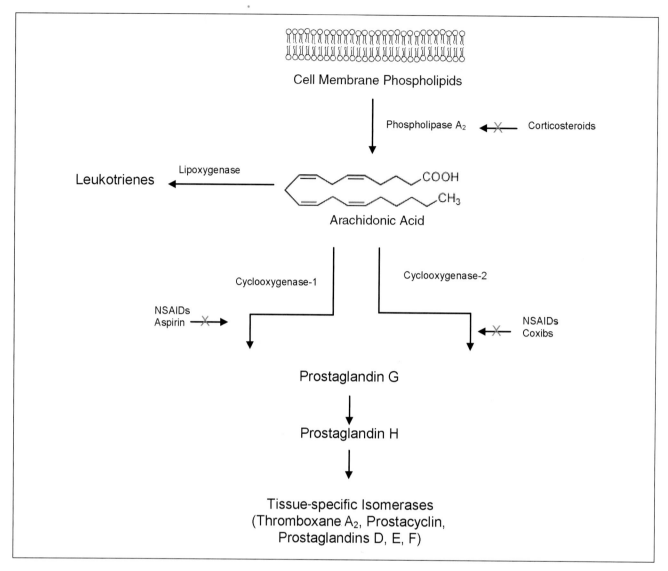

Figure 1   Effectors of inflammation on the arachidonic acid metabolic pathway.

Anticoagulation

Venous thromboembolic disease (VTE) encompasses a broad spectrum of clinical entities including pulmonary embolism (PE), deep venous thrombosis (DVT), and phlebitic syndrome. DVT is diagnosed in approximately 2 million patients each year in the United States; 200,000 to 600,000 of these patients will subsequently develop PE. It is well accepted that untreated patients undergoing elective total joint arthroplasty or skeletal trauma surgery have a high likelihood of developing some manifestation of VTE.

A venous thrombus is composed mostly of fibrin and red blood cells, mixed with platelets and white blood cells. Fibrin is the end product of the coagulation cascade. Agents for preventing and treating DVT take aim at the components of the clot and steps along the clotting cascade. Several pharmacologic options exist, with the most

common including aspirin, warfarin, low-dose heparin, adjusted-dose heparin, and low molecular weight heparin (LMWH). Newer agents such as factor Xa inhibitor and direct thrombin inhibitors have recently been investigated in orthopaedic patients for the prevention of VTE.

The ideal chemical prophylaxis has yet to be identified. It is difficult to draw meaningful conclusions from the available literature. For example, clinical trials that compare the different anticoagulation drugs often omit data such as patient compliance or supplementation with non-pharmacologic interventions in an uncontrolled fashion. Also, the duration of treatment and timing of surveillance following surgery is extremely variable in published studies, reflecting a lack of uniform biologic end points. As with any scientific investigation, critical analysis of the literature is encouraged to determine the most appropriate treatment strategy for a given patient.

Table 2   Prevention of DVT Following Total Hip Arthroplasty

Prophylaxis	No. of Trials	Combined Enrollment	Total DVT %	RRR %	Proximal DVT %	RRR %
Control	12	626	54	–	27	–
Aspirin	6	473	40	26	11	57
Warfarin	13	1828	22	59	5	80
LDH	11	1016	30	45	19	27
LMWH	30	6216	16	70	6	78

DVT = deep venous thrombosis, RRR = relative risk reduction, LDH = low-dose heparin; LMWH = low molecular weight heparin
Modified with permission from Geerts W et al: Prevention of venous thromboembolism. Chest 2001;119(1 suppl):132S-175S.

Table 3   Prevention of DVT Following Total Knee Arthroplasty

Prophylaxis	No. of Trials	Combined Enrollment	Total DVT %	RRR %	Proximal DVT %	RRR %
Control	6	199	64	–	15	–
Aspirin	6	443	56	13	9	42
Warfarin	9	1294	47	27	10	35
LDH	2	236	43	33	11	25
LMWH	13	1740	31	52	6	63

DVT = deep venous thrombosis, RRR = relative risk reduction, LDH = low-dose heparin; LMWH = low molecular weight heparin
Modified with permission from Geerts W et al: Prevention of venous thromboembolism. Chest 2001;119(1 suppl):1325S-1755S.

Aspirin

The best characterized mechanism of action for aspirin involves inhibition of prostaglandin synthesis. Prostaglandins are potent chemical messengers that are members of the 20-carbon eicosanoid lipid class. Prostaglandins are found in virtually all tissue types and have different physiologic effects depending on the location. They are synthesized from the free fatty acid arachidonic acid, which itself is created by the action of phospholipase A_2 in the cell membrane in response to specific stimuli. Arachidonic acid then proceeds down the lipoxygenase pathway to form leukotrienes, or the cyclooxygenase pathway to form prostaglandins (**Figure 1**).

Aspirin irreversibly binds COX-1 and COX-2. COX-1, a 578 amino acid protein that is encoded by a gene located on chromosome 9, is constitutively expressed, and is responsible for the baseline levels of prostaglandins. In contrast, COX-2, a 516 amino acid protein encoded by chromosome 1, is the product of an inducible gene and is only expressed in certain cells following stimulation. Although the two COX enzymes are 62% homologous, the structural difference is enough such that aspirin has a 50- to 100-fold more potent effect on COX-1 over COX-2. Aspirin causes acetylation of a serine residue at position 529 on COX-1, thereby inactivating the enzyme and halting the production of all downstream mediators. In platelets,

this action results in the suppression of thromboxane A_2 production, which in turn prevents platelet aggregation. Thromboxane A_2 activates phospholipase C within the cell, causing second messengers to trigger a rise in intracellular calcium, which in turn triggers platelet aggregation. In addition, aspirin exerts several nonprostaglandin-mediated effects by directly interacting with numerous substances involved in the clotting cascade, including fibrinogen, thrombin, and vitamin K, all of which play an interconnected role in thromboembolic disease.

Clinically, aspirin is still used for the prevention of DVT following minor orthopaedic procedures. In patients who have undergone total joint arthroplasty, although aspirin is superior to placebo, other agents have demonstrated greater efficacy in the prevention and treatment of thromboembolic disease (**Tables 2 and 3**).

Because most hip fractures occur in elderly patients and aspirin has been shown to be cardioprotective, the multi-institutional Pulmonary Embolism Prevention (PEP) Trial was performed to assess the use of aspirin in this specific patient population. The PEP trial included more than 3,000 patients given either 160 mg enteric-coated aspirin or placebo. For every 1,000 patients, there were 9 fewer VTE events, including 4 fewer fatal PEs in those treated with aspirin. There were also significant increases in wound complications, gastrointestinal bleeds, and blood transfusion requirements. The net mortality difference was zero.

Table 4 Known Drugs That Interact With Warfarin	
Agonists	**Antagonists**
Allopurinol	Antacids
Anabolic steroids	Antihistamines
Cephalosporins	Barbiturates
Cimetidine	Carbamazepine
Cyclic antidepressants	Corticosteroids
Erythromycin	Griseofulvin
Ethanol	Oral contraceptives
Fluconazole	Phenytoin
Ketonazole	Rifampin
Metronidazole	
NSAIDs	
Omeprazole	
Sulfonylureas	
Thyroxine	
Trimethoprim-sulfamethoxazole	

NSAIDs = nonsteroidal anti-inflammatory drugs

Warfarin

Warfarin, a synthetic derivative of coumarin, is the most widely used prophylactic agent following orthopaedic procedures. Warfarin is a vitamin K antagonist and exerts its effectiveness by blocking vitamin K 2,3-epoxide reductase, the enzyme needed for the reduction of vitamin K epoxide back to its active form. Active vitamin K is required for the postribosomal synthesis of active coagulation factors II, VII, IX, and X, as well as proteins S and C. Activation of these factors involves the carboxylation of specific n-terminal glutamic acid residues in the liver that occurs via a vitamin K-dependent oxidation-reduction reaction. In the absence of the reduced or active form of vitamin K, dysfunctional decarboxylated clotting factors accumulate, leading to decreased activation of prothrombin. In the presence of thromboplastin, prothrombin is cleaved to thrombin, which alters the solubility of fibrinogen in blood, causing it to clot.

The dose response of warfarin can be difficult to predict and is influenced by several intrinsic and extrinsic factors. The half-life of the affected clotting factors ranges from 4 to 60 hours. As a result, there is a significant delay in the action of warfarin with the full effect not observed for several days. In addition, several drug interactions with warfarin exist, causing both acceleration and inhibition of its metabolism (Table 4). Frequent phlebotomy is initially required, although careful monitoring is necessary throughout the patient's course of treatment.

The anticoagulation effect of warfarin is measured by the prothrombin time (PT) and international normalized ratio (INR), a reflection of the extrinsic clotting cascade. In these tests, thromboplastin is mixed with the patient's plasma and calcium. The length of time it takes for a clot to form is termed the PT. Because various preparations of thromboplastin exist, the patient's PT is then compared with that of a laboratory control and corrected by the International Sensitivity Index for thromboplastin. This process yields the INR. The normal range of the INR is 0.9 to 1.2.

The clinical efficacy of warfarin following total joint arthroplasty is summarized in Tables 2 and 3. Warfarin therapy remains very popular because of its lengthy track record following orthopaedic procedures. A target INR of 2.0 to 3.0 seems to be the most effective. Lower INRs are often maintained, although it is unclear if they are as effective in preventing VTE and do not necessarily decrease the risk of bleeding complications.

The most common adverse event associated with warfarin treatment is hemorrhage. In the event of unwanted bleeding or an excessively elevated INR, the action of warfarin can be reversed with 5 to 10 mg of vitamin K1 administration. Oral, intravenous, and subcutaneous vitamin K preparations are available depending on the severity of the situation. The second most common adverse event following warfarin treatment is skin necrosis. This complication usually occurs 3 to 8 days after treatment and is believed to be attributed to vascular thromboses in the subcutaneous fat.

Heparin

Heparin is a heterogeneous mixture of sulfated mucopolysaccharide chains composed of alternating residues of glucosamine and uronic acid. These chains vary in molecular weight, averaging about 15,000 d. Unfractionated heparin is commercially available heparin extracted from bovine and porcine tissues. Its biologic activity results from several mechanisms; the most important of these is dependent on pentasaccharide sequences randomly distributed along the heparin chain. The pentasaccharide sequence binds a lysine residue on a regulatory molecule called antithrombin (also called antithrombin III) and causes a conformational change in the structure of antithrombin, exposing its active site (arginine). By exposing its active site, the affinity of antithrombin for the proteases that convert inactive clotting factors to active clotting factors increases its binding 1,000-fold. The heparin/antithrombin complex inactivates factors IIa (thrombin), Xa, IXa, XIa, and XIIa. Of these, thrombin and factor Xa are the most sensitive to inhibition, with thrombin being 10 times more sensitive than factor Xa. By inhibiting the proteases, there is decreased production of factor Xa and thrombin and hence decreased fibrin production and clot formation. By this mechanism, heparin is not a direct antithrombotic but rather an indirect anticoagulant as it helps antithrombin to inhibit thrombin and factor Xa. In addition, heparin molecules with sufficient length (greater than 18 saccharides) have the ability to bind thrombin

Table 5   FDA Approved Low Molecular Weight Heparins

Generic	Trade Name	Indications
Dalteparin	Fragmin (Pharmacia-Upjohn, Peapack, NJ)	DVT prevention in THA
Enoxaparin	Lovenox (Sanofi-aventis, Bridgewater, NJ)	DVT prevention in THA and TKA DVT treatment ± PE
Tinzaparin	Innohep (LEO Pharma, Ballerup, Denmark)	DVT treatment ± PE
Nadroparin	Several	DVT prevention Clot prevention during extracorporeal circulation
Danaparoid (heparinoid)	Orgaran (Organon, Roseland, NJ)	DVT prevention in THA

DVT = deep venous thrombosis, THA = total hip arthroplasty, TKA = total knee arthroplasty

directly via a nonspecific charge effect. By binding thrombin, not only is fibrin formation diminished, but thrombin-induced activation of platelets and factors V and VIII is also affected.

Heparin displays extremely unpredictable pharmacokinetics for several reasons: (1) only one third of prepared heparin molecules contain the pentasaccharide sequence; (2) renal clearance is based on chain length; (3) heparin has a high affinity for other circulating proteins; and (4) it can induce or inhibit platelet function depending on surrounding conditions. In addition to its anticoagulant effects, heparin can also increase vessel wall permeability, suppress the proliferation of vascular smooth muscle cells, and induce osteopenia by suppressing osteoblast formation and activating osteoclasts. Heparin-induced thrombocytopenia is a well-recognized complication of heparin therapy, caused by antibody development against heparin complexed to platelet factor 4. Simultaneously, circulating platelets are inactivated and release procoagulant substances such that patients become thrombocytopenic and prothrombotic simultaneously. A 50% decrease in platelet count should raise the suspicion for heparin-induced thrombocytopenia. Treatment requires discontinuing heparin (including LMWH) but treating the risk of thrombosis. Two direct thrombin inhibitors, argatroban and lepirudin, are approved by the Food and Drug Administration (FDA) for this indication.

Unfractionated heparin is administered in an adjusted dose or a fixed low dose. Fixed low-dose heparin is typically given as 5,000 U every 8 to 12 hours. Although its efficacy in the general surgical population has been well established, fixed-dose heparin has failed to provide comparable thromboembolic protection in orthopaedic patients. Adjusted-dose heparin seems to provide thromboembolic protection, but its use is impractical because alternative anticoagulation methods can result in fewer bleeding complications and permit greater ease of use.

The action of unfractionated heparin can be reversed by the administration of an intravenous bolus of protamine. Protamine is a basic protein that binds heparin to form a stable salt. One milligram of protamine will neutralize approximately 100 units of heparin.

Low Molecular Weight Heparin

The existence of naturally-occurring LMWH fractions has been known for some time. Synthetic preparations were developed in the 1970s when it was discovered that LMWH was a more effective mediator of inhibiting factor Xa activity compared with unfractionated heparin. LMWH is derived from unfractionated heparin by chemical or enzymatic depolymerization resulting in chains averaging 5,000 d. Like heparin, LMWH exerts its major anticoagulation effect by binding antithrombin via the pentasaccharide sequence and inhibiting factor Xa production. Unlike heparin, LMWH has relatively low inhibitory activity against thrombin because it lacks the length to bind thrombin. LMWH also has a decreased propensity to bind other plasma proteins, platelets, macrophages, and other cells. These properties result in predictable pharmacokinetic properties, so much so that it is largely unnecessary to monitor the anticoagulation effect of LMWH. Because LMWH is cleared primarily by the renal route, its biologic activity is prolonged in patients with renal failure and hence monitoring may be required in this patient population.

Several LMWHs are FDA approved for clinical use and have proved to be safe and effective for DVT prophylaxis following orthopaedic procedures (Table 5). In patients who have undergone total hip and knee arthroplasty, LMWHs are superior in preventing DVT in comparison with aspirin and low-dose and adjusted-dose heparin preparations. Compared with warfarin, LMWH is at least as effective in the prevention of DVT in total hip arthroplasty patients and superior to warfarin in the prevention of the number of total DVTs (although not proximal DVTs) in total knee arthroplasty patients. A slight increase in postoperative bleeding with the use of LMWH in comparison with warfarin has been reported. This increase was attributed to therapy that was begun earlier than recommended. A recent meta-analysis failed to demonstrate any increased risk of bleeding with the use of LMWH in total knee arthroplasty patients. LMWH has been shown to decrease DVT rates in patients who have had hip fracture surgery, and those who have experienced acute spinal cord injury and polytrauma.

No antidote is known that completely neutralizes LMWH. Protamine, the unfractionated heparin antagonist, can neutralize 50% to 60% of LMWH. Recombinant activated factor VII appears to be effective in patients with severe postoperative bleeding.

Newer Agents

The limitations of currently available oral and parenteral anticoagulants have spawned interest in the development of novel agents. Several new anticoagulation drugs are currently under investigation. This section will focus on drugs that have already gained FDA approval or are currently in phase III orthopaedic trials.

Fondaparinux is FDA approved for the prevention of DVT in arthroplasty and hip fracture patients. It is a synthetic analog of the active pentasaccharide sequence found on heparin and LMWH and hence works as an indirect factor Xa inhibitor. In plasma, fondaparinux binds antithrombin without any appreciable binding of any other proteins, allowing for a long half-life (about 17 hours) and hence once-a-day subcutaneous dosing. It does not appear to bind platelets or platelet factor 4 and therefore is not implicated in heparin-induced thrombocytopenia. In phase III trials, it appears to be superior to LMWH (enoxaparin), although it is associated with increased bleeding complications. Although the incidence of death or hemorrhage requiring reoperation was similar between the two groups, important implications exist because no antidote for fondaparinux is known. Should uncontrolled bleeding occur, recombinant factor VIIa may be effective although it is not available in all hospitals, is extremely expensive, and can cause its own set of thrombotic complications.

Idraparinux is a sulfated derivative of fondaparinux. It binds antithrombin with such high affinity that its half-life is 130 hours, allowing for weekly subcutaneous dosing. Phase II trials revealed similar efficacy compared with warfarin and showed similar dose-related major bleeding, with fatal bleeding occurring in doses of 5 mg and higher. Based on these results, a 2.5-mg weekly dose is under investigation in phase III trials.

Hirudin and argatroban are direct thrombin inhibitors that are FDA approved for patients undergoing cardiac surgery with heparin-induced thrombocytopenia. Direct thrombin inhibitors work by directly binding thrombin, preventing the conversion of fibrinogen to fibrin. Hirudin is a recombinant form of the 65-amino acid polypeptide originally isolated from the salivary glands of the medicinal leech *Hirudo medicinalis*. The hirudin/thrombin complex is an irreversible interaction, an obvious potential drawback as there is no known antidote. For venous thromboprophylaxis in patients undergoing total hip arthroplasty, phase III trials comparing hirudin with LMWH (enoxaparin) demonstrated decreased rates of DVT in the hirudin group with comparable rates of major bleeding for the two groups. Despite these data, hirudin has not been approved for this indication.

The prodrug ximelagatran is an oral direct thrombin inhibitor that once ingested is metabolized to its active form, melagatran. Ximelagatran is currently under investigation for DVT prophylaxis. It has a half-life of about 4 hours and is administered twice daily. To date, no foods or drugs have been documented to influence its absorption and it does not require coagulation monitoring. Phase III trials suggest that a single subcutaneous preoperative dose of melagatran followed by oral ximelagatran postoperatively is more effective than enoxaparin and is as effective as warfarin. Bleeding complications appear to be slightly higher in patients receiving ximelagatran.

Regulators of Bone Metabolism

Approximately 98% of all calcium and 85% of phosphorus in the adult human is found in bone. Because these are two of the most important minerals for general cellular function, abnormalities in bone homeostasis not only cause disturbances in structural support of the body (osteoporotic fractures) but also cellular dysfunction (such as muscle weakness and coma). Disorders of skeletal homeostasis caused by impairment of hormonal control of bone formation, mineralization, or remodeling are termed metabolic bone diseases. Common conditions associated with abnormal bone metabolism include osteoporosis, Paget's disease, metastatic disease, corticosteroid usage, rickets, osteomalacia, and renal osteodystrophy. Of these, osteoporosis is the most common and serves as an excellent model to evaluate potential pharmacologic interventions for disorders of bone turnover. Numerous treatments of postmenopausal osteoporosis exist that either stimulate bone production or prevent bone loss. They include estrogens, selective estrogen-receptor modulators, calcitonin, bisphosphonates, vitamin D, calcium, and parathyroid hormone (PTH).

Bisphosphonates

Bisphosphonates represent the most clinically important class of antiresorptive agents available to treat diseases characterized by osteoclast-mediated bone resorption. They are synthetic, metabolically stable analogs of inorganic pyrophosphate in which the P-O-P bond has been replaced with a nonhydrolyzable P-C-P bond. The diphosphate configuration of both P-O-P and P-C-P contributes to a three-dimensional structure capable of binding divalent ions such as Ca^{2+} and is the basis for the bone targeting property of these compounds. Currently, seven bisphosphonates have FDA approval for use in various bone resorptive diseases (**Table 6**). Because of intense clinical interest and several compelling preclinical investigations, several bisphosphonates are also used off-label for a variety of skeletal conditions.

The mechanism of action of the bisphosphonates is largely dependent on the chemical structure, which can be

Table 6   FDA Approved Bisphosphonates

Generic Name	Proprietary Name	Route of Administration	R1	R2	FDA Approved Uses
Etidronate	Didronel (P&G Pharmaceuticals, Cincinnati, OH)	oral	-OH	-CH$_3$	Heterotopic ossification, hypercalcemia of malignancy, Paget's disease
Tiludronate	Skelid (Sanofi-aventis, Bridgewater, NJ)	oral	-H	-S- ⬡ -Cl	Paget's disease
Alendronate	Fosamax (Merck, Whitehouse Station, NJ)	oral	-OH	-(CH$_2$)$_3$-NH$_2$	Osteoporosis, Paget's disease
Pamidronate	Aredia (Novartis, East Hanover, NJ)	IV	-OH	-(CH$_2$)$_2$-NH$_2$	Paget's disease, hypercalcemia of malignancy, metastatic osteolysis
Risedronate	Actonel (P&G Pharmaceuticals)	oral	-OH	-CH$_2$- ⬡	Osteoporosis, Paget's disease
Ibandronate	Bondronat (Roche, Basel, Switzerland)	IV	-OH	-(CH$_2$)$_2$- N(CH$_3$)- (CH$_2$)$_4$CH$_3$	Osteoporosis
	Boniva (Hoffman-LaRoche, Nutley, NJ)	oral			
Zoledronic Acid	Zometa (Novartis)	IV	-OH	-CH^2- ⬠N	Hypercalcemia of malignancy, metastatic osteolysis

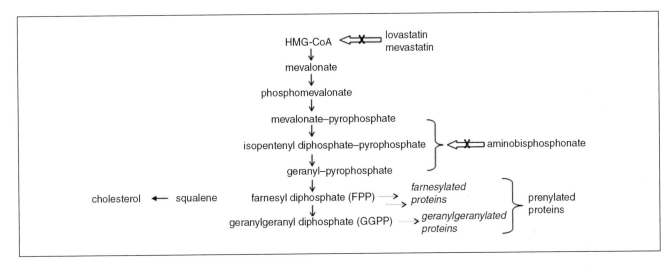

Figure 2   The mevalonate pathway.

grouped into two major pharmacologic classes: nitrogen-containing and non–nitrogen-containing compounds.

The initial compounds such as etidronate and clodronate possess simple, non-nitrogen containing substituents (-OH, -H, CH$_3$) and are metabolized into nonhydrolyzable analogs of adenosine triphosphate (ATP). The bisphosphonate preferentially binds to the mineral phase of bone exposed by osteoclasts during normal or pathologic bone resorption. Because osteoclasts have high endocytic activity, these cells resorb both the bone and the bound bisphosphonate or rather the ATP analog. These cytotoxic ATP analogs are then believed to accumulate intracellularly, inhibiting osteoclast function and inducing apoptosis.

A newer class of bisphosphonates developed by modifying the R2 side chain to include an amino group was found to be up to 1,000-fold more potent with respect to antiresorptive activity. Further modification of the primary amine has led to the development of even more po-

tent bisphosphonates. Collectively, these are called the nitrogen-containing bisphosphonates and include the commonly used drugs pamidronate, zoledronic acid, alendronate, and risedronate. They exert their effects by inhibiting components of the intracellular mevalonate pathway (**Figure 2**). The mevalonate pathway is the biosynthetic pathway responsible for cholesterol production and perhaps best known for 3-hydroxy-3-methylglutaryl-coenzyme A reductase inhibition by several cholesterol-lowering statin drugs such as lovastatin and mevastatin. The mevalonate pathway results in the production of the isoprenoid lipids such as farnesyl diphosphate and geranylgeranyl diphosphate, which are cholesterol precursors. Farnesyl diphosphate and geranylgeranyl diphosphate also are responsible for transferring their respective lipid group (farnesyl or geranylgeranyl) onto the cysteine residue of a protein. This process is called protein prenylation. Guanosine triphosphatase (GTPase), an important signaling protein, is formed by protein prenylation. The nitrogen-containing bisphosphonates inhibit protein prenylation and thus GTPase formation by inhibiting enzymes that have yet to be fully identified. The loss of GTP prenylation leads to a loss of osteoclast regulation including control of cell morphology, disruption of integrin signaling, altered membrane protein trafficking, loss of membrane ruffling and cytoskeleton disruption, and induction of apoptosis. Several basic investigations support the hypothesis that inhibition of protein prenylation is the major molecular mechanism by which the nitrogen-containing bisphosphonates inhibit bone resorption.

Oral alendronate was the subject of the multi-institutional randomized Fracture Intervention Trial (FIT). The 10-year follow-up data from the FIT study demonstrated the efficacy of alendronate at reducing vertebral, hip, and wrist fractures compared with placebo. Both 10 mg daily and 70 mg weekly dosing schedules appear to be equally effective. In patients with Paget's disease, both intravenous and oral preparations have a role in disease management depending on the severity of symptoms as evidenced by pain and alkaline phosphatase levels. In a recent randomized trial, a single 15-minute infusion of zoledronic acid was shown to be more effective than oral risedronate at producing a more rapid, complete, and sustainable response. Intravenous pamidronate and zoledronate have become standard therapy in patients with almost any metastatic disease to bone. In addition to managing hypercalcemia and decreasing the number of symptomatic skeletal events, there is evidence suggesting that bisphosphonates may actually exert direct antitumor activity against a variety of cancers and act synergistically with anticancer agents. Bisphosphonates are also used for several off-label indications, such as to manage osteogenesis imperfecta and fibrous dysplasia. More investigative clinical applications such as for periprosthetic loosening and osteonecrosis are gaining momentum.

The clinical manifestations of sustained bisphosphonate treatment are only beginning to emerge. There have been case reports of oversuppression of bone turnover in patients on long-term therapy, resulting in increased brittleness of bones with associated susceptibility of spontaneous fractures. Bisphosphonate-associated osteonecrosis of the jaw has been recently reported by numerous authors, with the number of cases increasing each year. The most common clinical scenario involves cancer patients being treated with pamidronate or zoledronic acid for skeletal metastases who undergo a dental procedure. Spontaneous osteonecrosis has been reported in these patients as well as in patients receiving oral bisphosphonate treatment (alendronate and risedronate) for noncancer conditions. The underlying mechanism accounting for this observation is not defined and there is no consensus to the clinical or radiographic characteristics. There are also no standard treatment recommendations at this time, as the literature contains almost exclusively retrospective analyses. In response to the surge of case reports on bisphosphonate-associated osteonecrosis of the jaw, the package inserts for both intravenous and oral bisphosphonates now contain information addressing the potential association.

Calcitonin

Calcitonin is a single chain 32-amino acid polypeptide hormone produced by the parafollicular cells of the thyroid gland. Its principal effect is to lower serum calcium and phosphate by its action on bone and kidney. Calcitonin inhibits osteoclastic resorption in bone through its receptors, inducing changes in the cytoskeleton. This action is accomplished by disruption of actin rings, structures that correspond to the clear zone in vivo and are responsible for the formation of bone resorption pits, or Howship's lacunae. In addition to inhibiting bone resorption, calcitonin is a powerful analgesic, stimulating the secretion of the natural opiate β-endorphin. In certain circumstances, it has been reported to be up to 50 times more potent than morphine.

Several molecular forms of calcitonin are available for therapeutic use. Salmon calcitonin is more potent than human calcitonin, although the two differ by just one amino acid. Although this difference is significant enough to be immunogenic, true allergic reactions consisting of anaphylaxis and urticaria are rare with the use of salmon calcitonin. Antibodies do develop in a significant number of patients undergoing long-term treatment with salmon calcitonin but without significant clinical consequences. Test dosing has been shown to be unnecessary because anaphylaxis is rare.

The traditional route of administration of calcitonin has been via subcutaneous or intramuscular injection. Recent formulations for intranasal delivery are available. Both the injectable and nasal preparations are FDA approved for the treatment of Paget's disease and osteoporosis. The FDA approved doses are 100 units per day for injection and 200 units per day for nasal spray. Animal studies have demonstrated comparable activity of both forms. Patients who receive nasal calcitonin seem to have better tolerance and fewer adverse effects than those receiving the injectable form, as evidenced by the number of patients who discontinue therapy (a small fraction of nasal calcitonin recipients, compared with up to one third of injectable calcitonin recipients.) Adverse effects, which seem to be dose related, include gastrointestinal disturbance, vascular flushing, and local rash or nasal irritation. Calcitonin has been shown to be effective in relieving osteoporosis-associated fracture pain, increasing bone density, and decreasing fracture rate. Several studies have demonstrated a range of responses in bone density in postmenopausal women ranging from maintained bone mineral density to up to 10% increased bone mineral density over 2 years of therapy. Benefits have been seen as early as 3 months after initiating therapy. Fracture rates have been shown to be reduced in postmenopausal women treated with calcitonin. The prevalence of lumbar vertebral fractures decreased in women with established osteoporosis when both injectable and nasal preparations of calcitonin were used. The data on hip fractures suggest a similar trend. The long-term effects of calcitonin in the treatment of osteoporosis are not well established, with the longest controlled study being 3 years.

For patients with Paget's disease, calcitonin has been effective in decreasing bone pain but ineffective in treating the pain of associated joint disease. Calcitonin has been shown to help improve neurologic symptoms in spinal stenosis by decreasing soft-tissue vascularity and edema, as opposed to affecting bony structures. Calcitonin has not been shown to be effective in improving the radiographic appearance (increased mineralization on radiographs) of lytic lesions. There has been some suggestion of the benefits of perioperative calcitonin, particularly as it pertains to reducing blood loss associated with highly vascular pagetic bone. Dosing is dependent on the severity of symptoms.

Parathyroid Hormone

PTH is an anabolic agent that enhances osteoblastic bone formation on both cortical and cancellous surfaces. It is synthesized in the parathyroid glands as a 115-amino acid precursor and is rapidly cleaved to its active, secreted 84-amino acid form. The biologic activity of PTH is found within amino acids 1 to 34 at the N-terminal. Teriparatide, a synthetic form of the hormone made from recombinant human PTH (rhPTH) that contains the active 34-amino acid sequence, is FDA approved for the treatment of osteoporosis in women and men. It is administered as a 20-μg subcutaneous daily injection.

PTH exerts its effectiveness by binding G protein coupled cell surface receptors on bone and kidney. The G protein stimulates adenyl cyclase, which in turn catalyzes the formation of the second messenger cyclic adenosine monophosphate, which mediates PTH action. PTH causes bone formation and bone resorption. Osteoblasts are the primary target cells for PTH. Once bound, PTH stimulates the osteoblast to produce receptor activator of nuclear factor-κB ligand (RANKL) and interleukin (IL)-6. Both of these proteins stimulate the proliferation and maturation of osteoclasts resulting in increased bone resorption.

Because of this coupled remodeling process, the timing and duration of PTH treatment have a profound impact on the net metabolic bone effect, leading to the following observations: (1) daily PTH injections increase bone mass; (2) continuous infusions lead to bone resorption; (3) Dosing should not continue beyond 2 years; and (4) the beneficial effects of PTH treatment might best be preserved by combining treatment with an antiresorptive agent such as a bisphosphonate. In the clinical trial that

led to FDA approval of teriparatide, 1,637 postmenopausal women were randomized to receive placebo, 20 μg of PTH, or 40 μg of PTH. A clear benefit was seen in the treatment groups as demonstrated by an increase in bone mineral density of the spine and a reduction in vertebral fracture risk by more than 60% over an 18-month period. One condition for FDA approval was that teriparatide should not be continued past 2 years. Animal studies demonstrated that following PTH cessation, gains in bone mineral density were lost. These observations led to consideration of the addition of bisphosphonates in an attempt to preserve bone mass. PTH treatment combined with alendronate in both a concomitant and sequential fashion has been investigated. Preliminary reports suggest that the addition of bisphosphonates appears to preserve and in some instances enhance bone mineral density in patients previously receiving PTH. The protective advantage of concurrent treatment with alendronate and PTH is not as obvious. This observation is believed to be the result of underappreciated changes in the bone microenvironment caused by the bisphosphonates, which may in turn affect PTH interactions at this level.

PTH therapy is not recommended for everyone. Although it is approved for women and men with osteoporosis, it is usually reserved for individuals at very high risk for fracture or those in whom other therapies have failed. In addition, PTH is not appropriate for patients at increased risk for osteogenic sarcoma, including those patients with Paget's disease, those who have previously undergone radiation, or the skeletally immature. In an animal carcinogenicity bioassay, osteosarcomas developed in rats that received supratherapeutic doses of rhPTH. Similar findings were not observed in monkeys receiving 4 to 10 times the maximal dose and have not been observed in patients previously enrolled in clinical trials.

Enhancers of Bone Repair

Bone repair mimics embryonic bone development such that actual bone tissue regenerates instead of forming scar tissue. Several growth factors implicated in the skeletal regeneration process have been investigated as therapeutic agents in the treatment of skeletal injuries. Of these, the bone morphogenetic proteins (BMPs) are the most studied and most promising. In 1965, Urist described ectopic bone formation in rodents after intramuscular transplantation of demineralized bone matrix. Further investigation identified BMP as the substance responsible for bone regeneration. In the late 1980s, BMP was sequenced and since then 16 isoforms have been identified (BMP-1 to BMP-16). With current technology, it is possible to produce recombinant forms of the protein (rh-BMP), creating an opportunity to assess the material properties devoid of impurities and without the potential risk of xenograft reaction during human use. To date, two BMPs have gained FDA approval: rh-BMP-7, also termed OP-1 or osteogenic protein-1, and rh-BMP-2. The BMPs are the only factors known to induce bone formation heterotopically by inducing undifferentiated mesenchymal cells to differentiate into osteoblasts.

With the exception of BMP-1, the BMPs are members of the transforming growth factor-β (TGF-β) superfamily. This superfamily of proteins contains five isoforms of TGF-β: the BMPs, growth differentiation factors, activins, inhibins, and müllerian inhibiting substance. These proteins regulate several cellular activities, including growth, differentiation, and extracellular matrix formation. BMP is the largest subgroup belonging to the TGF-β superfamily.

The BMPs act via a mechanism common to the growth factors in the TGF-β family. They bind to specific target cell transmembrane receptors that in turn induce an intracellular signal to act on the nucleus to produce a biologic response. Specifically, BMP binds a characteristic combination of type I and type II serine/threonine kinase receptors, which assemble a phosphorylated complex. This complex activates transcription factors called SMADs, which act on the nucleus to activate or suppress a given target gene. Eight different SMADs have been identified, each of which affects a different cellular response. Although this basic BMP receptor model has been identified, the manner in which these signaling pathways regulate bone repair are poorly understood.

For the BMPs to be clinically effective, they must be delivered to the local bone defect by a carrier. The carrier must be capable of adequate temporal distribution (retaining a critical threshold concentration of BMP at the implantation site for the required period); acting as a scaffold over which bone growth can occur; and spatial containment (contain the BMP at the localized site and prevent extraneous bone formation). To that end, several potential carriers have been investigated, including natural polymers, synthetic polymers, ceramics, and even gene therapy. Of these, an absorbable collagen sponge reconstituted from bovine tendon, and a collagen-based matrix derived from extracted bovine bone, are the two most common delivery materials currently being used for rh-BMP-2 and rh-BMP-7 respectively.

Several randomized trials have demonstrated clinical efficacy in the treatment of tibial fractures and spinal fusions. The BMP-2 Evaluation in Surgery for Tibial Trauma trial demonstrated that patients with tibial fracture treated with surgery plus local delivery of rh-BMP-2 were less likely to require a second procedure to achieve healing (compared with patients treated with surgery alone) and healed within a shorter period of time. Rh-BMP-7 has also been shown to accomplish similar results in patients with open tibial shaft fractures. Rh-BMP-7 has also been investigated in the treatment of established tibial nonunions. Equivalent clinical efficacy to autologous bone grafting was established.

For posterior lumbar spinal fusion, two separate clinical trials have shown rh-BMP-2 to be as effective as autologous bone grafting, demonstrating potential for elimination of graft harvesting. Rh-BMP-7 has also been demonstrated to be capable of achieving similar fusion rates in lumbar spine fusion. One of the major concerns in this specific clinical setting is the potential for bone overgrowth, leading to spinal or foraminal stenosis. As such, BMPs are often delivered within a spinal fusion cage to facilitate proper containment. In at least one animal study, no evidence of abnormal mineralization of the spinal cord has been found after treatment of laminectomy defects with rh-BMP-2. Although there is much to be learned before the maximal clinical benefit of BMPs can be exploited, the discovery of these molecules offers an intriguing addition to the armamentarium of bone graft alternatives. The initial clinical trials evaluating BMP-2 and BMP-7 are promising and are likely to open the door for a new surgical approach in the treatment of skeletal defects.

Anti-Inflammatory Agents
Corticosteroids

Corticosteroids are naturally occurring 21-carbon steroid hormones produced by the adrenal glands. Technically they include glucocorticoids and mineralocorticoids, although the former is most often used synonymously with corticosteroids. Glucocorticoids and mineralocorticoids are distinguished from each other by their specific receptors, target cells, and effects. Glucocorticoids are mediators of metabolism and inflammation, whereas mineralocorticoids control electrolyte and water balance. Most corticosteroids act via a glucocorticoid pathway, although some also have mineralocorticoid activity reflecting a wide range of pharmacokinetics. The most important corticosteroid is cortisol (or the synthetic form, hydrocortisone).

Corticosteroids influence all types of inflammatory events regardless of the inciting event. The anti-inflammatory signaling mechanisms are quite complex and fairly well described. The glucocorticoid receptor is a member of the steroid hormone-receptor family of proteins found in the cytosol. Once bound, the corticosteroid-receptor complex moves to the nucleus where it binds DNA sequences in the promotor region of target genes called glucocorticoid-responsive elements. This binding subsequently recruits other proteins and transcription factors that modify the structure of the chromatin, which in turn alters the transcription machinery. The net effect can be either an increase in the transcription of target genes (transactivation) or a decrease in target gene transcription (transrepression). One such gene that is activated by the corticosteroids is *annexin I* (also called *lipocortin-1*). Annexin I is an anti-inflammatory protein that binds to cell membranes and physically interacts with phospholipase A_2, preventing it from coming into contact with arachidonic acid. By inhibiting arachidonic acid

Table 7   Commonly Used Injectable Steroids

Solubility	Generic Name	Trade Name	Equivalent Dose, mg*
Most soluble	Betamethasone sodium phosphate	Celestone (Schering-Plough, Kenilworth, NJ)	0.6
Soluble	Dexamethasone sodium phosphate	Decadron (Merck, Whitehouse Station, NJ)	0.75
	Prednisolone sodium phosphate	Hydeltrasol (Merck)	5
Slightly soluble	Prednisolone tebutate	Hydeltra-TBA (Merck)	5
	Triamcinolone diacetate	Aristospan Forte (Sandoz, Princeton, NJ)	4
	Methylprednisolone acetate	Depo-Medrol (Pfizer, New York, NY)	4
Relatively insoluble	Dexamethasone acetate	Decadron-LA (Merck)	0.75
	Hydrocortisone acetate	Hydrocortisone	20
	Prednisolone acetate	Prednalone	5
	Triamcinolone acetonide	Kenalog	4
	Triamcinolone hexacetonide	Aristospan (Sandoz)	4
Combination	Betamethasone sodium phosphate-betamethasone acetate	Celestone Soluspan (Schering-Plough)	0.6

* For example, 0.6 mg of betamethasone sodium phosphate is equivalent to 0.75 mg of dexamethasone sodium phosphate, which is equivalent to 5 mg of prednisolone.

from being metabolized by phospholipase A_2, the production of prostaglandins and other eicosanoids is blocked (**Figure 1**).

In orthopaedic practice, synthetic corticosteroids are most often used as anti-inflammatory drugs to treat conditions such as arthritis and tendinitis.

Several injectable corticosteroids of varying solubility and half-life are commercially available (**Table 7**). Corticosteroid injections can be administered in an intra-articular, intrabursal, and intratendon sheath fashion. There are no firm guidelines with regard to choice and dosage of steroids. Choice is largely determined by the clinician's previous experience or office inventory. In general, short- or intermediate-acting preparations (more water soluble) may be selected for acute conditions, whereas longer-acting preparations (water insoluble) are preferred for chronic conditions. A mixture of both short- and long-acting compounds is often administered regardless of the type of inflammatory process.

Dosage is commonly chosen based on the surface area that will receive the injection with a dose-equivalent amount of a specific steroid. For estimating dosage, a useful guide is as follows (using prednisolone tebutate suspension as a reference): for small joints of the hand and foot, 2.5 to 10 mg; for medium-sized joints such as the elbow and wrist, 10 to 25 mg; for the knee, ankle, and shoulder, 20 to 50 mg; and for the hip, 25 to 40 mg. The longer the time between dosing intervals, the better. A minimum of 4 weeks between intra-articular injections is usually recommended.

Adverse effects associated with injectable steroids include corticosteroid arthropathy, adrenal suppression, ligament and tendon ruptures, iatrogenic infection, and skin atrophy and hyperpigmentation.

Nonsteroidal Anti-Inflammatory Drugs

Under certain proinflammatory conditions, arachidonic acid, a metabolite of membrane lipids, can be metabolized to effector molecules capable of regulating pain and inflammation. These effector molecules, the prostanoids, are a family of mediators that coordinate cell-cell communication by interaction with specific cell membrane receptors belonging to the G-protein-coupled rhodopsin-type family. The prostanoids implicated in inflammation include prostaglandins and thromboxanes. The enzyme that initiates and controls the production of the prostanoids is cyclooxygenase or COX. Up until 1991, it was believed that there was only one COX enzyme. A second form of the enzyme was reported, confirming that COX comprises a pair of isoenzymes, COX-1 and COX-2. COX-1 is constitutively expressed in almost all tissues and is responsible for regulating normal or "housekeeping" physiologic functions, most notably cytoprotection of the gastrointestinal mucosa, regulation of renal hemodynamics, and maintenance of normal hemostasis by stimulating platelet aggregation. COX-2 is an inducible enzyme activated during inflammatory states (such as arthritis and malignancy) leading to the production of prostaglandins, which mediate inflammation, pain, and fever.

Nonsteroidal anti-inflammatory drugs (NSAIDs) control pain and inflammation by inhibiting cyclooxygenase (**Figure 1**). These drugs are heterogeneous in their chemical structure and fall into three basic categories—traditional NSAIDs, COX-2 inhibitors, and salicylates. All NSAIDs inhibit both COX-1 and COX-2 to varying degrees, although they tend to preferentially inhibit one form more than another. Currently available NSAIDs are listed in **Table 8**. NSAIDs are probably the most frequently prescribed medications, accounting for about 4.5% of all prescriptions written in the United States.

Table 8 Dosage Data of Currently Available NSAIDs

Generic Name	Proprietary Name	Largest Unit Dose	Half-Life (h)	Dosing Frequency*
Aspirin	***	325 mg	0.25	2 q4h
Diclofenac	Voltaren (Novartis Ophthalmics, Duluth, GA)	75 mg	2	bid
Diflunisal	Dolobid (Merck, Whitehouse Station, NJ)	500 mg	19	bid
Etodolac	Lodine (Wyeth-Ayerst, Philadelphia, PA)	300 mg	6	qid
Fenoprofen	Nalfon (Pedinol, Farmingdale, NY)	600 mg	2-3	qid
Flurbiprofen	Ansaid (Pfizer, New York, NY)	100 mg	6	tid
Ibuprofen	Motrin (McNeil, Fort Washington, PA)	800 mg	2	qid
Indomethacin	Indocin (Merck)	50 mg	4	tid
Ketoprofen	Orudis (Wyeth, Madison, NJ)	75 mg	3	tid
Ketorolac	Toradol (A.G. Scientific, San Diego, CA)	10 mg	5	qid
Meclofenamate	Meclomen (Mylan, Canonsburg, PA)	100 mg	2	tid
Nabumetone	Relafen (Glaxo Smith Kline, Philadelphia, PA)	500 mg	20-30	2 qd
Naproxen	Naprosyn (Roche, Basel, Switzerland)	500 mg	14	bid
Oxaprozin	Daypro (GD Searle, New York, NY)	600 mg	40-50	2 qd
Piroxicam	Feldene (CIPLA, Mumbai, India)	20 mg	30-86	qd
Salicylsalicylic acid	Disalcid (3M Pharmaceuticals, St. Paul, MN)	750 mg	1	qid
Sodium salicylate	***	650 mg	0.5	q4h
Sulindac	Clinoril (Merck)	200 mg	8-14	bid
Tolmetin	Tolectin (McNeil)	400 mg	1-2	tid

* Dosage required for treatment of inflammation. Abbreviations: bid = twice a day; qd = each day; q4h = every 4 hours; qid = four times a day; tid = three times a day

(Adapted from Berger RG: Nonsteroidal anti-inflammatory drugs: Making the right choices. J Am Acad Orthop Surg 1994; 2:255-260.)

The traditional NSAIDs such as ibuprofen are reversible competitive inhibitors of COX. They block the active site of the enzyme by blocking the channel (COX channel) that leads to the active site. The traditional NSAIDs vary in their duration of action and potency because of variations in their COX-1 to COX-2 specificity ratio. The evidence to support the efficacy of NSAIDs is overwhelming when compared against placebo in acute or chronic conditions. The major limitation of the traditional NSAIDs is the associated toxicities, namely gastrointestinal disturbance. Several trials using upper endoscopy as an assessment tool have demonstrated a gastroduodenal ulcer incidence ranging from 15% to 40% with the use of traditional NSAIDs. The pathophysiology of NSAID-associated side effects is more complex than just COX-1 inhibition. The central event in the initiation of gastrointestinal damage involves uncoupling mitochondrial oxidative phosphorylation in the absorbing enterocyte. The enterocyte becomes adenosine triphosphate-deficient, which in turn sets off a cascade of detrimental events that, when combined with the lack of protection induced by COX-1 inhibition, leads to focal ischemia, increased intestinal permeability, acid back-diffusion, and hence ulceration. Several meta-analyses have verified that patients taking traditional NSAIDs are more likely to experience hospitalization or death as a result of gastrointestinal ulceration and bleeding.

Because COX-2 is upregulated in arthritis and responsible for the accompanying symptoms, drugs that suppress its activity without interfering with the homeostatic functions of COX-1 are theoretically beneficial. This realization led to the development of the COX-2 inhibitors, or coxibs. Several randomized clinical trials have demonstrated that COX-2 inhibitors are more effective than placebo and as effective as the traditional NSAIDs in decreasing the symptoms of arthritis. Furthermore, the studies effectively confirmed that the incidence of gastrointestinal adverse effects were similar to those associated with placebo and lower than with the use of traditional NSAIDs.

Until recently, three drugs that specifically inhibited COX-2 had FDA approval: valdecoxib, celecoxib, and rofecoxib. In 2004, data from controlled clinical trials revealed that the COX-2 selective agents might be associated with an increased risk of serious cardiovascular events (heart attack and stroke) secondary to increased thrombosis, especially when they are used for long periods of time or in very high risk settings (immediately after heart surgery). These findings led to the withdrawal of rofecoxib from the United States market and issuance of "black box" warnings for the other COX-2 inhibitors as well as several traditional NSAIDs. The investigation is ongoing and the interpretation and implications of the COX-2 data have yet to be fully understood.

Arthritis Medications

Cartilage is composed largely of extracellular matrix and chondrocytes. The extracellular matrix primarily consists of water, proteoglycans, collagens, and other proteins. The proteoglycans are complex macromolecules that consist of glycosaminoglycans attached to a central protein core. Most proteoglycans are of the large, aggregating type called aggrecan. At the N-terminal end of the protein core, there is a specific binding domain for hyaluronan, a stabilizing polysaccharide capable of binding many aggrecan molecules forming the so-called proteoglycan aggregates. The proteoglycans provide a framework for collagen and have a high affinity for water, which largely gives cartilage its biomechanical properties and helps in the formation of a viscous, elastic layer that lubricates and protects cartilage. The functional integrity of articular cartilage is maintained by a metabolic balance between extracellular matrix degradation and biosynthesis in the chondrocyte. Osteoarthritis results when the scale is tipped in the direction of extracellular matrix destruction, resulting in a relative decrease of proteoglycans and hence a decrease in water affinity, which has a negative impact on the biomechanical properties. Theoretically, if the proteoglycans could be replaced, perhaps the imbalance would be corrected and the properties of cartilage preserved. Such thinking led to the development of structure-modifying drugs capable of directly interfering with the disease process. These new chondroprotective supplements have generated great interest and equally great controversy.

Glucosamine and Chondroitin Sulfate

The most common glycosaminoglycans that comprise proteoglycans in cartilage are keratan sulfate, dermatan sulfate, and chondroitin sulfate; chondroitin sulfate is the most prevalent. Hyaluronate is also a common glycosaminoglycan but is not bound to a protein core and technically not part of the proteoglycan family.

Glucosamine (2-amino-2-deoxy-α-D-glucose) is a popular nutritional supplement for osteoarthritis that displays excellent bioavailability. It can be derived from the naturally occurring polymer chitin or produced by synthetic means. It is available alone or in preparations with vitamins and minerals or in combination with chondroitin sulfate. In vitro experiments demonstrate that the administration of glucosamine to cultured human chondrocytes promotes proteoglycan and glycosaminoglycan production. Glucosamine is believed to serve as a substrate for chondroitin sulfate and hyaluronate biosynthesis. In a meta-analysis of 1,020 patients receiving a minimum of 1,500 mg glucosamine daily, there was objective slowing of the degenerative process of articular cartilage as measured by radiographic joint space narrowing and Western Ontario McMaster University Osteoarthritis Index scores. Adverse drug reactions were infrequent.

Chondroitin sulfate is the major component of aggrecan. In vitro experiments have demonstrated that when it is added to cultured human chondrocytes, proteoglycan production increases and the collagenolytic activity is inhibited. The metabolic uptake of oral chondroitin sulfate is unclear. Several bioavailability studies have failed to demonstrate significant serum concentrations of the substance following oral ingestion. Some authors have suggested that the clinical findings after chondroitin sulfate treatment are related to the stabilization properties of the sulfur. In a meta-analysis of 775 patients, chondroitin sulfate demonstrated significant efficacy as measured by the Lequesne Index, visual analog scale pain, and mobility. Adverse drug reactions were infrequent. Most clinical studies have supported the effectiveness of glucosamine and chondroitin sulfate in relieving the symptoms associated with osteoarthritis. However, numerous concerns remain regarding the long-term efficacy and the optimal dosage and delivery route. The mechanism of action remains controversial.

Hyaluronic Acid Injection

Hyaluronic acid is a polysaccharide consisting of repeating disaccharide units of N-acetylglucosamine and glucuronic acid. It is synthesized and secreted into the joint space by type B synovial cells. A nonarthritic human knee contains approximately 2.5 to 4.0 mg/mL of high molecular weight (5×10^6 d) hyaluronic acid whereas an osteoarthritic knee contains less that half of the normal concentration. In addition, the molecular size of hyaluronic acid is reduced in arthritic joints, thereby decreasing its viscous and elastic properties.

Injectable intra-articular hyaluronic acid, termed viscosupplementation, theoretically supplements the reduced concentrations of hyaluronic acid, thereby improving the viscoelasticity properties of the cartilage. Currently, two preparations are FDA approved for the treatment of symptomatic osteoarthritis: Hyalgan (Sanofi-aventis, Bridgewater, NJ) and Synvisc (Genzyme, Cambridge, MA). Several mechanisms of action have been proposed for its effectiveness. Anti-inflammatory action has been observed in vitro and in vivo as evidenced by modification of leukocyte activity and the reduction of inflammatory mediators such as prostaglandins and cyclic adenosine monophosphate in the synovial fluid. In addition, direct analgesic effects by modulating pain perception have been suggested, which are believed to be accomplished by inhibition of nociceptor or binding of substance P (a pain signal peptide). Disease-modifying chondroprotective effects and physical alterations of the viscoelastic properties of the synovial fluid are believed to play a role in the efficacy of hyaluronate but are not well proven.

Hyaluronic acid is typically given as a series of three and five weekly injections. Aspiration of an effusion before injection is recommended if it is present. Several randomized trials comparing hyaluronic acid versus placebo have demonstrated a significant reduction in pain in the hyaluronic acid group over periods of 60 days to 1 year. Most of these trials excluded patients with severe osteoarthritis. Fewer trials have examined actual structural modification. One randomized controlled trial used arthroscopic changes at 1 year compared with baseline and found less deterioration in the hyaluronic acid group in comparison with those receiving a placebo. There is good evidence to support the use of hyaluronic acid for knee arthritis to improve pain and function. There is scant evidence to support the role of hyaluronic acid in disease modification.

Summary

This chapter highlights the pertinent basic science and translation principles behind the most commonly used drugs prescribed in orthopaedic practice. Because so many orthopaedic conditions are amenable to pharmacologic intervention, it will remain a constant challenge during the orthopaedist's professional career to balance the benefits of pharmacologic treatment with potential adverse affects including those that have yet to fully emerge. Because of the rapid nature at which new drugs become available, in-depth critical reviews of up-to-date literature are encouraged to ensure maximum patient safety.

Selected Bibliography

Antibiotics
Hanssen AD, Osmon DR: The use of prophylactic antimicrobial agents during and after hip arthroplasty. *Clin Orthop Relat Res* 1999;369:124-138.

Heitmann C, Patzakis M, Tetsworth K, Levin L: Musculoskeletal sepsis: Principles of treatment. *Instr Course Lect* 2003;52:733-743.

Perry CR: *Bone and Joint Infections*. St. Louis, MO, Mosby, 1996.

Anticoagulation
Della Valle C, Steiger D, Di Cesare P: Thromboembolism after hip and knee arthroplasty: Diagnosis and treatment. *J Am Acad Orthop Surg* 1998;6:327-336.

Geerts W, Pineo G, Heit J, et al: Prevention of venous thromboembolism: The Seventh ACCP Conference on Antithrombotic and Thrombolytic Therapy. *Chest* 2004;126:338S-400S.

Regulators of Bone Metabolism
Bamais A, Kastriris E, Bamia C, et al: Osteonecrosis of the jaw in cancer after treatment with bisphosphonates: Incidence and risk factors. *J Clin Oncol* 2005;23:8580-8587.

Lane N, Morris S: New perspectives on parathyroid hormone therapy. *Curr Opin Rheumatol* 2005;17:467-474.

Morris C, Einhorn T: Bisphosphonates in orthopaedic surgery. *J Bone Joint Surg Am* 2005;87:1609-1618.

Rodan G, Martin T: Therapeutic approaches to bone diseases. *Science* 2000;289:1508-1514.

Enhancers of Bone Repair
Hannouche D, Petite H, Sedel L: Current trends in the enhancement of fracture healing. *J Bone Joint Surg Br* 2001;83:157-164.

Lieberman J, Daluiski A, Einhorn T: The role of growth factors in the repair of bone: Biology and clinical applications. *J Bone Joint Surg Am* 2002;84:1032-1044.

Termaat M, Den Boer F, Bakker F, Patka P, Haarman H: Bone morphogenetic proteins: Development and clinical efficacy in the treatment of fractures and bone defects. *J Bone Joint Surg Am* 2005;87:1367-1378.

Anti-Inflammatory Agents
Capone M, Tacconeeli S, Sciulli M, Patrignani P: Clinical pharmacology of selective COX-2 inhibitors. *Int J Immunopathol Pharmacol* 2003;16:49-58.

Cole B, Schumacher H: Injectable corticosteroids in modern practice. *J Am Acad Orthop Surg* 2005;13:37-46.

Ekman EF Koman LA: Acute pain following musculoskeletal injuries and orthopaedic surgery: Mechanisms and management. *Instr Course Lect* 2005;54:21-33.

Arthritis Medications
Brief A, Maurer S, DiCesare P: Use of glucosamine and chondroitin sulfate in the management of osteoarthritis. *J Am Acad Orthop Surg* 2001;9:71-78.

Jordan KM, Arden NK, Doherty M, et al: EULAR recommendations 2003: An evidenced based approach to the management of knee osteoarthritis: Report of a Task Force of the Standing Committee for International Clinical Studies Including Therapeutic Trials (ESCISIT). *Ann Rheum Dis* 2003;62:1145-1155.

Richy F, Bruyere O, Ethgen O, Cucherat M, Henrotin Y, Reginster J: Structural and symptomatic efficacy of glucosamine and chondroitin in knee osteoarhtritis: A comprehensive meta-analysis. *Arch Intern Med* 2003;163:1514-1522.

Chapter 18

Bone Injury, Regeneration, and Repair

Theodore Miclau III, MD
Kevin J. Bozic, MD, MBA
Bobby Tay, MD
Hubert T. Kim, MD, PhD
Celine Colnot, PhD
Christian M. Puttlitz, PhD
Jean C. Gan, PhD
Barbara D. Boyan, PhD
B. Frank Eames, PhD
Jill A. Helms, DDS, PhD

Introduction

Bone formation begins during fetal development and continues throughout life in the form of regeneration or repair. Bone is a remarkable tissue that possesses an astounding regenerative potential and adaptive capacity. Unlike other tissues that heal through the development of scar tissue, bone heals by forming new bone that is indistinguishable from the adjacent, uninjured tissue. As bone is a structural organ, the processes of bone development, repair, and remodeling are intricately related to the mechanical environment.

Bone injury can result from multiple causes and conditions, including traumatic, infectious, oncologic, and metabolic insults. These injuries damage cell viability and integrity, and initiate a regenerative process to restore the overall structure of the tissue. Bone development and repair share common pathways, possibly accounting for similarities between the processes. The purpose of this chapter is to review the underlying biologic and mechanical processes of bone regeneration and repair in response to injury.

Osteonecrosis

Osteonecrosis (ON) has been defined as the in situ death of cells within bone as a result of vascular compromise. These cell populations include osteocytes and hematopoietic and fatty marrow precursor cells. The organic and inorganic matrices, containing collagen, proteoglycans, noncollagenous proteins, and minerals, generally are not affected by ON unless secondary effects occur. The term osteonecrosis is preferred to "avascular necrosis" or "aseptic necrosis" because it does not imply a specific etiology.

Etiology

ON can be broadly categorized as traumatic or nontraumatic. Although it is generally accepted that traumatic ON is caused by a traumatic event that leads to transient or permanent ischemia to the bone, the etiology of nontraumatic ON is less well understood. However, regardless of the classification, the final common pathway leading to cellular death in ON is vascular compromise of the bone. Possible mechanisms of vascular compromise include: (1) mechanical disruption of the vessels, (2) arterial vessel occlusion, (3) injury to or pressure on the arterial wall, and (4) venous outflow occlusion. Mechanical disruption of the vessels can occur with both traumatic (fracture or dislocation) and nontraumatic (stress or fatigue fracture) ON. Arterial occlusion can occur from embolic or thrombotic phenomena, nitrogen bubbles, or cells with abnormal morphology (such as sickle cells). Injury to or pressure on the vessel wall can result from either extramural sources (such as blood, fat, or marrow contents) or sources internal to the vessel or the vessel wall, such as in vasculitis, angiospasm, or radiation injury. Finally, venous occlusion can occur with any condition that causes venous pressure to rise above arterial pressure.

Jones has suggested that a combination of three factors result in microcirculatory thrombus leading to ON:

Traumatic
Femoral neck fracture
Hip dislocation
Slipped capital femoral epiphysis
Humeral head fracture

Nontraumatic
Cortico-steroid use
Excessive alcohol consumption
Cigarette smoking
Dysbaric phenomenon (for example, Caisson's disease)
Systemic lupus erythematosus
Sickle cell disease/hemoglobinopathies
Familial thrombophilia
Gaucher's disease
Organ transplantation
Inflammatory bowel disease
Pregnancy

(Data from Vail TP, Covington DB: The incidence of osteonecrosis, in Urbaniak JR, Jones JP Jr (eds): Osteonecrosis: Etiology, Diagnosis, and Treatment. Rosemont, IL, American Academy of Orthopaedic Surgeons, 1997, pp 43-49.

stasis, hypercoagulability, and endothelial damage. The microvascular anatomy of susceptible bones (such as the femoral head, talus, and carpal bones) facilitates vascular stasis, including terminal arterioles with few collateral vessels and long, narrow arcades of end capillaries. A hypercoagulable state can be caused by increased procoagulants and activated coagulants, decreased natural anticoagulants (especially proteins C and S), vasoconstriction of the subchondral arteriolar bed, or decreased endogenous fibrinolysis. Endothelial damage results in exposure of procoagulant subendothelial collagen, leading to platelet aggregation and fibrin thrombosis. Exposure of circulating blood to tissue factors in the endothelial walls results in activation of both the intrinsic and the extrinsic clotting pathways, ultimately leading to subchondral thrombosis, and end-organ (in this case, subchondral bone) ischemia.

Fat embolism has been widely reported to be associated with ON. Although the mechanism is not completely understood, in vitro and in vivo studies suggest that platelet aggregation occurs over the surface of intravascular fat globules, which then leads to the formation of fibrin thrombi. Fat emboli are associated with a fatty liver, destabilization and coalescence of plasma lipoproteins, and/or disruption of fatty bone marrow or other adipose tissue depots.

Intraosseous hypertension, another etiologic factor associated with ON, can occur as a result of excessive medullary venous stasis. However, controversy exists over whether intraosseous hypertension and impaired marrow

perfusion are a cause or an effect of ON. Some investigators believe this phenomenon may occur secondary to generalized thrombosis of the marrow vasculature.

Histopathologic Changes
Regardless of the etiology, there are characteristic histopathologic changes that occur with ON. Animal studies have shown that histologic changes begin 10 to 14 days following the precipitating event. Early changes consist of necrosis of the marrow contents, including hematopoietic cells, capillary endothelial cells, and lipocytes. Osteocyte cell death leads to characteristic empty lacunae. Necrosis of the marrow contents is associated with increased water content, which is distinctly different from normal fatty marrow, which contains little water. These changes can be seen on MRI as increased signal on T2-weighted images, and decreased signal on T1-weighted images.

Following necrosis of the bone, bone remodeling occurs. These changes mimic those that occur with fracture healing and/or bone graft incorporation. The first step in the reparative process is a reactive hyperemia and ingress of a vascularized fibrous tissue. The process of "creeping substitution" then begins with revascularization of necrotic bone from the adjacent fibrous tissue. Vessels carrying primitive mesenchymal cells, which differentiate into osteoblasts and osteoclasts, grow into the medullary canal and the haversian canals to revascularize the cancellous and cortical bone, respectively. In cancellous bone, osteoid is then laid down on the scaffolding of the necrotic trabeculae. In necrotic cortical bone, primitive mesenchymal cells differentiate into osteoclasts or "cutting cones" that aid in resorption of necrotic haversian bone. Once most of the haversian bone has been resorbed, osteoblasts begin the process of replacing haversian systems.

Associated Risk Factors
Although vascular compromise is the final common pathway leading to bone death in ON, other etiologic risk factors often trigger this event (**Table 1**). Bacterial endotoxins have been reported to cause a so-called Shwartzman reaction, with disseminated intravascular coagulation, hyperlipemia, systemic fat embolism, and fibrin thrombosis. The hypercoagulable state that results from the Schwartzman reaction can lead to ON. The Shwartzman phenomenon has also been reported to be associated with solid organ transplantation, as part of the hyperacute rejection syndrome.

Deep sea divers who experience dysbaric phenomena have demonstrated an abnormally high incidence of ON. The mechanism could be multifactorial, and likely involves both direct effects of nitrogen bubbles on the osseous vasculature, and secondary injury to the marrow adipose tissue by rapidly expanding nitrogen gas that triggers focal and systemic intravascular coagulation.

Table 2 Ficat and Arlet Radiographic Classification of Osteonecrosis of the Femoral Head			
Stage	Radiograph	Bone Scan	MRI
0* (Preclinical)	Normal	Normal	Normal
I (Preradiographic)	Normal	Nondiagnostic	Early changes
II	Osteopenia/sclerosis; head spherical	Positive	Positive
III	Flattened head/crescent sign	Positive	Positive
IV	Secondary degenerative changes	Positive	Positive

*The original Ficat and Arlet classification did not include stage 0. Stage 1 was preradiographic and known as the 'silent hip'.

(Modified with permission from http://www.orthoteers.co.uk/Nrujp~ij33lm/Orthboneon.htm.)

ON frequently occurs seen in patients with hemoglobinopathies, such as sickle cell disease and thalassemia. Patients with the hemoglobin SS genotype and α-thalassemia and those with frequent painful crises are at highest risk for developing ON. ON may occur in these patients as a result of abnormally-shaped cells that can lead to local vascular stasis as well as endothelial damage.

The effect of exogenous glucocorticoids on bone metabolism has been studied extensively both in vivo and in vitro. Despite many theories that have been proposed as a result of these studies, the precise mechanism of steroid-induced ON remains elusive. Some authors have suggested that steroid use can cause ON through effects on the marrow blood supply, such as intraosseous hypertension, intravascular fat emboli and coagulation, or compression of vessels by progressive accumulation of marrow fat stores. Others have suggested that steroid-induced osteonecrosis occurs as a result of direct cytotoxic effects on cells. Still other investigators have reported that increased fat cell size and volume, which are side effects of steroid use, might be the mechanism of osteonecrosis.

Excessive alcohol use has also been associated with the development of ON. Proposed mechanisms include fat emboli, cortisol release, and altered lipid metabolism. Animal models have also been used to demonstrate that alcohol can directly induce adipogenesis, decrease osteogenesis in bone marrow stroma, and produce intracellular lipid deposits resulting in the death of osteocytes that could lead to ON.

Clinical Sequelae

ON is an important cause of morbidity of the skeleton that can have devastating clinical implications because of its propensity to affect young people. ON can occur in any bone that relies on intraosseous circulation for its blood supply. However, the most common sites of ON in adults are the hip, shoulder, talus, hand/wrist, and knee. The magnitude of clinical symptoms and extent of disability caused by ON is related to the size and the location of the lesion.

ON of the hip can lead to secondary osteoarthritis, and is responsible for up to 18% of total hip arthroplas-

ties performed in the United States and Western Europe. The most commonly used staging system for ON of the femoral head is that of Ficat and Arlet (Table 2). This staging system is based primarily on plain radiographic changes that occur as a result of bone necrosis, reparative change, collapse of the femoral head, and degeneration.

Radiographic Findings

The histologic changes that occur during bone necrosis and bone remodeling are associated with characteristic findings on MRI and plain radiographs. When necrosis of the marrow contents occurs, the normal fatty marrow is replaced with water, which is detectable as decreased signal on T1-weighted MRI images (Figure 1, A). These changes can occur before the onset of symptoms. Early in the bone remodeling process, the subchondral cyst formation seen on plain radiographs represents the increased size of the individual trabeculae. Over time, sclerotic changes are seen as a result of thickening of the trabeculae and calcification of the necrotic marrow. The characteristic crescent sign and subchondral collapse that is seen in later stages of ON of the femoral head is a result of necrosis of the subchondral bone, ultimately leading to collapse of a portion of the femoral head (Figure 1, B). Finally, changes on the acetabular side begin to appear later as a result of incongruency of the flattened femoral head articulating with the acetabulum (Figure 1, C).

Biology of Fracture Healing

Fracture healing involves a unique, highly integrated sequence of events where bone is restored to its preinjured condition. This capacity for bone to regenerate into tissue identical to the preinjured bone may be secondary to similarities in the programs between skeletal formation and regeneration; the events that transpire during the maturation of a fracture callus into bone closely resemble those that occur during development and in the growth plate. Fracture repair is clearly related to external factors, including the mechanical environment at the fracture site. Motion at the fracture site results in healing primarily through cartilage formation (endochondral ossification), and stability favors the direct formation of bone (in-

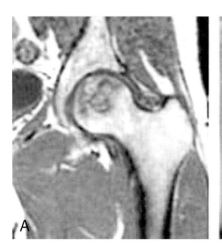 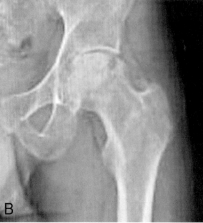 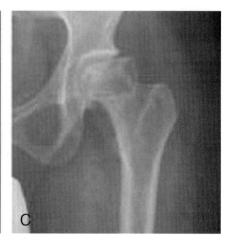

Figure 1   Characteristic findings of bone necrosis on MRI and plain radiographs. **A,** T1-weighted MRI demonstrating the replacement of normal fatty marrow with water, which appears as decreased signal on the T1 image. **B,** AP radiograph of the hip demonstrating collapse of the subchondral bone in the femoral head (Ficat III). **C,** AP radiograph of the hip demonstrating arthrosis secondary to joint incongruity related to ON and collapse of the femoral head (Ficat IV). *(Reproduced with permission from http:// www.orthoteers.co.uk/Nrujp~ij33lm/Orthboneon.htm)*

tramembranous ossification) (**Figures 2 and 3**). Most fractures heal through a combination of intramembranous and endochondral ossification.

After a fracture occurs, the architecture and vascular supply of the preinjured bone are disrupted. This results in a loss of mechanical stability, a decrease in the local oxygen and nutrients, and a release of various factors into the site of injury. An inflammatory response (inflammatory stage of repair) is initiated, and macrophages and degranulating platelets infiltrate the fracture site, releasing cytokines that include platelet-derived growth factor (PDGF), transforming growth factor-β (TGF-β), interleukins-1 and -6, and prostaglandin E_2 (PGE2). These factors likely play a key role in the initiation of the repair process by acting on a variety of cells in the bone marrow, periosteum, and cell populations in the fracture hematoma.

Early postfracture, periosteal preosteoblasts and local osteoblasts, characterized by the expression of the osteocalcin gene, differentiate into new bone. There is an increase in mesenchymal cell proliferation, a phenomenon that is associated with factors such as acidic fibroblast growth factor (aFGF, or FGF-1) and basic fibroblast growth factor (bFGF, or FGF-2). These factors have angiogenic effects on endothelial cells, as well as mitogenic effects on fibroblasts, chondrocytes, and osteoblasts. Coincident with the formation of early new bone, mesenchymal cells and fibroblasts proliferate and eventually replace the fracture hematoma. Primitive mesenchymal and osteoprogenitor cells also express several of the bone morphogenetic proteins (BMPs), members of the subfamily of the TGF-β superfamily of polypeptides that play key roles in cell growth, differentiation, and apoptosis (programmed cell death). Stem cells likely originate from a variety of sources, including the bone marrow, the periosteum, the

local muscle and soft tissues, and the vasculature.

As the fracture hematoma matures, the network of new blood vessels into the healing fracture callus grows. New blood vessels likely provide a source of progenitor cells and growth factors that influence the differentiation of mesenchymal cells. The fracture hematoma develops a collagenous matrix, composed of various collagen isotypes, which may be important for presenting cytokines such as TGF-β, PDGF, bFGF, and BMPs to receptive cells. Collagens type I and type II, the major collagens, contribute to the integrity of the noncartilaginous and cartilaginous extracellular matrix (ECM), respectively. Mesenchymal cells form aggregates, expressing factors such as *sox9* that upregulate the expression of cartilage specific genes, such as *col2*. These cells differentiate into chondrocytes (soft callus phase of repair), which stabilize the fracture through the formation of a cartilaginous callus. Shortly after the induction of *col2*, the chondrocytes proliferate and differentiate, expressing other genes, such as indian hedgehog (*Ihh*), which influences these activities. As chondrocytes mature and progress to hypertrophy, the cells begin to express collagen type X and release proteases that degrade the ECM. Hypertrophic chondrocytes also express factors such as runx2, a transcription factor that affects cell differentiation by regulating ECM proteins, such as osteocalcin and osteopontin, that are essential for ossification.

The conversion of the hypertrophic cartilage to bone is a complex, spatially organized phenomenon involving the coordination of terminal chondrocyte differentiation, apoptosis, ECM degradation, angiogenesis, and osteogenesis. As hypertrophic chondrocytes terminally differentiate, cartilage calcifies at the junction of the maturing cartilage and newly formed woven bone (hard callus stage of fracture repair). Once hypertrophic chondrocytes reach terminal differentiation, the cells undergo apoptosis, the

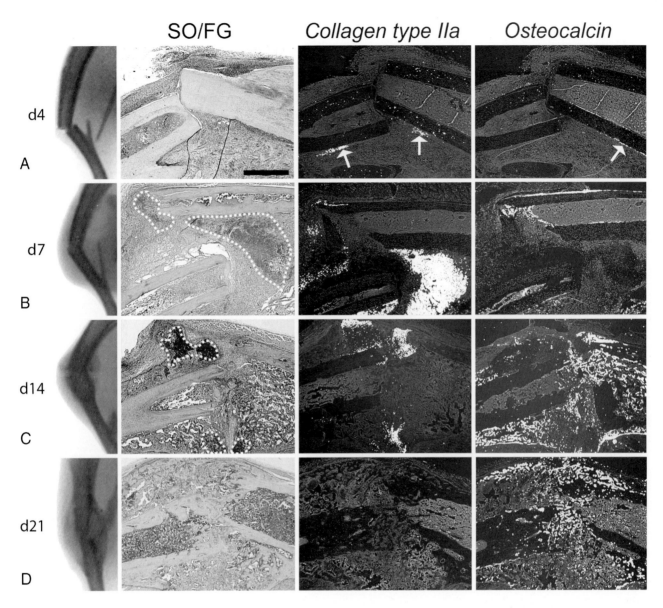

Figure 2   Nonstabilized fractures heal through endochondral ossification. **A,** Radiographs taken on day 4 show misaligned bone segments caused by the lack of stabilization following fracture. Safranin O-fast green (SO/FG) staining does not indicate the formation of cartilage or bone; however, collagen type IIa (*col2a*) expression indicates that some cells are differentiating along a chondrogenic lineage (arrows). *Osteocalcin* expression reveals a small amount of new bone forming along the periosteum (arrow). **B,** By day 7, radiographs show an enlarged callus at the fracture site. SO/FG staining shows abundant cartilage (outlined areas) at the site of the fracture, and a small amount of new bone forming along the periosteum. These histologic observations are confirmed by the widespread, strong expression of *col2a* (bright signal) throughout the callus, and the limited expression of *osteocalcin* (bright signal) along the periosteum. **C,** By day 14, radiographs indicate the presence of a radiopaque tissue, which has formed at the fracture site. SO/FG staining indicates that this radiopaque tissue is predominantly bone replacing the cartilage callus (outlined areas). *Col2a* (bright signal) transcripts continue to be detected in the fracture callus, although at much lower levels than observed at day 7. *Osteocalcin* (bright signal) is expressed throughout the callus tissues, bridging the bone segments. **D,** By day 21, radiographs indicate the bone ends are aligned to a greater extent, suggesting that the callus is undergoing remodeling. SO/FG staining indicates that most cartilage has been replaced by bone during this phase of healing. The lack of *col2a* expression indicates the absence of chondrocytes. *Osteocalcin* (bright signal) is expressed throughout the callus, albeit at lower levels than observed at day 14. Scale bar = 1 mm. (*Reproduced with permission from Thompson Z, Miclau T, Hu D, Helms JA: A model for intramembranous ossification during fracture healing.* J Orthop Res *2002;20:1091-1098.*)

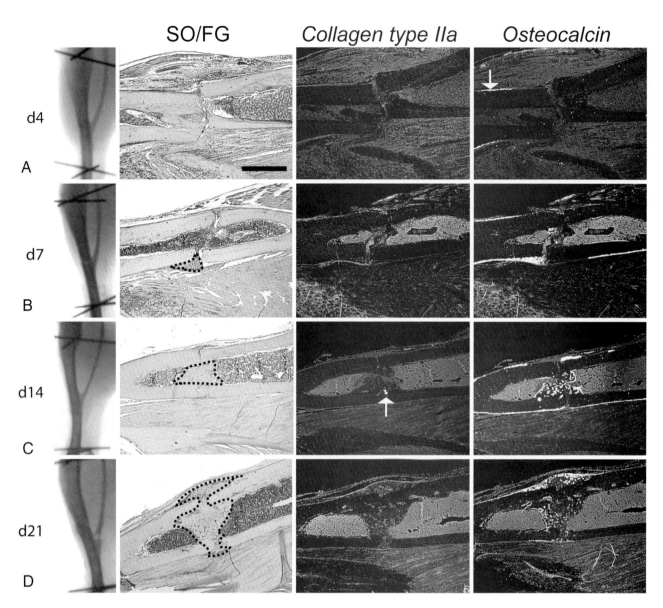

Figure 3   Stabilized fractures heal through intramembranous ossification. **A,** Radiographs taken 4 days after murine tibial fracture reveal no evidence of callus formation. Safranin O-fast green (SO/FG) staining confirms the lack of cartilage in the callus tissues. Collagen type IIa (*Col2a*) transcripts are undetectable in the fracture site. In an adjacent section, *osteocalcin* transcripts (bright signal) are detected in the periosteum (arrow). **B,** Seven days after fracture, radiographs fail to reveal a callus at the site of fracture. SO/FG staining of the callus tissues shows no evidence of cartilage, and some new bone (outlined area) at the fracture site. The lack of *col2a* expression confirms the absence of cartilage from the stabilized fracture callus, and *osteocalcin* expression (bright signal) shows that new bone has been generated in the form of a periosteal wedge. **C,** At day 14, radiographs indicate a small bone callus at the fracture site. SO/FG staining reveals new bone forming in the medullary canal (outlined area), and a lack of cartilage. There is an extremely small region of *col2a* expression (arrow) detectable on the posterior aspect of some fracture calluses. The lack of pro-teoglycan staining in SO/FG staining indicates that these cells have not progressed to differentiated cartilage. *Osteocalcin* expression (bright signal) shows evidence of new bone that is bridging the fracture gap, as well as new bone in the medullary canal. **D,** By day 21, radiographs indicate that the fracture is almost healed. SO/FG staining confirms these radiographic data, as new bone (outlined area) bridges both anterior and posterior cortices. *Col2a* is not expressed at the fracture site, whereas *osteocalcin* transcripts (bright signal) indicate new bone on the anterior and posterior aspects of the fracture callus. Scale bar = 1 mm. *(Reproduced with permission from Thompson Z, Miclau T, Hu D, Helms JA: A model for intramembranous ossification during fracture healing.* J Orthop Res *2002; 20:1091-1098.)*

Table 3 Molecules Involved in Bone Formation	Chondrogenic	Osteogenic	Angiogenic
Secreted proteins and their receptors			
Bone morphogenetic proteins (BMPs)	+	+	+
Transforming growth factor-β (TGF-β)	+	+	+
Growth differentiation factors (GDFs)	+	+	+
Platelet derived growth factor (PDGF)	+	+	+
Fibroblast growth factors (FGFs)	+	+	+
Insulin growth factor (IGF)	+	+	+
Vascular endothelial growth factor (VEGF)	anti/-	+	+
Growth hormone (GH)	+	+	+
Parathyroid hormone (PTH)	+	+	+
PG (prostaglandin)	+	+	+
Hedgehog (hh)	+	+	+
Wnt	+	?	?
Transcription factors			
Runx2	-	+	+
Sox	+	anti	possibly
Hox	+	anti/-	+
Osterix (osx)	?	+	?

(+) - molecules having a positive effect on chondrogenesis, osteogenesis and/or angiogenesis; (-) - molecules having no positive effect; (anti) molecules having a negative effect; (?) - molecules having an unknown effect.

ECM degrades, and new blood vessels invade the interface. The events of hypertrophic chondrocyte apoptosis and vascular invasion appear to be tightly coupled.

As hypertrophic cartilage continues to be replaced by bone, a variety of osteoblast- (BMPs, TGF-β, insulin growth factors (IGFs), and osteocalcin) and collagen-related genes (including types I, V, and XI) continue to be expressed widely in the callus. The newly formed woven bone eventually remodels through organized osteoblast and osteoclast activity (remodeling stage of repair). Ultimately, the mature bone is indistinguishable from the surrounding bone and contains a host of growth factors, including TGF-β, BMPs, and IGFs.

Biologic Requirement for Skeletal Tissue Repair

From a biologic perspective, there are clear requirements for skeletal tissue formation, whether it occurs during development or adult fracture repair: (1) skeletal progenitor cells are present at the right time and in the correct place to receive molecular signals and mechanical stimuli that will induce their differentiation into cartilage or bone; (2) an appropriate ECM is available to serve not only as a scaffold upon which skeletal progenitor cells can adhere, but also as a repository for growth factors and cytokines that play important and sometimes critical roles in stem cell differentiation; (3) a cadre of molecules and their downstream effectors are present at the site of skeletogen-

esis (**Table 3**); and (4) an intact vasculature is present to deliver oxygen and other essential nutrients (growth factors, hormones, cytokines), as well as progenitor cells, to the site where skeletal development will ensue.

Skeletal Progenitor Cells

Most knowledge of bone repair comes from analyses of long bone fractures. During adult bone fracture healing, mesenchymal cells from the surrounding tissues invade the wound site, where they proliferate, condense, and differentiate into cartilage or bone. Some evidence suggests that, in response to growth factors and cytokines produced by the neighboring tissues, pluripotent mesenchymal stem cells are recruited from the surrounding soft tissues and hematopoietic system. Despite considerable interest, the origins of these stem cells still remain uncertain. Although stromal cells isolated from bone marrow can participate in skeletal tissue regeneration, it is unclear the extent to which they contribute to the various phases of normal repair, or even if they contribute equally to the repair of different skeletal elements. The periosteum is another rich source of stem cells, which participate in reparative events.

The Extracellular Matrix

The major role of ECM molecules is to maintain structural integrity and define the physical properties of cartilage and bone tissues. However, it is becoming clear that the role of the ECM is more than structural. The ECM is a dynamic structure. Throughout the process of bone regeneration, changes in its composition influence the recruitment and differentiation of skeletal progenitor cells.

Collagens are the major structural molecules of the ECM of cartilage and bone. Collagen types II, IX, XI, and X are the main components of the cartilage matrix, whereas collagen types I and VI are found in the bone matrix. Proteoglycans are other important components of the pericellular and extracellular matrices. Aggrecan, perlecan, and syndecans are found in cartilage, and syndecans are also found in bone. Proteoglycans have the ability to bind and store growth factors, such as FGFs, which allows these molecules to be protected from proteolysis and possibly modulate the bioavailability of signaling molecules. The hedgehog and *wnt* signaling pathways, implicated in skeletal tissue formation, are known to be affected by proteoglycan glycosylation. Another group of ECM molecules from cartilage and bone are glycoproteins such as fibronectin, laminin, tenascin-C, thrombospondins, osteocalcin, osteopontin, and osteonectin. Many of these glycoproteins can bind to other ECM components and to the cell surface via specific receptors. For example, fibronectin may regulate chondrocyte and osteoblast differentiation through integrin signaling. Integrins are cell surface receptor-like molecules that are connected to the intracellular actin cytoskeleton and activate intracellular signaling pathways.

The ECM is constantly remodeled during bone repair. Endochondral ossification represents the most dramatic example of tissue remodeling, where one tissue (cartilage) is completely replaced by another (bone). Because of their ability to cleave most components of the ECMs of cartilage and bone, it is not surprising that matrix-degrading enzymes such as matrix metalloproteinases (MMPs) play a major role in bone formation. The main groups of MMPs are the collagenases, gelatinases, and stomelysins, which respectively cleave preferentially native collagens, denatured collagens, and noncollagenous substrates. Other matrix-degrading enzymes involved in bone formation are members of the ADAM (A Desintegrin and Metalloprotease domain) family, which cleave various substrates including aminoprocollagen and proteoglycans, and the cathepsin families, which are predominantly found in lysosomes but may also participate in ECM remodeling by cleaving collagen fragments.

During skeletal repair, MMPs may act on cell migration, proliferation, death, and morphogenesis. By degrading the ECM, MMPs may also modulate the activities of other molecules, such as releasing sequestered signaling factors, and regulate indirectly matrix mineralization. For example, mutant mice lacking *MMP9* develop nonunions and delayed unions of their fractures because of persistent cartilage at the injury site.

Molecules Involved in Chondrogenesis and Osteogenesis

The molecular programs regulating chondrogenesis and osteogenesis during skeletal development and repair appear to be highly conserved. Two bodies of knowledge regarding the molecular regulation of skeletogenesis are beginning to merge. Transcription factors that dictate cell fate decisions are being associated with signaling pathways that encourage skeletal cell differentiation.

The key transcription factors that mediate commitment to a chondrogenic phenotype are members of the Sox family of transcription factors, a fact appreciated following the identification of *sox9* mutations in the human skeletal syndrome camptomelic dysplasia. Cells participating in cartilage formation express *sox5, 6*, and *9*, and Sox proteins directly regulate the expression of several collagen genes including *collagen type II, IX, and XI*. *Runx2*, a transcription factor directing osteoblast differentiation (see below), also plays an essential role in chondrocyte maturation. In *runx2$^{-/-}$* mice, most cartilages fail to express *col10, ihh, BMP6*, and bone sialoprotein (*bsp*) and to undergo hypertrophy and mineralization.

The identification of *runx2* mutations in patients with the human skeletal syndrome cleidocranial dysplasia led to the realization of its central importance to osteoblast differentiation. *Runx2* (also called *cbfa1, OSF2, AML3*, and *PEBP2αA*) is a transcription factor that can directly activate expression of *col1, osteopontin*, and *osteocalcin*. Other DNA binding proteins also participate in osteogenesis. For example, the zinc-finger transcription factor osterix (Osx) is required for the differentiation of osteogenic condensations.

Previous in vitro data using progenitor mesenchymal cell lines indicate that a variety of factors, such as TGF-βs, IGFs, and BMPs, can act to promote osteoblast differentiation. Expression of these molecules in and near developing bone in vivo has been widely reported. FGFs can initiate precocious osteogenesis of calvarial sutures in vivo. The links from growth factor to transcription factor are beginning to be revealed. A common target of BMP2, as well as TGF-β1, is *runx2*. Noggin, a secreted decoy receptor that binds BMPs and blocks their activity, inhibits cartilage formation in the cranial base. In contrast, BMP4 causes an upregulation of *sox9* and *col2*, and promotes chondrocyte proliferation and cartilage formation. FGFs can also upregulate *runx2*. Expression of *sox9* in undifferentiated mesenchyme and chondrocytes can be induced by BMPs and FGFs.

Vasculature

The importance of blood supply for bone formation is well established. However, the cellular and molecular interactions between endothelial cells and osteoblasts are still not fully understood. Skeletal injuries are generally associated with disruption of blood vessels; therefore, the repair process requires angiogenesis. During endochondral ossification, hypertrophic cartilage must become vascularized to be replaced by bone tissue. Many molecules that play a role in bone repair are indeed angiogenic regulators such as vascular endothelial growth factor (VEGF), parathyroid hormone, and members of the TGF, BMP, FGF, IGF, and PDGF families. VEGF acts directly on endothelial cells and bone cells to regulate fracture healing. Other factors such as BMPs enhance angiogenesis indirectly via the upregulation of VEGF.

A key factor of vascular invasion in many physiologic processes, including bone healing, is the increase in the activity of matrix degrading enzymes such as MMPs. Mutations in *MMP9*, *MMP13*, and membrane type 1-MMP affect vascular invasion during long bone and cranial skeletal development. In some instances, such as with the *MMP9* mutant mouse, these vascular defects are also observed during skeletal tissue healing. Injection of VEGF at the fracture site of *MMP9* mutant mice can overcome and compensate for the healing defect present in *MMP9* mutant mice. Thus, there is rescue of the delay in hypertrophic cartilage degradation and vascularization. This supports the hypothesis that MMPs act in part by regulating the availability of growth factors that are required for bone formation.

Biomechanics of Bone Fracture and Fixation

Fracture Fixation

The development of various fracture fixation devices has provided the clinician with an array of techniques to treat each clinical situation. Understanding the relative strengths and weaknesses of each type of fixation design is important in the selection of a treatment method. Clearly, fracture healing is affected by motion present at the fracture site; a certain degree of interfragmentary motion will stimulate the initiation and progression of the healing process. However, it is still unclear how much motion is optimal, and the best time for definitive fixation. What is known is that the mechanism of repair is partially governed by the interfragmentary strain imposed on the callus tissue. The degree of motion across the fracture fragments is a function of the overall construct rigidity (bone and hardware). A great number of in vitro mechanical studies on osteotomized cadaveric or synthetic bone have been performed to determine the load-displacement behavior of bone-implant-bone preparations to determine the stability achieved with different fixation methods. The resultant data are usually reported in terms of the bending, axial, and torsional stiffness.

Intramedullary Nails

An intramedullary (IM) nail essentially acts as an internal splint that shares the load with the native bone. IM nails provide good bone alignment and allow for earlier return to weight bearing. Clinically, IM nails have provided excellent results, and can be inserted at a site distant to the injured tissue, thereby avoiding additional surgical soft-tissue disruption at the fracture site.

An important aspect of IM nail design is the interfacial relationship between the bone and the nail. Of prime importance is the degree of bone-nail contact, which is related to whether the nail is inserted into a canal that is reamed or unreamed.

The inherent mechanical properties of the IM nails are essentially dependent on two parameters: geometry and material composition. These factors affect the nail's ability to resist torsion, bending, and axial loads. Bending rigidity is directly proportional to the nail's radius to the fourth power. Thus, small increases in rod diameter can provide significant gains in the bone-nail construct's ability to resist large bending forces. From a mechanical standpoint, reaming and large nail insertion should provide the most stable construct. However, excessive reaming may significantly impair healing by altering the vascular supply to the healing bone.

IM nails with longitudinal slots have also been developed. During insertion, the slot is compressed radially throughout the cross-section of the nail. The nail provides equal and opposite forces against the endosteal surface of the bone, resulting in greater bone-nail purchase. The disadvantage of slotted IM nails is that they are weak in torsion, with a more than 400-fold decrease in torsional rigidity. Twisting of the nails during insertion because of their low torsional stiffness can complicate the subsequent insertion of locking screws.

An important mechanical concept relevant to the use of IM nails is unsupported length. This parameter is the actual distance that the IM nail must span the fracture fragments. Unsupported length is highly dependent on the type of fracture that is being treated. For simple transverse fractures, where there is full cortex to cortex apposition, this distance is typically nominal. However, in highly comminuted fractures or with bone loss, this length can be relatively large. As the amount of interfragmentary strain is proportional to the square of the unsupported length, even small increases in the distance between opposing cortices can have a dramatic effect on the amount of strain at the fracture site. Consequently, the type of bone healing obtained may be affected. Given the low inherent stability afforded by IM rods in torsion, the concept of unsupported length is critical.

Although it has been shown that locking mechanisms provide large gains in torsional resistance, they also greatly affect the bone-nail construct's ability to resist axial compression forces. Statically placed distal and proximal locking screws provide resistance of the IM nail to axially translate within the canal. Oval proximal interlocking screw holes, or dynamic interlocking screw holes, allow for axial compression that resists rotation. The effectiveness of these mechanisms is largely dependent on bone quality. When the bone quality is normal, then cancellous bone purchase is sufficient for the proper function of interlocking screws. However, cortical purchase is essential for osteoporotic bone.

Inadequate rigidity, improper IM nail fit, and inability of the nail to resist torsional forces are all possible mechanical complications that can lead to deleterious outcomes. These failures are usually manifested as implant breakage, permanent alteration in the implant's shape (permanent deformation), and/or translation of the rod within the canal. Many newer designs have been advocated for promoting better IM nail-canal purchase including Poller or blocking screws placed adjacent to the nail, wings or miniscrews, and a fluted and textured surface.

Bone Plates

Bone plates represent a class of fracture fixation devices that allow for load sharing between the native bone and the implant. There are three distinct interfaces that affect the mechanics of the bone-plate construct: the screw-bone interface, the screw-plate interface, and the plate-bone interface. Any alteration in these interfaces can significantly change the mechanical behavior of the plated bone. For example, corrosion between the screw and plate can result in loss of adequate screw head compression, leading to micromotion at the plate-bone interface, and subsequent, loss of fracture fixation.

The individual components of the screw-plate-bone construct each play a significant role in overall fixation stability. Many plates are used to fix fractures of long bones, whereby significant bending stresses need to be resisted. The bending rigidity of the plate can be greatly increased by relatively small changes in the plate's thickness. Specifically, the bending stiffness of the plate is proportional to the third power of the plate's thickness, whereas the bending rigidity is linearly proportional to the elastic modulus and other plate dimensions. Similarly, the quality of the bone affects the screw-bone and plate-bone interfaces. Plating of osteoporotic or osteopenic bone produces higher demands on the plate because it must assume a greater percentage of the load. In addition, adequate screw purchase in low-density bone can be difficult to achieve. Fatigue loosening of the screw as a result of local material failure of the bone can produce a loss of adequate plate fixation to the fracture site, resulting in nonunion.

The concept of working length also applies to plated bone. In this instance, the working length is the distance between screws that are on opposite sides of the fracture site. Thus, the working length can be reduced as screw purchase is achieved as close as possible to the fracture. Bending deformation of the plate is proportional to the square of the working length, and is decreased if screws are placed close to the fracture site.

One critical factor associated with the use of bone plates involves the optimal circumferential placement. As stated earlier, many of these plates are used when significant bending loads need to be resisted. In bending across an open gap (fracture site), the tensile side tends to open up (distance between fracture ends increases) and the compressive side is further reduced. It is important that the plate be placed on the tensile (convex) side of the bending axis. Resistance of the tensile load provides for continuous fracture end contact, resulting in the best opportunity for full union healing. This concept is called the tension band effect and has been advocated for achieving primary bone healing between opposing cortices.

One important outcome of rigid compression plating is osteopenia below the surface of the bone plates. After healing, the bone does not bear the normal magnitude of load that it would had a plate not been present. The plate still bears a significant amount of the load, essentially (stress) shielding the bone from its normal load bearing. The natural response of the bone is to reduce its mass and geometry, effectively decreasing its mechanical properties. Animal models have shown that plated bones achieve 80% of the intact bone strength after 20 weeks, after which the bone strength decreases to about 60% of the intact condition. If the plates are removed after 20 weeks, then the bones are able to attain equivalent strength to the intact condition after an additional 8 weeks. These data clearly demonstrate that there can be deleterious effects of plating after full osseous healing has occurred.

External Fixation

External fixation provides a versatile way to treat problem fractures because of the almost endless combinations of different configurations. The use of different frames, pins, and wires allows the treating physician to create custom configurations that will provide the needed stability while minimizing the number of components. In addition, the degree of fixation can be changed during the course of the healing period. External fixation also allows fracture reduction as well as limb lengthening (distraction osteogenesis). When there is direct bone contact, the fixator bears only part of the load and the bone construct stiffness is relatively high. When the fracture cannot be reduced, as in comminuted fractures, the external fixator must assume the entire load. Thus, it is important to understand the different techniques that allow for increased or decreased construct rigidity.

The rigidity offered by external fixation is multifactorial. Although the material properties of the implant hardware are extremely important, the geometric configuration of the fixation construct is also an essential variable. Pins and wires are usually considered the weakest link in any external fixator configuration, because of their diameter. These components experience high bending stresses as they are oriented perpendicular to the long axis

Table 4   Bone Graft Substitute Properties

Class	Example	Osteoconductive	Osteoinductive	Structural Support	Remodels
Allograft	Structural, particulate, DBM	+	Variable	Variable	Variable
Calcium sulfate	Osteoset*	+	-	-	Resorbs
Calcium phosphate	Norian SRS,* α-BSM*	+	-	Variable	+
Collagen-calcium phosphate composite	Healos*, Collagraft*	+	-	-	+
Polymer	IMMIX* Cortoss+	+	-	+	Variable
BMP with matrix carrier	BMP-2*, BMP-7/OP-1‡	+	+	-	+

*Approved for use by FDA

+Investigational device

‡Available under FDA Humanitarian Device Exemption

DBM = demineralized bone matrix; BMP = bone morphogenic protein; Osteoset (Wright Medical Technology, Arlington, TN.)

of the bone. Bending rigidity is related to the fourth power of the pin diameter; increasing the size of the pins can have a dramatic effect on their ability to resist these bending forces. High bending stresses can lead to loss of good pin fixation (loosening). This is a common clinical issue and is related to bone resorption at the pin-bone interface. Another important geometric concern is the distance between the longitudinal external fixation bar and the bone (sidebar-to-bone distance). As this distance is decreased, there are large resultant decreases in pin deflection, and ultimately the axial stiffness of the construct.

Many fixator designs allow a certain amount of axial telescoping of the hardware, or dynamization. Dynamization can deliver a prescribed amount of strain to the healing callus, promoting micromotion between the fracture ends. It has been shown that increases in fracture site micromotion (25%) result in significant increases in the callus volume as well as in regional blood supply (up to 400%).

Bone Graft Substitutes and Growth Factors

Historically, autogenous bone graft from the iliac crest or other local sources has been the material of choice for the treatment of significant bone loss, delayed unions and nonunions, and to promote bone healing after arthrodesis. Autogenous bone grafting, however, is limited by the amount of bone available and by donor site morbidity that approaches 30%. These limitations have prompted the development and use of materials to replace or reduce the need for autograft bone.

Current understanding of the material, chemical, and biologic properties of living bone has led to the development of materials that mimic the properties of autogenous bone graft. The ideal bone graft substitute is: (1) osteogenic, (2) biocompatible, (3) bioabsorbable, (4) able to provide structural support when necessary, (5) easy to use clinically, and (6) cost effective. Depending on where it is

used, one or more of these properties may be more desirable than the others (**Table 4**). For instance, the requirements for a material used to fill a metaphyseal bone defect are much different biologically and mechanically than for a material used in the treatment of a fracture nonunion or a spine fusion. With metaphyseal bone defects, a purely osteoconductive material in concert with internal or external fixation may provide the transient scaffold necessary to complete the patient's natural healing process. Treatment of nonunion, in contrast, requires stimulation of bone growth above and beyond that of simple osteoconduction.

This section will focus on the materials most commonly used to address bone stock deficiency in orthopaedic surgery: allograft bone, calcium sulfate bone graft substitutes, tricalcium phosphate ceramics and calcium phosphate cements, collagen-ceramic composites, polylactic acid and polyglycolic acid polymers, and bioactive glasses. The role of growth factors, and specifically BMPs, as bone graft substitute enhancers also will be discussed.

Human Allograft

More than 35% of all bone transplantations involve the use of human allograft tissues. Allograft that is used in orthopaedic applications is usually fresh frozen, freeze dried, or demineralized. The mechanical and biologic properties of allograft bone depend on its method of preparation. Fresh frozen allografts retain much of their original mechanical strength but are more immunogenic. In contrast, freeze-drying reduces graft immunogenicity but also reduces graft strength by up to 50%. Disease transmission from donor to recipient is a concern with human allografts. The principal pathogens include the human immunodeficiency virus, hepatitis viruses B and C, and prions. Most allografts are now screened for these agents (except for prions) using polymerase chain reaction testing in accordance to standards set by the American Association of Tissue Bank and good tissue practices.

Allograft bone retains most of the organic phase of

bone but lacks the cellular constituents. Mineralized allograft is primarily osteoconductive and has weak osteoinductive properties. In the absence of a strong osteoinductive or osteogenic agent, the successful application of allograft tissue is dependent on the biologic capacity of the host environment into which the graft is placed. The host bed must provide the cellular and hormonal components of the osteogenic process as well as vascularity and mechanical stability.

Allograft is available in particulate and structural forms. Particulate allograft can be obtained as cancellous allograft or crushed cortical allograft. Particulate allograft adds little structural stability but has a higher rate of incorporation than structural allografts. New bone formation occurs around the individual bony particles with relatively rapid revascularization, and, in some instances, total remodeling into host bone. In contrast, cortical allograft incorporation occurs slowly. In massive cortical structural allografts, as used in oncologic surgeries, remodeling of the cortical bone is limited to 1 to 2 mm of the host-graft junction. Although in some instances a small amount of periosteal bone may form along the allograft surface, the bulk of the graft fails to remodel and remains devascularized. This is the reason that these structural grafts are prone to stress fracture, which ultimately occurs in one fourth of structural grafts used in tumor surgeries.

Demineralized allograft bone can be prepared in a powder form or, more commonly, mixed with a carrier compound to produce a demineralized bone matrix (DBM). Common carriers include hyaluronic acid, glycerol, and gelatin. The process of demineralization releases matrix-bound osteoinductive glycoproteins (including BMPs) that can then activate host bone-forming cells. Approximately 20 µg of osteoinductive protein can be extracted from 10 kg of bovine cortical bone. Bone that is induced by DBM follows an endochondral pathway in subcutaneous and submuscular implants. In calvarial defects, DBM directly induces resident mesenchymal stem cells to differentiate into osteoblast, and bone formation occurs without a cartilage intermediate. In the past, demineralized preparations of allograft bone possessed no intrinsic structural properties. Technical advances in surface demineralization of structural allografts will potentially provide the osteoinductive advantages of DBM with the mechanical strength of structural allograft.

Calcium Sulfate

Calcium sulfate dihydrate, or plaster of Paris, has long been used in vivo and is highly biocompatible. Mixing gypsum powder with water initiates an exothermic reaction that leads to recrystallization of the calcium sulfate into the solid form of plaster. However, the recrystallization process randomly produces crystals of varying sizes

and shapes, and multiple defects occur within the crystalline structure. The inconsistency in the crystalline structure causes significant variability in solubility, mechanical properties, and porosity. Thus, the traditional preparation is too heterogeneous to provide the consistent results required for widespread use. In addition, nonmedical grade calcium sulfate may reabsorb too rapidly, leading to fibrous ingrowth instead of bone substitution.

Newer forms of calcium sulfate are crystallized in highly controlled environments, producing very regularly shaped crystals of similar size and shape. The material that is produced possesses slower and more predictable solubility and resorption. Medical grade calcium sulfate bone graft substitute and bone void filler is commercially available and can be found in the form of pellets, functioning as a bone void filler and providing an osteoconductive matrix for bone substitution. The proprietary processing methods produce a highly consistent material that typically dissolves in vivo within 30 to 60 days depending on the volume and location. However, the relatively rapid rate of dissolution precludes its use in situations where structural support is critical.

Osteoblasts attach to calcium sulfate, and osteoclasts actively reabsorb calcium sulfate, forming lacunae in a manner similar to what is seen in normal bone. The dissolution of calcium sulfate produces an acidic microenvironment (pH 5.6) that may help limit bacterial activity. Despite this local dissolution, the breakdown of the graft material does not appear to lead to any appreciable increase in systemic serum calcium levels.

Numerous animal studies have shown the material's efficacy as a bone void filler. In a rat femoral defect model, calcium sulfate pellets were comparable with fresh frozen corticocancellous allograft in healing rates and mechanical strength at 2, 4, and 5 weeks. Canine humeral cavitary defects packed with this calcium sulfate material show equal healing rates compared with autograft bone. Similarly, in a rabbit spinal fusion model, this material was shown to be comparable to autograft.

More recently, the manufacturer has introduced several composite grafts that combine its proprietary calcium sulfate with DBM or DBM plus cancellous allograft. These materials are available in an injectable form as well in a moldable putty form. Theoretically, these composites will enhance osteoinductive properties in addition to providing a good osteoconductive scaffold for bone healing.

Tricalcium Phosphate Ceramics, Calcium Phosphate Cements, and Collagen-Ceramic Composites

The earliest application of calcium phosphate salts was in the form of powders. Early studies used tricalcium phosphate ($Ca_3[PO_4]_2$) as a stimulus for osteogenesis in rabbit bone with a positive effect on healing. However, this material had limited structural integrity until the ceramic form became available in the 1960s. The most commonly used calcium phosphate ceramics are hydroxyapatite and tricalcium phosphate, which are most commonly used as implant coatings and defect fillers. These materials require high temperature and often high-pressure processing to produce dense, highly crystalline, bioinert ceramics. These ceramics are not moldable intraoperatively and have poor fatigue characteristics.

More recently, in situ-setting calcium phosphate cements have become commercially available or are in the final stages of Food and Drug Administration (FDA) approval. They have the advantage of excellent biocompatibility as well as in situ setting without heat generation or shrinkage. Norian Skeletal Repair System (SRS, Synthes, West Chester, PA) is a combination of monocalcium phosphate, tricalcium phosphate, calcium carbonate, and a sodium phosphate solution mixed into an injectable paste. Under physiologic conditions, the material hardens into a dahllite (carbonated hydroxyapatite) in a nonexothermic reaction. It reaches 85% to 95% of completion within 12 hours. Additional studies showed that the chemical composition and crystallinity of the material are similar to that of the mineral phase of bone. This osteoconductive material appears to undergo the same in vivo remodeling as normal bone; it undergoes cell-mediated osteoclast resorption and replacement with osteoblast-mediated mineralized tissue formation to reestablish bone morphology and strength. This material can be used to augment fixation during the healing process as noted in increased strength when used with sliding hip screw fixation, pedicle screw fixation, and femoral neck fractures.

α-BSM Bone Substitute Material (ETEX Corporation, Cambridge, MA; DePuy, Warsaw, IN), another recently introduced calcium phosphate cement, provides a crystalline calcium phosphate apatite with a favorable absorption profile and good handling characteristics. It is composed of a calcium phosphate material that can be hydrated with saline to form a workable paste. This paste remains formable for hours at room temperature, but hardens within 20 minutes at physiologic body temperature (37°C) and can be prepared to harden to a variety of compressive strengths (5 to 40 MPa). The setting reaction is also endothermic, avoiding the thermal damage seen with exothermic cements such as polymethylmethacrylate. The crystalline nature of the cement closely mimics the mineral phase of bone, thus providing an excellent osteoconductive scaffold for cell-mediated absorption and remodeling into natural host bone. The setting reaction of α-BSM takes place at relatively neutral pH and is compatible with a variety of buffers including human serum. The lack of heat generation also minimizes denaturing of protein structure, and unconfirmed proprietary studies have verified the maintenance of incorporated protein bioactivity. Consequently, this material also appears quite well suited to incorporation of antibiotics or other bioactive agents.

To overcome some of the disadvantages associated with calcium phosphate ceramics, companies have engineered composite grafts of calcium phosphate and collagen matrices. One such product, Healos (DePuy Spine, Raynham, MA) is synthesized from bovine type I collagen and is coated with a thin soluble layer of hydroxyapatite and tricalcium phosphate. The coated collagen fibers are then formed into a sponge-like material with good handling properties. A second product, Collagraft (Zimmer, Warsaw, IN), is a composite of fibrillar collagen and a porous calcium phosphate ceramic. These engineered matrices, when combined with an osteoinductive agent or autogenous bone marrow, show promise as effective bone graft extenders or substitutes.

Polymers and Bioactive Glass

Polylactic acid and polyglycolic acid polymers are osteoconductive materials that can be molded into almost any shape. Their stoichiometry can be engineered to alter the rate of resorption that occurs through hydrolysis into carbon dioxide and water. Currently, their use has been limited to resorbable fixation devices such as suture anchors and screws and spinal interbody fusion cages. In the spine, these materials can provide structural support and an osteoconductive environment, whereas bone fusion occurs through use of an adjunctive osteogenic or osteoinductive agent (autogenous bone graft, DBM, or a cytokine). Early preparations of polylactic acid and especially polyglycolic acid used in resorbable pins and screws exhibited relatively rapid hydrolysis after application, leading to sterile sinus formation. The polymers that are currently in use have a much more gradual rate of resorption, and sterile sinus formation has not been a problem. IMMIX Extenders (Osteobiologics, Inc, San Antonio, TX) are small particles that are manufactured from an amorphous ration of 75%/25% D,L-polylactide-co-glycolide. Designed as a fully resorbing bone graft substitute or extender, this material has been shown to be an effective carrier for recombinant BMP using a mouse intramuscular implantation model. However, the efficacy of these materials as bone graft substitutes in humans has not been established.

Other types of polymers may offer specific advantages in particular applications. For example, CORTOSS (Orthovita, Malvern, PA) is a high-strength, self-setting composite resin engineered specifically to mimic the characteristics of human cortical bone. Although available for use in Europe for vertebral augmentation, it is not yet approved for use in the United States. Bioactive glasses are surface-active silica-based synthetic materials. In addition to silica, these glasses contain sodium oxide, calcium oxide, and phosphate as major components. The term bioactive refers to the in vivo formation of a superficial zone of biologically active hydroxyapatite that allows for direct bonding to bone. The surface reactivity of these materials can be altered by modification of their composition. Recent studies using a rabbit model of spine fusion suggested that bioactive glass may be used successfully as a bone graft extender. However, the brittleness of this material currently limits its use to applications that do not require it to provide structural support.

Growth Factors

Since the initial studies by Urist in the 1960s, the potential use of BMPs in orthopaedic surgery has been enthusiastically pursued. Over 20 different BMPs have been discovered. The first of these cytokines to be considered for human use include BMP-2, BMP-7, and BMP-14 (also known as growth differentiation factor-5 [GDF-5] and cartilage-derived morphogenic protein-1 [CDMR-1]). BMP-2, -7, and GDF-5 are members of the TGF-β supergene family. These proteins are secreted as inactive dimmers that are activated by proteolytic cleavage. Activated BMPs bind specific cell surface receptors which then phosphorylate a group of proteins called SMADs. Once phosphorylated, SMADs form heteromeric complexes that translocate into the cell's nucleus and activate specific genes that lead to osteoblast activation and differentiation.

BMP-2 and BMP-7 appear to be more osteogenic than GDF-5. In animal models, GDF-5 appears to play more of an "upstream" regulatory role in osteogenesis and chondrogenesis than BMP-2 and -7. In small animal models of fracture healing and spinal fusion, BMP-2 has been shown to be superior to autogenous bone graft in terms of osteogenesis. However, in nonhuman primates, extremely high doses and concentrations of BMP-2 are necessary to achieve solid arthrodesis, especially in the posterolateral intertransverse fusion bed. BMP-7 appears to behave much like BMP-2 in that the dose required for effective osteogenesis are many orders of magnitude higher than that produced endogenously. These findings suggest that bone formation likely involves the interaction of multiple morphogens acting in concert instead of just one acting alone. Recent work comparing the relative efficacy of the BMPs in a series of in vitro and in vivo animal studies showed that BMP-9 had the most bone-inducing potential. However, BMP-9 is not currently in clinical use.

Recombinant human BMP-2 (rhBMP-2) has been evaluated in two prospective randomized clinical trials. The first study compared rhBMP-2 to autologous iliac crest graft for anterior interbody lumbar spine fusions using cages. One hundred forty-three patients received rhBMP-2 on an absorbable collagen sponge; 136 patients received iliac crest graft. Twenty-four months after surgery, the BMP-2 treated group had a fusion rate of 94.5% compared with 88.7% in the iliac crest group. Clinical outcomes were similar for both groups. The second trial evaluated the effects of rhBMP-2 in the treatment of open tibia fractures. Four hundred fifty patients were randomized to receive "standard of care" treatment with or without rhBMP-2 (0.75 mg/mL or 1.5 mg/mL) on an absorbable collagen sponge. Patients who received the higher dose of rhBMP-2 had a 44% reduction in the need for secondary intervention to treat delayed unions in comparison with controls. These patients also had earlier fracture healing, fewer infections, and faster wound healing. The dose and effectiveness of rhBMP-2 in promoting spinal fusion in the posterolateral space is still under investigation. In this more stringent environment, the dosage and the type of carrier matrix that is used in combination with the cytokine appears to play a significant role in the formation of a fusion mass. Recombinant human BMP-7 (rhBMP-7) has also been evaluated in a prospective randomized trial involving 124 tibial nonunions. Patients underwent intramedullary nailing with the addition of either rhBMP-7 on a collagen sponge carrier or autologous bone graft. Although there was a trend toward superior results in the treatment group, no statistically significant differences were found in regard to clinical or radiographic healing. Currently, BMP-7 is available only under FDA Humanitarian Device Exemption.

In summary, cytokine-matrix composites are at the forefront of new technologies designed to promote osseous healing and fusion. These agents have been shown to be efficacious in lower animals and in primates, albeit at extremely high doses. They hold great promise for situations where a high degree of osteoinduction is necessary, when sufficient autogenous bone is not available, and/or when there is a need to avoid donor site morbidity. Initial clinical trials have demonstrated the efficacy of RhBMPs in certain clinical applications. However, their eventual role in clinical practice remains to be defined, and additional well-designed controlled studies should be forthcoming. In particular, cost-benefit analyses and data from long-term follow-up will be necessary before broader use of these agents can be recommended.

Adjunctive Therapies
Electrical Stimulation and Ultrasound

The basis for the use of electrical stimulation for bone healing first came from observations by Bassett and Becker. They observed the generation of electric fields in bone under mechanical strain. These strain-generated, endogenous electric fields are believed to underlie the mechanism by which bone remodels in response to mechanical stimuli (Wolff's law). Cells are triggered to lay down bone in the electronegative regions in areas of compression, while bone resorption occurs in the electropositive regions in areas of tension. Electric fields are also generated at sites of soft-tissue and bone trauma (injury-induced potentials) and in areas of rapid bone formation (biopotentials), such as at the growth plates of developing skeletal structures. Strain-generated potentials in bone originate from the piezoelectric properties of the collagen matrix and the electrokinetic effects of streaming poten-

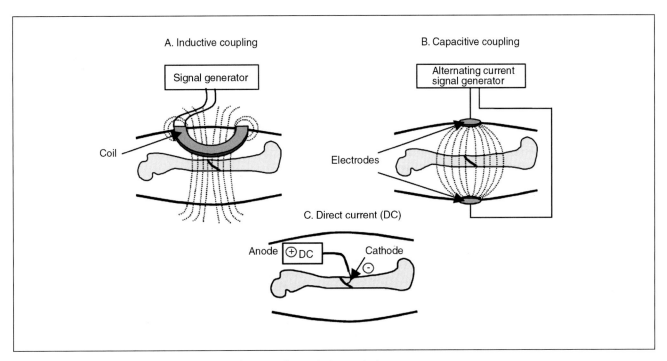

Figure 4   **A** through **C**, Schematic diagrams of electrical stimulation techniques.

tials, whereas injury-induced potentials and biopotentials are metabolically driven processes.

Because these endogenous electric fields can modulate bone cell activities, electrical stimulation devices have been designed to simulate these fields for therapeutic use. The types of electrical stimulation devices available include inductive coupling (IC), such as pulsed electromagnetic fields and combined magnetic fields, as well as capacitive coupling (CC) and direct current. All have been FDA-cleared for treating nonunions and spinal fusions. The pulsed electromagnetic field devices are also indicated for treating failed fusions and congenital pseudarthroses in the appendicular system.

IC and CC stimulation are noninvasive methods of generating electric fields in the bone and tissue. In IC, the external current-carrying coils, driven by a signal generator, produce a magnetic field that induces a secondary electric field at the fracture site (**Figure 4,** *A*). When placed over a cast, the magnetic field goes through the cast without attenuation, inducing an electric field in the bone and tissue. IC positively affects the various stages of bone healing by promoting angiogenesis, chondrogenesis, and osteogenesis. Recent studies indicate that the mechanism behind the effectiveness of IC involves the upregulation of normal physiologic regulators of bone healing such as TGF-β1, FGF-2, IGF-II, and BMP-2, -4, -5, and -7. In addition, biophysical stimulation affects prostaglandin production necessary for osteogenesis, and modulates expression of receptors for factors involved in the bone healing process. Cell culture studies show that cells at all stages in the osteoblast lineage, from progenitor cells to terminally differ-

entiated osteocytes, respond to biophysical stimulation. Similar mechanisms appear to be involved when cells from chronic nonunion tissues are exposed to IC stimulation.

In noninvasive CC stimulation, the electrodes with conductive gel are placed on the skin and connected to an external alternating current signal generator to produce an electric field at the fracture site (**Figure 4,** *B*). The mechanism of action of CC stimulation involves transmembrane calcium translocation via voltage-gated calcium channels, subsequent activation of calmodulin, and upregulation of factors that modulate normal bone healing such as TGF-β1, BMP-2, BMP-6, FGF-2 and PGE$_2$, resulting in enhanced bone formation.

Direct current stimulation produces a localized electric current at the fracture site via surgically implanted electrodes, with the cathode placed at the fracture site and the anode in the soft tissue (**Figure 4,** *C*). The electrochemical reaction at the cathode reduces oxygen concentration and increases tissue pH, factors that have been found to stimulate osteoblastic activity. An increase in pH also decreases osteoclastic activity. In addition, in vivo studies have shown that direct current stimulation upregulates several osteoinductive growth factors including BMP-2 and -7 and the BMP receptor activin receptor-like kinase 2.

Ultrasound, another type of treatment, is based on transmitting mechanical energy in the form of high-frequency acoustical pressure waves to the bone. Low-intensity ultrasound is FDA-cleared for treatment of nonunions and specific types of fresh fractures, that is, fresh, closed, posteriorly displaced distal radius fractures and fresh, closed, or grade I open tibial diaphysis fractures in skeletally mature individuals when these fractures are orthopaedically managed by closed reduction and cast immobilization. Low-intensity ultrasound is transmitted to the fracture site via an ultrasound transducer and coupling gel placed on the skin. The ultrasonic energy is absorbed at a rate proportional to tissue density, thus targeting the energy to bone, but also attenuating the ultrasound as it passes through tissue. Low-intensity ultrasound has been found to reduce the healing time of tibial fractures and distal radial fractures when treated with a cast. However, a clinical trial with IM fixed tibial fractures showed that ultrasound has no effect on the healing time of IM fixed tibial fractures. The presence of metal in the fracture area was indicated as a possible factor contributing to the negative results. The mechanism of action of ultrasound involves the response of bone to mechanical stimuli (Wolff's law). Wolff has demonstrated that bone structure adapts to the mechanical environment by remodeling to accommodate the applied forces. It has thus been suggested that bone would similarly respond to the acoustical pressure wave form of mechanical energy of ultrasound. In vitro studies with ultrasound have also shown increased expressions of TGF-β1, PGE$_2$, and PDGF-AB.

There are numerous studies investigating the effects and mechanisms of action of electrical stimulation and ultrasound on bone healing. Both internal and external treatments are available for clinical use, and can also be used as adjuncts to bone grafts. Consideration of the benefits and shortcomings of the devices would determine use in specific applications.

Summary

More than 6 million fractures are sustained annually in the United States. It is estimated that approximately 10% of fractures have impaired healing. Over the past decade, significant progress has been made in fracture treatment. The cellular and molecular events that govern the repair and regeneration of osseous tissue following injury are better understood. Techniques that stimulate bone repair, including bone graft substitutes, growth factors, and adjunctive therapies have been further developed. Fracture fixation techniques and bone implants have been designed to minimize further damage to the injured bone and surrounding soft tissues. The next decade will bring further advances in bone healing as understanding of the basic elements of the repair process continue to be revealed, and important emerging technologies continue to develop.

Selected Bibliography

Osteonecrosis

Cruess RL: Osteonecrosis of bone: Current concepts as to etiology and pathogenesis. *Clin Orthop Relat Res* 1986;208:30-39.

Ficat RP: Idiopathic bone necrosis of the femoral head: Early diagnosis and treatment. *J Bone Joint Surg Br* 1985;67:3-9.

Hutter CD: Dysbaric osteonecrosis: A reassessment and hypothesis. *Med Hypotheses* 2000;54:585-590.

Jones JP Jr: Concepts of etiology and early pathogenesis of osteonecrosis. *Instr Course Lect* 1994;43:499-512.

Mankin HJ: Nontraumatic necrosis of bone (osteonecrosis). *N Engl J Med* 1992;326:1473-1479.

Matsuo K, Hirohata T, Sugioka Y: Influence of alcohol intake, cigarett smoking, and occupational status on idiopathic osteonecrosis of the femoral head. *Clin Orthop Relat Res* 1988;234:115-123.

Vail TP, Covington DB: The incidence of osteonecrosis, in Urbaniak JR, Jones JP Jr (eds): *Osteonecrosis: Etiology, Diagnosis, and Treatment.* Rosemont, IL, 1997, pp 43-50.

Wang GJ, Cui Q, Balian G: The pathogenesis and prevention of steroid induced osteonecrosis. *Clin Orthop Relat Res* 2000;370:295-310.

Wang Y, Li Y, Mao K, Li J, Cui Q, Wang GJ: Alcohol-induced adipogenesis in bone and marrow: A possible mechanism for osteonecrosis. *Clin Orthop Relat Res* 2003;410:213-224.

Biologic Requirements for Skeletal Tissue Repair

Andreshak JL, Rabin SI, Patwardhan AG, Wezeman FH: Tibial segmental defect repair: Chondrogenesis and biomechanical strength modulated by basic fibroblast growth factor. *Anat Rec* 1997;248:198-204.

Barnes GL, Kostenuik PJ, Gerstenfeld LC, Einhorn TA: Growth factor regulation of fracture repair. *J Bone Miner Res* 1999;14:1805-1815.

Bi W, Deng JM, Zhang Z, Behringer RR, de Crombrugghe B: Sox9 is required for cartilage formation. *Nat Genet* 1999;22:85-89.

Bruder SP, Fink DJ, Caplan AI: Mesenchymal stem cells in bone development, bone repair, and skeletal regeneration therapy. *J Cell Biochem* 1994;56:283-294.

Buxton P, Edwards C, Archer CW, Francis-West P: Growth/differentiation factor-5 (GDF-5) and skeletal development. *J Bone Joint Surg Am* 2001;83-A(suppl 1):S23-S30.

Carano RA, Filvaroff EH: Angiogenesis and bone repair. *Drug Discov Today* 2003;8:980-989.

Colnot C, Thompson Z, Miclau T, Werb Z, Helms JA: Altered fracture repair in the absence of MMP9. *Development* 2003;130:4123-4133.

Deckers MM, van Bezooijen RL, van der Horst G, et al: Bone morphogenetic proteins stimulate angiogenesis through osteoblast-derived vascular endothelial growth factor A. *Endocrinology* 2002;143:1545-1553.

Devine MJ, Mierisch CM, Jang E, Anderson PC, Balian G: Transplanted bone marrow cells localize to fracture callus in a mouse model. *J Orthop Res* 2002;20:1232-1239.

Ducy P, Zhang R, Geoffroy V, Ridall AL, Karsenty G: Osf2/Cbfa1: A transcriptional activator of osteoblast differentiation. *Cell* 1997;89:747-754.

Einhorn TA, Majeska RJ, Rush EB, Levine PM, Horowitz MC: The expression of cytokine activity by fracture callus. *J Bone Miner Res* 1995;10:1272-1281.

Enomoto-Iwamoto M, Nakamura T, Aikawa T, et al: Hedgehog proteins stimulate chondrogenic cell differentiation and cartilage formation. *J Bone Miner Res* 2000;15:1659-1668.

Ferguson C, Alpern E, Miclau T, Helms JA: Does adult fracture repair recapitulate embryonic skeletal formation? *Mech Dev* 1999;87:57-66.

Gerber HP, Vu TH, Ryan AM, Kowalski J, Werb Z, Ferrara N: VEGF couples hypertrophic cartilage remodeling, ossification and angiogenesis during endochondral bone formation. *Nat Med* 1999;5:623-628.

Haynesworth SE, Goshima J, Goldberg VM, Caplan AI: Characterization of cells with osteogenic potential from human marrow. *Bone* 1992;13:81-88.

Kang Q, Sun MH, Cheng H, et al: Characterization of the distinct orthotopic bone-forming activity of 14 BMPs using recombinant adenovirus-mediated gene delivery. *Gene Ther* 2004;11:1312-1320.

Linkhart TA, Mohan S, Baylink DJ: Growth factors for bone growth and repair: IGF, TGF beta and BMP. *Bone* 1996;19:1S-12S.

Pola R, Ling LE, Silver M, et al: The morphogen Sonic hedgehog is an indirect angiogenic agent upregulating two families of angiogenic growth factors. *Nat Med* 2001;7:706-711.

Biomechanics of Bone Fracture and Fixation
Hayes WC: Biomechanics of fracture healing, in Heppenstall RB (ed): *Fracture Treatment and Healing.* Philadelphia, PA, WB Saunders, 1980, pp 124-172.

Hipp JA, Hayes WC: Biomechanics of fractures, in Browner B, Jupiter J, Levine A, Trafton P: *Skeletal Trauma: Basic Science, Management, and Reconstruction.* Philadelphia, PA, WB Saunders, 2003.

Mow VC, Hayes HC: *Basic Orthopaedic Biomechanics,* ed 2. New York, NY, Lippincott-Raven Press, 1971.

Perren SM: Physical and biological aspects of fracture healing with special reference to internal fixation. *Clin Orthop Relat Res* 1979;138:175-196.

Perren SM, Cordey J, Rahn BA, Gautier E, Schneider E: Early temporary porosis of bone induced by internal fixation implants: A reaction to necrosis, not to stress protection? *Clin Orthop Relat Res* 1988;232:139-151.

Rhinelander FW: Effects of medullary nailing on the normal blood supply of diaphyseal cortex. *Instr Course Lect* 1973;22:161-187.

Weber BG: On the biomechanics of external fixation, in Weber BG, Magerl G (eds): *The External Fixator: AO/ASIF-Threaded Rod System Spine-Fixator.* Berlin, Germany, Springer-Verlag, 1985, pp 27-53.

White AA, Panjabi MM, Southwick WO: The four biomechanical stages of fracture repair. *J Bone Joint Surg Am* 1977;59:188-192.

Bone Graft Substitutes and Growth Factors
Bruder SP, Kraus KH, Goldberg VM, Kadiyala S: The effect of implants loaded with autologous mesenchymal stem cells on the healing of canine segmental bone defects. *J Bone Joint Surg Am* 1998;80:985-895.

Chapman MW, Bucholz R, Cornell C: Treatment of acute fractures with a collagen-calcium phosphate graft material: A randomized clinical trial. *J Bone Joint Surg Am* 1997;79:495-502.

Connolly JF, Guse R, Tiedeman J, Dehne R: Autologous bone marrow injection as a substitute for operative bone grafting of tibial nonunions. *Clin Orthop Relat Res* 1991;266:259-270.

Geesink RG, Hoefnagels NH, Bulstra SK: Osteogenic activity of OP-1 bone morphogenetic protein (BMP-7) in a human fibular defect. *J Bone Joint Surg Br* 1999; 81:710-718.

Govender S, Csimma C, Genant HK, Valentic-Opran A: Recombinant human bone morphogenetic protein-2 for treatment of open tibial fractures: A prospective, controlled, randomized study of four hundred and fifty patients. *J Bone Joint Surg Am* 2002;84-A: 2123-2134.

Muschler GF, Boehm C, Easley K: Aspiration to obtain osteoblast progenitor cells from human bone marrow: The influence of aspirate volume. *J Bone Joint Surg Am* 1997;79:1699-1708.

Tiedeman JJ, Connolly JF, Strates BS, Lippiello L: Treatment of nonunion by percutaneous injection of bone marrow and demineralized bone matrix: An ex-perimental study in dogs. *Clin Orthop Relat Res* 1991; 268:294-302.

Adjunctive Therapies

Anglen J: The clinical use of bone stimulators. *J South Orthop Assoc* 2003;12:46-54.

Bassett CA, Becker RO: Generation of electric potentials by bone in response to mechanical stress. *Science* 1962;137:1063-1064.

Guerkov HH, Lohmann CH, Liu Y, et al: Pulsed electromagnetic fields increase growth factor release by nonunion cells. *Clin Orthop Relat Res* 2001;384:265-279.

Rubin C, Bolander M, Ryaby JP, Hadjiargyrou M: The use of low-intensity ultrasound to accelerate the healing of fractures. *J Bone Joint Surg Am* 2001;83-A:259-270.

Chapter 19

Articular Cartilage Repair

Shawn W. O'Driscoll, PhD, MD
Daniël B.F. Saris, MD, PhD

Introduction

The field of cartilage repair has experienced rapid and dramatic changes over the past 10 years. The challenge of treating articular cartilage defects in an already significant and continuously growing population of young adults with cartilage damage remains considerable. The outcomes of surgery and other treatments for cartilage repair are variable and in most instances additional questions have been raised about the clinical dilemma of damaged articular cartilage and its limited capacity for natural healing. In a young, active patient, damage to the articular surface may lead to an increased incidence of cartilage degeneration and eventual osteoarthritis. Elderly patients with arthritis can experience dramatic relief from pain and restoration of function after total joint arthroplasty. However, total joint arthroplasties have higher rates of failure in young and early middle-aged patients than in elderly patients. Various surgical and nonsurgical treatment methods are being investigated with the goal of restoring or maintaining the articular surface and normalizing joint function. The implications of such possibilities are great in terms of the number of patients affected, quality of life, and ultimately the decrease in long-term health care costs related to joint arthroplasty and multiple revisions. Thus, a method for biologic healing and repair of cartilage is needed to prevent arthritis in patients with cartilage injuries and disorders. The possibility for repair of cartilage, an objective that has been elusive for so many years, has recently generated a great deal of interest. This chapter discusses the goals, results, and limitations of clinical cartilage repair as well as future developments.

Articular Cartilage Damage

Patients seeking medical attention for recent trauma or joint dysfunction related to articular cartilage damage are often young and active, and have functional limitations to some extent because of their symptoms. Cartilage defects larger than 2 mm in diameter rarely heal. In one study, 63% of 31,500 patients undergoing arthroscopy had some form of cartilage damage. Up to 15% of patients with hemarthrosis caused by knee trauma have a relevant cartilage defect. It has been estimated that the incidence of articular cartilage defects is 2.6 patients per 1,000 adults; persistent defects frequently progress to joint degeneration. Cartilage damage most frequently occurs in the knee, as a result of trauma (**Figure 1**), ligament instability, malalignment of the extremity, meniscectomy, or osteochondritis dissecans. In most instances, accompanying ligament or meniscal damage may exist and the diagnosis of a solitary cartilage lesion is not made during primary evaluation.

Healthy hyaline cartilage contributes to a smooth articular surface and is essential for proper joint function. Articular cartilage provides the joint with a low friction surface that under normal conditions has unsurpassed wear resistance and a high compressive stiffness. These characteristics are secondary to the unique biologic and biochemical composition of articular cartilage, which is composed of a type II collagen sponge supported by water that is held in place by an extracellular matrix rich in glycosaminoglycans. Under normal conditions, articular cartilage can perform its required function for a lifetime, although some age-related degenerative alterations occur. Nevertheless, in the absence of joint trauma, articular cartilage is well designed to tolerate a lifetime of use.

In adults, articular cartilage has neither a blood supply nor lymphatic drainage. No neural elements connect it to the remainder of the homeostatic systems within the body. In fact, after being surrounded by an extracellular matrix, articular chondrocytes are sheltered even from immunologic recognition. Although the cells continue to produce new extracellular matrix throughout life, they are ineffective in responding to injury.

Natural Healing Response

Spontaneous repair of all musculoskeletal tissue begins with an inflammatory response. Injured cells and platelets

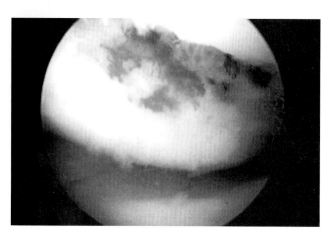

Figure 1 Arthroscopic view of a fresh traumatic cartilage defect in the right medial femoral condyle. This defect extends to the calcified cartilage layer with areas of subchondral perforation. Initial spontaneous bleeding can be seen from the subchondral bone. This lesion was treated by microfracture of the delaminated region with limited weight bearing postoperatively.

release mediators that promote the vascular response to injury. Inflammatory cells help remove necrotic tissue and release mediators that stimulate migration and proliferation of mesenchymal stem cells. The occurrence of these events during inflammation is critical for initiation of effective tissue repair. In the nonvascular articular cartilage surface the vascular and inflammatory responses are blunted, and superficial cartilage injuries do not heal. Wounds that are limited to the cartilage itself, without penetration of the subchondral bone, stimulate only a slight reaction in the adjacent chondrocytes. Cell replication and increased matrix turnover are briefly induced.

In full-thickness defects that penetrate the calcified cartilage and subchondral bone, cells enter the injury site from the bone marrow space. This action initiates a classic wound repair reaction with a combination of mesenchymal stem cells from the bone marrow and inflammatory cells, which produce and organize a tissue that fills the defect. Shapiro and associates extensively described the cell origin and differentiation during natural repair of full-thickness articular cartilage defects in the rabbit knee. Fibrous arcades that fill the defects in the first week of repair (**Figure 2,** *A)* span the defect and provide a scaffold on which mesenchymal stem cell ingrowth can occur. Cartilage matrix synthesis was seen as early as 10 days after repair and increased during a 6- to 8-week period as seen on safranin O staining (**Figure 2,** *B)*. At the base of the defect, mesenchymal stem cells differentiate into osteoblasts and reconstitute the tidemark by 24 weeks. In the repaired tissue, cartilage thickness is only half of the original depth (**Figure 2,** *C)*. Early traces of degeneration were observed in many defects as soon as 12 weeks into the repair, increasing by 24 to 48 weeks (**Figure 2,** *D)*. Polarized light microscopy demonstrated failure of the newly synthesized repair matrix to become adherent to and integrate with the

cartilage immediately adjacent to the defect. Attempts at spontaneous repair do not consistently restore the surface with a tissue that has the unique composition, structure, and material properties of normal articular cartilage. The only cell type found in articular cartilage, the highly differentiated chondrocyte, has limited capacity for proliferation or migration. In normal mature cartilage, chondrocytes synthesize sufficient matrix macromolecules to maintain the matrix, and they can increase their rate of matrix synthesis in response to injury or osteoarthritic changes. However, chondrocytes synthesize insufficient matrix to repair large tissue defects. The extent to which the newly formed tissue resembles articular cartilage depends on the age and species of the host as well as the size and location of the defect (**Figure 3**). However, durable and complete restoration of the hyaline articular cartilage and the subchondral bone to a normal status rarely occurs.

The Concept of Joint Homeostasis

An articulating joint has a complex design, with many essential components such as synovium, cartilage, menisci, synovial fluid, ligaments, and subchondral bone; a multitude of interactions occur among these components. These anatomic structures are influenced by factors such as motion, loading, alignment, weight, age, and hormonal influences. It is evident that this complex environment must be rigorously regulated. Furthermore, metabolic control must be flexible because the external environment to which cells are exposed is not constant. Studies of a wide range of organisms have shown that several mechanisms are responsible for the control of physiologic equilibrium (homeostasis) (**Figure 4**). The basic scientific concept of homeostasis should be implemented when the clinical problem of restoring a damaged articulation is addressed. Normal joint homeostasis refers to the stable equilibrium of synovium and cartilage matrix in a well-functioning articulation devoid of inflammatory activity. When joint homeostasis is disturbed, as in damaged cartilage, this equilibrium is altered and intra-articular factors such as inflammatory, molecular, or cellular components come into play. It was recently demonstrated that old defects in a state of disturbed homeostasis have a significantly worse outcome after surgical restoration attempts than fresh defects in an otherwise normal knee treated similarly.

Treatment Options for Damaged or Lost Cartilage

It is important to discern the difference between achieving symptomatic relief and good functional outcome for the patient within a reasonably short period of time versus the 'ultimate goal' of delaying osteoarthritis, and truly striving to restore full articular function for the remaining life span of the patient.

Various treatment options exist, from conservative measures such as functional adaptation, physiotherapy,

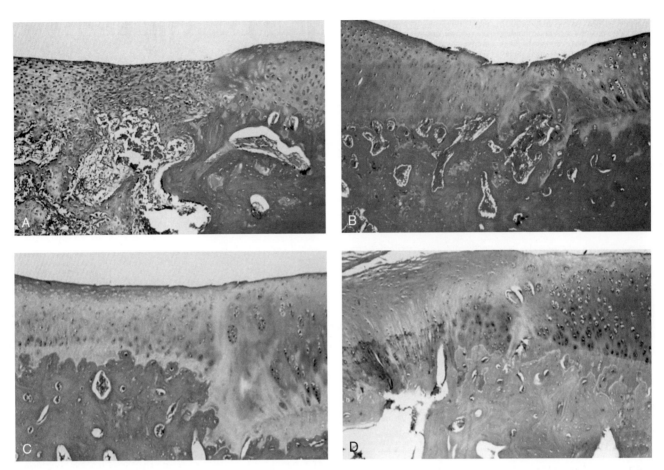

Figure 2   Histologic examples of repair in a 3-mm experimental defect in the rabbit knee. *(Reproduced with permission from Shapiro F, Koide S, Glimcher MJ: Cell origin and differentiation in the repair of full-thickness defects of articular cartilage.* J Bone Joint Surg Am. *1993;75A:532-553.* **A,** Repair tissue closely adherent to residual cartilage at 2 weeks. Empty chondrocyte lacuna at the edge of the defect indicate cell death in association with trauma. Most tissue is still composed of undifferentiated mesenchymal cells, with early evidence of cartilage formation. Proteoglycan content of the residual cartilage near the defect is already markedly diminished in comparison to the staining at the far right. **B,** Repair tissue at the right, residual tissue at the left, at 6 weeks. Tidemark persists on left but is not yet reestablished on the right. The repair bone has been synthesized to fill the adequate depth. Superficial tissue is cartilaginous. The repair tissue is hypercellular compared with residual cartilage. Proteoglycan content of the repair tissue is excellent. **C,** A higher power photomicrograph of the junction between repair and residual cartilage at 24 weeks after creation of the defect is shown. Continuity of the cartilaginous tissue is good. The bulk of the repair cartilage is characterized by orthochromatic staining (dark) indicative of proteoglycan synthesis and retention. The tidemark has been reestablished; however, the original cartilage is twice as thick as the repair cartilage. **D,** Follow-up at 48 weeks shows extensive degenerative changes. The superficial fibrillation is accompanied by hypocellular regions in the repair cartilage.

and medication to surgical intervention ranging from arthroscopic or minimally invasive procedures to joint arthroplasty. Whole tissue transplants and tissue engineering have been considered for biologic regeneration of the cartilage surface. The selected method depends on the presenting symptoms and findings at physical examination and diagnostic imaging, patient age, defect characteristics, and surgeon preference.

Conservative Measures

A meta-analysis of 10 studies compared patient education with medication. The patient education group experienced a significant reduction in pain scores but no improvement in function over the medication group. Studies

indicate that physiotherapy, adaptation of lifestyle, and education can provide considerable symptomatic relief and are important adjuncts in perioperative management.

Nonsteroidal anti-inflammatory drugs (NSAIDs) are used to decrease pain and reduce synovitis. There is evidence suggesting that NSAIDs may inhibit chondrogenesis and cartilage metabolism; therefore, their use in postoperative pain management in patients undergoing joint repair procedures should be carefully considered. Studies have shown that improvement of pain and function is better with NSAID use compared with placebo, but NSAIDs also have been shown to have no lasting effect after 2 years. To address adverse effects of NSAIDs and retain a similar level of pain relief, cyclooxygenase-2

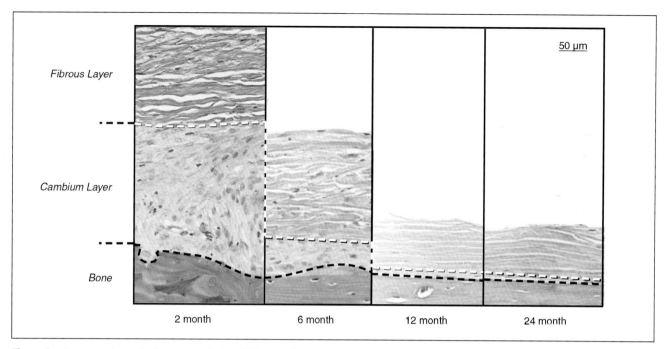

Figure 3   An age-related decline occurs in the thickness of the periosteal cambium layer and the number of mesenchymal stem cells. This composite photomicrograph of intact periosteum along the rabbit tibial surface shows how both the cambium and fibrous layers become thinner with age. Most notable is the marked reduction in total cell number in the cambium layer, which contains chondrocyte precursors.

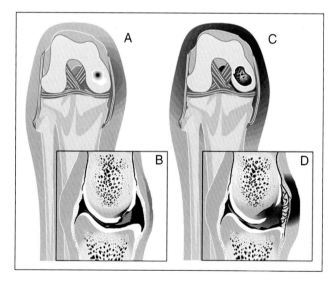

Figure 4   **A,** In normal joint homeostasis, a healthy equilibrium exists between smooth cartilage, subchondral bone, synovial fluid, intact menisci, and ligaments. **B,** A cartilage defect is not only a local problem. Once present it will begin to influence the surrounding joint. **C,** After a cartilage defect occurs, equilibrium is disturbed and homeostasis is altered. This environment with matrix degradation, synovial thickening, effusion and subchondral sclerosis constitutes a very different environment in which tissue-engineered cartilage repair is attempted. **D,** Now the defect is part of an altered intra-articular environment for which it has been shown that cartilage repair is significantly inhibited when compared with repair using the same technique in a fresh defect.

(COX-2) inhibitors were introduced. These agents have a therapeutic result similar to NSAIDs for pain relief, with the possible benefit that gastrointestinal ulcers may be less likely to occur. Recent developments have indicated that cardiovascular complications may be related to long-term use of COX-2 inhibitors, a cause for considerable concern and debate on the use of these medications for musculoskeletal pain relief.

Food supplements such as chondroitin sulfate and glucosamine are available and in use predominantly in the United States. Although some beneficial effects have been shown, the efficacy of dietary supplementation of these cartilage matrix proteins is currently under investigation in randomized trials. Intra-articular injections are used more often to treat osteoarthritis when signs of effusion or synovitis are present. Corticosteroids have been shown to provide significant pain relief and reduction of effusion for 4 to 6 weeks. Because intra-articular injections can have a negative effect on cartilage metabolism and acceleration of cartilage damage, it is suggested that these injections should not be the only therapeutic strategy. Hyaluronic acid is a polysaccharide present in normal synovial fluid that provides lubrication and shock absorption and plays an important role in embryonic joint formation where it regulates joint cavitation (separation of the cartilage into two articulating surfaces). In synovial fluid from osteoarthritic joints, there is a reduction in hyaluronan levels. Randomized controlled trials have shown pain relief superior to placebo, comparable to the use of corticosteroids but lasting longer. The exact roles and cost effectiveness of these therapies within a treatment algorithm remain to be determined. In the current treatment of cartilage defects, injection therapy is not used because these patients are young and have localized cartilage disease as opposed to arthritic changes throughout the involved joint.

Strategies for Cartilage Repair

Surgical strategies for cartilage repair are divided into three categories: enhancement of the natural healing of cartilage (and subchondral bone), implantation of cells (or tissues) and/or synthetic materials into a defect, and placement of osteochondral grafts or transplants into the defect.

Enhancement of Natural Healing of Cartilage and Subchondral Bone

Cartilage has a limited capacity to heal, and only after the subchondral bone has been perforated and contact with the marrow cavity is established does the natural healing response of musculoskeletal tissue occur.

Natural repair of all musculoskeletal tissue begins with an inflammatory response. Injured cells and platelets release mediators that promote the vascular response to injury. Inflammatory cells help remove necrotic tissue and release mediators that stimulate migration and proliferation of mesenchymal cells. These inflammatory events are critical for initiation of effective tissue repair. Abrasion chondroplasty and microfracture/drilling (**Figure 5**) are cartilage repair methods based on this principle. Perforation of the subchondral bone opens the marrow cavity and provides a source of undifferentiated stem cells that have osteochondrogenic potential.

Abrasion Arthroplasty

Abrasion arthroplasty is an arthroscopic technique that combines lavage, removal of loose bodies, and the resection of unstable cartilage at the defect rim with abrasion of the subchondral bone at the base of the defect with a burr. This technique stimulates a cartilage healing response that results in a fibrocartilage rather than a hyaline cartilage matrix, but provides relief in 60% to 70% of patients at 6 months to 1 year after treatment of a full-thickness cartilage defect of the knee. The results were better in patients younger than 40 years of age. Rand reported on 28 patients who had exposed bone. At an average of 3.8 years after an abrasion arthroplasty, 11 patients had improvement, 8 had no change, and 9 experienced worsening of their condition. Fourteen patients had total knee arthroplasty an average of 3 years after the abrasion procedure. In a retrospective, comparative study of 126 patients, Bert and Maschka reported an average of 60 months of follow-up on either débridement with abrasion arthroplasty or arthroscopic débridement only for treatment of unicompartmental gonarthrosis. Of 59 patients treated with débridement and abrasion, 51% had good to excellent results, 16% had fair results, and 33% had a poor result. Of the 67 patients in the débridement alone group, results were good to excellent in 66%, fair in 13%, and poor in 21% of patients. Twelve of the knees in which results were poor became worse after débridement and arthroplasty was required. For patients with osteoarthritis, the effect of an osteotomy was compared with that of concomitant abrasion chondroplasty and osteotomy. Patients treated using the combined approach had a significantly higher proportion of hyaline-like cartilage repair tissue and had a lower incidence of tissue degeneration 12 months after surgery than did those who received an osteotomy only. However, the repair was not durable and outcome became less satisfactory over time.

Microfracture Technique

Steadman popularized a technique in which multiple small holes and subchondral bone "microfractures" (**Figure 5**) are made by hand using small picks rather than drills or pins. The holes are small, numerous, and very close together. Calcified cartilage, but not the subchondral bone, is removed with a curet. Under the stimulus of continuous passive motion and regulated load bearing, bone marrow cells in the clot on the surface of the exposed bone undergo metaplasia to fibrocartilage. This technique is based on the theory that impaction with an awl results in microfracture of the trabeculae and signals the initiation of a healing response in the defect as well as in the surrounding bone. Moreover, heat necrosis is avoided. The mechanical properties of the subchondral bone layer are altered to a different extent than by drilling. The newly formed cartilage tissue no longer rests on a sclerotic bed but on a remodeled bone layer that may possess more optimal mechanical characteristics for longer term survival of a covering cartilage layer. The microfracture technique requires less equipment, is easier to perform, and is considered as effective as drilling; however, data from comparative studies, which are not yet available, are needed to confirm or refute the technique's efficacy. The indications for intervention and techniques used vary considerably, which creates difficulty in comparing the outcome of such procedures in the literature. Beneficial outcomes have been reported in 75% to 100% of patients. Most authors agree that these methods may provide relief for up to 3 to 5 years, but long-term benefits seem less likely.

The relative effectiveness of using the various techniques for penetration of subchondral bone is controversial. However, these treatment options have little likelihood of making symptoms worse, and symptoms are improved in most patients. Based on current knowledge, microfracture is a reasonable first step in the management of a patient who has a previously untreated cartilage defect.

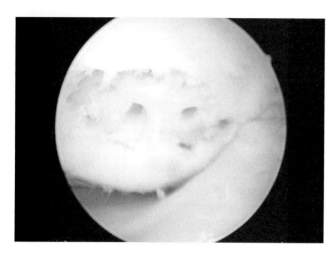

Figure 5 This arthroscopic view of the right knee shows the medial femoral condyle with a grade IV cartilage defect that has been cleaned up to the subchondral bone. Perforation of the subchondral bone plate was done by microfracture to permit an influx of mesenchymal stem cells from the bone marrow. Microfracture also influences the mechanical characteristics of the subchondral plate, which in cartilage defects is frequently sclerotic (hard).

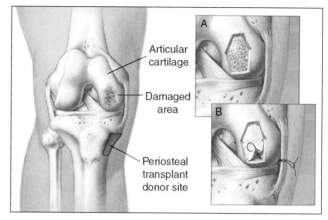

Figure 6 Cartilage repair is possible with periosteal grafting. After preparation of the lesion down to the subchondral bone (**A**), periosteum from the proximal medial tibia is sutured into the bottom of the defect with the cambium layer facing up into the joint space (**B**).

Implantation of Cells, Tissue, and/or Synthetic Materials

Because of the limited capacity of cartilage to heal, even with the type of stimulation previously described, recent research has been directed toward repair of the damaged joint surface by grafting or transplanting cells or a tissue with chondrogenic potential into the joint.

Whole Tissue Grafts (Periosteum/Perichondrium)

In procedures such as perichondral and periosteal grafting, the defect is cleaned and extended into the subchondral region. Tissue is obtained from the rib bone-cartilage interface or from the proximal medial tibia and sutured into the bottom of the defect through bone tunnels, usually with the cambium layer facing outward into the joint (**Figure 6**). The mesenchymal stem cells in the cambium layer initiate a chondrogenic and osteogenic process that restores both the cartilage surface and the subchondral bone. With this method, localized defects and larger areas of cartilage damage may be treated. Using perichondrium, Homminga described good initial results in 85% of patients. However, recent reevaluation of this group at almost 10-year follow-up noted a decline in good results to 38%; there was no difference in good results between the patients treated with a perichondral graft and a matched group of patients treated with arthroscopic drilling. Using periosteal grafts, Engkvist observed symptomatic relief in patients with arthritic joints. Angermann described 14 consecutive periosteal transplantations evaluated 1 year postoperatively; 9 knees were pain-free, but after 6 to 9 years of follow-up, only 2 knees were pain-free. Arthritis developed in six knees. Hyaline-like cartilage was docu-

mented in 1 patient and assessed as possible in another, but in 10 patients the tissue that formed in the defects was not hyaline cartilage. In experiments using a large animal defect in a goat model, the chronicity of the cartilage defect was shown to be of significant influence on the outcome of repair (**Figure 7**). Fresh defects healed well when treated with periosteal grafting, whereas a poor repair with hypertrophy, calcification, and incomplete filling was seen when older defects were treated. This could be an explanation for the discrepancy between results of animal studies and the observed clinical outcome of cartilage defect repair using these methods. Since 1986, one of the authors has performed periosteal transplantation in approximately 40 patients (SW O'Driscoll, MD, unpublished data). Twenty-three of the 40 patients who were so managed had osteochondral defects in the knee; the others had defects that involved the elbow, ankle, shoulder, or hand. The defects ranged in size from 1.5 x 1.5 cm to 4 x 10 cm and were as deep as 2 cm, but generally they were large and full-thickness, penetrating the subchondral bone. Some defects were treated with bone grafting simultaneously. The success rate of the procedure was disappointing, particularly given the optimism created by basic scientific data on periosteal chondrogenesis and results in animals. The lack of convincing positive evidence for the efficacy of whole tissue grafts has led to the use of these techniques in only selected indications.

Autologous Chondrocyte Transplantation

Bentley and Greer are believed to be the first to show that chondrocytes could be transplanted into articular cartilage defects and improve healing. Isolated chondrocytes are expanded in cell culture, making it possible to start with a relatively small quantity of tissue as a source of cells (**Figure 8**). Expanded populations of chondrocytes are implanted using arthrotomy and are placed under peri-

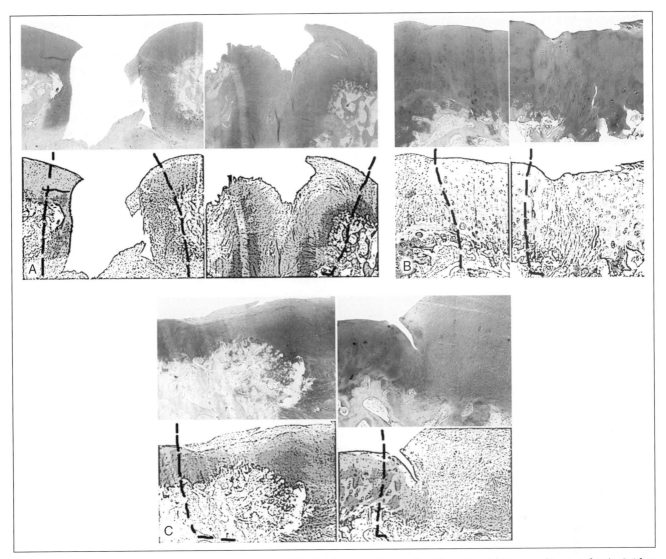

Figure 7   **A,** Top row: histologic sections of an untreated defect in a goat knee after 10 weeks of follow-up (3 µm, safranin O / fast green, magnification x200). Bottom row: schematic representation of the sections depicting the location of the original defect. These two typical samples demonstrate that the cartilage defects that were left untreated either remained unchanged as on the left, or had some degree of filling with fibrocartilage or extruding cartilage from the normal cartilage rim as on the right. **B,** Top row: histologic sections demonstrating the outcome of cartilage repair in an experimental cartilage defect in the untreated goat defect immediately after creation (3 µm, safranin O / fast green, magnification x200). Bottom row: schematic representation of the sections depicting original defect. These two typical samples show how the fresh cartilage defect, which was treated early by using a periosteal graft, showed a marked repair of the cartilage surface with a tissue resembling hyaline cartilage. There are some chondrocyte clusters and nearly normal proteoglycan staining throughout the matrix. Some remodeling of the subchondral bone is seen. **C,** Top row: histologic sections of defects that were treated after 10 weeks of 'natural healing' identical to the situation of a defect treated late (3 µm, safranin O / fast green, magnification x200). Bottom row: schematic representation of the sections depicting the location of the original defect. These two typical samples from the 'late treatment' group demonstrate an identical full-thickness defect as in the previous groups but were treated with a periosteal graft after 10 weeks of motion and loading on the previous superficial cartilage defect. There is irregular fibrocartilage filling and hypertrophy with uneven staining of the matrix. Also, signs of delamination and sidewall fissures were seen more frequently than in the 'early treatment' group.

osteal tissue or under a collagen sheet that is sutured in place. This covering is sutured into the defect rim with resorbable suture material and sealed with fibrin glue (**Figure 9**). The cultured cells are injected into the area under the flap. In vitro studies have shown no negative or added effect from the glue on the cells. The sutures, however, do have a negative effect on the cartilage surrounding the de-

fect; increased cell death and matrix alterations have been noted shortly after the procedure. There are two additional technical challenges to this approach. The first is to ensure that the explanted chondrocytes maintain a chondrocyte phenotype in cell culture and after transplantation. There is a strong tendency for fibroblastic dedifferentiation. The second challenge is maintaining the transplanted cells in the damaged area following implantation; this is more difficult with uncontained defects, large defects, or whole joint surfaces than it is with small, confined lesions. Finally, the periosteal covering provides growth factors and contains cells that can contribute to the repair, but also can calcify or hypertrophy. As many as 10% to 40% of patients undergo a second surgery to treat symptoms attributable to hypertrophy of the graft associated with mechanical impediment.

Short-term to mid-term follow-up in animal experiments evaluating the percentage of defect filling, quality of cartilage, and incorporation show good results in 70% to 85% of patients. The clinical results described by Brittberg and associates in a 10-year follow-up study of more than 100 patients are encouraging. In patients with isolated femoral condyle lesions, 92% had good to excellent clinical results. Furthermore, there was a correlation between the quality of the repair tissue and the clinical results. Mechanical testing with an arthroscopic indentation measurement device in eight patients revealed the stiffness of the repair tissue to be at least 90% of normal.

Knutsen and associates compared arthroscopic microfracture and autologous chondrocyte implantation in a group of 80 patients with a solitary cartilage defect of the knee. International Cartilage Repair Society, Lysholm, Short Form-36, and Tegner scores as well as the visual analog scale for pain and biopsy specimens in 84% of patients were evaluated at 2-year follow-up. Both treatments resulted in similar decreases in pain and functional improvement. International Cartilage Repair Society macroscopic cartilage scores at second-look arthroscopy were similar and graded as nearly normal in both groups. Arthroscopic débridement was performed at second-look arthroscopy in 25% of autologous cartilage implantation patients and 10% of microfracture patients. Histologic evaluation did not show a statistical difference between

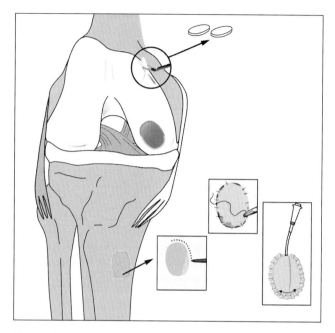

Figure 8 Autologous chondrocyte transplantation involves taking a small cartilage biopsy during an arthroscopic procedure. The chondrocytes are released from the matrix and cultured/expanded. After a period of approximately 4 weeks, an arthrotomy is performed and a periosteal soft-tissue covering or collagen sheath is sutured over the defect and sealed with fiber and glue. The cultured chondrocytes are injected into the defect under the cover.

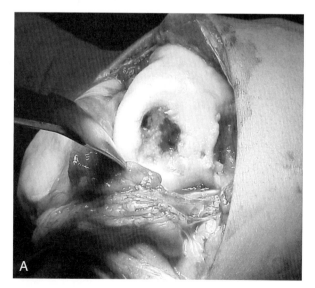
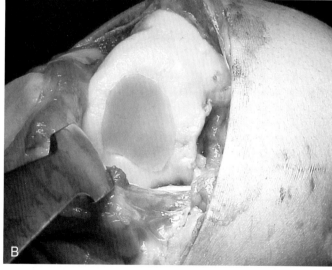

Figure 9 Surgical view of an autologous chondrocyte implantation using a matrix seeded with precultured chondrocytes. The defect in the lateral femoral condyle of the left knee is approached by arthrotomy using a previous scar **(A)**. The defect is cleaned, taking care not to perforate the calcified cartilage layer. The collagen scaffold is contoured to fit the defect **(B)**. The sidewalls are 'sealed' with fibrin glue. Depending on location and aspect of the fit, some sutures may be added to support the matrix during the first period of repair.

the groups. However, more autologous chondrocyte implantation patients had either a hyaline or a fibrohyaline cartilage repair. In contrast, most of the microfracture patients had fibrocartilage or no repair tissue (Figure 10). Knutsen and associates concluded that both techniques have acceptable short-term results. Younger patients have better results regardless of treatment choice. Short Form-36 scores were better in the microfracture patients. No relation between treatment and histologic outcome or with clinical outcome was found.

The United Kingdom Midlands development evaluation report reviewed 37 reports on autologous chondrocyte transplantation in the literature. Twenty-four could not be included, 15 of these because they were reviews or news features; the remainder lacked relevant data or contained duplicate data. All included reports were case series with a variable duration of follow-up. With one exception, patient improvement was reported (typically with a follow-up period of less than 2 years). The overall outcome of autologous chondrocyte transplantation surgery was rated 'good' or 'excellent' in approximately 70% of patients over a 2-year period, in the largest patient series. On average, 15% of patients required further arthroscopic surgical procedures. Treatment was considered a failure in 3% to 7% of patients. For comparative treatments, in 80% to 95% of patients, results were rated 'good' or 'excellent' over a 2-year period. Absenteeism and disability costs were dramatically reduced in a cohort of patients undergoing autologous chondrocyte transplantation. However, over 10 years the expected cost of treating patients with autologous chondrocyte transplantation was estimated at $16,500 compared with $4,700 for cartilage defect treatments. An estimate of the expected cost per quality-adjusted life years gained with autologous chondrocyte transplantation was $14,250 (best case $2,700, worst case $21,800).

Unsolved biologic issues associated with this approach include incomplete differentiation, lack of healing to adjacent joint cartilage, and periosteal hypertrophy or calcification, which are serious drawbacks to full regeneration of a functional articulation. Meaningful outcomes of clinical cartilage repair require 5 to 10 years of follow-up, making outcome studies more challenging, and are in conflict with the health insurers and biotechnology and pharmaceutical companies. Currently, first-generation products consist of cultured cells placed under a periosteal flap or collagen sheath. Second-generation products are in development and use a tissue engineering approach in which cells are implanted in a mechanically solid matrix, which enables minimally invasive or even arthroscopic implantation. Biotechnology companies are investigating methods to maintain implanted chondrocytes in the defect using a scaffold or injectable gel so sutures are not required during arthroscopic implantation. Alternative sources of mesenchymal stem cells are being investigated, including bone marrow, peripheral blood-derived

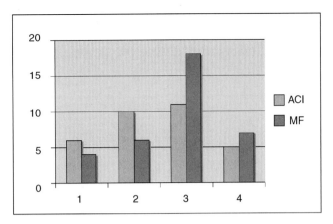

Figure 10   In a comparison of patients who underwent microfracture (MF) or autologous chondrocyte implantation (ACI), histologic scores were no different at an average of 24 months after initial surgery. Eighty-four percent of patients were available for second-look arthroscopy and histologic biopsy. A higher number of patients from the microfracture group are in the category in which mainly fibrotic tissue was seen, or no significant repair tissue was found, whereas more autologous cartilage implantation patients were scored as having hyaline or partial hyaline filling. The histologic category is represented at the x axis on the figure (group 1, predominantly hyaline; group 2, fibrocartilage hyaline mixture; group 3, fibrocartilage; group 4, no repair tissue or inadequate biopsy). (From Knutsen G, Engebretsen L, Ludvigsen, et al: Autologous chondrocyte implantation compared with microfracture in the knee: A randomized trial. J Bone and Joint Surg Am 2004;86:455-464.)

stem cell populations, and even adipose tissue. This research offers the hope of ready-to-implant materials containing a matrix and cells produced in vitro. The advantage to the patient it that only one surgical procedure needs to be performed and there is no additional intraarticular damage from a cartilage biopsy.

Tissue Engineering

For the purpose of this discussion, tissue engineering is defined as a combination of engineering science, cell biology, molecular biology, and technology. It is widely believed that biomaterials science, scaffolds or matrices for delivery of bioactive agents, and transplantation of cells will play a fundamental role in the development of tissue engineering for restoration of the cartilage and the joint surface. Tissue engineering in cartilage repair focuses on improving incorporation to the native cartilage, optimizing cartilage quality, and facilitating surgical technique by developing scaffolds and matrices that can retain and sustain the cultured cells during initial chondrogenesis and will allow arthroscopic implantation. Furthermore, bioactive factors are being explored to normalize the intraarticular environment to improve matrix synthesis and regulate ossification. Two examples of such novel developments are a resorbable scaffold for arthroscopic implantation that is impregnated with growth and differentiation factors aimed at retaining bone marrow stem cell influx initiated by microfracturing. The defect is treated by microfracture as currently performed and the implant is inserted. Cells that subsequently fill the scaffold are retained in the defect, thereby allowing the predetermined growth and differentiation factors and native platelet-derived growth factors to interact and improve cartilage repair.

Another novel concept is to mix native chondrocytes derived from the rim of the defect with marrow-derived stem cells and growth and differentiation factors in the operating room. This cell paste is immediately reimplanted into the defect using a biodegradable scaffold that provides initial biomechanical strength. In vivo and in vitro investigations of this system have shown interactions between the two cell populations and improved cartilage volume. These examples illustrate the general trend toward one-step surgical solutions.

Additional advances in cartilage repair may come from a growing understanding of the cell and tissue response to intra-articular damage. Based on the hypothesis that proteoglycans prevent mesenchymal cells from adhering to and migrating over the surfaces of partial-thickness defects, Hunziker and associates used a fibrin clot containing growth factors (basic fibroblast growth factor, transforming growth factor-β1, epidermal growth factor, insulin-like growth factor-1, and growth hormone) to furnish a matrix or scaffold for cell migration. Combining this method with enzymatic treatment of partial-thickness cartilage defects with chondroitinase resulted in an initial increase in mesenchymal cell recruitment, presumably from the synovial tissue.

Recombinant human bone morphogenetic protein-2 was examined in full-thickness osteochondral defects in adult rabbits. This treatment accelerated the reformation of subchondral bone and substantially improved the histologic appearance of the overlying articular cartilage. At 24 weeks, the thickness of the healing cartilage was 70% of that of the normal adjacent cartilage, and a new tidemark had formed between the repaired cartilage and the underlying subchondral bone.

The implantation of chondrocyte-seeded collagen scaffolds using fibrin glue is being studied in clinical practice. Solid synthetic degradable carriers are under development along with injectable biogels that may serve as cell carriers. Much attention is focused on biomaterial properties, fixation techniques, glues, and press-fit arthroscopic surgical implantation instruments. Biologic and technical approaches currently under study include the targeting of cells in specific zones (cartilage and subchondral bone) in a vertical organization with different growth factors and with the timed release of the growth factors. The concept of a two-phase scaffold (collagen matrix or copolymer) containing growth factors or chondrocytes for the healing of articular defects has been investigated; the objective is to separately influence the restoration of the subchondral bone and the cartilage.

Synthetic Implants

Would it be possible to repair an articular surface by simply filling the defect with a synthetic material? This question remains relevant because lasting biologic repair has not been achieved. As a model, dental implants show that a nonbiologic substance may provide an excellent replacement with years of adequate function in a hostile environment with extensive mechanical requirements. Scaffolds have been used alone and in combination with growth factors or cells to heal joint defects. The many substances tested include nonabsorbable materials such as carbon fiber, Dacron, and Teflon, porous metal plugs, absorbable polymers, fibrin, and collagen. Most carbon plugs or comparable materials have failed and created cartilage erosion and synovitis. Metallic and ceramic implants have been developed to fill solitary condylar defects and are under experimental use. It is conceivable that an osteochondral defect could be treated similar to dental caries with cleaning and preparation of the host tissue bed followed by filling with an implant that is molded into the defect.

Osteochondral Grafts/Transplants

Osteochondral techniques involve transplanting multiple autologous plugs from less loaded areas or whole osteochondral allografts from donors. Conceptually these techniques are straightforward; a substitute can be fitted into the defect that fills the lesion: either partially, with a series of small plugs (mosaicplasty), or completely, with a matched transplant.

Mosaicplasty

Mosaicplasty can be performed arthroscopically or in an open surgical procedure. Multiple plugs are harvested and inserted perpendicular to the joint surface (Figure 11). Hangody and associates reported on the results of 831 mosaicplasties; good to excellent results were noted in 92% of patients treated for a femoral defect, 87% for those with a tibial defect, 79% in those with patellar and trochlear defects, and 94% for patients who underwent talar procedures. Sixty-nine of 83 patients who had a subsequent arthroscopy had a congruent gliding surface, with histologic evidence of the transplant survival and filling of the donor defects with fibrous tissue. Autografts can only be harvested from a limited area within the knee, and although the authors did describe donor-related complications, this issue remains a concern (Figure 12). The donor site is usually located at the edge of the patellar groove in the region just proximal to the intercondylar notch. In cases involving reconstruction of joints other than the knee, some surgeons believe it is safe to harvest plugs from the normal knee. At this time, there are no studies demonstrating the safety of this procedure or long-term outcome of the tissue harvest. Animal studies and MRI evaluation in humans show rapid and reliable integration of the bone cylinders into the surrounding subchondral bone. The overlying

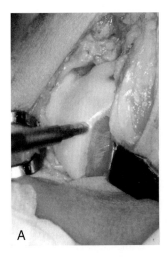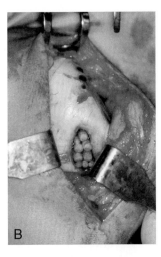

Figure 11 Surgical view of an open mosaicplasty procedure. The cylindrical osteocartilaginous plugs are harvested from a region of the knee that bears less weight, the medial femoral ridge shown here (**A**). It is imperative to align the instruments at exactly 90° angles to the articulating surface for both harvest and docking procedures to regain normal articulating surface geometry (**B**). A mosaic of osteocartilaginous plugs is made to fill the defect in the load-bearing region of the medial femoral condyle. The voids are filled by stem cells which regenerate a fibrous interface between plugs. (*Photographs courtesy of Dr J.L.C. van Susante*).

cartilage remains viable and filling between cylinders is incomplete, with clefts or fissures remaining. Sizing and depth as well as axial orientation are important and malpositioned plugs will cause early symptoms of pain, effusions, and loosening or degeneration. Outerbridge and associates reported that 10 patients with a large osteochondral defect of the weight-bearing surface of the femoral condyle had successful treatment with use of an autogenous osteochondral graft obtained from the lateral facet of the patella. At an average of 6.5 years after surgery, six patients had no symptoms and four had mild anterior knee pain. Small osteophytes were present in five patients, and two patients had mild patellofemoral incongruity. This procedure is probably useful only in carefully selected patients because of the structural alterations created at the donor site.

Allograft Osteochondral Transplants

Allograft osteochondral transplants provide the advantage of matching size and geometry of the full defect. Animal experiments on fresh osteochondral allografts have shown good repair, prolonged viability, and incorporation of the osseous and to some extent even the chondral component of the transplant. Clinical results in focal posttraumatic defects were described as good to excellent in 27 of 31 patients with a follow-up of 2 to 10 years and successful in 75% of patients at 5 years, 64% at 10 years, and 63% at 14 years. Ghazavi and associates reported clinical success in 85% of 126 knees at an average of 7.5 years after trans-

plantation of a posttraumatic osteochondral defect. Survivorship analysis revealed a 95% rate of graft survival at 5 years, an 80% rate at 10 years, a 65% rate at 15 years, and a 46% rate at 20 years. The criteria for success included patient age of 50 years or younger, a unipolar defect (involving only one side of the articulation), and normal alignment or unloading by means of an osteotomy.

Chondrocyte viability was demonstrated in fresh articular cartilage following refrigeration for 24 to 48 hours and in retrieved specimens at a maximum of 12 years after transplantation of fresh allografts. However, fresh allografts have a greater immune response compared with frozen allografts in dog experiments. Replacement of a missing portion of the joint surface with a small-fragment osteochondral allograft is a good option for significant osteochondral defects. Harvesting and storage of allografts and potential for disease transmission are challenges to widespread use.

Current understanding of cartilage repair techniques is hindered by a lack of well controlled prospective clinical trials that compare the various treatments. Minimally invasive techniques such as microfracture are the most widely accepted first-line treatment option and are the standard to surpass in developing new strategies. More advanced techniques, such as autologous chondrocyte transplantation and mosaicplasty, should be reserved for patients in whom the lower risk/morbidity first-line options fail. More conclusive efficacy data are needed before these more advanced techniques can be used with regularity.

A final approach is to perform periarticular osteotomy to improve the mechanical alignment of the joint and to unload areas of arthritic degeneration. Factors predictive of poor outcome are older age, obesity, ligament instability, overcorrection or undercorrection, and severe degeneration. In patients undergoing valgus-producing tibial osteotomies, 73% to 86% good results were observed for a 6- to 10-year period. Osteotomy is generally indicated in patients too young for arthroplasty, with angular deformities of more than 5°, limited walking distance, and pain at rest. From a review of reports of fresh osteochondral allografts performed in concert with osteotomy it is not possible to distinguish the beneficial effects of the osteotomy from those of the allograft.

Evaluation of Treatment Outcomes

Reliable treatment choices should be based on validated outcome measures and well-designed clinical trials.

Clinical Evaluation

Standards for the evaluation of a joint surface (cartilage and subchondral bone) have been developed by the International Cartilage Repair Society (http://www.cartilage.org/). The traditional knee evaluation systems have been developed and validated for the assessment of

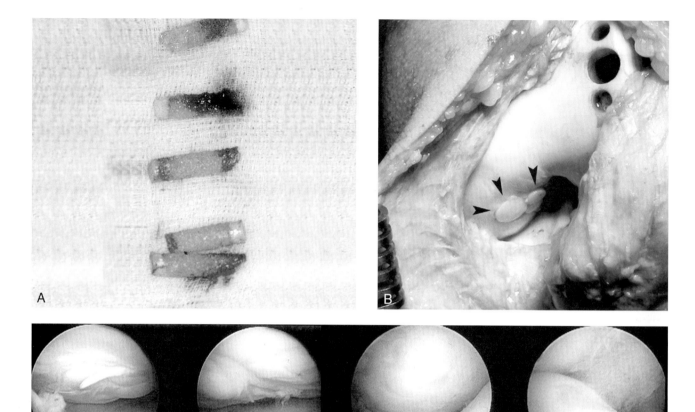

Figure 12 The technique of mosaicplasty involves harvesting various sizes of cylindrical plugs from a region that is believed to bear less weight. **A,** These plugs are inserted into the prepared region of the defect to reconstitute the weight-bearing femoral condyle, similar to the look of a cobblestone road. The bone cylinders undergo rather quick integration into the surrounding bone and fixation is mechanically sound. However, the fate of the donor region should be monitored carefully because inherent to this technique, another set of cartilage lesions is created that may contribute to disturbing joint homeostasis in this articulation and could be the cause of future degenerative disease. **B,** The donor region of the plugs were inserted to reconstruct the medial femoral condyle. The arrows indicate where the defect is surgically filled, whereas donor site-related postoperative complications could be frequently underestimated. **C,** Arthroscopic view shows the aspect of the repair and the cobblestone appearance of the articulating surface and relatively nice filling of the donor site.

osteoarthritis and knee surgery rather than for focal defects and cartilage repair. Thus it was necessary to establish specific cartilage defect scores. Until recently, the best-known arthroscopic cartilage lesion evaluation had been the Outerbridge system, which is simple but does not account for the defect depth. The goal of the International Cartilage Repair Society score is to provide a simple system that is descriptive and enables prognostic assessment of the injured cartilage. Furthermore, it allows uniform documentation of the surgical technique and other parameters that now are still quite variably reported (**Table 1**). It would be valuable if all information for classification and follow-up of patients treated for a cartilage lesion were collected using this tool.

Imaging

Radiography is required for preoperative planning and can provide valuable information about loose bodies, evi-

dence of osteoarthritis, and the loading axis of the extremity. MRI is the most suitable noninvasive imaging modality. Newer MRI techniques have proved to have more than 95% sensitivity for detecting focal cartilage lesions. Abnormalities are evident in the contrast between normal and damaged tissue and MRI detects the high water content in normal cartilage. Brittberg and Winalski previously recommended fast spin-echo (with or without fat suppression) and/or fat-suppressed (or water-selective excitation) spoiled gradient echo image acquisitions, which should be combined with high spatial resolution acquisition parameters because the tissue is thin, usually less than 4 mm, and the articular surfaces are curved, leading to "partial volume" artifacts. Even with the improved resolution through increased magnet strength and use of better detection coils, the ability to accurately measure articular cartilage thickness, the depth or size of a defect, or the presence of a fissure in clinical practice is

Table 1   International Cartilage Repair Society Grading Scale for Cartilage Repair Surgery

Criteria	Degree of Defect Repair	Points
I Protocol A*	In level with surrounding cartilage	4
	75% repair of defect depth	3
	50% repair of defect depth	2
	25% repair of defect depth	1
	0% repair of defect depth	0
I Protocol B†	100% survival of initially grafted surface	4
	75% survival of initially grafted surface	3
	50% survival of initially grafted surface	2
	25% survival of initially grafted surface	1
	0% survival of initially grafted surface	0
II Integration to Border Zone	Complete integration with surrounding cartilage	4
	Demarcating border < 1 mm	3
	¾ of graft integrated, ¼ with a notable border > 1 mm width	2
	½ of graft integrated with surrounding cartilage, ½ with a notable border > 1 mm	1
	From no contact to ¼ of graft integrated with surrounding cartilage	0
III Macroscopic Appearance	Intact smooth surface	4
	Fibrillated surface	3
	Small, scattered fissures or cracks	2
	Several, small or few but large fissures	1
	Total degeneration of grafted area	0
Overall Repair Assessment	Grade I = Normal	12 P
	Grade II = Nearly normal	11-8 P
	Grade III = Abnormal	7-4 P
	Grade IV = Severely abnormal	3-1 P

* Protocol A: cartilage biopsy location: autologous chondrocyte implantation; periosteal or perichondrial transplantation; subchondral drilling; microfracturing; carbon fiber implants; others
† Protocol B: cartilage biopsy location: mosaicplasty; OAT; osteochondral allografts; others
(Reproduced with permission from International Cartilage Repair Society.)

somewhat limited. However, these techniques are available in research settings and, based on previous developments, are likely to be used clinically. Future evolution of MRI protocols and postprocessing computer power may allow the capability to image cartilage at the cellular level. These techniques provide tools to determine zonal characteristics within the cartilage and visualize collagen fibril organization. Biochemical composition and the special distribution of matrix composition can be made accessible for evaluation. Morphologic aspects such as cartilage volume, curvature, and thickness can be measured, and changes over time or following interventions also can be measured. MRI technology may alter the approach to cartilage repair by detecting subclinical changes and enabling earlier decisions regarding treatment.

Arthroscopic Evaluation

Arthroscopic examination permits assessment of the anatomic integrity of the joint. Interobserver and intraobserver variability was shown to be considerable even for parameters such as defect size and volume. Tools including mechanical indentation, electrical deformation, high-resolution B-mode ultrasound, and optical coherence

tomography were developed to permit more objective measurements to quantify cartilage degeneration and repair. Measurements of electrical streaming potentials or mechanical properties of the cartilage can be related to the status of the matrix and its functional integrity. It is hoped that refinement and standardization of these instruments and the determination of normal values would eventually provide a method to determine the quality of damaged or repaired cartilage and correlate these data to a clinical prognosis and treatment strategy. Currently there is no consensus or common practice on mechanical indentation or other methods of evaluating mechanical integrity of the repair tissue.

Histologic Evaluation

There is controversy regarding the relationship between the histologic appearance of the repair tissue and clinical outcome. This controversy is not surprising considering the unpredictable relationship between the radiographic appearance of a damaged joint surface and clinical symptoms. However, a better understanding will develop from the uniform application of validated parameters for histologic assessment of cartilage repair. Many cartilage repair scoring systems have been described; the score by O'Driscoll is frequently used albeit with some modifications. It was shown to have high intraobserver and inter-observer reliability and is relatively simple to use. An added advantage is the ability to analyze subsets of evaluation categories. Reproducibility and objectivity of histologic evaluation may be improved by semiautomated histomorphometric analysis, which has proven feasible with a standardized (safranin O / fast green) staining technique. The criteria are being developed by the International Cartilage Repair Society and is expected to become standard in the near future (**Table 2**).

Table 2   Cartilage Repair Score by O'Driscoll and Associates

Characteristics	Score
Nature of Predominant Tissue	
Cellular morphology	
Hyaline articular cartilage	4
Incompletely differentiated mesenchyme	2
Fibrous tissue or bone	0
Safranin O staining of the matrix	
Normal or nearly normal	3
Moderate	2
Slight	1
None	0
Structural Characteristics	
Surface regularity	
Smooth and intact	3
Superficial horizontal lamination	2
Fissures 25% to 100% of the thickness	1
Severe disruption, including fibrillation	0
Structural integrity	
Normal	2
Slight disruption, including cysts	1
Severe disintegration	0
Thickness	
100% of normal adjacent cartilage	2
50% to 100% of normal cartilage	1
0% to 50% of normal cartilage	0
Bonding to the adjacent cartilage	
Bonded at both ends of graft	2
Bonded at one end, or partially at both ends	1
Not bonded	0
Freedom From Cellular Changes of Degeneration	
Hypocellularity	
Normal cellularity	3
Slight hypocellularity	2
Moderate hypocellularity	1
Severe hypocellularity	0
Chondrocyte clustering	
No clusters	2
< 25% of the cells	1
25% to 100% of the cells	0
Freedom From Degenerative Changes in Adjacent Cartilage	
Normal cellularity, no clusters, normal staining	3
Normal cellularity, mild clusters, moderate staining	2
Mild or moderate hypocellularity, slight staining	1
Severe hypocellularity, poor or no staining	0

(Copyright Shawn W. O'Driscoll, PhD, MD.)

Summary

The field of cartilage repair has witnessed a revolutionary expansion of activity over the past 10 years. Because of advances in tissue engineering, there is optimism about ongoing improvements in patient care. Current methods such as microfracture, chondrocyte transplantation and mosaicplasty improve patient outcome. However, carefully designed and executed clinical trials comparing the results of different treatments are lacking, as are long-term follow-up studies. Major advances in cartilage repair may take many years to either develop or to have their respective roles determined. Physicians should exercise caution and patience in the pursuit of the long-term goal of cartilage repair and prevention of arthritis, while realizing the immediate concern is relief of pain and suffering.

Selected Bibliography

Articular Cartilage Damage

Bobic V, Noble J: Articular cartilage: To repair or not to repair. *J Bone Joint Surg Br* 2000;82:165-166.

Buckwalter JA: Articular cartilage injuries. *Clin Orthop Relat Res* 2002;402:21-37.

Buckwalter JA: Integration of science into orthopaedic practice: Implications for solving the problem of articular cartilage repair. *J Bone Joint Surg Am* 2003; 85-A(suppl 2):1-7.

Jackson DW, Lalor PA, Aberman HM, Simon TM: Spontaneous repair of full-thickness defects of articular cartilage in a goat model: A preliminary study. *J Bone Joint Surg Am* 2001;83-A:53-64.

Jakob RP, Mainil-Varlet P, Gautier E: Isolated articular cartilage lesion: Repair or regeneration. *Osteoarthritis Cartilage* 2001;9(suppl A):S3-S5.

Kurz B, Jin M, Patwari P, Cheng DM, Lark MW, Grodzinsky AJ: Biosynthetic response and mechanical properties of articular cartilage after injurious compression. *J Orthop Res* 2001;19:1140-1146.

O'Driscoll SW: Preclinical cartilage repair: Current status and future perspectives. *Clin Orthop Relat Res* 2001;(suppl 391):S397-S401.

Walker EA, Verner A, Flannery CR, Archer CW: Cellular responses of embryonic hyaline cartilage to experimental wounding in vitro. *J Orthop Res* 2000;18:25-34.

Natural Healing Response

Buckwalter JA, Mankin H: Articular cartilage: Degeneration and osteoarthrosis, repair, regeneration, and transplantation. *Instr Course Lect* 1998;47:487-504.

Buckwalter JA, Mankin HJ: Articular cartilage: Tissue design and chondrocyte-matrix interactions. *Instr Course Lect* 1998;47:477-486.

Frisbie DD, Oxford JT, Southwood L, et al: Early events in cartilage repair after subchondral bone microfracture. *Clin Orthop Relat Res* 2003;407:215-227.

Hunziker E, Quinn T: Surgical removal of articular cartilage leads to loss of chondrocytes from cartilage bordering the wound edge. *J Bone Joint Surg Am* 2003;85-A(suppl 2):85-92.

Hunziker EB, Driesang IM, Morris EA: Chondrogenesis in cartilage repair is induced by members of the transforming growth factor-beta superfamily. *Clin Orthop Relat Res* 2001;(suppl 391):S171-S181.

Martin J, Buckwalter J: The role of chondrocyte senescence in the pathogenesis of osteoarthritis and in limiting cartilage repair. *J Bone Joint Surg Am* 2003;85-A(suppl 2):106-110.

Shapiro F, Koide S, Glimcher MJ: Cell origin and differentiation in the repair of full-thickness defects of articular cartilage. *J Bone Joint Surg Am* 1993;75:532-533.

The Concept of Joint Homeostasis

Buschmann MD, Kim YJ, Wong M, Frank E, Hunziker EB, Grodzinsky AJ: Stimulation of aggrecan synthesis in cartilage explants by cyclic loading is localized to regions of high interstitial fluid flow. *Arch Biochem Biophys* 1999;366:1-7.

Dye SF: The knee as a biologic transmission with an envelope of function: A theory. *Clin Orthop Relat Res* 1996;(suppl 325):10-18.

Guilak F, Butler DL, Goldstein SA: Functional tissue engineering: The role of biomechanics in articular cartilage repair. *Clin Orthop Relat Res* 2001;(suppl 391):S295-S305.

Hogervorst T, Pels Rijcken TH, Rucker D, van der Hart CP, Taconis WK: Changes in bone scans after anterior cruciate ligament reconstruction: A prospective study. *Am J Sports Med* 2002;30:823-833.

Rodrigo JJ, Steadman JR, Syftestad G, Benton H, Silliman J: Effects of human knee synovial fluid on chondrogenesis in vitro. *Am J Knee Surg* 1995;8:124-129.

Saris DB, Dhert WJ, Verbout AJ: Joint homeostasis: The discrepancy between old and fresh defects in cartilage repair. *J Bone Joint Surg Br* 2003;85:1067-1076.

Yang KG, Saris DB, Geuze RE, et al: Altered in vitro chondrogenic properties of chondrocytes harvested from unaffected cartilage in osteoarthritic joints. *Osteoarthritis Cartilage* 2006;14:561-570.

Treatment Options for Damaged or Lost Cartilage

Ahsan T, Sah R: Biomechanics of integrative cartilage repair. *Osteoarthritis Cartilage* 1999;7:29-40.

Fond J, Rodin D, Ahmad S, Nirschl RP: Arthroscopic debridement for the treatment of osteoarthritis of the knee: 2- and 5-year results. *Arthroscopy* 2002;18:829-834.

Grande DA, Halberstadt C, Naughton G, Schwartz R, Manji R: Evaluation of matrix scaffolds for tissue engineering of articular cartilage grafts. *J Biomed Mater Res* 1997;34:211-220.

Gross AE: Repair of cartilage defects in the knee. *J Knee Surg* 2002;15:167-169.

Hangody L, Feczko P, Bartha L, Bodo G, Kish G: Mosaicplasty for the treatment of articular defects of the knee and ankle. *Clin Orthop Relat Res* 2001;(suppl 391):S328-S336.

Peterson L, Minas T, Brittberg M, Nilsson A, Sjogren-Jansson E, Lindahl A: Two- to 9-year outcome after autologous chondrocyte transplantation of the knee. *Clin Orthop Relat Res* 2000;374:212-234.

Wakitani S, Imoto K, Yamamoto T, Saito M, Murata N, Yoneda M: Human autologous culture expanded bone marrow mesenchymal cell transplantation for repair of cartilage defects in osteoarthritic knees. *Osteoarthritis Cartilage* 2002;10:199-206.

Strategies for Cartilage Repair

Angermann P, Riegels-Nielsen P, Pederson H: Osteochondritis dissecans of the femoral condyle treated with periosteal transplantation: Poor outcome in 14 patients followed for 6-9 years. *Acta Orthop Scand* 1998; 69:595-597.

Bentley G, Greer RB III: Homotransplantation of isolated epiphyseal and articular cartilage chondrocytes into joint surfaces of rabbits. *Nature* 1971;230:385-388.

Bert JM, Maschka K: The arthroscopic treatment of unicompartmental gonarthrosis: A five-year follow-up study of abrasion arthroplasty plus arthroscopic debridement and arthroscopic debridement alone. *Arthroscopy* 1989;5:25-32

Brittberg M, Tallheden T, Sjogren-Jansson B, Lindahl A, Peterson L: Autologous chondrocytes used for articular cartilage repair: An update. *Clin Orthop Relat Res* 2001;(suppl 391):S337-S348.

Engkvist O, Johansson SH, Ohlsen L, Skoog T: Reconstruction of articular cartilage using autologous perichondrial grafts: A preliminary report. *Scand J Plast Reconstr Surg* 1975;9:203-206.

Ghazavi MT, Pritzker KP, Davis AM, Gross AE: Fresh osteochondral allografts for post-traumatic osteochondral defects of the knee. *J Bone Joint Surg Br* 1997;79: 1008-1013.

Hangody L, Fules P: Autologous osteochondral mosaicplasty for the treatment of full-thickness defects of weight-bearing joints. *J Bone Joint Surg Am* 2003; 85-A(suppl 2):25-32.

Homminga GN, Bulstra SK, Bouwmeester PS, van der Linden AG: Perichondral grafting for cartilage lesions of the knee. *J Bone Joint Surg Br* 1990;72:1003-1007.

Hunziker EB: Articular cartilage repair: Basic science and clinical progress. A review of the current status and prospects. *Osteoarthritis Cartilage* 2002;10:432-463.

Knutsen G, Engerbretsen L, Ludvigsen TC, et al: Autologous chondrocyte implantation compared with microfracture in the knee: A randomized trial. *J Bone Joint Surg Am* 2004;86:455-464.

Outerbridge HK, Outerbridge RE, Smith DE: Osteochondral defects in the knee: A treatment using lateral patella autografts. *Clin Orthop Relat Res* 2000;377:145-151.

Rand JA: The role of arthroscopy in osteoarthritis of the knee. *Arthroscopy* 1991;7:358-363.

Steadman JR, Briggs KK, Rodrigo JJ, Kocher MS, Gill TJ, Rodkey WG: Outcomes of microfracture for traumatic chondral defects of the knee: Average 11-year follow-up. *Arthroscopy* 2003;19:477-484.

Evaluation of Treatment Outcomes

Brittberg M, Winalski C: Evaluation of cartilage injuries and repair. *J Bone Joint Surg Am* 2003;85-A (suppl 2):58-69.

Bouwmeester PS, Kuijer R, Homminga GN, Bulstra SK, Geesink RG: A retrospective analysis of two independent prospective cartilage repair studies: Autogenous perichondral grafting versus subchondral drilling 10 years post-surgery. *J Orthop Res* 2002;20:267-273.

Burstein D, Gray M: New MRI techniques for imaging cartilage. *J Bone Joint Surg Am* 2003;85-A(suppl 2):70-77.

Lammentausta E, Kiviranta P, Nissi MJ, et al: T2 relaxation time and delayed gadolinium-enhanced MRI of cartilage (dGEMRIC) of human patellar cartilage at 1.5 T and 9.4 T: Relationships with tissue mechanical properties. *J Orthop Res* 2006;24:366-374.

Lee CR, Grodzinsky AJ, Hsu HP, Martin SD, Spector M: Effects of harvest and selected cartilage repair procedures on the physical and biochemical properties of articular cartilage in the canine knee. *J Orthop Res* 2000;18:790-799.

Mainil-Varlet P, Aigner T, Brittberg M, et al: Histological assessment of cartilage repair. *J Bone Joint Surg Am* 2003;85-A(suppl 2):45-57.

Moojen DJ, Saris DB, Auw Yang KG, Dhert WJ, Verbout AJ: The correlation and reproducibility of histological scoring systems in cartilage repair. *Tissue Eng* 2002;8:627-634.

Potter HG, Linklater JM, Allen AA, Hannafin JA, Haas SB: Magnetic resonance imaging of articular cartilage in the knee: An evaluation with use of fast-spin-echo imaging. *J Bone Joint Surg Am* 1998;80:1276-1284.

Steadman JR, Rodkey WG, Briggs KK: Microfracture to treat full-thickness chondral defects: Surgical technique, rehabilitation, and outcomes. *J Knee Surg* 2002;15:170-176.

Chapter 20

The Biologic Response to Orthopaedic Implants

Yousef Abu-Amer, PhD
John C. Clohisy, MD

Introduction

Total joint arthroplasty for end-stage degenerative disease of the joints is an extremely effective surgical intervention. Unfortunately, wear debris, primarily generated from the prosthetic joint articular surface, is the major factor that limits the survivorship of joint implants. Wear debris results in the subtle progression of bone destruction around the implant that typically produces no clinical signs and symptoms until the late stages of failure. Although the basis of tissue destruction is accepted as the biologic response to implant debris, this response is the outcome of multiple factors, including physical and biologic components. This chapter focuses on the makeup of the biologic response. The acute and chronic biology of implant fixation and the effects of implant debris both locally and systemically are reviewed. Emphasis is given to host response, inflammatory processes, and mediators of the response. Therapeutic approaches to address certain aspects of this biologic and inflammatory response following reconstructive surgery are also summarized.

Implant Fixation and Osteointegration

The initial or early aspects of implant fixation are critical in establishing a durable interface with host bone that will withstand physical and biologic demands over long periods. As total joint arthroplasty surgery is used to treat younger, more active patients, these demands continue to

increase for improving implant fixation and longevity. Clearly, the local biology at the implant-bone interface is extremely important in optimizing implant stability and durability of fixation. The two major modes of implant fixation with respect to arthroplasty surgery include cemented fixation, in which polymethylmethacrylate (PMMA) acts as an adhesive between prosthesis and bone, and cementless fixation, in which bony ingrowth and/or ongrowth provides biologic attachment to the skeleton. There are several factors involved in the integrity and longevity of cemented and cementless fixation, including host bone quality, surgical technique, implant alignment, implant characteristics, implant wear issues, adaptive remodeling around the prosthesis, and the local biology associated with the implant-bone interface. Primary implant fixation is achieved at the time of implant insertion, and secondary fixation results from repair and bone remodeling similar to fracture healing. With respect to implant fixation, three phases of healing have been described, including an initial phase of injury or destruction, a repair phase characterized by osteointegration, and a phase of stabilization at the bone-implant interface. The final phase of stabilization is dynamic in that this interface is subject to alterations from load transfer and the local biologic consequences of implant particulate debris over long periods.

At the local level, preparation of bone for prosthetic implantation and cement application results in a series of biologic events that characterize the acute or injury phase at the bone-cement interface. In addition to the initial mechanical and vascular injury of prosthetic implantation and cementation, thermal and chemical insult from PMMA polymerization may also contribute to the initial tissue necrosis. Thus, the biology of early cemented implant fixation is characterized by an injury phase resulting from implant bed preparation and the application of bone cement. The mechanical, vascular, thermal, and chemical aspects of this injury phase lead to local tissue necrosis at the cement-bone interface. In the repair phase, a fibrous membrane is formed at the interface, vascularization is re-established, and tissue regeneration, including osteointegration, progresses. After maturation of initial osteointegration at the cement-bone interface, the quality and integrity of this interface is modulated by various factors, including patient and host bone characteristics, component design, cement technique, and implant wear debris.

In long-term fixation, the mechanical environment of periprosthetic bone after component implantation is altered and can result in secondary bone adaptation. This biologic response of surrounding bone to the prosthesis is called adaptive remodeling. Bone remodeling around well-fixed cemented implants has been described via autopsy retrieval studies. The findings were characterized by direct apposition of host bone to the cement and rare intervening fibrous tissue. A dense shell of bone or new cortex formed around the cement mantle and was attached to the surrounding cortical bone by trabecular struts. There was substantial osteoporosis and thinning of the adjacent femoral cortex. Despite osteointegration of the cement mantle, debonding of the femoral stem and cement mantle fractures were evident. These findings suggest that mechanical failure at the implant-cement interface is an important factor in late aseptic loosening of femoral implants. This major periprosthetic bone remodeling combined with mechanical failure at the implant-cement interface are clinically relevant and make the periprosthetic bone more susceptible to late mechanical failure and implant particle-driven osteolysis.

In addition to adaptive bone remodeling around cemented prostheses, implant wear and particulate debris generation assume a major role in the pathophysiology of aseptic loosening. This has been delineated in studies with cemented acetabular components that defined late aseptic loosening as a progressive three-dimensional resorption of bone at the cement-bone interface. This progressive resorption of bone is associated with particulate debris and a macrophage inflammatory response that results in resorption of bone at the cement-bone interface. This resorption can compromise the mechanical stability of the implant. Thus, long-term fixation of cemented implants can be compromised by a combination of mechanisms, including adaptive bone remodeling, mechanical failure of the implant-cement interface, and progressive implant debris-induced bone resorption at the cement-bone interface.

Although cemented implant fixation continues to be an extremely effective option for hip and knee replacements, certain cemented designs have resulted in aseptic implant loosening over time. In the 1980s, various cementless designs were introduced in an attempt to improve the durability and longevity of total joint arthroplasty fixation. Cementless implants are designed to achieve fixation by osseous ingrowth and/or ongrowth to the prosthesis. Theoretically, this type of biologic fixation should surpass that obtained with cemented implants by establishing a living, functional interface between the implant and bone. The quality of biologic fixation with a cementless implant is dependent on various factors, including surgical technique, implant design, initial implant stability, bone quality, and patient-related factors. The initial or early biologic response around the implant is extremely important in establishing bony ingrowth and implant stability for long-term fixation.

As with cemented implants, the early phase of cementless fixation is characterized by initial injury and repair. After initial injury, the implant-bone interface undergoes intramembranous bone formation and under favorable conditions results in osteointegration of the implant. The implant material composition, ingrowth surface pore size (or surface characteristics), initial implant stability, and bony apposition are all important factors in optimizing osteointegration. Additionally, more recent efforts have focused on enhancing cementless fixation with the application of osteoinductive bioactive factors, osteoconductive inorganic matrix, and the use of novel biomaterials.

Various ingrowth surfaces and materials have been used for cementless fixation. The most commonly used implants have included cobalt-chromium and titanium sintered beads, titanium fiber metal, titanium plasma spray, and diffusion-bonded titanium. In general, these implant surfaces have provided osseous ingrowth or ongrowth and can provide biologic fixation and good clinical function at midterm to long-term follow-up.

Factors Enhancing Implant Osteointegration

Pore size of the bone ingrowth surface is an important factor in optimizing the osteointegration potential of an implant. Various studies have shown that a pore size of 100 to 500 µm results in consistent bony ingrowth and a relatively rapid enhancement of fixation strength. Small-pore bony ingrowth surfaces did not allow for uniform tissue calcification, whereas large-pore bony ingrowth surfaces resulted in more areas of a persistent fibrous membrane. In addition to pore size, initial implant stability and bone apposition are essential for reliable bone ingrowth. Excessive micromotion at the implant-bone interface has a negative impact on osteointegration. The literature suggests that micromotion of 150 µm or more is likely to result in a fibrous tissue ingrowth with suboptimal biologic fixation.

Apposition of the implant to host bone is an important determinant of osteointegration. Animal studies assessing fixation strength and bone ingrowth using uncoated and hydroxyapatite-coated implants showed that interface attachment strength and bone ingrowth were positively correlated with decreasing initial gap size (< 1.0 mm). In humans, the biologic capacity to fill gaps with ingrowth may not be as great. In one study, patients undergoing staged bilateral total knee arthroplasty had porous cylindrical implants placed in the contralateral knee at the time of the first replacement. The implants were either titanium control or hydroxyapatite-coated. During the staged, contralateral replacement, the implants were harvested and subsequently analyzed at an average of 7 weeks. Although short term, these experiments suggest that porous-coated and porous with hydroxyapatite-coated implants placed in the distal femur frequently fail to fill 50- to 500-µm gaps with bone ingrowth. These gaps were frequently ingrown with a fibrous connective tissue. Thus, in humans, osseous ingrowth spanning gaps greater than 50 µm may be unreliable.

Despite consistent ingrowth and good clinical function of contemporary cementless components, there is a need for improved implants that will enable a more rapid and extensive osteointegration. Thus, new biomaterials and alterations of current biomaterials to enhance implant fixation characteristics are continually being identified. Better implant design will result in more rapid and extensive ingrowth and should create an improved barrier to particulate debris migration. This will slow the process of secondary particle osteolysis and aseptic loosening.

Porous tantalum, a highly porous biomaterial with unique physical, mechanical, and tissue ingrowth properties, is a relatively new biomaterial that is composed of a low-density vitreous carbon skeleton with a repeating dodecahedron array of pores interconnected by smaller openings. Commercially pure tantalum is deposited on the carbon skeleton to create a porous metal construct. The porous tantalum is 75% to 80% porous by volume, and the average two-dimensional porosity is 430 µm. Most notably, this material has a microtexture that is conductive to bone formation, a low modulus of elasticity that is consistent with improved load transfer to bone, and a higher coefficient of friction for improved initial implant stability. The theoretic benefit of porous tantalum is an improved implant-bone interface that decreases the effective joint space, increases the resistance to the progression of particle osteolysis, and improves the load transfer to surrounding bone.

Corundum-blasted implants constitute another group of cementless components that have received more attention over the past decade. These titanium implants have a microtextured surface created by blasting with small particles similar to corundum. For total hip replacement implants, the surface roughness is usually in the range of 3 to 5 µm. These roughened titanium surfaces stimulate bone formation and directly activate osteoblast expression of prostaglandin E_2 (PGE_2) and transforming growth factor (TGF)-β1. Most importantly, rough titanium surfaces enhance osteoblast differentiation as evidenced by increased production of alkaline phosphatase and osteocal-

cin. In addition to osteointegration by direct bone ongrowth, the femoral implants are made with a double-wedge taper design that achieves initial implant stability.

As potentially advantageous biomaterials continue to be developed and investigated, bioactive surfaces and bioactive factors are also being developed to accelerate and amplify osteointegration of orthopaedic implants. Perhaps the most extensively studied surface augmentation technique is hydroxyapatite coating of the implants. Treatment of implants with an osteoconductive coating of hydroxyapatite has been shown to be efficacious in experimental as well as midterm clinical studies. Various animal models have demonstrated improved ingrowth capacity of hydroxyapatite-coated implant surfaces when compared with that of noncoated implants. Clinically, hydroxyapatite coating of cementless femoral stems has provided consistent ingrowth and good function in midterm follow-up studies.

In addition to improving the osteoconductive characteristics of implants, increasing the bone-forming capacity of the implant-bone microenvironment is another strategy that is being developed to improve osteointegration. Theoretically, increasing the number of osteoprogenitor cells will enhance bone ingrowth at this interface. In experimental models, cell-coated implants demonstrated more rapid and more extensive ingrowth into implant channels when compared with that of noncoated implants. Therefore, cellular augmentation of implant surfaces for enhanced biologic activity is an alternative biotechnology that deserves additional investigation.

As the availability of recombinant proteins becomes more commonplace, osteoinductive factors will be used to enhance implant-bone osseointegration. In this regard, studies have shown that TGF-β1 and bone morphogenetic proteins (BMPs) exert osteoinductive activity at the implant interface. Specifically, human recombinant BMP-2 has been shown to enhance the osteointegration of ectopic porous-coated titanium implants in rat and rabbit models. Thus, biologic factors can be successfully applied to implant surfaces for enhanced osteointegration and fixation in experimental models. The clinical application of these technologies will likely be investigated over the next decade.

Adaptive Bone Loss and Potential Therapies

Adaptive bone loss refers to changes in bone mass and geometry in response to alterations in mechanical forces and environment. Body disuse that results in bone loss or increased bone mass following exercise is a representative example.

During growth and development, the skeleton optimizes its architecture by subtle adaptations to mechanical loads. The mechanisms for adaptation involve a multistep process of cellular mechanotransduction including mechanocoupling (the conversion of mechanical forces into local mechanical signals such as fluid shear stresses that initiate a response by bone cells), biochemical coupling (the transduction of a mechanical signal to a biochemical response involving pathways within the cell membrane and cytoskeleton), cell-to-cell signaling from the sensor cells (probably osteocytes and bone lining cells) to effector cells (osteoblasts or osteoclasts) using signaling molecules such as prostaglandins and nitric oxide, and the effector response (bone formation or resorption to cause appropriate architectural changes).

Structural changes can be predicted based on three fundamental rules: (1) bone adaptation is driven by dynamic rather than static loading, (2) extending the loading duration has a diminishing effect on further bone adaptation, and (3) bone cells accommodate to a mechanical loading environment that makes them less responsive to routine or customary loading signals.

Exercise helps maintain bone mass and counter osteoporosis, but the relationship between mechanical force and bone formation is complex. In this respect, short periods of exercise, with 4 to 8 hours of rest between them, provide a more effective osteogenic stimulus than a single sustained session of exercise. Several studies concluded that low-magnitude, high-frequency mechanical stimuli are anabolic as demonstrated in trabecular bone in children and by prevention of postmenopausal bone loss. However, studies also suggest that the repetitive coordinated bone loading associated with habitual activity may have little effect on the preservation of bone mass and may even reduce the osteogenic potential of an otherwise highly osteogenic stimulus.

Implants introduced into the skeleton often alter the mechanical properties of bone and ultimately change the load to the host bone. These changes have been called stress shielding and are believed to contribute to net bone loss. The severity of stress shielding is determined by the relative stiffness of the implant and the host bone. The geometry and material properties of the implant and host bone are the factors that determine the degree of stress shielding. Cobalt-chromium alloy implants have a higher modulus of elasticity and cause more stress shielding than similarly shaped titanium alloy implants. Additionally, the relative placement of the implant within the host bone and the diameter of implant relative to host bone play a crucial role in determining the severity of stress shielding. Implants placed centrally and small diameter implants cause less stress shielding.

It appears that adaptive bone remodeling or loss is not influenced by the type of porous coating. In fact, proximally coated implants do not appear to protect against bone loss when compared with fully coated implants; moreover, noncoated implants cause as much proximal bone loss over time as coated implants. It can be deduced, therefore, that an effective method to protect against long-term bone loss after total hip arthroplasty requires the reduction of stress shielding by reducing the stiffness of the implant. Conversely, loading and osteogenic methods could be applied to increase the structural stiffness of the host bone and thereby improve its biologic compatibility with the implant.

Bone is a living tissue that undergoes changes reflective of cellular processes that dictate these alterations. It should be recognized that adaptive bone responses to mechanical and other stresses are governed by cellular responses. Cells of the osteocyte/osteoblast (mesenchymal) and osteoclast (hematopoietic) networks are best placed to appreciate mechanical strain. Strain-related responses induce major changes in the function and fate of these cells, which vary as a result of bone formation, bone resorption, and a reduced rate of apoptosis. Thus, attention should be given to the mechanistic regulation of these cells under bone-adaptive processes. Alternatively, the inhibition of bone loss and remodeling could be achieved through inhibition of osteoclasts. In addition to bisphosphonates, a new generation of osteoclast inhibitors, such as osteoprotegerin (OPG), receptor activator of nuclear factor-kappaB (RANK)-Fc, etanercept, and selective inhibitors of tyrosine kinases are now available. These agents have been shown to be effective in animal models, and some have shown promise in arresting bone loss in humans.

Response to Implant Debris and Inflammatory Bone Loss
Factors Perpetuating Periprosthetic Bone Resorption

Although implants are believed to be biologically inert, the soft tissue surrounding or in the vicinity of the implant is impacted by the foreign body. Generation of wear debris occurs immediately and long after implant insertion. The causes for this particle accumulation vary from micromotion to corrosion and oxidative reactions. In general, the initial response is a localized anti-inflammatory response that is characterized by the formation of fibrous tissue that encapsulates the implant. Often, synovial fluid and a thick synovial lining membrane is formed, and a granulomatous tissue is established. Immunohistochemical studies of these tissues show an abundance of macrophages, fibroblasts, and lymphocytes. However, aseptic loosening is characterized by poorly vascularized connective tissue dominated by fibroblasts and macrophages. Subsequently, secretion of proinflammatory factors, gelatinases, and proteases contribute to periprosthetic osteolysis and failure of the joint implant (**Figure 1**).

Wear debris is formed at normal joint articulations, modular interfaces, and nonarticulating interfaces. Although a wide range of particles has been identified, most particles are less than 5 μm in diameter and randomly shaped. Different studies have suggested that the cellular response to particles may vary with size, shape, composi-

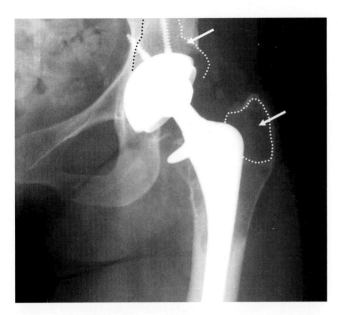

Figure 1 AP radiograph of the right hip of a 60-year-old woman 7 years after undergoing cementless primary total hip replacement shows inflammatory osteolysis; the periarticular and femoral bone loss (dotted lines and arrows) is the result of polyethylene wear and particle activation of the osteolytic cascade.

tion, charge, and number of particles. Furthermore, it was proposed that particle phagocytosis constitutes an important component of the cellular response to implants; hence, the size of these particles is significant. In this regard, several reports have estimated that particles ranging from 0.2 to 10 μm in diameter are phagocytized by macrophages. In vitro studies with macrophage cultures have clearly indicated that smaller PMMA (< 20 μm) and polyethylene particles elicited a significantly greater inflammatory cytokine response, which is evident by increased release of tumor necrosis factor (TNF), interleukin (IL)-1, IL-6, PGE_2, matrix metalloproteinases, and other factors. Although particle phagocytosis has been emphasized as a critical component of this biologic response, recent studies indicate that direct particle-cell surface interactions are adequate to activate osteoclastogenic signaling pathways in human macrophages.

The rate at which particles accumulate is also considered an important factor for the occurrence of osteolysis. Osteolysis was found in different studies to be associated with increasing wear rates. Specifically, areas of increased lysis were found to contain significantly larger concentrations of particles (of similar size and shape) when compared with nonosteolytic regions of the loosened implant at revision. These observations were further supported by findings from in vitro studies in which the induction of transcriptional activity and cytokine release were particle-dose–dependent. The effect of particle concentration on various cell types was also reported. In primary human monocytes, the release of cytokines, PGE_2, and hexosaminidase depended on the size, concentration, and

surface area of particles. Other studies using macrophage cell lines reported dose-dependent apoptosis of the cells when treated with ceramic and polyethylene particles. Toxic effects were reported in studies using other cells such as synovial fibroblasts and chondrocytes treated with increasing doses of cobalt and vanadium. Clearly, the particulate debris load and particle composition are important factors in the osteolytic process. Therefore, ongoing investigations and clinical use of alternative bearing surfaces are critical for identifying optimal bearing materials that will minimize particle generation over time. Ceramic, highly cross-linked polyethylene and metal-on-metal articulations have shown promise for markedly reducing the production of wear particles.

Biologic and mechanical factors have been suggested in the early and late stages of the development of osteolysis after joint arthroplasty. Inflammatory reactions develop at early stages as part of the healing process, including primarily increased circulation and elevated fluid levels toward the affected tissue. In addition, host defense mechanisms, which include massive recruitment of macrophages and lymphocytes, are summoned to the injury site. Perhaps the most complicating aspect of this reaction is secretion of a variety of cytokines and factors by these and other cells, leading to adverse effects over time. The cellular and associated inflammatory responses are not restricted to the initial healing process, but seem to occur during progression and late stages of periprosthetic osteolysis.

Several cofactors have been described to facilitate propagation of inflammatory and eventual osteolytic events. One major component relates to poor implant fixation and subsequent motion. In this regard, ample evidence indicates that the loosening of implants is associated with excessive motion and physical strains, which result in accelerated release of particulate debris. This is evident by the progressive nature of bone resorption around loose screws that is associated with wear debris. Compelling findings in recent years indicate that the release of such debris leads to inflammatory responses that ultimately result in bone loss. Evidence implicating particulate debris as a major component of osteolysis is derived from studies with animal models exposed to particulate debris, studies with macrophages and osteoclasts in vitro and in vivo, and evaluation of osteolysis and cofactors using clinically successful and failed total joint prostheses. The amounts of particulate debris around implants usually provide a fair correlation with the degree of aseptic loosening. However, particles have been identified in remote tissues as well. Factors that contribute to such distribution include (but are not limited to) particle number and size, fluid flow, implant design, and joint space.

Biology of the Osteolytic Cascade

The cellular response, although vastly governed by phagocytes and macrophages, involves different types of cells

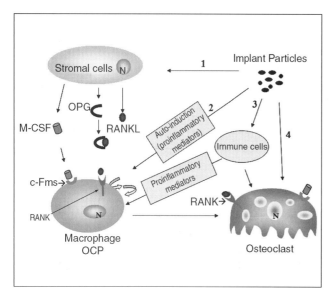

Figure 2   Illustration of the cellular targets of particles. Implant particles may affect osteoclastogenesis and induce osteolysis by acting via several possible cellular targets. Implant particles can stimulate stromal cells/synovial-like fibroblasts to secrete RANKL and OPG, through a mechanism possibly involving PGE$_2$ and other factors (1); RANKL and OPG regulate osteoclast differentiation and survival. Implant particles can also target macrophage/osteoclast precursors (2), which lead to stimulation and secretion of inflammatory mediators and establishment of an inductive loop that augments the inflammatory response. Additionally, implant particles can target cells of the immune system resulting in secretion of inflammatory factors that activate osteoclasts and osteoclast precursors (3). Finally, implant particles can directly activate mature osteoclasts (4) and enhance their resorbing activity. M-CSF = macrophage colony-stimulating factor; OCP = osteoclast precursor.

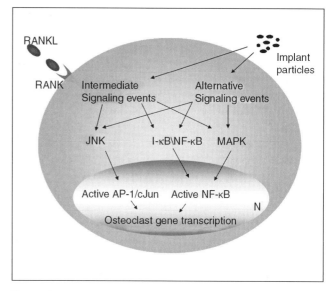

Figure 3   Molecular mechanisms of implant particle-induction of osteoclastogenesis and osteolysis. Implant particles intersect with intermediate signaling events transmitted by TNF family members, especially TNF and RANKL. This convergence leads to further activation of molecules and transcription factors, such as NF-κB, cJun/AP-1, and mitogen-activated protein kinases, (MAPK) which regulate osteoclast target genes. Alternatively, implant particles may directly activate osteoclast relevant pathways by unidentified mechanisms.

such as osteoclasts, fibroblasts, and osteoblasts/stromal cells (**Figure 2**). This is evident by the wide array of secreted products by various cells, which includes cytokines, growth factors, metalloproteinases, prostanoids, lysosomal enzymes, and others. The mechanisms underlying particle induction of cellular responses and osteolysis are under vigorous investigation. It is believed that recognition of particles relies on phagocytosis of small particles by macrophages and by unidentified cell surface interaction. The latter interaction may include nonspecific physical induction of transmembranal proteins or recognition of cell surface molecules by particles or proteins/factors adherent to their surface. Both animal and human studies suggest that endotoxin, a bacterial protein, becomes concentrated on the surface of particles and induces inflammatory reactions in immune cells. However, the exact nature and a comprehensive understanding of the stimulation of cells by particles remain unknown. It is unanimously accepted that host defense cells, which constitute the core of the inflammatory reaction, recognize particles and release significantly large quantities of proinflammatory cytokines and factors. These include TNF-α, IL-1α and -1β, IL-6, recep-

tor activator of nuclear factor-kappaB ligand (RANKL), and PGE$_2$. Studies with animal models and with in vitro cell cultures have shown that TNF plays a crucial role as a mediator of particle-induced osteoclastogenic and osteolytic events. In this regard, PMMA particles fail to promote aggressive osteolysis in TNF-α-receptor null animals or in the presence of TNF-α-neutralizing agents, such as various soluble TNF-α-binding proteins. Likewise, animals lacking RANK or RANKL resist particle induction of osteolysis. This is not unexpected, considering that members of the TNF-α family, especially RANKL, are prerequisites for osteoclast formation. The molecular details of TNF-α and RANKL as essential mediators of particle-induced osteolysis are described elsewhere in this chapter.

Additional downstream signaling by wear particles, not surprisingly, overlaps that of TNF-α and RANKL. In this regard, activation of kinases and recruitment of molecules essential for osteoclast differentiation and activation have been documented. Notably, particle-induced pathways lead to activation of kinases and transcription factors essential for osteoclastogenesis. Among these are activation of the tyrosine kinase c-src, mitogen-activated protein kinases, and the nuclear factor kappaB (NF-κB) cascade. Although activation of these pathways might be secondary to other events, selective blockade of these downstream pathways reduces particle-transmitted effects (**Figure 3**).

Potential Therapies for Inflammatory Bone Loss

Molecular Approaches to Arrest Osteoclast Activity

It is accepted that osteoclasts execute the final destructive phase of bone loss in wear debris-mediated inflammatory osteolysis, which makes osteoclasts the prime target for therapeutic intervention. To design precise antiosteoclastic therapies, certain key steps that are essential for osteoclast differentiation and activation must be recognized. Differentiation of bone marrow macrophages (osteoclast precursors) into mature osteoclasts requires recognition and binding of the osteoblast and T cell-secreted factor RANKL by its cognate receptor, RANK, which is expressed on the surface of osteoclast precursors. This process is regulated by another osteoblast-secreted factor, OPG, which acts as a decoy receptor by binding to RANKL and reducing its bioavailability. Recent studies suggest that the synovial fibroblast-like cells present in the inflammatory membrane surrounding loose implants secrete RANKL. Synovial fibroblasts increase RANKL expression in response to the inflammatory mediator PGE$_2$ and thus these cells, which previously have received less attention, may be important targets.

The binding of RANKL to RANK prompts induction of several intracellular pathways by this receptor, leading to activation of key transcription factors, most notably NF-κB. It has been mentioned that this family of transcription factors is central to pathologic responses and essential for osteoclast differentiation. It consists of several family members that primarily form heterodimers. These dimers are found bound to an inhibitory κB (I-κB) protein that under unstimulated conditions retains the complex in the cytoplasm. Stimulation by RANKL or other specific stimuli leads to activation of upstream I-κB kinases (IKKs), which in turn phosphorylate I-κB, leading to its dissociation from the NF-κB complex and eventually to its degradation by the proteosome system. I-κB–liberated NF-κB then translocates to the nucleus, binds to specific DNA sites, and induces gene transcription.

Based on the details of NF-κB activation mechanisms that eventually lead to osteoclast formation and, when induced by other factors such as TNF and PMMA particles, exacerbate osteoclastogenesis and inflammatory responses, several approaches were designed to perturb this pathway and alleviate the deleterious effects of inflammatory osteolysis. Several approaches must be considered regarding osteoclast-based therapy: first, by targeting osteoclast precursor cells, which are recruited to inflammatory sites by circulating cytokines; second, by targeting precursors, which are stimulated by the particle-mediated cellular response to differentiate and form bone-resorbing osteoclasts; and third, by targeting activation mechanisms of mature osteoclasts. To inhibit the differentiation-based arm, multiple approaches are available. First and foremost, direct inhibition of osteoclast differentiation may be achieved by the application of the RANKL decoy molecules, OPG, or a soluble receptor fusion protein, RANK-Fc. Indeed, studies with animal models and with in vitro osteoclast cultures have shown significant inhibition of osteoclastogenesis and reduced osteolysis.

Other possible approaches target key intracellular signal transduction pathways essential for osteoclast differentiation and exacerbation of the inflammatory process. Specifically, the transcription factor NF-κB is essential for both the inflammatory and osteolytic responses. Because inhibition depends on disrupting its translocation to the nucleus, overexpression of a dominant-negative form of the NF-κB inhibitory protein, I-κB, which retains NF-κB in the cytoplasm, is sufficient to block osteoclast formation and activity. Another approach is to block activation of the upstream IKK complex that is responsible for phosphorylation of I-κB and subsequent activation of NF-κB. Introduction of a small peptide that perturbs assembly of the IKK complex attenuates NF-κB activation. Application of the dominant-negative I-κB protein or the IKK inhibitory small peptide to mice significantly blocks bone erosion associated with inflammatory arthritis and particle-induced osteolysis.

Several genes and gene products have been shown to be critical for osteoclast differentiation, including c-fms, c-fos, RANKL, NF-κB, c-src, and the protein adenosine triphosphatase. Recent studies have shown that proinflammatory cytokines, such as TNF-α, act directly on some of these genes and their products, in particular c-src and NF-κB, to accelerate osteoclast formation and cause a potent osteoclastic response. Selective inhibitors of the c-src tyrosine kinase show great promise in halting osteoclast activity, and future studies should be geared toward testing the effect of such inhibitors on inflammatory osteolysis.

Another potential approach is the use of bisphosphonates. Bisphosphonates inhibit osteoclast function and induce its apoptosis. In a canine total hip replacement model, administration of an oral bisphosphonate reduced wear debris-mediated bone resorption, in spite of the finding that the levels of PGE$_2$ and IL-1 remained elevated in tissue cultures from these implants. In another animal study, bone loss around implants caused by the intra-articular injection of polyethylene particles was prevented and treated using alendronate. Thus, bisphosphonates may be useful in preventing particle-induced osteolysis around total joint implants. These studies have served as the basis for ongoing clinical trials using alendronate in patients with radiographically evident osteolytic lesions.

Anti-Inflammatory Strategies

Inhibition of recruitment of precursor and other cells to the inflammatory site involves anti-inflammatory approaches to neutralize mediators such as TNF, IL-1, and

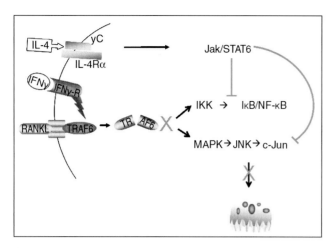

Figure 4   Mechanisms of osteoclast inhibition by IL-4 and IFN-γ. The anti-inflammatory cytokine IL-4 binds to its receptor and induces tyrosine phosphorylation of the transcription factor STAT6 by Jak3 tyrosine kinase. Phosphorylated STAT6 (STAT-p) dimerizes and partially inhibits activation of the MAP kinase c-Jun-N-terminal kinase (JNK) and NF-κB nuclear translocation in the cytoplasm. Activated STAT6 dimers also translocate to the nucleus and block DNA binding of the NF-κB transcription factor to DNA. The inflammatory cytokine IFN-γ inhibits RANKL/RANK signaling by targeting the adaptor protein TRAF6. Thus, IFN-γ causes degradation of TRAF6 and attenuates down stream signaling including arresting NF-κB and JNK pathway activation.

IL-6. Pharmacologic interventions targeting the macrophage may provide a means to slow the response to wear debris. Local cytokine inhibition has the potential to reduce inflammation in the periprosthetic tissue. IL-1 receptor antagonist protein (IL-1Ra) has been successful in reducing inflammation, and the anti-inflammatory cytokine, IL-10, appears to possess the capacity to reduce cell-mediated reactions in inflammation. Using particle-stimulated murine air pouch and calvarial models to evaluate the potential for gene therapy to treat inflammation provoked by orthopaedic wear debris, it has been shown that retroviral vectors encoding human IL-1Ra, human TNF receptor, or viral IL-10 (vIL-10) lead to a marked decrease in inflammation, decreased pouch fluid accumulation, and lowered macrophage influx. Histologic analysis revealed that air pouches transduced with vIL-10 or IL-1Ra have a 40% reduction in the inflammatory cell infiltration. In calvaria models, gene delivery of vIL-10 inhibited three processes critically involved in periprosthetic osteolysis: wear debris–induced proinflammatory cytokine production, osteoclastogenesis, and osteolysis.

In addition to IL-10, IL-4 and interferon (IFN)-γ are also secreted by T lymphocytes and are effective in antagonizing proinflammatory cytokine actions. In addition, they inhibit osteoclast formation and have the potential to inhibit bone resorption in inflammatory bone diseases. The finding that activated T1 helper cells (which secrete RANKL and proinflammatory cytokines) and T2 helper cells (which secrete IL-4) are present in the synovium

strongly implicates the immune system as a key regulator of inflammatory bone diseases. Recently, IL-4 messenger RNA was found more frequently in patients with nonerosive than erosive disease (38% versus 15%). These findings provide indirect evidence that IL-4 has bone-sparing effects in vivo. Additionally, IL-4 adenoviral gene therapy reduced inflammation, inhibited proinflammatory cytokine secretion, and spared bone destruction in a mouse model of adjuvant-induced arthritis. Clarifying the molecular mechanisms underlying the antiosteoclastogenic action of these anti-inflammatory cytokines may provide useful molecular targets.

IFN-γ is another major product of immune cells that potently inhibits bone resorption. IFN-γ interferes with the RANK\RANKL signal transduction in osteoclasts and their precursors. It induces rapid degradation of tumor necrosis factor receptor-associated factor 6 (TRAF6), a RANK adaptor protein (**Figure 4**). This action results in failure to activate RANK downstream signals such as NF-κB and cJun/JNK pathways. It has also been shown that RANKL-induced secretion of IFN-β by osteoclast precursors blocks osteoclastogenesis and reduces bone resorption in an autoregulatory fashion. Although a direct role of interferons in particle-induced inflammatory osteolysis has not yet been established, the possibility that these cytokines will block bone loss associated with this disease is worthy of further investigation.

Metal Ion Release, Sensitivity, Immune Response, and Compatibility

Achieving optimal biocompatibility between host and implants is ultimately a primary factor for the success rate of orthopaedic implants. This approach, however, can be compromised by long-term adverse effects emanating from the implant material properties. One such complicating factor is corrosion debris derived from metal implants. Electrochemical corrosion occurs when metal interacts with biologically active material leading to formation of metal ions, which in turn may form complexes with host proteins and induce the immune system.

Metals used in implants such as titanium, aluminum, vanadium, cobalt, chromium, and nickel are potentially toxic. Toxicity can range from altering normal cellular responses to immunologic responses and carcinogenesis. Metal ions can reside in tissues adjacent to the implant and may also bind to circulating factors and proteins and be distributed systemically through the bloodstream. Clearly, the adverse reaction mounted by the host stands in direct correlation with metal quantity, tissue distribution, and metal properties. In this regard, nickel, cobalt, and chromium are considered the most reactive metals. In excessive amounts, these metal ions can lead to a wide range of toxic reactions, including hypothyroidism, cardiomyopathy, carcinogenesis, nephropathy, hypersensitivity, and dermatitis. Nevertheless, the clinical relevance and incidence of toxicity from implant-derived metal ions remains controversial. A detrimental response to metal ions in some patients is hypersensitivity, which can be an immediate humoral and/or a delayed cell-mediated response. This is further supported by evidence that more patients with loose implants exhibit hypersensitivity than those with well-fixed implants. This cell-mediated response is characterized by antigen activation of immune cells of the T lymphocyte lineage. Activated T lymphocytes secrete a wide range of cytokines including TNF-α, IL-1, IL-2, and granulocyte-macrophage colony-stimulating factor. These cytokines recruit and activate inflammatory cells such as monocytes/macrophages, leukocytes, and neutrophils. These events are continuous and form positive feedback loops that can exacerbate immunopathologic cycles, resulting in greater tissue damage.

Other reactions reported in the literature include the ability of metals to cross-link cell-surface thiols and receptors, which are capable of activating T lymphocytes and provoking immunologic responses. Overall, the literature is conflicting regarding the role of specific immune responses in aseptic loosening and osteolysis. Early reports suggested that an immune response may contribute to aseptic loosening. These reports were based on the finding that 9 of 14 patients with loose metal-on-metal implants had cutaneous sensitivity to one or more of the components of the alloys. The clinical observation that different individuals may respond differently to what presumably are similar particulate burdens has led to speculation that there is a genetically mediated host variability in the reaction to particulate degradation products. In agreement with this hypothesis, one recent study examined 19 metal-on-metal articulations that failed prematurely and demonstrated histologic changes consistent with a cell-mediated immune response. These data suggest that enhanced hypersensitivity to metal ions may predispose certain patients to early clinical failure if treated with metal-on-metal bearing surfaces.

In a study of in vitro cellular immune responses to particulate cobalt-chromium alloy and PMMA in patients before and after surgery, specific cellular responses to PMMA, cobalt-chromium alloy particles, or both were associated with loose or painful prostheses. Altogether, these observations underscore the potential role of immune responses to implants. In contrast, other studies dispute the significance of immunologic responses against orthopaedic implants. A study using peripheral blood mononuclear cells cultured with large PMMA particles that preclude phagocytosis concluded that PMMA essentially was immunologically inert. In a subsequent study, nonphagocytosable ultra-high molecular weight polyethylene particles, although inducing a foreign-body reaction, were relatively immunologically inert. Conflicting results were also observed in a study investigating lymphocyte-mediated immune response to PMMA in patients with failed ce-

mented total hip arthroplasties. In these experiments, patch tests for PMMA were positive in 50% (13 of 26) of these patients. However, no differences were found in patch test reactivity between granulomatous and nongranulomatous loosening patterns.

The reasons for such discrepancies are not clear; however, data suggest that phagocytosable particles may be more relevant than particles that are not phagocytosable. It should be noted that strong immune responses are largely directed against cellular components such as proteins and antigens. Thus, implants carrying significant amounts of allogenic cells or proteins are prone to trigger a substantial immune response. In contrast, hypersensitivity is a generalized response to metal ions that can occur following allogenic and autogenic grafts alike.

Response to Autograft and Allograft

Bone grafts provide mechanical support, act as weight-bearing space fillers, and can act as osteoconductive/osteoinductive agents to enhance osseous healing. Grafted bone is incorporated into host bone during the weeks and months after surgery. The incorporation of bone graft occurs in five distinct stages. In the first stage, an acute inflammatory cellular response occurs as a result of recruitment of inflammatory cells to the grafted area within the first week after surgery. This is followed by vascularization and osteoinduction, two meaningful biologic processes that take place simultaneously and are highlighted by recruitment of osteoprogenitor cells and factors essential for osteointegration. Exposure to host factors may lead at this stage to development of an immune response typical of allografts. Expansion of the host response to the graft at various levels leads to graft incorporation otherwise known as osteoconduction. The length of this process depends vastly on the type of grafted material used, whether the bone is cancellous or cortical, and whether allograft or autograft is used, and could last months and/or years. The final stage in graft incorporation is remodeling, a process that is characterized by gradual resorption by osteoclasts and new bone formation by host osteoblasts. This phase is prolonged, may last several months, and provides stability and skeletal integrity.

Autografts

Cancellous autograft is highly osteogenic, readily revascularizes, and integrates rapidly in host tissue. This type of autograft lacks any significant structural support; however, it induces rapid new bone formation that contributes to rapid stability of the bone-healing site. This unique function of autografts harvested from the iliac crest is attributed to its histocompatibility and its large content of osteoblasts and osteogenic precursor cells. Although a large number of cells that cover the autograft die following surgical procedures, a reservoir of osteoblasts remains along the surface to produce new bone. The porosity of cancellous autografts further facilitates rapid vascular and cellular invasion by the host and accelerates graft resorption, new bone formation, and bone remodeling.

Nonvascularized and vascularized cortical autografts provide structural support and are variably osteogenic. Delayed vascularization in the nonvascularized cortical autograft may be attributed to the structure of the cortical bone that awaits osteoclastic resorption for vascular invasion. As a result, cortical bone becomes radiolucent, and the graft becomes significantly weaker than normal bone. Successful vascularized cortical autografts, which are implanted with functional blood supply, heal quickly and do not rely entirely on local tissue or on local vascular invasion for survival. Likewise, its incorporation is not dependent on local supply of vascular buds. Under these conditions, most osteocytes as well as other cellular components survive the procedure, thus contributing to rapid host-graft union. The sources of vascularized bone autografts are generally the fibula, iliac crest, and ribs, all of which can be grafted with vessels, veins, and arteries. These grafts undergo remodeling following mechanical loading.

Allografts

Unlike live autografts in which cells from both the graft and the host participate in bone union, healing of an allograft is solely mediated by invasion of the graft by host tissues because allografts remain inert. The entire union process is critically dependent on remodeling and new bone formation and mineralization, events that are mediated by vascularization and recruitment of appropriate cells. These events are compromised in allografts, thereby contributing to failure of such implants when compared with autografts.

Several types of allografts are available and include allogeneic demineralized bone matrix, morcellized and cancellous bone, and corticocancellous and cortical grafts. Allogeneic demineralized bone matrix revascularizes relatively quickly and is moderately osteoinductive. The implantation process is followed by an inflammatory process governed by recruitment of hematopoietic cells. This phase is followed by recruitment of mesenchymal cells that bind to the implanted matrix and undergo differentiation to support bone mineralization. Consequently, vascular invasion and osteoblast recruitment occur and new bone formation and remodeling processes proceed.

The osteoinductivity of the demineralized bone matrix has direct correlation with its source and processing procedures. Improper storage conditions (nonfrozen bone) and sterilization methods may impact the osteoinductivity of bone matrix. Morcellized and cancellous allogeneic bone grafts are normally derived from cancellous or cortical bone and processed to yield chips in the low-

millimeter diameter range. These grafts are porous; thus, they physically favor ingrowth of vessels and provide limited mechanical support. A better structural support and some osteoconductivity are achieved with corticocancellous and cortical allografts. These allografts are usually derived from the ilium, distal femur, and proximal tibia. Cortical cancellous grafts are typically thoroughly washed and processed and have a limited potential for immune response. In contrast, some structural allografts, particularly those that maintain soft-tissue attachments, are fresh frozen and maintain potential for immunologic responses. Processing of these grafts normally involves deep freezing at −70°C, and they contain residual amounts of protein and nonviable cells. Altogether, these responses lead to decreased revascularization and delayed osteoinduction of allografts and ultimately delayed osteointegration.

The host response to allografts typically entails mounting an immune response based on specific histocompatibility antigen reaction, and controversy exists over the potential role this plays in allograft incorporation. An immune response may reduce revascularization and remodeling of cortical grafts. However, a recent study cast doubt over lack of allograft revitalization as a consequence of an immune response, but rather because of lack of appropriate signals that stimulate bone remodeling and vascularization.

Summary

Once the general concepts of implant fixation and bone loss associated with implants are understood, it is apparent that future investigations should focus on three main areas of research. First, innovative implant design should be investigated to enhance implant fixation and reduce adaptive reactions. Second, efforts should be focused on the development of alternative joint bearings to reduce the generation of particulate debris and secondary inflammatory bone loss. Third, investigative efforts to delineate the molecular mechanisms underlying inflammatory bone loss and design-specific and efficacious inhibitory therapies should continue. Similarly, more complete understanding of the molecular, cell, and tissue responses to bone grafts will improve incorporation and patient outcomes.

Acknowledgments

The authors are supported by NIH grants DE13754, AR47443 (YA), and AR47096 (JCC); by a grant from the Shriners Hospital for Children (YA), and by an Arthritis Foundation Award (YA).

Selected Bibliography

Implant Fixation and Osteointegration
Bobyn JD, Pilliar RM, Cameron H, Weatherly GC: The optimum pore size for the fixation of porous-surfaced

metal implants by the ingrowth of bone. *Clin Orthop Relat Res* 1980;150:263-270.

Clohisy JC, Harris WH: The Harris-Galante porous-coated acetabular component with screw fixation: An average ten-year follow-up study. *J Bone Joint Surg Am* 1999;81:66-73.

Dalton JE, Cook SD, Thomas KA, Kay JF: The effect of operative fit and hydroxyapatite coating on the mechanical and biological response to porous implants. *J Bone Joint Surg Am* 1995;77:97-110.

D'Antonio JA, Capello WN, Manley MT, Geesink R: Hydroxyapatite femoral stems for total hip arthroplasty: A 10- to 13-year followup. *Clin Orthop Relat Res* 2001;393:101-111.

Frosch KH, Sondergeld I, Dresing K, et al: Autologous osteoblasts enhance osseointegration of porous titanium implants. *J Orthop Res* 2003;21:213-223.

Hacking SA, Bobyn JD, Tanzer M, Krygier JJ: The osseous response to corundum blasted implant surfaces in a canine hip model. *Clin Orthop Relat Res* 1999;364:240-253.

Lincks J, Boyan BD, Blanchard CR, et al: Response of MG63 osteoblast-like cells to titanium and titanium alloy is dependent on surface roughness and composition. *Biomaterials* 1998;19:2219-2232.

Petty W: Methyl methacrylate concentrations in tissues adjacent to bone cement. *J Biomed Mater Res* 1980;14:427-434.

Pilliar RM, Lee JM, Maniatopolous C: Observations on the effect of movement on bone ingrowth into porous-surfaced implants. *Clin Orthop Relat Res* 1986;208:108-113.

Sumner DR, Turner TM, Urban RM, et al: Locally delivered rhTGF-beta2 enhances bone ingrowth and bone regeneration at local and remote sites of skeletal injury. *J Orthop Res* 2001;19:85-94.

Sychterz CJ, Claus AM, Engh CA: What we have learned about long-term cementless fixation from autopsy retrievals. *Clin Orthop Relat Res* 2002;405:79-91.

Urban RM, Jacobs JJ, Sumner DR, Peters CL, Voss FR, Galante JO: The bone-implant interface of femoral stems with non-circumferential porous coating. *J Bone Joint Surg Am* 1996;78:1068-1081.

Adaptive Bone Loss and Potential Therapies

Huiskes R: Bone remodeling around implants can be explained as an effect of mechanical adaptation, in Galante JO, Rosenberg AG, Callaghan JJ (eds): *Total Hip Revision Surgery*. New York, NY, Raven Press, 1995, pp 159-171.

Maloney WJ, Sychterz C, Bragdon C, et al: Skeletal response to well fixed femoral components inserted with and without cement. *Clin Orthop Relat Res* 1996;333:15-26.

Sandborn PM, Cook SD, Spires WP, Kester MA: Tissue response to porous-coated implants lacking initial bone apposition. *J Arthroplasty* 1988;3:337-346.

Sychterz CJ, Engh CA: The influence of clinical factors on periprosthetic bone remodeling. *Clin Orthop Relat Res* 1996;322:285-292.

Turner CH, Robling AG: Exercise as an anabolic stimulus for bone. *Curr Pharm Des* 2004;10:2629-2641.

Response to Implant Debris and Inflammatory Bone Loss

Abu-Amer Y, Tondravi MM: NF-kappaB and bone: The breaking point. *Nat Med* 1997;3:1189-1190.

Abu-Amer Y: Mechanisms of inflammatory mediators in bone loss diseases, in Rosier RN, Evans CH (eds): *Molecular Biology in Orthopaedics*. Rosemont, IL, American Academy of Orthopaedic Surgeons, 2003, pp 229-239.

Abbas S, Clohisy JC, Abu-Amer Y: Mitogen-activated protein (MAP) kinases mediate PMMA-induction of osteoclasts. *J Orthop Res* 2003;21:1041-1048.

Archibeck MJ, Jacobs JJ, Roebuck KA, Glant TT: The basic science of periprosthetic osteolysis. *J Bone Joint Surg Am* 2000;82:1478-1489.

Aspenberg P, Herbertsson P: Periprosthetic bone resorption: Particles versus movement. *J Bone Joint Surg Br* 1996;78:641-646.

Bauer TW: Particles and periimplant bone resorption. *Clin Orthop Relat Res* 2002;405:138-143.

Bechtold JE, Kubic V, Soballe K: Bone ingrowth in the presence of particulate polyethylene: Synergy between interface motion and particulate polyethylene in periprosthetic tissue response. *J Bone Joint Surg Br* 2002;84:915-919.

Clohisy JC, Frazier E, Hirayama T, Abu-Amer Y: RANKL is an essential cytokine mediator of polymethylmethacrylate particle-induced osteoclastogenesis. *J Orthop Res* 2003;21:202-212.

Clohisy JC, Teitelbaum SL, Chen S, Erdmann J, Abu-Amer Y: Tumor necrosis factor-alpha mediates polymethylmethacrylate particle-induced NF-kB activation in osteoclast precursor cells. *J Orthop Res* 2002;20:174-181.

Greenfield EM, Bi Y, Ragab AA, Goldberg VM, Nalepka JL, Seabold JM: Does endotoxin contribute to aseptic loosening of orthopedic implants? *J Biomed Mater Res B Appl Biomater* 2005;72:179-185.

Hicks DG, Judkins AR, Sickel JZ, Rosier RN, Puzas JE, O'Keefe RJ: Granular histiocytosis of pelvic lymph nodes following total hip arthroplasty: The presence of wear debris, cytokine production, and immunologically activated macrophages. *J Bone Joint Surg Am* 1996;78:482-496.

Jacobs JJ, Roebuck KA, Archibeck M, Hallab NJ, Glant TT: Osteolysis: Basic science. *Clin Orthop Relat Res* 2001;393:71-77.

Maloney WJ, Smith RL: Periprosthetic osteolysis in total hip arthroplasty: The role of particulate wear debris. *J Bone Joint Surg Am* 1995;77:1448-1461.

Merkel KD, Erdmann JM, McHugh KP, Abu-Amer Y, Ross FP, Teitelbaum SL: Tumor necrosis factor-a mediates orthopedic implant osteolysis. *Am J Pathol* 1999;154:203-210.

Schwarz EM, Lu AP, Goater JJ, et al: Tumor necrosis factor-alpha/nuclear transcription factor-kappaB signaling in periprosthetic osteolysis. *J Orthop Res* 2000;18:472-480.

Wooley PH, Fitzgerald RH Jr, Song Z, et al: Proteins bound to polyethylene components in patients who have aseptic loosening after total joint arthroplasty: A preliminary report. *J Bone Joint Surg Am* 1999;81:616-623.

Potential Therapies for Inflammatory Bone Loss

Childs LM, Goater JJ, O'Keefe RJ, Schwarz EM: Effect of anti-tumor necrosis factor-α gene therapy on wear debris-induced osteolysis. *J Bone Joint Surg Am* 2001;83:1789-1797.

Childs LM, Goater JJ, O'Keefe RJ, Schwarz EM: Efficacy of etanercept for wear debris-induced osteolysis. *J Bone Miner Res* 2001;16:338-347.

Haynes DR, Rogers SD, Howie DW, Pearcy MJ, Vernon-Roberts B: Drug inhibition of the macrophage response to metal wear particles in vitro. *Clin Orthop Relat Res* 1996;323:316-326.

Itonaga I, Sabokbar A, Murray DW, Athanasou NA: Effect of osteoprotegerin and osteoprotegerin ligand on osteoclast formation by arthroplasty membrane derived macrophages. *Ann Rheum Dis* 2000;59:26-31.

Lark MW, James IE: Novel bone antiresorptive approaches. *Curr Opin Pharmacol* 2002;2:330-337.

Millett PJ, Allen MJ, Vet MB, Bostron MP: Effects of alendronate on particle-induced osteolysis in a rat model. *J Bone Joint Surg* 2002;84:236-249.

Ulrich-Vinther M, Carmody EE, Goater JJ: S balle K, O'Keefe RJ, Schwarz EM: Recombinant adeno-associated virus-mediated osteoprotegerin gene therapy inhibits wear debris-induced osteolysis. *J Bone Joint Surg Am* 2002;84:1405-1412.

Wooley PH, Schwarz EM: Aseptic loosening. *Gene Ther* 2004;11:402-407.

Metal Ion Release, Sensitivity, Immune Response, and Compatibility

Black J, Sherk H, Bonini J, Rostoker WR, Schajowicz F, Galante JO: Metallosis associated with a stable titanium-alloy femoral component in total hip replacement: A case report. *J Bone Joint Surg Am* 1990;72:126-130.

Hallab N, Merritt K, Jacobs JJ: Metal sensitivity in patients with orthopaedic implants. *J Bone Joint Surg Am* 2001;83(3):428-436.

Jacobs JJ, Silverton C, Hallab NJ, et al: Metal release and excretion from cementless titanium alloy total knee replacements. *Clin Orthop Relat Res* 1999;358:173-180.

Jacobs JJ, Skipor AK, Patterson LM, et al: Metal release in patients who have had a primary total hip arthroplasty: A prospective, controlled, longitudinal study. *J Bone Joint Surg Am* 1998;80:1447-1458.

Jacobs JJ, Urban RM, Gilbert JL, et al: Local and distant products from modularity. *Clin Orthop Relat Res* 1995;319:94-105.

Jiranek W, Jasty M, Wang JT, et al: Tissue response to particulate polymethylmethacrylate in mice with various immune deficiencies. *J Bone Joint Surg Am* 1995; 77:1650-1661.

Konttinen YT, Takagi M, Mandelin J, et al: Acid attack and cathepsin K in bone resorption around total hip replacement prosthesis. *J Bone Miner Res* 2001;16: 1780-1786.

Lee SH, Brennan FR, Jacobs JJ, Urban RM, Ragasa DR, Glant TT: Human monocyte/ macrophage response to cobalt-chromium corrosion products and titanium particles in patients with total joint replacements. *J Orthop Res* 1997;15:40-49.

Merritt K, Rodrigo JJ: Immune response to synthetic materials: Sensitization of patients receiving orthopaedic implants. *Clin Orthop Relat Res* 1996;326:71-79.

Nakashima Y, Sun DH, Trindade MC, et al: Signaling pathways for tumor necrosis factor-alpha and interleukin-6 expression in human macrophages exposed to titanium-alloy particulate debris in vitro. *J Bone Joint Surg Am* 1999;81:603-615.

Stulberg BN, Merritt K, Bauer TW: Metallic wear debris in metal-backed patellar failure. *J Appl Biomat* 1994;5:9-16.

Urban RM, Jacobs JJ, Gilbert JL, Galante JO: Migration of corrosion products from modular hip prostheses: Particle microanalysis and histopathological findings. *J Bone Joint Surg Am* 1994;76:1345-1359.

Wang JY, Wicklund BH, Gustilo RB, Tsukayama DT: Prosthetic metals impair murine immune response and cytokine release in vivo and in vitro. *J Orthop Res* 1997;15:688-699.

Willert HG, Buchhorn GH, Fayyazi A, et al: Metal on metal bearings and hypersensitivity in patients with artificial hip joints: A clinical and histomorphological study. *J Bone Joint Surg Am* 2005;87:28-36.

Response to Autograft and Allograft
Buddecke DE Jr, Lile LN, Barp EA: Bone grafting: Principles and applications in the lower extremity. *Clin Podiatr Med Surg* 2001;18:109-145.

Chandler HP, Tigges RG: The role of allografts in the treatment of periprosthetic femoral fractures. *J Bone Joint Surg Am* 1997;79:1422-1432.

Horowitz MC, Friedlaender GE: Induction of specific T cell responsiveness to allogeneic bone. *J Bone Joint Surg Am* 1991;73:1157-1168.

Ito H, Koefoed M, Tiyapatanaputi P, et al: Remodeling of cortical bone allografts mediated by adherent rAAV-RANKL and VEGF gene therapy. *Nat Med* 2005;11:291-297.

Kerry RM, Masri BA, Garbuz DS, Czitrom A, Duncan CP: The biology of bone grafting. *Instr Course Lect* 1999;48:645-652.

Malloy KM, Hilibrand AS: Autograft versus allograft in degenerative cervical disease. *Clin Orthop Relat Res* 2002;394:27-38.

Pelker RR, Friedlaender GE, Markham TC: Biomechanical properties of bone allografts. *Clin Orthop Relat Res* 1983;174:54-57.

Stevenson S: Enhancement of fracture healing with autogenous and allogeneic bone grafts. *Clin Orthop Relat Res* 1998;(suppl 355):S239-S246.

Chapter 21

Molecular Basis of Cancer

Jun Yuan, MD, PhD
Bruno Fuchs, MD, PhD
Sean P. Scully, MD, PhD

Hallmarks of Cancer

The molecular process of carcinogenesis is complex, although much has been learned in recent years. There appears to be a small number of molecular, biochemical, and cellular traits that are shared by most or even all types of human cancer. Hanahan and Weinberg recently described the hallmarks of cancer, which represent the fundamental concepts that govern the development of malignant transformation. It is hypothesized that a developing malignant cancer cell may represent the interplay between these fundamental concepts.

Unlimited replicative potential is the first hallmark. Cancer cells can switch on a protein component of telomerase that allows them to maintain their telomeres and to divide indefinitely. The avoidance of various mechanisms that lead to apoptosis is the second hallmark. Third, a malignant cell needs to have the capacity to mimic extracellular growth signals, for example by activating mutations, to make self-sufficient proliferation possible. Fourth, tumors need to produce their own blood supply if they are to grow beyond a certain size. The nature of the so-called angiogenic switch is yet unclear, but endothelial cells must be recruited, grow, divide, and invade the tumor to form blood vessels. Fifth, a malignant cell acquires the potential to break away from the original tumor mass and travel through extracellular matrix into blood or lymphatic vessels to repopulate and survive in a distant organ. During this process, the cancer cell is able to remodel the extracellular matrix. These fundamental concepts of the process of carcinogenesis will help in the understanding of the complexity of such a disease in terms of a relatively small number of underlying molecular principles. It is important to understand that these hallmarks represent a model and that sometimes all of them or a combination of some of them can be found in a tumor. An emerging understanding is that this set of principles has a specific mechanism for each tumor type, so that each tumor bears its own molecular circuitry that needs to be characterized individually.

Overview of the Cell Cycle

For a cancer cell to grow indefinitely, it must divide. Cell division is characterized by the cell cycle. Understanding the cell cycle is therefore important because ultimately all genetic changes impinge on this process. The cell cycle consists of four distinct phases: initial growth (G_1), DNA replication (S), a gap (G_2) and mitosis (M) (**Figure 1**). The G_1 and G_2 phases of the cell cycle represent the "gaps" or growth phases in the cell cycle that occur between DNA synthesis and mitosis. G_0 cells are in a stable state and have not entered the cell cycle. During the S phase, the DNA is synthesized and replicated. During the M phase or mitosis, all genetic material divides into two daughter cells. The cell cycle represents the interplay of highly complicated biologic processes coordinated by various proteins.

Cyclin/CDK Complex

Many regulatory networks in the cell are activated by the addition of a phosphate group by specific protein kinases. Cell cycle transitions are controlled by cyclins and cyclin-dependent serine/threonine kinases (CDKs). The cyclin-CKD complexes are activated by phosphorylation via upstream acting cyclin-activating kinases. As the name implies, the activation level of the cyclins varies with the cell cycle phase, and each cyclin is not only specific for a particular part of the cell cycle phase, but it also associates with a particular CDK to exert its specific effect during the cell cycle (**Figure 1**).

Internal demands or external mitogenic stimuli such as growth factors promote nondividing, quiescent G_0 cells into the G_1 phase of the cell cycle. Cyclin D is then expressed and binds to CDK4 and/or CDK6 depending on the particular cell type. The cyclin D/CDK4 or 6 and cyclin E/CDK2 complexes activate the Rb/E2F pathway to promote the cell from G_1 to S phase (**Figure 2**). Then, cyclins A and E bind and activate CDK2 and this allows the cell to traverse the S phase. Cyclin A/CDK2 then facilitates the transition from the S to G_2 phase; the cyclin B/CDK1

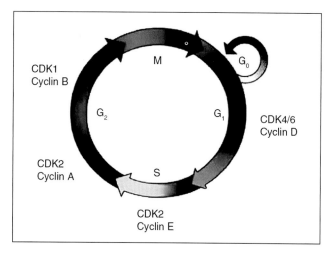

Figure 1   Schematic overview of the cell cycle. Following mitogenic signals that promote entry into early G_1 phase, progression through the cell cycle is regulated by sequential activation of cell phase-specific cyclins and CDKs. Activation of CDK4 and CDK6 by cyclin D propels the cell through G_1 phase. Activated CDK2 is required for progression through the S phase into G_2 phase, where CDK1/cyclin B complex then facilitates its passage into M phase.

complex accumulates in late G_2 phase, which is required for progression of the cell through the M phase. Following the completion of anaphase, cyclin B is degraded, allowing the cell to return to the G_1 phase, which, in the presence of maintained growth factor stimulation, proceeds to successive rounds of cell division.

The Restriction Point and Checkpoints

The cell cycle is a collection of highly ordered biochemical processes. The cell has developed safeguards to ensure the proper unidirectional functioning of the cell cycle, namely the restriction point and the cell cycle checkpoints. The restriction point is the moment in G_1 after which cells no longer respond to withdrawal of growth factors, thereby defining the G_1/S transition. This restriction point, which is largely regulated by Rb, is a point of no return, and the cell is committed to cycle (**Figure 2**).

Cell cycle checkpoints ensure the dependence of all unrelated biochemical processes during the cell cycle. Included are the transitions of G_1/S phase, G_2/S phase, spindle duplication, and spindle function checkpoints. For example, the cell must make sure that DNA replication is completed before the chromosomes are separated. Or, if some DNA is damaged, cell cycle arrest must occur to facilitate repair before the DNA is replicated and distributed to the daughter cells. Cell cycle arrest is produced by

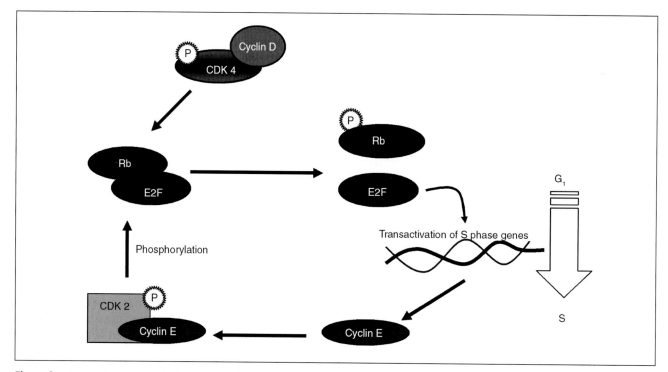

Figure 2   The pathway of Rb/E2F complexes in the G_1 to S transition. Cells enter the cycle by expressing cyclin D at G_1, which binds to CDK4/6 to form a catalytic complex involved in the phosphorylation of the retinoblastoma protein (Rb). The latter acts as a suppressor of the E2F family of transcription factors. Phosphorylation of Rb leads to the dissociation of E2F. E2F then binds to DNA and promotes the expression of a variety of genes important for S phase entry. One of the genes upregulated by E2F is cyclin E. This protein, when associated with CDK2, further hyperphosphorylates Rb to "drive" cells into S phase.

Table 1 Oncogenes and Tumor Suppressor Genes in Bone and Soft-Tissue Tumors

Oncogenes/Tumor Suppressor Genes	Normal Cell Cycle Function	Oncogenic Alteration	Disease
p53	Promotes G_1 arrest after DNA damage	Mutation	Malignant fibrous histiocytoma (MFH), leiomyosarcoma, rhabdomyosarcoma, angiosarcoma, fibrosarcoma, liposarcoma, osteosarcoma, chondrosarcoma, Ewing's sarcoma, synovial sarcoma
Rb	Restriction point regulator	Deletion	MFH, leiomyosarcoma, rhabdomyosarcoma, fibrosarcoma, liposarcoma, osteosarcoma, chondrosarcoma, Ewing's sarcoma
p16 (suppressor)	Inactivates G_1 cyclin-CDK complexes and inhibits Rb phosphorylation	Mutation or deletion	Leiomyosarcoma, osteosarcoma
p18 (suppressor)	Inactivates G_1 cyclin D/CDK4/6 complexes	Mutation	Leiomyosarcoma
p21 (WAF1/CIP1)	Inactivates CDK activity		Leiomyosarcoma
MDM2	Overrides p53 transcriptional activity	Gene amplification or enhanced mRNA translation	Sarcomas
Sarcoma-amplified sequence (SAS)	Regulated growth-related cellular process	Gene amplification	MFH and liposarcoma
c-myc (oncogene)	Stimulate cell proliferation	Gene amplification, alteration, or overexpression	MFH and osteosarcoma
Ras family	Regulate gene transcription	Mutation	MFH, leiomyosarcoma, rhabdomyosarcoma

a variety of factors that may be intrinsic or extrinsic and may affect several different checkpoints. Checkpoint loss results in genomic instability and has been implicated in the transformation of normal cells into cancer cells.

Oncogenes and Tumor Suppressor Genes

Oncogenes are genes whose products have the ability to transform eukaryotic cells to effect growth as tumor cells. A proto-oncogene is a gene that has the potential to induce transformation if it sustains genetic damage. For example, growth factors may act as dominant proto-oncogenes that can cause neoplasia if only one copy of this gene is abnormal. Tumor suppressor genes are genes whose encoded protein directly or indirectly inhibits progression through the cell cycle and in which a mutation that causes loss of function is oncogenic. Inheritance of a single mutant allele of many tumor suppressor genes greatly increases the risk for developing certain types of cancer. Table 1 summarizes the oncogenes and tumor suppressor genes, classified by mechanism of alteration, and the roles of oncoproteins and tumor suppressors encoded by these genes in bone and soft-tissue tumors.

The p53 Tumor Suppressor Gene

p53 is the most widely studied tumor suppressor gene. It acts as a transcription factor and is mainly regulated by

MDM2. The biologic functions of p53 include cell cycle and/or growth arrest, and maintenance of genetic stability by modulation of DNA repair, replication, and recombination (Figure 3). It is also possible for cells under growth arrest to undergo apoptosis. However, cells defective for p53 do not respond to irradiation normally and have reduced apoptosis and decreased G_1 growth arrest. Mutated p53 is no longer able to control cell proliferation in cancerous cells, which then results in inefficient DNA repair and genetically unstable cells.

Mutations in p53 are found in all major histogenetic groups, including cancers of the colon (60%), stomach (60%), breast (20%), lung (70%), brain (40%), and esophagus (60%). Therefore, it is estimated that p53 mutations are the most frequent genetic event in human cancers, accounting for more than 50% of cases. These mutations have also been associated with clinical outcome for various cancer types.

Retinoblastoma Gene

The retinoblastoma susceptibility gene (Rb) was the first tumor suppressor gene to be identified. It belongs to the Rb gene family, which also includes two related proteins, pRb2/p130 and pRb2/p107. These proteins are similar in structure and function. The three Rb family members show growth-suppressive properties, although the growth arrest mediated by each is not identical. Thus, although the three members complement each other, they are not functionally redundant.

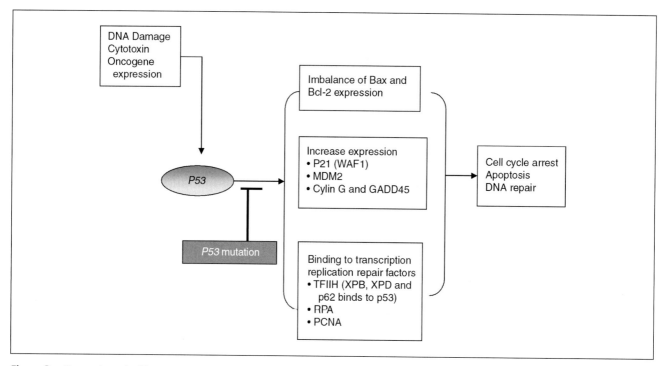

Figure 3   Expression of *p53* tumor suppressor gene activates a series of genes involved in cell cycle regulation. *p53* as a transcription factor activates genes controlling the cell cycle, apoptosis, and DNA repairs. RPA = replication protein A; PCNA = proliferating cell nuclear antigen.

Rb is the most prominent member of this family. It forms a complex with the transcription factor E2F and acts as an inhibitor of the G_1/S transition. The function of *Rb* is negatively regulated by a cell-cycle dependent phosphorylation catalyzed by CDKs in late G_1. Thus, phosphorylated Rb is inactive. If *Rb* function is absent, E2F is unbound and is free to initiate transcription of genes important for cell proliferation. As a consequence, cells pass their restriction point and progress through the cell cycle. The absence of *Rb* results in improper responses to mitogenic signals, which ultimately leads to abnormal cell proliferation. The *Rb* alterations most commonly associated with human neoplasia are deletions and missense mutations that result in a truncated, nonfunctional *Rb* or complete loss of *Rb*.

Genetic Abnormalities Associated With Musculoskeletal Tumors

Over the past decades, genetic alterations have been associated with numerous diseases and have yielded valuable insights into tumor pathogenesis and prognosis. There are numerous specific genetic alterations in cancer (**Figure 4**), which range from subtle changes in methylation status of individual nucleotides to multiple genetic alterations such as chromosomal abnormalities or abnormalities in genes that control DNA repair and genomic instability. The silencing of tumor suppressor genes by CpG island promoter hypermethylation is the most studied change of

DNA methylation in neoplasms. This results in silencing of genes such as *p16(INK4a)*, *BRCA1*, and *hMLH1*, which are important tumor suppressor genes. A large proportion of cancers show the chromosome-instability phenotype, in which many chromosome abnormalities are present. This is believed to be the result of mutations that disrupt chromosome maintenance, but the causative mutations are not known. The increasing application of molecular techniques to the study of cancer has contributed greatly to the understanding of mechanisms controlling cell growth.

Chromosomal Translocation and Chimeric Proteins

Translocation of a portion of one chromosome to another or rearrangement within a single chromosome can produce a new genetic structure that may act as a potential oncogene. The new chromosomal structure can place a growth-promoting gene near a strong or constitutively active transcriptional promoter. Alternatively, it can unite the introns of two different genes (most often, transcription factors) so that the spliced transcripts of the rearranged site now will produce a fusion of peptide domains, creating a novel chimeric protein. In many musculoskeletal tumors, the translocation is the major cytogenetic abnormality, indicating the probable causative role in the genesis of these tumors (**Table 2**). These translocations serve as a basis of molecular diagnosis as well as potential therapeutic products.

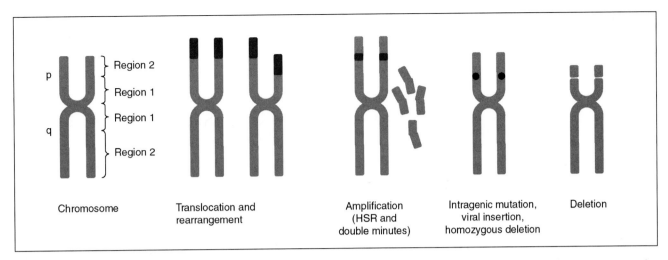

Figure 4 Schematic illustration of normal chromosome and genetic chromosomal abnormalities. The normal chromosome contains arms (p and q), regions (1 and 2), and bands. Chromosome translocation is the exchange of a portion of one chromosome between two chromosomes, whereas rearrangement occurs within a single chromosome. Small portions of a chromosome, or a complex rearrangement of multiple chromosomes, can result in a dramatic increase in copy number, a process termed gene amplification. Intragenic mutation is a small mutation that affects the function of only a single gene. Deletion can manifest as loss of the entire chromosome or as translocation or rearrangement, or can be cytogenetically undetectable. HSR = homogeneously staining region. Double minutes refers to multiple subchromosomal fragments.

Table 2 Specific Chromosome Translocations Established Cytogenetically and Corresponding Fusion Proteins in Musculoskeletal Cancers

Tumor	Translocation	Fusion Protein
Ewing's sarcoma	t(11;22)(q24;q12)	EWS-FLI1
	t(21;22)(q22;q12)	EWS-ERG
	t(7;22)(p22;q12)	EWS-ETV1
	t(17;22)(q21;q12)	EWS-ETV4
	t(2;22)q(33;q12)	EWS-FEV
Clear cell sarcoma	t(12;22)(q13-q14;q12)	EWS-ATF1
Desmoplastic small round-cell tumor	T(11;22)(p13;q12)	EWS-WT1
Myxoid liposarcoma	t(12;16)(q13;p11)	TLS(FUS)-CHOP
	t(2;22)(q13;q12)	EWS-CHOP
	t(12;22;20)(q13;q12;q11)	EWS-CHOP
Extraskeletal myxoid chondrosarcoma	t(9;22)(q22;q12)	EWS-CHN (TEC)
	t(9;17)(q22;q11.2)	RBP56 (HTAF1168)-CHN(TEC)
Alveolar rhabdomyosarcoma	t(2;13)(q35;q14)	PAX3-FOXO1A
	t(1;13)(p36;q14)	PAX7-FOXO1A
Synovial sarcoma	t(X;18)(p11.2;q11.2)	SYT-SSX1 or SSX2
Dermatofibrosarcoma protuberans	t(17;22)(q22;q13)	COL1A1-PDGFB
Congenital fibrosarcoma	t(12;15)(p13;q25)	ETV6-NTRK3
Alveolar soft-part sarcoma	t(X;17)(p11.2;q25)	ASPL-TFE3

Ewing's Sarcoma Family of Tumors

Ewing's sarcoma is the prototype of a translocation-associated musculoskeletal tumor. Seven translocation products have been reported in Ewing's sarcoma. The translocation results in a chimeric protein composed of an ETS component and an EWS component. ETS family transcription factors, characterized by an evolutionarily conserved ETS domain, play important roles in cell development, cell differentiation, cell proliferation, apoptosis, and tissue remodeling. The translocation is the result of a fusion of the *EWS* gene, which constitutes the 5' portion of the fusion transcript, and one of five *ETS* genes, representing the 3' portion of the fusion transcript. The *EWS* gene encodes an RNA-binding protein of yet poorly characterized function, but mainly acts as a transcriptional activator. The most prominent rearrangements are t(11;

22)(q24;p12) or EWS-FLI1, which is observed in more than 85% of all Ewing's sarcomas. The EWS-FLI1 fusion protein consists of several subtypes, which differ in the precise location of its breakpoints in central introns, resulting in subtle sequence changes. There are 12 different EWS/FLI1 fusions known, each with variable combinations of exons flanking the fusion point. More recent studies suggest that structurally different EWS/FLI1 fusions may have prognostic significance. There are other, less frequent fusion proteins described in Ewing's sarcoma, such as EWS-ERG, EWS-ETV1, EWS-FEV, and EWS-E1AF. Because this family of chimeric proteins is found almost exclusively in Ewing's sarcoma, it is hypothesized that they share not only structural but also common biologic sequelae. The EWS-ETS fusion proteins act as aberrant transcription factors and cause transformation. Although EWS-ETS oncoproteins are uniquely associated with a particular cancer, tumor growth is not abrogated by blocking its function, thereby implying that other mechanisms that contribute to tumorigenesis remain present but are still unknown. Considering that some ETS transcription factors are involved in malignant transformation and tumor progression, including invasion, metastasis, and neoangiogenesis through the activation of cancer-related genes, the chimeric proteins could be potential molecular targets for selective cancer therapy.

Myxoid Liposarcoma

Seventy-five percent of myxoid liposarcomas contain a t(12;16)(q13;p11) translocation, resulting in the fusion of the CCAAT-enhancer binding homologous protein gene (CHOP) on chromosome 12 with the translocated liposarcoma gene (TLS, otherwise known as FUS fusion) on chromosome 16. The CHOP/TLS fusion is specific for myxoid liposarcoma and appears to act as an aberrant transcription factor, similar to the EWS/ETS fusion products in Ewing's sarcoma.

Synovial Sarcoma

Cytogenetic analysis revealed a nonrandom and highly specific t(X;18)(p11;q11) translocation in 90% to 95% of all synovial sarcomas. The translocation generates a fusion between the synovial sarcoma translocation gene (SYT) on chromosome 18 and the synovial sarcoma X breakpoint 1 or 2 genes (SSX1 or SSX2), two highly homologous genes on band Xp11. Histologic grade, but not SYT-SSX fusion type or biphasic/monophasic histology, is a strong predictor of survival. The presence of this chimeric protein in synovial sarcoma has led to attempts at novel therapy by vaccination with a nine-amino-acid peptide located at the junction. Although safety and induction of an immunologic response have been demonstrated, efficacy is currently unclear. The genotype of synovial sarcomas (SYT/SSX1 or SYT/SSX2) has inconsistently been correlated with biphasic or monophasic histology.

Chromosome Abnormalities Not Associated With Specific Translocation

There are many musculoskeletal tumors with genetic abnormalities other than translocations. The most common genetic event is loss of heterozygosity (LOH) occurring in tumor suppressor genes. LOH, or allelic imbalance, is generally defined as inactivation of the wild-type copy of a tumor suppressor gene by deletion, gene conversion, mitotic recombination (rearrangement), or loss of an entire chromosome. Studies showing localization of LOH to a particular genomic region may serve as an indicator that the region contains an important tumor suppressor gene. Tumor suppressor genes act recessively at a cellular level, meaning that alterations in both alleles are necessary to cause loss of normal function of the tumor suppressor, which dysregulates normal cellular growth and proliferation. Such regions are likely to harbor genes involved in the onset and/or progression of cancer. Regions of LOH can also occur because of regional amplification, in which tumorigenesis may be related to duplication of oncogenes. However, it seems that each tumor has its own molecular signature; therefore, the genetic findings vary from patient to patient. **Table 3** summarizes some of the cytogenetic abnormalities in musculoskeletal tumors not associated with translocations.

Osteosarcoma

Genetic abnormalities in osteosarcoma are usually complex with extensive numerical and structural changes, particularly in high-grade tumors. The highest frequencies of LOH were found on chromosomes 3q, 13q, 17p, and 18q. The most frequent aberrations include copy number increases at 1q21 and 8q (8q21.3-q22) and 8cen-q13, followed by 14q24-qter and Xp11.2-p21. The most common losses are detected at 6q16 and 6q21-q22. Patients with copy number increases at 8q21.3-q22, 1q21, and 8cen-q13 appear to have diminished distant disease-free survival and show a trend toward short-term overall survival.

Genomic alterations of oncogenes and tumor suppressor genes that deregulate the G_1/S transition play a key role in the pathogenesis of osteosarcoma. Examples include Li-Fraumeni syndrome, which is characterized by a defect in p53 (17q13). The Rothmund-Thomson and the Bloom syndromes are characterized by a mutation in the RECQL4 DNA helicase gene (8q24.3) and (15q26.1), respectively. Many other genetic alterations were also associated and correlated with the outcome of patients with osteosarcoma. For example, overexpression of c-erbB2, a cellular growth factor, is observed in approximately 40% of osteosarcomas and correlates with decreased 4-year survival, early pulmonary metastases, and poor survival. The term gene amplification refers to an increase in the number of copies of a specific gene in an organism. This increase can lead to the production of a corresponding protein at elevated levels. Increased amounts of MDM2

Table 3   Genetic Abnormalities Without Specific Translocation in Some Musculoskeletal Tumors

Tumor	Chromosomal Gain	Chromosomal Loss	Loss of Heterozygosity (LOH)
Osteosarcoma	1q21, (8q21.3-q22), 8-q1314, q24; Xp11.2-p21; 1p21-31; 3q25; 6p12-21; 8q12; 12p11-12; 12q12-15; 0q12; 20p; 8q24.1	6q16; 6q21-q22; 3p; 10q; 11p; 13	3q; 13q; 17p; 18q; Xq21; 6-q22; 18-q11.2
Chondrosarcoma	20q; 17p; 20p; 1-q24; 14q23; 6-q22; 7; 5q14-q32; 6p; 12q; 20q12; 20q; 8q24.1	X-q21; 6-q22; 18-q11.2	9p21; 10; 59-61 13q14; 17p13
Malignant fibrous histiocytoma	7q32; 1p31; 12q13-q14; 12q12-q15; 3; 4q31; 5p; 6; 7; 14q22; 1q21-q22; 17q28; 20q; 7p15r	9p21; 10q; 11q23; 13q10-q31; 13q21; 13q22	
Leiomyosarcoma		10	
Chondromyxoid fibroma	Inv(6)(p25q13)		
Chordoma	Dic(1;9)(p36.1;p21)	1p	1p36

and its homologous sarcoma-amplified-sequence (*SAS*) genes are found in the surface osteosarcoma. Alterations in the *c-fos* gene occur more frequently in patients with recurrent or metastatic disease, and LOH of *Rb* has been identified as a negative prognostic marker. Alterations of the *c-myc*, *N-myc*, *p53*, *p16*, and *p19* genes are also common. In conjunction with these gene alterations, inactivation of *Rb* has been reported in up to 80% of patients with osteosarcoma.

Cartilaginous Tumors

Chondrosarcoma may arise centrally in bone (central chondrosarcoma) or in a secondary location within the cartilaginous cap of a hereditary or sporadic exostosis (peripheral chondrosarcoma) or osteochondroma. The genetic abnormalities of central chondrosarcoma include changes in 9p21, 10, 13q14, and 17p13. Well differentiated (grade I) chondrosarcoma shows numerous structural chromosome aberrations and a striking degree of genetic instability. In one study, genetic aberrations were found in 72% of chondrosarcomas and amplifications of small chromosome regions in only 17% of patients. Although amplification of *c-myc* has rarely been observed, the *fos/jun* oncogene has recently been implicated in the pathogenesis of chondrosarcoma. Recent work is beginning to indicate that *p53* mutations may be correlated with increasing histologic grade.

Extraskeletal myxoid chondrosarcoma is a rare entity comprising approximately 2.3% of soft-tissue sarcomas. Cytogenetic studies have demonstrated the presence of a recurrent translocation t(9;22)(q22;q12) in myxoid chondrosarcoma that results in the fusion of the *EWSR1* gene on chromosome 22 with *NR4A3* (*TEC, CHN*, or *NOR1*) gene on chromosome 9. The diagnostic and therapeutic implications of this translocation are currently unknown.

Abnormalities in cell differentiation can effect devel-

opment of malignancy. Enchondromatosis is seen in Ollier's disease and Maffucci's syndrome, conditions that have been associated with an increased rate of malignant transformation. Parathyroid hormone-related protein delays the hypertrophic differentiation of growth plate chondrocytes. Recently a mutation in the parathyroid hormone-related protein type 1 receptor resulting from a single amino acid substitution has been identified and has been associated with enchondromatosis. This results in a constitutively active receptor that results in enchondromatosis when placed into transgenic mice.

Other abnormalities in chondrosarcoma may predispose an individual to metastasis. It has been reported that matrix metalloproteinase-1 (MMP-1) is a prognostic factor in cancer recurrence for patients with chondrosarcoma. Others have reported increased MMP-1 immunostaining at the periphery of chondrosarcoma lobules, lending credence to the idea that this molecule facilitates cell egress from the tumor. A single nucleotide polymorphism in the promoter of MMP-1 that results in the presence of an ETS binding site does not correlate with survival in chondrosarcoma as it has in other malignancies.

Other Soft-Tissue Tumors

Multiple structural and numerical aberrations in chromosomes (for example, marker chromosomes, translation, telomeric associations, double minutes, and ring chromosomes) were reported in soft-tissue tumors such as malignant fibrous histiocytoma (MFH), leiomyosarcoma, rhabdomyosarcoma, fibrosarcoma, and liposarcoma. The amplification unit 12q13-q14, which contains *SAS* gene, was observed in many soft-tissue tumors. Other chromosome alterations such as 7q32 and 1p31 were associated with a worse prognosis and a higher relapse rate. In patients with leiomyosarcomas, for example, almost 60% show LOH for at least one marker on chromosome 10.

Despite the recent progress, further analyses need to be performed to establish the clinical and potential prognostic relevance of specific genetic alterations in soft-tissue tumors.

Moving Toward Molecular Diagnosis

Cytogenetic and molecular biologic techniques have already become indispensable for the routine clinical practice of tumor diagnoses. Although the histologic analysis is and will remain the mainstay of diagnosis, there are certain instances when histology is not precise enough to establish an accurate and reliable diagnosis. For example, histology often does not allow differentiation among the family of small round blue cell tumors, namely Ewing's sarcoma, embryonal rhabdomyosarcoma, non-Hodgkin's lymphoma, malignant hemangiopericytoma, and neuroblastoma. However, precise diagnosis is absolutely essential for the selection of the appropriate therapy, which may vary significantly in this group. Most recently, microarrays have been used to establish a molecular profile of specific diseases. Analyzing several different cancers such as non-Hodgkin's lymphoma, breast cancer, or prostate cancer, it has been shown that the molecular expression profile allows precise distinction between subtypes of these cancers in a manner not possible merely using histology. Microarray analyses recently revealed that a specific genetic profile can be attributed to each of the family members of the small round blue cell tumors, allowing accurate separation and thereby establishing the exact diagnosis. Reverse transcriptase polymerase chain reaction is another molecular method useful for diagnosis. This technique takes advantage of the fact that many musculoskeletal tumors have specific mutations that are tumor-specific. With reverse transcriptase polymerase chain reaction, the messenger RNA of specific genetic rearrangements can easily and specifically be detected to establish an accurate diagnosis. It is expected that the use of molecular techniques and their application in clinical practice will be more commonplace.

Principles of Chemotherapy and Resistance

The term chemotherapy most traditionally refers to the use of conventional cytotoxic drugs but also includes hormonal or endocrine drug therapy to treat patients diagnosed with cancer. Many of these chemotherapeutic agents cause DNA damage through interaction with their intracellular targets. As a consequence, such damage may prevent the cell from cycling and may lead to its death.

It has been observed that many cancers initially respond well to chemotherapy. However, the occurrence of cellular drug resistance remains a major adverse effect of chemotherapy that ultimately may lead to treatment failure. Using in vitro cell lines made resistant against different classes of anticancer agents, a large variety of drug resistance mechanisms such as alterations in target proteins, carrier mediated drug uptake, drug metabolism, cellular repair mechanisms, and cellular drug efflux, can cause anticancer drug resistance in vivo. Although in vitro results indicating sensitivity to chemotherapy have been interpreted carefully, they are often not observed in vivo. More precise definition of molecular mechanisms of resistance carries a great potential to improve or overcome the drug resistance problem.

Chemotherapy Approaches

The timing of chemotherapy with respect to other treatment modalities is important. "Adjuvant" chemotherapy refers to chemotherapy administered postoperatively to treat presumed micrometastases. "Neoadjuvant" chemotherapy refers to chemotherapy administered before the surgical resection of the primary tumor. The rationale for the success of chemotherapy has been the eradication of subclinical pulmonary micrometastases at the time of presentation. Neoadjuvant chemotherapy in patients with osteosarcoma or Ewing's sarcoma has the additional advantage of tumor and edema shrinking, thereby facilitating surgical resection.

Despite intensive investigations, only four drugs showed reproducible single-agent activity with a response better than 15% to 20% in patients with osteosarcoma and Ewing's sarcoma. These include the anthracyclines doxorubicin and epirubicin, ifosfamide, and dacarbazine. For these reasons, nearly all treatment protocols use a combination chemotherapy consisting of doxorubicin with dacarbazine, or a four-drug regimen (Cy-VADIC), consisting of cyclophosphamide, vincristine, doxorubicin, and dacarbazine, or a combination of an anthracycline with ifosfamide plus or minus dacarbazine. With the use of modern chemotherapy protocols, the current 5-year survival rate for localized high-grade osteosarcoma and Ewing's sarcoma is approximately 70%. Similarly, chemotherapy plays a role in the treatment of soft-tissue tumors such as MFH, or rhabdomyosarcoma. Although its precise role for many other malignancies needs to be clearly established, chemotherapy is not useful for cartilaginous lesions and most low-grade malignancies.

The emergence of tumor cell populations resistant to multiple anticancer drugs represents a major obstacle in cancer chemotherapy. One form of resistance is characterized by an active, energy-dependent removal of a variety of chemically unrelated cytotoxic agents by membrane transporter protein (P-glycoprotein), which is encoded by the multidrug resistant gene (MDR-1). P-glycoprotein pumps cytotoxic drugs rapidly out of the cell, keeping the amount of drug in the cytoplasm below the toxic level. P-glycoprotein was earlier believed to be one of the key molecules that cause multidrug resistance. However, the expression of P-glycoprotein was not correlated with sensitivity to chemotherapy or survival in patients with osteosarcoma in a recent multicenter prospective trial.

Tyrosine Kinase Inhibitors

The protein tyrosine kinases constitute a large and diverse family of homologous proteins that serve as important regulators of intracellular signal transduction pathways. Their activities control a range of fundamental cellular processes including growth, metabolism, differentiation, adhesion, and apoptosis. The deregulation of protein tyrosine kinase activity was shown to play a central role in the pathogenesis of human cancer. In particular, the molecular pathogenesis of chronic myelogenous leukemia depends on the formation of the *bcr-abl* oncogene, leading to constitutive expression of the tyrosine kinase fusion protein, Bcr-Abl. Imatinib was originally developed as a specific inhibitor of the Bcr-Abl protein tyrosine kinase. Imatinib competes with adenosine triphosphate for its specific binding site in the kinase domain and was shown to be highly active in the treatment of chronic myelogenous leukemia (Figure 5). The development of this inhibitor has established a new standard for targeted cancer therapy. Recent clinical studies show that the drug might also be useful for the treatment of soft-tissue sarcomas. The presence of the *c-kit* mutation was examined in patients with leiomyosarcomas. *c-kit* expression was identified in 24 of 25 tumors but a mutation in exon 11 or 17 was present in only one sample, making it unlikely that leiomyosarcomas will respond to this drug. The concept of "designer drugs" specifically targeted to molecular abnormalities of tumors is still in its early stages of development.

Tumor Metastasis

Metastasis describes a process in which a tumor cell leaves the primary tumor, finds access to the circulatory system, travels to a distant site, extravasates into the surrounding tissues, and establishes a secondary tumor. Certain tumors, including breast, prostate, thyroid, kidney, and lung, preferentially metastasize to bone. Metastases in general are the leading cause of cancer death, and bone metastases in particular significantly impact health status because of the potential for loss of ambulation and function.

Over the past decade, as genomics and proteomics have evolved, tumors such as breast cancer have been evaluated for gene signatures that prognosticate metastasis. Using genomic and proteomic technologies, it is now possible to identify some patients with an inherited risk of developing breast cancer, and to more accurately assess the prognosis of others with the disease. Various techniques are also available or under investigation to identify patients who are most likely to respond to various treatments. Analysis of 1,975 published microarrays spanning 22 tumor types has recently been published. The authors

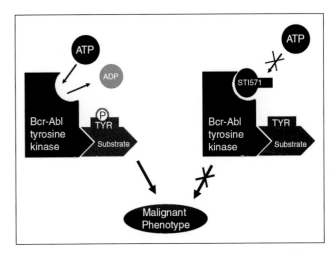

Figure 5 Mechanism of action of tyrosine kinase inhibitors. The Bcr-Abl tyrosine kinase is a constitutively active kinase that functions by binding adenosine triphosphate (ATP) and transferring phosphate from ATP to tyrosine residues on various substrates. This activity causes the malignant phenotype. STI571 functions by blocking the binding of ATP to the Bcr-Abl tyrosine kinase, thus inhibiting the activity of the kinase. In the absence of tyrosine kinase activity, substrates required for Bcr-Abl function cannot be phosphorylated. ADP = adenosine diphosphate.

describe expression profiles in different tumors as subclasses of genes with similar functions. Using these methods, there appears to be a shared mechanism for both primary tumor proliferation and metastasis to bone among many tumors.

More than 100 years ago, Paget first launched the "seed and soil" hypothesis, which posed the following question: "What is it that decides what organ shall suffer in a case of disseminated cancer?" His answer is basically still valid: "The microenvironment of each organ (the soil) influences the survival and growth of tumor cells (the seed)."

Over the past few years, many researchers have made valuable contributions to the understanding of the pathogenesis of metastasis, detailing the molecular aspects of the interaction between the migrating cancer cells and local homeostatic factors. Fidler redefined the "seed and soil" hypothesis, which consists of three principles. First, tumors contain not only cancer cells but also host cells. Host cells include fibroblastic cells, epithelial cells, endothelial cells, and infiltrating leukocytes. Moreover, neoplasms are biologically heterogeneous and contain genotypically and phenotypically diverse subpopulations of tumor cells, each of which have the potential to complete some but not all of the steps in the metastatic process. Second, the process of metastasis is selective for cells that succeed in invasion, embolization, survival in the circulation, arrest in a distant capillary, and extravasation into and multiplication within the organ parenchyma. Although some of the steps in this process contain stochastic elements, as a whole, metastasis favors the survival and growth of a few subpopulations of cells that probably preexist within the parent neoplasm. Thus, metastases can have a clonal origin, and different metastases can originate from the proliferation of different single cells. Third, the outcome of metastasis depends on multiple interactions (cross-talk) of metastatic cells with the host homeostatic mechanisms. Therefore, the therapy of metastatic foci should not only be targeted against tumor cells but also against the local homeostatic factors that promote tumor cell growth, survival, angiogenesis, invasion, and metastasis.

Angiogenesis

Blood and lymph vessels provide tumors with nutrients necessary for growth and invasion. They provide the routes for systemic spread of cancer cells, and they mediate the communication between the primary tumor and its metastasis. The process of angiogenesis can be divided into the following three steps that parallel those required for the invasion of tumor cells: (1) proliferation of endothelial cells, (2) breakdown of the extracellular matrix, and (3) migration of endothelial cells. These steps can be promoted by growth factors secreted by tumor cells. These growth factors are termed angiogenic factors and include the heparin-binding growth factor or fibroblast growth factor family, transforming growth factor, angiogenin, vascular permeability growth factor, and vascular endothelial growth factor, the most potent of these growth factors. The production of these growth factors leads to tumor growth and causes a concomitant increase in vascularization. Angiogenesis requires an interaction of tumor cells, endothelial cells, and the extracellular matrix. The enzymes that mediate these interactions are serine proteases and metalloproteinases. The expression of these enzymes in turn are under the control of angiogenic factors.

Invasion

Tumor invasion is an active process that requires the sequential processes of cell attachment, local proteolysis of the extracellular matrix, and cell migration. In vivo, these processes are interrelated and cannot be separated from each other.

It is still poorly understood how a migrating cancer cell is able to attach and extravasate at a specific location. This process involves a very complex interplay between tumor cells and local host cells, and is modulated by the cells from the immune system, which attempt to reject the tumor. Other cell types are recruited to the site of metastasis to support either invasion (by the tumor cell) or killing the tumor cell (by host cells) (**Figure 6**). For example, cancer cells produce chemokines, which attract host leukocytes. Leukocytes produce matrix-degrading proteinases that support the growth of the invading cancer cell and facilitate angiogenesis, and augment the process of invasion. The integrin receptor family also has a critical role in tumor invasion. Integrins are transmembrane receptors that bind to a variety of extracellular matrix molecules including laminin, fibronectin, vitronectin, and collagens. They are involved in cell signaling pathways through association with cytoskeletal components inside the cell. Specific integrins have been recognized to play an important role in the metastasis of tumor cells to bone by serving as attachment factors and through stimulation of tumor cells.

Degradation of the extracellular matrix is another crucial activity of invasive cells. Extracellular matrix frequently contains stored latent proteinases that can be activated by the invading cell pseudopodia and contributes to matrix turnover. The MMP family are important proteases whose expression levels are correlated with invasiveness. MMPs are associated with disease progression in many malignancies.

Active MMPs can be inhibited by a class of inhibitor proteins termed tissue inhibitor of metalloproteinase (TIMP). TIMPs bind stoichiometrically in the active site of target MMPs. In patients with esophageal carcinoma and squamous cell carcinoma, the *TIMP-3* gene has been shown to undergo methylation, which downregulates expression of the TIMP protein. Patients with *TIMP-3* gene methylation and silencing have a worse prognosis. In sarcomas, the role of TIMPs has been less well defined, but TIMP expressions are reportedly altered in soft-tissue sarcomas.

Various other factors contribute to metastasis by stimulation of motility. These factors can be divided into three groups. The first group consists of factors that are secreted by the tumor cells themselves, or autocrine motility factors, such as the hepatocyte growth factor/scatter factor, the insulin-like growth factor II, and autotaxin. The second group of motility factors corresponds to extracellular matrix proteins. Matrix proteins that can induce motility are vitronectin, fibronectin, laminin, type I collagen, type IV collagen, and thrombospondin. The third class of tumor motility factors is host-secreted growth factors such as insulin-like growth factor-I, interleukin-8, and histamine. Through a variety of mechanisms, motility factors may cause changes in cell shape, cytoskeletal rearrangements, and changes in cell adhesion and/or membrane fluidity.

Bone Metastasis

Tumor metastases in bone can be either lytic or osteoblastic (**Figure 7**). Most metastatic tumors cause bone lysis of the host bone. Multiple mechanisms may be involved in the process of osteolysis. In some instances, the tumor cell may secrete proteases that directly degrade bone matrix. Most often, however, tumor cells activate the host osteoclasts via complex signaling pathways to cause bone resorption. The central mechanism activating osteoclasts in cancers involving bone includes receptor activator of nuclear factor-kappaB (RANK) and its ligand RANKL

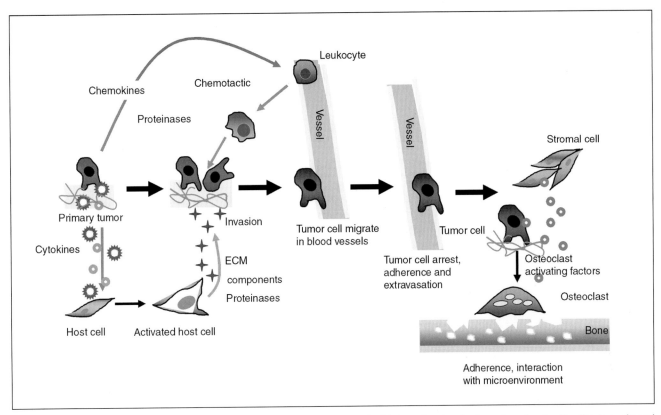

Figure 6   Schematic of tumor cell invasion. Cellular activities associated with invasion implicate reduced cell-cell adhesion, altered cell-matrix adhesion, migration, ectopic survival, and lysis of extracellular matrix (ECM). Most of these activities are modulated by the cross-talk between cancer cells, host cells, and host leukocytes which are activated by cytokines or chemotactic cytokines (called chemokines) released from the cancer cells. Cancer cells also release osteoclast activating factors, which may cause a breakdown of bone matrix.

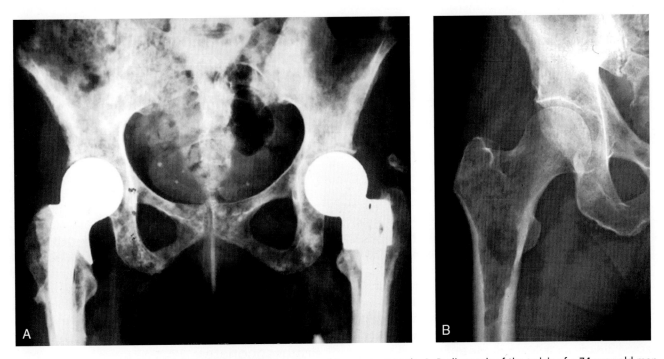

Figure 7   Radiographs show the lytic and osteoblastic lesions of tumor metastasis. **A,** Radiograph of the pelvis of a 74-year-old man shows osteoblastic lesions in the entire pelvis from prostate carcinoma. **B,** AP hip radiograph of a 65-year-old woman shows extensive lytic lesions in the proximal femur from breast carcinoma.

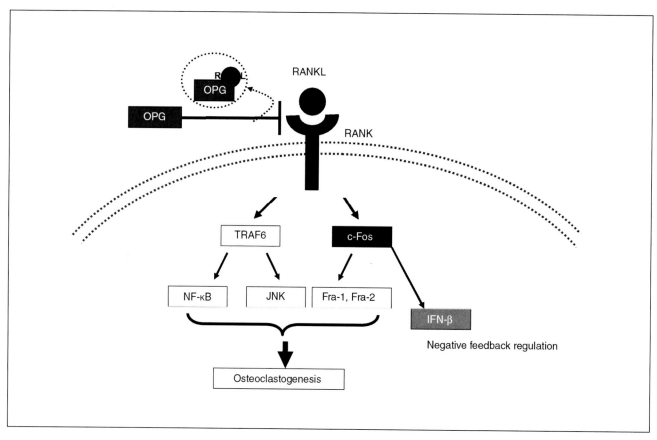

Figure 8   RANK and its signaling system in osteoclast. RANK signal transduction stimulates osteoclast development and activation. RANKL is a tumor necrosis factor-related cytokine that interacts specifically with RANK. OPG is a soluble decoy receptor that binds to RANKL and blocks its biologic activity. OPG = osteoprotegerin; TRAF6 = cytoplasmic factor; JNK = c-Jun N-terminal kinase; IFN-β = interferon-β.

(Figure 8). RANKL is able to directly activate osteoclast precursors and stimulate their differentiation into maturing bone-forming osteoclasts. In bone metastasis, RANKL comes from a combination of two potential sources. Many tumors make RANKL and thus can directly stimulate osteoclast formation. However, tumors secrete other factors, such as parathyroid hormone-related protein that cause RANKL expression by host stromal cells, and thus indirectly stimulate osteoclast formation. Several knockout studies found a pivotal role for the members of the RANK signaling cascade in bone homeostasis. Whereas parathyroid hormone-related protein was shown to be mainly responsible for causing lytic lesions, endothelin-1 was found to cause osteoblastic lesions in prostate carcinoma through yet undetermined mechanisms.

Occasionally, metastases lead to new bone formation at the site of tumor cell deposits, particularly in breast and prostate cancer. This may occur without prior osteoclastic resorption, and the newly formed bone may be placed directly on trabecular bone surfaces without a preceding resorptive episode. The mechanisms responsible for the osteoblastic metastasis are poorly understood, but are attracting great interest.

Principles of Medical Management of Metastases

Metastasis is the leading cause of death of cancer patients. Bone metastases in particular may lead to significant morbidity as a result of pain and skeletal compromise. The goal of systemic treatment of metastatic tumors is to improve the patient's quality of life. Surgical therapy is performed when mechanical reinforcement or reconstruction of the skeleton is necessary. Quality of life and overall survival of patients with metastases have been significantly improved by advances in chemotherapy, radiation therapy, immunotherapy, hormonal manipulation, and cryosurgery. New treatment modalities recently introduced include image-guided ablation with use of radiofrequency, other thermal energy sources, or high-intensity focused ultrasonography. Because these techniques can be minimally invasive with a low morbidity for the patient, these new strategies hold promise for the future.

Bisphosphonates

Over the past decade, bisphosphonates have been widely used to treat bone metastases because of their ability to alleviate pain and to inhibit osteoclast-mediated bone resorption. Bisphosphonates are effective in the treatment of tumor-induced hypercalcemia and prevent skeletal complications in patients with bone metastasis. Several mechanisms have been proposed to explain these observations in addition to the known effects that bisphosphonates have as inhibitors of osteoclast activity. Bisphosphonates directly inhibit proliferation and induce apoptosis of a variety of human tumor cell lines in vitro, including breast, myeloma, melanoma, and prostate. Bisphosphonates also inhibit the ability of breast and prostate cancer cells to adhere to and invade the extracellular matrix, and may have antiangiogenic effects in vivo. Three generations of bisphosphonates have entered clinical use. Zoledronate is significantly more active than pamidronate in prostate and other solid tumors. However, a retrospective analysis of patients with advanced renal cell carcinoma with multiple metastases enrolled in a multicenter, randomized, and placebo-controlled study has shown that bisphosphonates significantly reduce the percentage of patients who had skeletal-related events while having no effect on overall tumor survival. There has been antitumor activity and a delay of metastasis in patients with breast cancer treated with zoledronate.

Radiofrequency Ablation and Cryotherapy

Radiation remains an important adjuvant modality for the treatment of many bone metastases. It targets tumor cells via *p53*-induced DNA damage, and may lead to mineralization and pain alleviation. However, sometimes precise targeting and killing of the tumor cells is preferred, particularly in anatomically difficult regions. Radiofrequency ablation is an attractive new development in addressing this problem. Radiofrequency energy devices work by generating a high frequency of alternating electromagnetic current that flows from the tip of a probe into adjacent tissue, causing heat (90° C) and necrosis of the tumor cells. The potential advantages of radiofrequency include immediate cell death, accurate control of the size of the lesion, monitoring of the applied temperature, and precise placement of the electrode using a percutaneous image-guided procedure.

Cryosurgery is a therapeutic method for treating neoplastic tissue by freezing it in situ to achieve devitalization. The basic principles of cryosurgery include rapid freezing, slow thawing, and immediate repetition of the freezing and thawing cycle. The main mechanisms of cryosurgery-induced cell death include formation of intracellular ice crystals and membrane disruption, in conjunction with electrolyte changes, denaturation of cellular proteins, and microvascular failure. Cryosurgery is used with curative intention in the treatment of benign-aggressive and low-grade malignant bone tumors. It may also be used in metastatic disease to achieve local tumor control and to provide symptomatic pain relief.

Summary

Significant advances over the past few decades led to a greatly improved outlook for patients with musculoskeletal cancers. Surgical techniques were refined so that in most instances limb-sparing surgery is possible as opposed to amputation, a method that was the mainstay of treatment up to three decades ago. Without any doubt, however, the introduction of chemotherapy was the most significant improvement in the treatment of the most common musculoskeletal tumors. It led to a dramatic increase in survival of these patients. Despite a tremendous effort in modulating, adjusting, and defining new drug regimens, the survival rate of these patients has remained more or less stable over the past 15 years. Therefore, there is a great need for defining new avenues in the treatment of these cancers. The understanding of molecular carcinogenesis has greatly improved over the past few years, and knowledge of the molecular biology of cancer will in the future have a major impact on daily clinical practice. Additional studies are needed to more precisely elucidate and understand the underlying molecular mechanisms of each cancer before findings can be translated into widespread routine use in daily patient care.

Selected Bibliography

Hallmarks of Cancer

Hanahan D, Weinberg RA: The hallmarks of cancer. *Cell* 2000;100:57-70.

Overview of the Cell Cycle

Elledge SJ: Cell cycle checkpoints: Preventing an identity crisis. *Science* 1996;274:1664-1672.

Ford HL, Pardee AB: Cancer and the cell cycle. *J Cell Biochem* 1999;33:166-172.

Schafer KA: The cell cycle: A review. *Vet Pathol* 1998;35:461-478.

Sherr CJ: Cancer cell cycles. *Science* 1996;274:1672-1677.

Sherr CJ: The Pezcoller lecture: Cancer cell cycles revisited. *Cancer Res* 2000;60:3689-3695.

Oncogenes and Tumor Suppressor Genes

Esteller M: Aberrant DNA methylation as a cancer-inducing mechanism. *Annu Rev Pharmacol Toxicol* 2005;45:629-656.

Komarova NL, Sengupta A, Nowak MA: Mutation-selection networks of cancer initiation: Tumor suppressor genes and chromosomal instability. *J Theor Biol* 2003;223:433-450.

Krug U, Ganser A, Koeffler HP: Tumor suppressor genes in normal and malignant hematopoiesis. *Oncogene* 2002;21:3475-3495.

Tokino T, Nakamura Y: The role of p53-target genes in human cancer. *Crit Rev Oncol Hematol* 2000;33:1-6.

Wang XW, Harris CC: p53 tumor-suppressor gene: Clues to molecular carcinogenesis. *J Cell Physiol* 1997;173:247-255.

Zheng L, Lee WH: The retinoblastoma gene: A prototypic and multifunctional tumor suppressor. *Exp Cell Res* 2001;264:2-18.

Genetic Abnormalities Associated With Muscuoloskeletal Tumors

Arvand A, Denny CT: Biology of EWS/ETS fusions in Ewing's family tumors. *Oncogene* 2001;20:5747-5754.

Berend KR, Toth AP, Harrelson JM, Layfield LJ, Hey LA, Scully SP: Association between ratio of matrix metalloproteinase-1 to tissue inhibitor of metalloproteinase-1 and local recurrence, metastasis, and survival in human chondrosarcoma. *J Bone Joint Surg Am* 1998;80:11-17.

Fuchs B, Pritchard DJ: Etiology of osteosarcoma. *Clin Orthop Relat Res* 2002;397:40-52.

Guillou L, Benhattar J, Bonichon F, et al: Histologic grade, but not SYT-SSX fusion type, is an important prognostic factor in patients with synovial sarcoma: A multicenter, retrospective analysis. *J Clin Oncol* 2004;22:4040-4050.

Hopyan S, Gokgoz N, Poon R, et al: A mutant PTH/PTHrP type I receptor in enchondromatosis. *Nat Genet* 2002;30:306-310.

Ladanyi M: Fusions of the SYT and SSX genes in synovial sarcoma. *Oncogene* 2001;20:5755-5762.

Letson GD, Muro-Cacho CA: Genetic and molecular abnormalities in tumors of the bone and soft tissues. *Cancer Control* 2001;8:239-251.

Mendelsohn J, Howley PM, Israel M, Liotta L (eds): *The Molecular Basis of Cancer,* ed 2. Philadelphia, PA, Elsevier, 2001.

Sandberg AA: Cytogenetics and molecular genetics of bone and soft-tissue tumors. *Am J Med Genet* 2002;115:189-193.

Moving Toward Molecular Diagnosis

Bridge JA, Sandberg AA: Cytogenetic and molecular genetic techniques as adjunctive approaches in the diagnosis of bone and soft tissue tumors. *Skeletal Radiol* 2000;29:249-258.

Graadt van Roggen JF, Bovee JV, Morreau J, Hogendoorn PC: Diagnostic and prognostic implications of the unfolding molecular biology of bone and soft tissue tumours. *J Clin Pathol* 1999;52:481-489.

Oliveira AM, Nascimento AG: Grading in soft tissue tumors: Principles and problems. *Skeletal Radiol* 2001;30:543-559.

Uchida A, Seto M, Hashimoto N, Araki N: Molecular diagnosis and gene therapy in musculoskeletal tumors. *J Orthop Sci* 2000;5:418-423.

Principles of Chemotherapy and Resistance

Buchdunger E, O'Reilly T, Wood J: Pharmacology of imatinib (STI571). *Eur J Cancer* 2002;38(suppl 5):S28-S36.

Gottesman MM, Pastan I, Ambudkar SV: P-glycoprotein and multidrug resistance. *Curr Opin Genet Dev* 1996;6:610-617.

Terek RM, Schwartz GK, Devaney K, et al: Chemotherapy and P-glycoprotein expression in chondrosarcoma. *J Orthop Res* 1998;16:585-590.

Ueda K, Yoshida A, Amachi T: Recent progress in P-glycoprotein research. *Anticancer Drug Des* 1999;14:115-121.

Wunder JS, et al: MDR1 gene expression and outcome in osteosarcoma: A prospective, multicenter study. *J Clin Oncol* 2000;18:2685-2694.

Tumor Metastasis

De Wever O, Mareel M: Role of myofibroblasts at the invasion front. *Biol Chem* 2002;383:55-67.

Fidler IJ: The pathogenesis of cancer metastasis: The "seed and soil" hypothesis revisited. *Nat Rev Cancer* 2003;3:453-458.

Guise TA, Kozlow WM, Heras-Herzig A, Padalecki SS, Yin JJ, Chirgwin JM: Molecular mechanisms of breast cancer metastases to bone. *Clin Breast Cancer* 2005;5(suppl 2):S46-S53.

Lipton A: Management of bone metastases in breast cancer. *Curr Treat Options Oncol* 2005;6:161-171.

Mareel M, Leroy A: Clinical, cellular, and molecular aspects of cancer invasion. *Physiol Rev* 2003;83:337-376.

Paget S: The distribution of secondary growths in cancer of the breast. *Cancer Metastasis Rev* 1989;8:98-101.

Woodhouse EC, Chuaqui RF, Liotta LA: General mechanisms of metastasis. *Cancer* 1997;80(suppl 8):1529-1537.

Chapter 22

Osteoarthritis and Rheumatoid Arthritis

Theodore R. Oegema, PhD
Jack L. Lewis, PhD
Katalin Mikecz, MD, PhD
Istvan Gal, MD

Introduction

Osteoarthritis (OA) and inflammatory arthritis both cause significant disability because of synovial joint destruction, but the destruction occurs via different mechanisms (Figure 1). This chapter reviews the basic science of what is known about these disease processes. Rather than providing a brief summary of all inflammatory arthritic diseases, the focus is on rheumatoid arthritis (RA) as an archetype.

OA is defined with emphasis on the difference between structural and symptomatic disease, and its socioeconomic impact and incidence are discussed along with the risk factors identified from epidemiologic and clinical studies. The pathology section emphasizes that while in early disease, cartilage loss may be a central feature, as the disease progresses OA involves all aspects of the joint. Changes in the soft tissue and bone dominate the later pathology, contribute to pain, and compromise joint function. In the etiology of OA, genetic, biologic, and biomechanical contributions are discussed. Because cartilage destruction is a key characteristic of OA and the current strategies to find disease-modifying agents to slow progression are directed at preventing cartilage loss, the biology and biomechanics of OA cartilage are presented in detail.

The definition and pathology of RA are discussed, but major emphasis is placed on the complex interactions of the cells and cytokines that initiate and perpetuate the autoimmune process in the joint and the mechanisms of bone and cartilage destruction. The mechanisms of action of key drugs are presented later in this chapter.

Osteoarthritis

Socioeconomic Impact

OA has a significant socioeconomic impact. It is the leading cause of the loss of mobility in the elderly population and affects the quality of life and ability to perform activities of daily living. In 1990, it was estimated that there were 27 million Americans with OA. With the increase in the aging population by 2020, this number will increase to more than 47 million, with a cost to society of lost productivity and increased care estimated at 1% of the gross national product. OA of the knee, because of its frequency and impact on the quality of life, has the most significant socioeconomic impact of OA of any joint.

Definition

Although OA is a degenerative disease of the synovial joint that involves the progressive focal loss of the articular cartilage and includes extensive bone changes as prominent features, the disease involves all the joint structures. These changes, which include ligamentous laxity and joint deformity, contribute to the surgical challenge of reconstruction. Thus, OA can be defined as either structural or symptomatic.

Structural OA

Structural OA is defined by focal loss of articular cartilage, usually in a weight-bearing area, and includes the presence of osteophytes and other bone changes. Because of its general availability and relatively low cost, radiography is used to assess most patients with structural OA. The radiographic criteria for assessing joints, such as those described by the American College of Rheumatology, are used for

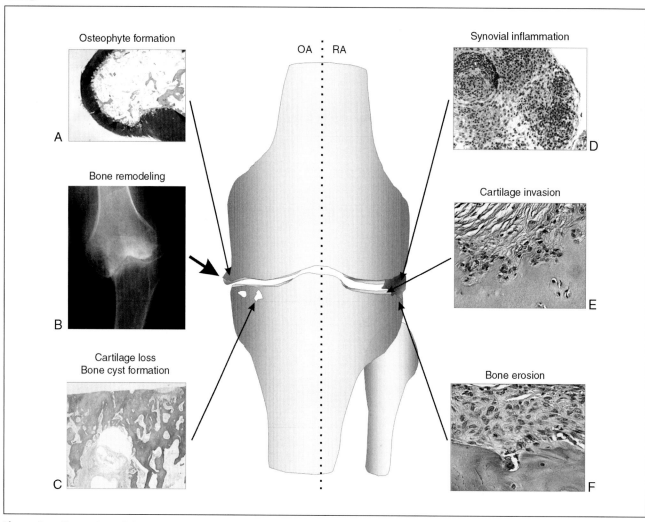

Figure 1   Illustration of the pathology of a synovial joint with OA or RA. **A,** Photomicrograph of a knee osteophyte. The original articular cartilage makes a smooth transition with the osteophytic cartilage (safranin O-fast green, original magnification ×2). **B,** Radiograph of knee with OA and extensive bone remodeling and instability. **C,** Photomicrograph of eburnated bone with a subchondral cyst and failed fibrocartilage outgrowth from subchondral bone (safranin O-fast green, original magnification ×10). **D,** Photomicrograph of rheumatoid synovium with a multilayered synovial lining and the presence of inflammatory cells (hematoxylin and eosin, original magnification ×20). **E,** Photomicrograph of rheumatoid pannus-cartilage interface (hematoxylin and eosin, original magnification ×60). **F,** Photomicrograph of rheumatoid pannus-bone interface (hematoxylin and eosin, original magnification ×60).

diagnosing structural OA. Joint-specific grading scales, such as the radiographic Kellgren-Lawrence scale for the knee, can be used to describe the impact of the overall changes on the joint. Because radiographs do not visualize soft tissues of the joint, these changes are unappreciated, and the radiographic criteria are based on bone changes, especially the presence of osteophytes and joint space narrowing, which is a surrogate for cartilage loss. In research studies in which progression of joint-space narrowing is assessed quantitatively, radiographs are obtained under carefully specified conditions and limb positioning. Structural OA can also be visualized by other methods, including arthroscopy and MRI, which visualize soft tissues and provide different perspectives of joint damage. For research of structural OA, arthroscopy is still the gold standard for documenting cartilage loss, surface fibrillation,

and the condition of ligaments and meniscus. Proton MRI with specific imaging sequences can provide detailed cartilage and soft-tissue images and cartilage volume as well as detect the presence of bone marrow edema.

MRI methods can provide additional detail of the cartilage structure. Using an anionic gadolinium complex as a contrast agent and a timed delay before imaging to allow the agent to diffuse into cartilage, delayed gadolinium-enhanced MRI of cartilage can be used to determine the negative image of the glycosaminoglycan distribution in cartilage. The negative image is generated because the anionic contrast agent is excluded from areas with high glycosaminoglycan content. Sodium is the major cation that provides the counter ion to the anionic glycosaminoglycans in cartilage; therefore, sodium MRI can also be used to obtain a positive image of glycosaminoglycan content.

Table 1 Factors Contributing to Secondary Arthritis

Systemic	Local

Growth Factors Dysregulation
  Acromegaly
  Hyperparathyroidism
	Disruption of joint continuity
	  Trauma to joint structures
	    (meniscus, ligaments,
	    cartilage, and bone)
	  Osteochondritis

Abnormal loading
  Ehlers-Danlos syndrome
  Hyperlaxity syndromes
	Abnormal loading
	  Developmental deformity
	  Neuropathic arthropathy

Metabolic defects
  Hemachromatosis
  Ochronosis
  Wilson's disease
  Amloidosis
	Cartilage damage
	  Septic arthritis
	  Rheumatoid arthritis
	  Gout
	  Chondrocalcinosis
	  Hemophilia

	Bone changes
	  Paget's disease
	  Osteonecrosis

Table 2 Risk Factors for Osteoarthritis

Systemic	Extrinsic Factors Acting on the Joint	Intrinsic Joint Vulnerabilities
Age Ethnicity Gender Hormonal status Bone density Nutritional factors Genetics	Obesity Injurious activities	Malalignment Proprioception Laxity Previous trauma Bridging muscle weakness

Both of these methods allow evidence of OA to be identified in its early stages.

Symptomatic OA

Symptomatic OA is defined by the criteria of the American College of Rheumatology. Symptomatic disease is easily documented by physical examination and radiography or, if needed, can be confirmed by arthroscopy. Clinical diagnosis requires not only changes in the synovial joint, but also the presence of symptoms that possibly include joint pain, decreased joint motion, joint effusion, crepitus with motion, and joint deformity. Additional goals of the diagnosis of symptomatic OA are to rule out RA and determine whether OA is a secondary complication of other possibly treatable causes (Table 1). Because there is frequently discordance between the various simple measures of incidence and the progression and response to treatment of symptomatic OA, multidimensional descriptors have been developed. These disease-specific questionnaires have been designed and validated for particular patient groups and joints. An example of such an instrument is the Western Ontario and McMaster Universities Osteoarthritis Index (WOMAC), with a recent addition of a knee injury and OA score (KOOS) module for patients who have higher expectations and are more active than those for whom the WOMAC was originally designed. Some of the instruments are primarily for research, but others may be useful in clinical practice.

Incidence

OA (the variable presence of inflammation, degenerative joint disease, or degenerative arthritis) can occur in all synovial joints. OA commonly occurs in order of preva-

lence in the first distal interphalangeal, first carpometacarpal, and proximal interphalangeal joints of the hand; the metatarsophalangeal joints of the feet; and the facet joints of the cervical and lumbar spine, knee, and hip. OA can occur in single joints or multiple joints. When multiple joints are involved, it is sometimes referred to as generalized OA and can be divided into patients with and without Heberden's nodes.

The incidence of OA in the general population depends on how it is measured (radiographic, self-reported, or symptomatic) and the cut-off criteria used to determine the presence of OA. However, the different measures follow the same trends. By any measure (the number of joints involved, the severity of the symptoms, or the incidence of self-reported occurrence), the incidence of OA increases with age. In a study of self-reported OA in any joint, the incidence was 10% to 15% in men and women in the age range of 34 to 44 years, but increased to 50% in those in the age range of 65 to 74 years. By age 70 years, virtually everyone will have a joint with structural OA. Radiographic evidence of OA occurs at the rate of 33% in the hand and 33% in the knee in individuals older than 60 years, but 40% to 50% of these individuals have no symptoms. Conversely, joint pain is common and does not always correspond to the presence of OA. Twenty-five percent of individuals older than 55 years have knee pain, but approximately half of them have radiographic evidence of OA. In extremely elderly individuals, the percentage of individuals with symptomatic OA may actually decline.

Epidemiologically and Clinically Identified Risk Factors

The risk factors for OA can be different for initiation and progression of the disease and for determining whether structural OA becomes symptomatic (Table 2). Additionally, the risk factors may be different for different joints. Although the impact of a single risk factor may be sufficient to initiate OA or cause progression, in most patients it is likely that several risk factors interact.

Systemic Factors

Age and Gender There are gender differences in occurrence, but these differences depend on the joint and sex. Males younger than 50 years experience more radiographic OA and those 50 years and older continue to have more hip OA than females, but females have a higher incidence in the knee and hand after age 50 years.

Ethnic Background There are racial differences in the prevalence of OA. In the United States, the occurrence of knee OA is roughly equivalent in Caucasians and African Americans; but African Americans typically have a more serious and disabling form of the disease. There are differences in the prevalence of OA in China and the United States; and although Chinese-surnamed Americans have a lower incidence of hip and hand OA, they have a higher incidence of knee OA than American Caucasians.

Hormonal Status All major tissues of the joint are responsive to sex hormones. Because of the increased prevalence of OA in women older than 50 years, hormonal status is believed to play a role in the development and/or progression of OA. However, the results of hormone replacement studies have yielded varied results and generally show little or no effect of hormone replacement on symptomatic OA.

Bone Density There is a long-standing hypothesis that increased bone density may predispose cartilage to damage and that osteoporosis may be protective. Increased bone density increases the risk of hand and knee structural OA. However, once OA is initiated, osteoporosis may increase the chance for progression possibly because it interferes with bone remodeling and repair.

Nutrition Little is known about the effect of nutrition on OA. In a cohort study, the consumption of vitamin C in the middle to upper tertile was noted to lower the risk of structural OA. When the vitamin D levels were in the middle and lower tertile, the risk of OA increased, which may be the result of the impact of vitamin D on bone metabolism.

Genetics Genetics contribute significantly to OA initiation and progression. The interactions are non-mendelian, multifactorial, and complex. For example, an individual with a family member with hip OA is three times more likely to develop hip OA. In twin studies of OA in the hand, spine, and hip, 60% to 70% of the variance is the result of genetic influences. In the knee, genetics are a significant factor, but account for only 30% to 40% of the variance.

Extrinsic Factors Acting on the Joint

Normal joints withstand the activities of daily life, and the movement provides important biomechanical feedback to the cells of all structures of the joints. When the mechanical forces of normal activity affect an abnormal joint, or excess forces act on a normal joint, injury and subsequent OA may occur. Work-related activities can require highly repetitive actions for many hours per day over many years and may result in motions and forces that exceed the normal protective mechanisms of the joint. For example, farmers have an increased incidence of hip OA, individuals in occupations requiring heavy lifting and carrying have an increased incidence of knee and spine OA, jackhammer operators have an increased incidence of elbow and shoulder OA, and dockyard workers have an increased incidence of knee and finger OA. In fact, knee bending while lifting or carrying may account for a substantial portion (10% to 15%) of knee OA in men that is not genetic. The repetitive motion of sports can provide the same type of motions and forces that damage joints when they are excessive, but this cause is not as strongly implicated as others. For example, runners are not at excessive risk for knee OA, but persons with hip OA are more likely to have been runners. The interaction of risk factors is demonstrated by the fact that runners with previous joint injuries are especially vulnerable to late OA in the knee.

Obesity is a risk factor for the initiation and progression of OA in the knee and to a lesser extent in the hip. Most of the effects of obesity are believed to be a result of increased force on the joints. For example, in a one-leg stance, forces increase by a factor of two; therefore, small differences in weight can have a significant impact. Not only does obesity contribute to OA, but losing as little as 20 lb will decrease the risk of radiographic OA by 50%, and weight loss will improve symptomatic OA. Because obese women with bilateral knee OA also have an increased incidence of hand OA, systemic factors related to obesity, such as leptin, may also contribute to the disease.

Local Biomechanical Factors

Joint Injury Acute trauma to the articular cartilage leads to different types of cartilage and bone damage, which probably pose different levels of risk for OA initiation and progression. At the time of joint arthroplasty, 10% to 15% of patients with hip or knee OA report an earlier significant incident of trauma. In the ankle, which is a joint that does not normally develop OA, acute trauma can lead to rapid joint destruction. Massive articular and bone fractures need to be reduced to less than 3 mm of displacement or there will be a rise in local contact stress that is sufficient to cause focal cartilage loss. Less severe traumatic forces can lead to bone bruises, with small subchondral bone fractures occurring through the zone of calcified cartilage, cracks occurring on the articular surface, and cell death occurring around the cracks. In weight-bearing areas, these injuries may rapidly result in further degeneration. Even low-impact loads can lead to surface cartilage cracks and cell death. It is not known whether these lesions progress.

Hip Dysplasia Hip dysplasia increases the risk for hip OA. The magnitude of articular cartilage contact stress increases because of abnormal joint shape and correlates with an increased risk of degeneration. This may be because there is a critical threshold of cumulative articular cartilage surface contact stress that, when exceeded, causes cartilage degeneration.

Knee Deformity Varus and valgus deformity of the knees are associated with increased risk of OA and OA progression because of abnormal loading.

Bridging Muscle Weakness In the knee, weakness of the quadriceps muscles has been found in both the involved and uninvolved knees of women with OA, suggesting that weakness may precede and contribute to the development and progression of OA. Additional evidence from genetic studies suggests that muscle weakness may predispose a normal joint to OA. Muscle strengthening and exercise have positive affects on symptomatic OA.

Joint Proprioception The conscious and unconscious perception of joint position and moment is essential for maintaining dynamic joint stabilization. Proprioception declines with age and is reduced in both the arthritic and nonarthritic joints of patients with OA, which suggests that the decline may precede the development of OA and contribute to increased risk of OA.

Joint Laxity In individuals with joint laxity in the knee, there is a displacement or rotation of the tibia with respect to the femur. Frontal plane or varus-valgus laxity increases with age, and the degree of this type of laxity is greater in women than men. Varus-valgus laxity may precede the development of OA and may predispose individuals to knee OA. Anteroposterior laxity may increase in persons with mild OA, but it may decline with advanced disease as the capsule thickens.

Joint Alignment
Joint alignment in the knee is related to the hip and ankle. The magnitude of torque that adducts the knee during the stance phase of gait is related to OA severity and may predict progression. Malalignment is associated with poor surgical outcomes.

Pain in Symptomatic OA
The synovial capsule, ligaments, synovium, periosteum, and subchondral bone are innervated with nerve endings that can respond to nociceptive stimuli. Both subchondral bone changes and synovitis in patients with OA correlates with the presence of pain; therefore, at least these two tis-

sues can generate pain in vivo. The normal joint is relatively resistant to generating pain probably because a low pain threshold can hinder the activities of daily living. Some evidence supports the presence of peripheral hyperalgesia in the OA joint that could be mediated by cytokines and nerve growth factors. Furthermore, there may be sensitization of the spinal cord and on the cortical level in the brain. There can also be a destruction feedback loop in which stimulation from neurogenic inflammation can cause the release of factors such as substance P and cytokines that interact with inflammatory pathways and further exacerbate joint pathology. The perception of pain can be modified by psychological, social, and contextual factors.

Because pain is the dominant characteristic in symptomatic OA that causes patients to seek treatment, understanding pain is a key element of treating symptomatic OA. Psychosocial risk factors for pain in patients with OA include some physical activities, health status, anxiety in women, psychological well-being, depression, hypochondria, and negative affect or emotion. In addition, health-seeking behavior, educational status, and ethnic background may modify pain reporting.

Pathology
A progressive loss of the articular surface occurs in OA (**Figure 2**), with sporadic (sometimes successful) attempts at repair, a remodeling of the subchondral bone with sclerosis, synovial and capsular thickening (sometimes with mild to moderate inflammation), the frequent occurrence of marginal osteophytes (**Figure 1**), and, especially in patients with end-stage disease, the presence of sclerotic bone cysts. As seen in radiographic, population-based studies, mild to severe degenerative changes are present in many joints, but most never progress to the point of symptomatic OA.

Articular Cartilage
In animal models, such as the canine anterior cruciate ligament resection model, and also believed to occur in human OA, initial changes involve damage to the tangential zone immediately below the articular surface, with disorganization of the collagen network, loss of proteoglycans, and swelling (**Figure 2**). This is followed by a hypertrophic repair response with increased synthesis and accumulation of proteoglycan. Eventually, the tissue begins to fail with the loss of surface integrity and fibrillation parallel to the surface. In the deeper layers, the fibrillation follows the alignment of the collagen fibrils and becomes perpendicular to the surface. In the regions of extensive damage, there is an accompanying generalized loss of cellularity and the sporadic formation of cell clusters or clones (**Figure 2**). Just above the tidemark, which was a functional growth plate in the immature joint, the cells again express a hypertrophic phenotype that produces alkaline phosphatase,

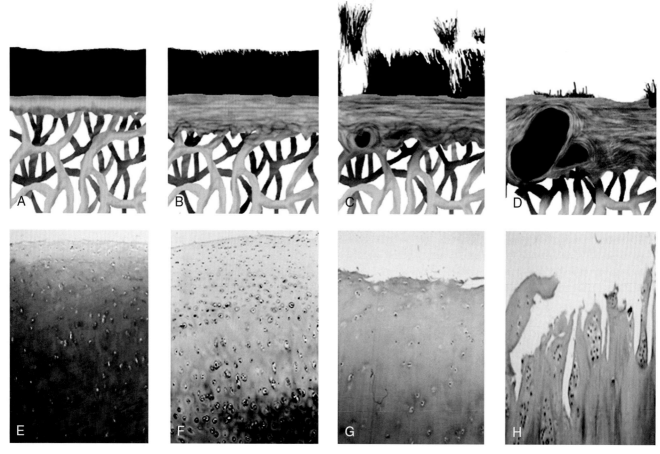

Figure 2   **A** through **D**, Schematic representation of osteoarthritic changes in subchondral bone and increasing cartilage fragmentation. **E** through **H**, Photomicrographs show human articular cartilage (stained with safranin O-fast green) with progressive loss of surface integrity and proteoglycan (darkest areas) followed by fibrillation with decreased cellularity and formation of clones. (Original magnification ×10).

type X collagen, and matrix vesicles. Multiple tidemarks are formed that suggest an active remodeling of the region. Catastrophic failure of the fibrillated cartilage leads to the presence of cartilage fragments in the joint. Although the loss of cartilage can be rapid, it usually occurs slowly, and there may be extended periods in which the loss is stabilized or even temporarily reversed by the repair process or replacement by fibrocartilage arising from the subchondral bone. Distinguishing slow from rapid cartilage loss is an area of active investigation and may be a key to effective early interventions. Because cartilage is a spacer between the bones, the consequences of the loss of cartilage are increased joint laxity and angular deformity.

Synovium and Capsule
In the early phases of OA, there are mild inflammatory changes in the synovium. Although inflammation is not a dominant characteristic in the early phases, even low levels of inflammatory cytokines can make the cartilage more vulnerable to degeneration. In the middle phases of OA, the synovium has moderate inflammatory changes focused

around the areas of cartilage destruction, and the synovium appears hypervascular. In the late phases of OA, there is increased evidence of inflammation. The synovium has multiple layers of lining cells, thickening, villus formation, and neovascularity. When ultrasound was used to identify joint infusion and inflamed synovium in patients with symptomatic OA, 60% had inflammation, and this was highly correlated with the presence of pain. With advancing OA, the joint capsule is usually thickened and may adhere to the underlying bone and limit movement.

Bone
Bone changes, especially in the subchondral plate, are an important part of the pathology of OA, and there is a complex relationship among cartilage pathology, changes in subchondral bone, and bone pathology and remodeling (**Figure 2**). For example, when there is rapid degradation in the overlying cartilage, elevated subchondral bone remodeling occurs, as detected using bone scintigraphy or by the presence of elevated markers of bone turnover such as type I collagen cross-links in the urine or osteocalcin in

the blood. There is a much debated proposal that bone changes may precede cartilage changes. In a rabbit model of impulse loading, subchondral bone damage precedes cartilage changes. However, there is little evidence that this is true in humans. Early on, there is a loss of subchondral bone possibly caused by altered loading, and then there is an increase in the subchondral plate thickness and sclerosis in later stages in most types of joints (Figure 2). This bone is hypomineralized and is less stiff than normal bone.

OA bone may also contain areas identified by MRI as bone marrow edema. These areas correspond to areas of high bone turnover detected by scintigraphic methods and lie below areas of cartilage damage. Histologically, the areas show little edema, but contain abnormal bone with excess fibrosis, small areas of necrosis, and areas consistent with ongoing extensive bony remodeling. In patients with knee OA, medial bone marrow lesions are associated with varus limbs, and lateral lesions are associated with valgus limbs. The presence of bone marrow edema is associated with pain and predicts increases in joint deformity and the risk of OA progression.

Frequently, cells from bone or marrow spaces generate fibrocartilage that can partially replace the function of articular cartilage for many years. When denuded bone surfaces are present, there may be areas of avascular necrotic bone mixed with hypervascularized bone and altered blood flow.

Bone cysts are a common late characteristic of OA. Bone cysts differ from those in RA in that they are lytic and have sclerotic edges (Figures 1 and 2). Bone cysts contain a viscous clear fluid and a fibrous tissue containing only a few cells that are capable of producing cytokines, prostaglandins, proteinases, metalloproteases, and nitric oxide. These cells can recruit and stimulate osteoclasts. In animal models of OA, areas that will become cysts are detected by MRI soon after early cartilage changes are observed. Once the cyst has formed, mechanical forces promote enlargement (as least in the knee), and their presence correlates with increased risk of knee pain.

Osteophytes

Osteophytes are frequently present in the OA joint (Figure 1). Although it has been suggested that osteophytes may be a mechanism for stabilizing the degenerative joint, this is unlikely because the new surfaces usually are not articulating. Osteophytes typically originate near the insertion of the synovium on the bone and arise from mesenchymal progenitor cells in the periosteum or synovium. Osteophytes require a complex set of growth factors to develop and mature, including insulin-like growth factor (IGF)-1 and bone morphogenetic proteins (BMPs). Transforming growth factor-β (TGF-β), which is present in high concentrations in the synovial fluid of patients with OA, is a potent inducer of osteophytes. The cells initiate a chondrogenic differentiation process in the fibrous connective tissue and form a fibrocartilage, the deep layers of which undergo endochondral ossification. The mature osteophyte has a well-developed hyaline cartilage surface that is easily confused with the articular cartilage (Figure 1). The bone in the osteophyte may have thickened cortices and vascular canals with prominent cement lines. Because osteophytes are easily recognized on radiographs, they are frequently used as an indicator for the presence of OA; however, in many joints the correlation of the presence, number, or size of osteophytes with the progression of OA is unclear.

Etiology

OA is not simply a wear and tear disease of articular cartilage, and many possible initiating events exist that lead to end-stage OA. Disease initiation and progression are separate processes, and each is probably controlled by different combinations of genetic, mechanical, and environmental factors. The relative importance of genetic, mechanical, and environmental factors may depend on the individual and may represent a continuous spectrum from a good joint in a bad environment to a bad joint in a good environment.

Age

Older individuals may be more prone to develop OA than younger individuals, but the age-related changes of cartilage are not part of the pathology of OA. Although a loss of cartilage height occurs at maturation, there is only a slow loss in cartilage height, hydration, and cellularity after maturation. In some joints, the surface cells are especially vulnerable to cell death by apoptosis. Chondrocytes also show signs of senescence, including telomere shortening. Telomeres are long repetitive DNA sequences that cap the ends of chromosomes and are required for chromosomal duplication. With each cell division, the telomeres shorten until they are too short to support cell duplication, and the cell enters senescence. Chondrocytes also have a slow loss of the redox potential, which results in decreased protection against oxidative species and leads to more mitochondrial damage.

In addition to the loss of water, other compositional changes occur. The type II collagen network is stable, but the dry weight of collagen content decreases because of the relative increase in other proteins. The proteoglycan content is relatively constant, but there is a shift to an aggrecan with high molecular weight, highly sulfated keratan sulfate and low molecular weight chondroitin sulfate (with more chondroitin-6 sulfate and less chondroitin-4 sulfate). There is an increase in aggrecan fragments with less hyaluronic acid binding. Hyaluronic acid content also increases with age, but decreases in size. Because there is less link protein, proteoglycan aggregates are less stable.

In immature cartilage, chondrocytes turn over both the interterritorial and territorial matrix components.

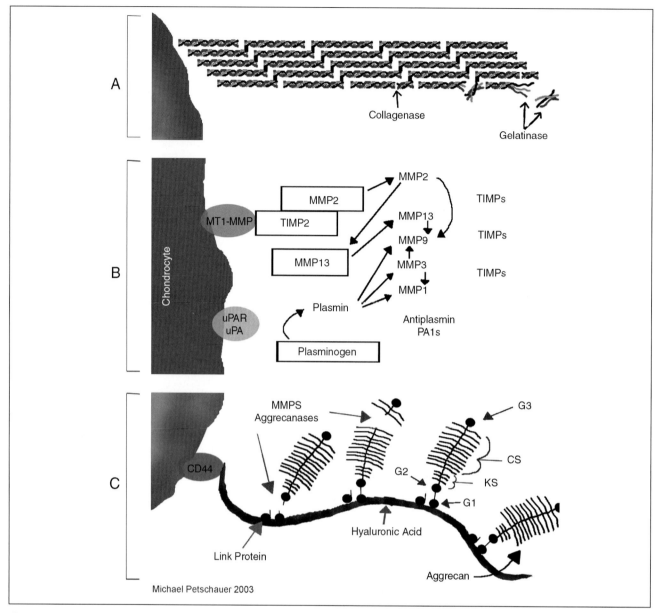

Michael Petschauer 2003

Figure 3   **A,** Illustration of type II collagen homotrimer in fibrils (type IX or XI collagen are omitted). The vertical bar represents a hydroxylpyridinium cross-link between collagen molecules. After collagenase digestion the three fourths and one fourth fragments both are retained in the fibril until removed by gelatinases. **B,** Illustration of the complex pathways of metalloprotease activation. The arrows indicate a protease activating a proform to give an active enzyme. The membrane protein membrane type 1 MMP (MT1-MMP) forms a complex with TIMP2 and pro-MMP-2 to activate the bound pro-MMP-2. TIMPs (1, 2, and 3) can then inhibit the active MMPs. Plasmin, which is activated by a plasminogen activator (uPA) in complex with an uPA receptor (uPAR), also activates some MMPs. Plasmin is inhibited by plasmin inhibitors. **C,** Aggrecan is organized into G1, G2, keratan sulfate-rich, CS-rich, and G3 domains and stabilized with link protein on HA. MMPs and aggrecanase(s) degrade aggrecan into fragments that still bind HA. PA = plasminogen activate; KS = keratan sulfate; CS = chondroitin sulfate

With age, cells experience a slow loss of synthetic capacity, and the rate of turnover declines, especially that of the interterritorial matrix. The collagen network barely turns over (a half-life of more than 100 years). Proteoglycan turnover slows and shifts primarily to the pericellular area. For example, aggrecan in the interterritorial matrix has a half-life of 30 years, but within the pericellular environment, it is 4 months. In mature and aging cartilage, turnover of aggrecan is controlled by proteases, and progressively shorter fragments of aggrecan that can bind hyaluronic acid (HA) are produced (**Figure 3**). These aggrecan fragments account for most of the noncollagenous proteins that accumulate in aging cartilage.

Old cartilage is beige in color because of the linear increase with age of "browning" produced by a nonenzymatic reaction of glucose with lysine and arginine side chains in proteins and subsequent rearrangement to advanced glycation end products, some of which (such as pentosidine) are colored. Chondrocytes in the glycated matrix produce less matrix molecules. Advanced glycation end products and lipid peroxidation products form cross-links between matrix components that lead to a stiffer and more brittle matrix. Some of the other mechanical properties of cartilage vary with age, but the compression stiffness is relatively unchanged. All of these changes make cartilage more vulnerable to developing OA.

Genetics

With the completion of the human genome project and large-scale human genetic studies such as the Icelandic and Finnish Studies, rapid progress is being made in understanding the genetic component of OA. Methods that have been applied to identify the genes responsible for OA include using markers of genetic polymorphism (such as polymorphic microsatellite markers) to find regions of interest that differ in individuals with OA and control subjects and using genes that are differentially expressed in OA chondrocytes and candidate gene screenings to screen for specific polymorphism.

Structural OA has a major genetic component that is transmitted in a nonmendelian complex manner. The genetic risk may vary with the site and between sexes. The genetic risk may also involve joint components other than cartilage because in individuals with knee OA, decreased muscle strength and decreased tibial bone area have both been identified as risk factors in genetic studies. Early studies focused on matrix proteins that are mutated in mendelian-inherited osteochondrodysplasia diseases and in patients with the rare early onset of OA and found mutations in type II collagen, type IX collagen, and cartilage oligomeric protein. Because of a low frequency of occurrence in the general population, there is no convincing evidence that specified mutations in these genes have spread into the general population and are major risk factors for monoarticular primary OA. Polymorphisms in the chondroitin sulfate repeat region of aggrecan, which results in different numbers of chondroitin sulfate chains per aggrecan, are associated with OA of the hand. This suggests other structural molecules may also be involved.

It has been suggested that many genes, each with diverse functions, contribute to primary OA; thus far, however, each of these candidate genes accounts for only a small percentage of OA and many are involved in signaling or inflammation. The vitamin D receptor, a silent mutation that does not cause loss of function, has been associated with OA. Similarly, estrogen receptor 1 variants are associated with an increased risk of OA. Several of the candidate genes are inflammatory cytokines or their receptors and include an interleukin (IL)-1 polymorphism, a risk factor for erosive hand OA, and an IL-4 receptor. Others include the matrix protein, matrilin 3; a developmental factor, frizzled-related protein 3, which is a chon-

drogenic regulator; asporin, a small leucine-rich protein that binds TGF-β; and BMP-5, which regulates cartilage development. Genes may affect different aspects of OA. BMP-2, a thrombospondin and collagen receptor, cyclooxygenase (COX)-2, and a nucleus receptor corepressor were identified as genetic risks factors for prevalence. In contrast, cartilage intermediate layer protein, osteoprotegerin, tetranectin, and estrogen receptor 1 were associated with progression. However, a disintegrin and metalloproteinase domain 12 gene, *ADAM-12*, was associated with both prevalence and progression.

Mediators

Proinflammatory cytokines produced by the synovium and the chondrocytes contribute to cartilage destruction, especially in the later stages of OA, the best characterized of which are IL-1β and tumor necrosis factor-α (TNF-α). Both cytokines are elevated in osteoarthritic synovial fluid and are produced by chondrocyte and synovial cells. The receptor for IL-1 is elevated in osteoarthritic chondrocytes, and the level of IL-1 receptor antagonist, a natural inhibitor, is lower. Similarly, TNF-α is elevated in late-stage osteoarthritic synovial fluid. Osteoarthritic chondrocytes produce TNF-α and elevated levels of one of the TNF-α receptors (TNF-α p55 receptor), localized to areas of matrix damage. TNF-α and IL-1 can synergize to promote matrix destruction via synthesis of matrix metalloproteinases (MMPs), inducible nitric oxide synthase, and COX-2. Additional cytokines such as oncostatin M, IL-8, and IL-6 have been found in osteoarthritic joints and can function as enhancers, inhibitors, or modulators of matrix synthesis and destruction.

Regarding tissue repair and synthesis, TGF-β is found in high concentrations in osteoarthritic synovial fluid, along with BMP-2, -4, -6, -7, -9, and -13 and growth and differentiation factor-5. Osteoarthritic chondrocytes, as with aging chondrocytes, are resistant to the anabolic effect of IGF-1, despite the presence of elevated levels of IGF-1, IGF-1 receptor, and IGF-binding proteins 2, 3, and 4.

Osteoarthritic Changes in Cartilage Biology and Biomechanics

Cell and Matrix

Chondrocyte proliferation, cell death, or loss of phenotype are dominant characteristics of early OA. In early OA, there is an upregulation of chondrocyte metabolism that reflects a response to the altered environment, with a less mature form of aggrecan with more chondroitin 4-sulfate and increases in type VI collagen and fibronectin. There is only a moderate loss in cellularity, with 1% to 3% of cells near the surface showing apoptotic markers. In the later stages of OA, there is limited proliferation in damaged areas, leading to cell clones. In these areas, a few chondrocytes also take a fibroblastic morphology and express abnormal matrix molecules such as type I and type III collagen, but this is not generalized. The deep chondrocytes become more hypertrophic, and this change may contribute to the pathology by altering mineralization and degradation.

Biomechanics

Normal-functioning cartilage has material properties within a narrow range; diseased cartilage has properties outside of this range. Diseased cartilage is generally less stiff, weaker, and has poorer energy dissipation than normal-functioning cartilage. Cartilage material properties are a consequence of microstructural composition and organization of the tissue. This microstructure is degraded by the disease process, resulting in softening and fibrillation of the tissue.

Normal-functioning cartilage has a rubbery feel and a glistening surface. As cartilage first begins to degenerate in OA, it becomes swollen, softer, and takes on a dull appearance. There is also a significant decrease in tensile stiffness of the surface layer that progresses to the deeper layers. This decrease correlates with collagen content and collagen damage. A probe pushed into the surface of degenerating cartilage leaves an impression, reflecting increased hydraulic permeability and decreased compressive stiffness. Microscopic surface disruptions result in the dull appearance of degenerating cartilage.

The disease process attacks critical elements of the load-carrying system. Early damage to the collagen network allows proteoglycans to expand and swell the tissue. The proteoglycan expansion is driven by the Donnan swelling pressure of the chondroitin sulfate and keratan sulfate. Later in the disease process, there is an increase of the hydraulic permeability because the lower concentration of glycosaminoglycans results in increased pore size in the tissue. The increase in water flow changes how the load is distributed in the tissue. In normal cartilage, 90% to 95% of the load is supported by pressurization of the trapped interstitial water. With increased water flow, this load is transferred to the collagen-proteoglycan matrix, which is no longer shielded from damage. More rapid water flow upsets the friction and energy dissipation mechanisms, causing increased friction and decreased ability to absorb impact energy. This can lead to the fibrillation that is typical of late-stage osteoarthritic lesions. It also causes more focal transfer of force to the adjacent bone.

Osteoarthritic Cartilage: Anabolism Versus Catabolism

In combination with mechanical factors, cell-mediated responses contribute significantly to matrix breakdown in OA. The loss of matrix is the result of a shift in the balance between anabolism and catabolism. Very early in the disease process, there is an elevation of matrix synthesis, including aggrecan, the small leucine-rich proteoglycans, decorin and biglycan, and the cartilage-specific isoform of

fibronectin. Although the messenger RNA for type II collagen is also greatly upregulated over levels normally found in mature cartilage, little of the major normal structural isoform of type IIA collagen is deposited into the matrix. In contrast, the type IIB collagen isoform that is normally produced during cartilage formation and binds BMPs is secreted into the matrix.

Even in the late stages of OA, there is a continued effort to produce matrix; however, as the disease progresses, catabolism predominates. The cartilage contains more fragments of matrix proteins, and these are released into the synovial fluid in elevated amounts. For example, cartilage oligomeric protein is a member of the thrombospondin family and helps stabilize the collagen matrix by Ca^{2+}-dependent binding to type II collagen and by forming bridges with type IX collagen. The appearance of proteolytic fragments of cartilage oligomeric protein in the synovial fluid is a sensitive marker of early damage. Some of the fragments, such as those generated from fibronectin and collagen, have biologic activities that are not exhibited by the parent molecule and can either inhibit synthesis or enhance catabolism.

Damage to the collagen network occurs early at the surface layer. This allows the proteoglycans to expand their domain, resulting in a 3% to 6% increase in water content. This early damage is believed to be the result of breaking connections between the fibrils. Subsequently, increased collagenase activity at the surface degrades the collagen molecules into three fourths to one fourth fragments that remain attached to fibrils via cross-links (**Figure 3**). Although MMP-1, MMP-8, MMP-13, and membrane type 1 MMP (MMP-14) can act as collagenases, MMP-13 shows the greatest increase in OA and has the highest activity for type II collagen. The denatured collagen fragments can be removed by many enzymes, but especially by the gelatinases, MMP-2 and MMP-9, as well as MMP-3 (stromelysin). Collagen damage increases in the late stages of OA and occurs deeper in the tissue; in end-stage OA, up to 50% of the collagen present in the tissue is partially degraded.

In the early stages of OA, aggrecan loss is more pronounced than collagen damage. A rebound in synthesis occurs in early lesions, resulting in normal or elevated concentrations of aggrecan that are rapidly turned over. With disease progression, catabolism becomes dominant, and aggrecan levels are reduced to less than 50% of the normal level. In aging cartilage, the predominant fragments of aggrecan are generated by MMPs (MMP-3 and membrane type 1 MMP [MMP-14]). In OA, the predominant cleavages are produced by ADAMTS-4 and ADAMTS-5, enzymes that were originally called aggrecanases and members of a family of proteases containing the disintegrin and metalloproteinase with thrombospondin motifs. A recent study shows that deletion of the *ADAMTS-5* gene slows the development of osteoarthritis in a mouse knee joint injury model. Thus, catabolic enzymes might be a target to modify the progression and development of OA.

There is no evidence of unique proteases being expressed only in OA, but there are differences in the amount and localization of the proteases. Stromelysin (MMP-3) expression is upregulated in early OA, but decreases in later stages of the diseases. The gelatinase MMP-9 and collagenase MMP-13 are highly upregulated in late stages of OA, as is membrane type 1 MMP. These enzymes are synthesized as inactive proforms that are then activated in complicated pathways (**Figure 3**). Because there is little change in the expression of tissue inhibitor of metalloproteinases (TIMPs) during OA, this could lead to increased proteolytic activity. Other families of proteases such as cathepsins and plasmins may also play a role.

Principles of Medical Therapy
Hyaluronic Acid
HA or hyaluronan is used clinically to decrease joint pain and improve function in patients with OA. HA is a normal constituent of synovial fluid that, because it is a high-molecular-weight linear glycosaminoglycan that is present in high concentrations, increases the viscosity of the fluid and forms a boundary layer at the synovial lining-synovial fluid interface that retards the flow of fluid. In osteoarthritic synovial fluid, the concentration and molecular weight of HA are slightly reduced, but not as much as in patients with RA. In some acute animal models of OA and in race horses with traumatic arthritis, HA injections decrease pain and improve gait. In the synovium, HA modifies many biologic responses via specific cellular receptors, such as CD44. Hyaluronan also modifies cell activities such as the stretch-mediated firing of afferent nociceptive fibers via its physical properties. Controversy exists regarding the clinical efficacy of intra-articular HA for patients with OA, but it may be useful in a subset of patients with early symptomatic OA.

Glucosamine
Glucosamine hydrochloride and glucosamine sulfate are popular over-the-counter dietary supplements usually used in combination for the treatment of OA, with a long history of effective symptomatic relief in dogs and horses. As a slow-acting compound with an unknown mechanism of action, some studies have shown glucosamine relieves pain in approximately 50% to 60% of patients with early symptomatic OA. Glucosamine may also be chondroprotective because it is a precursor for the synthesis of chondroitin sulfate and keratan sulfate components of aggrecan. Oral glucosamine substitutes for glucosamine that is normally synthesized intracellularly from glucose and glutamine, but the levels that reach the joint are low. Glucosamine is not a rate-limiting precursor in proteoglycan synthesis, except in actively repairing tissue; therefore, determining the mechanisms of action of oral glucosamine and whether it is chondroprotective is still an area of ac-

tive research, and may involve primary action on tissue near the gut and secondary action on the joint.

Chondroitin Sulfate
Glucosamine is frequently used in combination with chondroitin sulfate. How chondroitin sulfate works in vivo is unknown, but both human and animal studies have shown that it usually achieves a small but positive effect. Oversulfated chondroitin sulfate is an inhibitor of many metalloproteinases in vitro, and it alters the activity of some growth factors and cytokines. Because of its large size and negative charge, only a small amount of chondroitin sulfate is absorbed by the gut; correspondingly, serum levels are low and may not reach the joint at effective concentrations. Its action may involve tissue near the gut (such as nearby lymph nodes).

COX Inhibitors
COX-2 is the major isoform detected in the damaged joints of patients with OA. The use of selective COX-2 inhibitors has increased because these agents may decrease the rate of stomach ulcers caused by nonselective COX-1 and COX-2 inhibitors. Prostaglandin E2 (PGE2) is the major prostaglandin produced in the joint, and depending on the context, it can be either protective or destructive and contribute to pain. Inflammation is not as prominent in osteoarthritic joints as in rheumatoid arthritic joints; therefore, these issues must be considered when deciding to use COX-2 inhibitors, especially because their long-term use is associated with an increased risk of stroke and heart attack. COX-3 is a recently discovered isoform of COX that occurs in the brain and is sensitive to acetaminophen, which may explain the effectiveness of acetaminophen as a front-line drug in relieving pain associated with OA.

Rheumatoid Arthritis
The most common form of inflammatory arthritides is RA, a systemic, progressive inflammatory disease of the synovial joints. RA is characterized by leukocyte infiltration of the synovial tissue, synovial hyperplasia, erosion of articular cartilage, and localized bone resorption. The destructive inflammatory process causes severe pain and ultimately leads to deformities and loss of joint function. RA affects more than 1% of the general population and, as with OA, has a significant socioeconomic impact. RA affects the quality of life and the ability to perform the activities of daily life and decreases life expectancy. The economic cost of RA is approximately 1% of the gross national product in terms of loss of productivity and health care costs. The autoimmune character of RA is underscored by the presence of rheumatoid factor (RF), a set of self-reactive anti-immunoglobulin (Ig) G antibodies that are detectable in the serum of more than 80% of patients with RA. A strong correlation between disease susceptibil-

ity and expression of certain class II major histocompatibility complex (MHC) haplotypes such as HLA-DR4 and HLA-DR1 suggests a role for genetic factors in the etiology and pathogenesis of RA.

The so-called seronegative (RF-negative) forms of arthritis include a large number of inflammatory joint diseases such as ankylosing spondylitis, psoriatic arthritis, inflammatory bowel disease and lupus-associated arthritis, as well as a group of reactive arthritides (such as Reiter's syndrome and Lyme disease). These forms of arthritis or spondylarthropathy (not discussed in this chapter) are generally distinguished from RA by the lack of RF, their frequent association with the HLA-B27 haplotype, and in most instances by a less progressive clinical course.

Clinical and Morphologic Features

The prevalence of RA is three times higher in women than in men, and it typically affects individuals between 20 and 60 years of age, with a peak onset during the fourth and fifth decades of life. Clinically, the onset of RA is characterized by pain and swelling that in most but not all patients occurs first in small peripheral joints such as those of the wrist, ankle, and phalanges. Unlike in OA, the distal interphalangeal joints are spared in RA. As RA progresses, larger joints such as those of the knee, elbow, and shoulder, become inflamed—often symmetrically. Involvement of the axial skeleton is usually restricted to the upper cervical vertebrae. Radiographic changes detected in patients with advanced RA include joint-space narrowing (caused by cartilage loss); malalignment of the bones in the wrist (ulnar deviation), hands, or feet; focal bone erosion; and the frequent appearance of bone cysts in the epiphyseal regions. Osteophyte formation and reactive sclerosis, which are characteristic of OA (**Figure 1**), are uncommon in patients with RA.

Histopathology reveals leukocyte infiltration in the synovial tissue in patients with RA, with a prominent accumulation of mononuclear cells around blood vessels (**Figure 1**). Infiltrating B lymphocytes may form lymphoid follicles that are reminiscent of lymph node germinal centers. Hyperplasia of the synovial lining and neovascularization are characteristic features of rheumatoid synovitis. Expansion of the synovium results in the outgrowth of villous projections from the intimal surface (**Figure 1**). These synovial villi are composed of synovial lining cells, lymphocytes, macrophages, and blood vessels. Deposition of fibrin from serum may occur early, but synovial fibrosis (caused by enhanced production of collagen) develops late in the affected joints, usually after the articular cartilage has been destroyed and inflammatory cells are no longer present in the synovium.

One of the major destructive elements of the rheumatoid joint is the synovial pannus, an invasive granulation tissue that contains fibroblast-type synoviocytes but relatively few inflammatory cells (**Figure 1**). Synovial cells in the rheumatoid pannus exhibit a "transformed" phenotype (anchorage-independent growth and invasiveness) and are capable of directly attacking and destroying articular cartilage.

The synovial fluid of the rheumatoid joint appears turbid (in contrast to the clear fluid of a noninflamed joint) because of the presence of inflammatory cells, predominantly neutrophil leukocytes. Although the volume of the synovial fluid is increased in rheumatoid joints, the viscosity of the fluid is decreased. The decrease in viscosity results in a reduced ability of the joint fluid to lubricate and protect the opposing cartilage surfaces, thus further increasing the susceptibility of cartilage to pannus attachment and matrix damage.

Radiographic evidence of cartilage loss and erosion of subchondral bone can be found in more than 70% of patients with RA within 2 years after the onset of the disease. The contribution of chondrocytes to matrix degradation is less evident in patients with RA than it is in those with OA. Cartilage loss in RA results from both direct invasion by the synovial pannus and cleavage of matrix molecules by proteases released into the joint fluid by inflammatory leukocytes and synoviocytes. Once the cartilage is destroyed, the pannus, the joint capsule, and the adjacent ligaments and tendons undergo fibrosis. This results in ankylosis that marks the permanent loss of joint function that occurs in the final stage of RA.

Destruction of bone requires specialized cells that are able to remove the mineral component of bone matrix. Osteoclasts, the phagocytic cells specialized for bone destruction, are frequently found in "resorption pits" (**Figure 1**) located at the bone and soft-tissue interface.

Pathogenesis

According to current concepts of RA pathogenesis, the regulatory and effector cells of the adaptive and innate immune system act in concert to initiate and maintain a vicious cycle of events leading to chronic inflammation and targeted tissue destruction (**Figure 4**).

Adaptive Immune System: T and B Lymphocytes and Antigen-Presenting Cells

The most characteristic features of rheumatoid synovitis are the presence of T cells in the inflamed tissue and the paucity of lymphocytes at the invasion front and in the synovial fluid. Most T lymphocytes in the rheumatoid joint belong to the helper 1 (Th1) phenotype of memory cells. Cells that can present antigen to T lymphocytes (predominantly macrophages, B cells, and dendritic cells) exhibit a unique expression pattern of HLA class II molecules in RA. Several class II molecules, such as HLA-DRB*0401, DRB*0404, and DRB*0101, express a common sequence (QKRAA), also called the shared epitope. The locus containing the gene that encodes the DRB chain shows the strongest genetic link with RA. For example, in

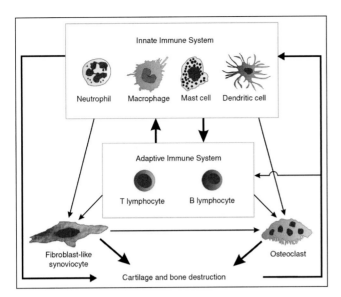

Figure 4   Illustration of the vicious cycle of inflammatory events and cells participating in immune/inflammatory reactions and joint destruction in RA.

the Caucasian population, the relative risk of developing a progressive disease is elevated in individuals carrying DRB*0401 or DRB*0404 alleles. The restricted pattern of HLA class II expression and the presence of the shared epitope suggest that the DRB molecules can present a select population of antigenic peptides to T cells. In vitro T cell stimulation assays and in vivo studies on animal models of RA have identified several autoantigens as candidate antigens that could be preferentially recognized by the T cells of RA. Strikingly, most (but not all) of these putative autoantigens are cartilage components such as type II collagen, aggrecan, cartilage link protein, and gp39. However, it is not clear whether T cell recognition of cartilage-specific antigens contributes to the induction or perpetuation of joint inflammation in RA.

T cells require multiple activation signals from antigen-presenting cells. One such signal is initiated on engagement of the T cell receptor/CD3 complex with the MHC class II molecule-antigenic peptide complex on the surface of the antigen-presenting cell. Costimulatory signals are provided through interactions of CD28 and CD152 (cytotoxic T lymphocyte antigen 4) on the T cells with their cognate ligands expressed on the antigen-presenting cells. Equally important is the binding of CD154 on activated T cells to CD40, expressed by B cells, macrophages, endothelial cells, or fibroblasts. CD154 expression is elevated in RA, and its amount shows a direct correlation with disease activity. Activated T cells normally undergo apoptosis (antigen-induced cell death), which is the primary mechanism of elimination of autoreactive T cells. T cells in RA exhibit increased resistance to apoptosis.

The absence of lymphocytes at the invading front of the inflamed pannus suggests a regulatory rather than a

true effector function for T cells in the rheumatoid synovium. Indeed, activated T cells produce several lymphokines (cytokines and chemokines) that regulate the immune response. Interferon γ (IFN-γ), produced by Th1 cells, enhances expression of MHC class I and class II molecules and induces the neoexpression of MHC class II molecules on RA synoviocytes and chondrocytes, thus enabling these cells to present antigen. Another product of activated Th1 cells is IL-2 that supports T and B cell proliferation. T cells can also stimulate macrophages in the synovium by either direct cell contact or through the release of proinflammatory mediators such as IFN-γ, IL-17, and IL-18. Th2 type T cells, which can downregulate the immune response, express anti-inflammatory cytokines such as IL-4 that inhibit Th1 cell activation but induce B cell differentiation and antibody production. Another Th2 cytokine, IL-10, inhibits both T cell proliferation and the synthesis of various proinflammatory cytokines. However, IL-10–producing Th2 cells are underrepresented in the RA synovium, which might account for the dominance of proinflammatory activities in the rheumatoid joint.

B cells and plasma cells are present in significant proportions in the rheumatoid synovium and often form cellular aggregates. These lymphoid follicles are similar to lymph nodes in structure and cellular organization and may contain clonally expanded B cells. One of the major functions attributed to these B cell follicles is the local production of RF. RFs are autoantibodies that recognize the Fc region of self-IgG molecules, and exist as IgG-IgG or IgM-IgG immune complexes. RFs and other autoantigen-containing immune complexes in the synovial fluid or deposited in joint tissues (frequently in cartilage) trigger phagocytic cells (neutrophils and macrophages) and activate the complement system, thus contributing to the perpetuation of the inflammatory response. The direct role of autoantibodies in tissue destruction, however, has not been clearly demonstrated. In addition to antibody production, activated B cells can promote T cell activation by serving as antigen-presenting cells.

Innate Immune System: Granulocytes, Macrophages, and Accessory Cells

Neutrophil granulocytes comprise the major leukocyte population in the synovial fluid of rheumatoid joints. As the most potent effector cells of the innate immune system, these cells have a remarkable capacity to inflict cartilage damage in patients with RA (**Figure 4**). Chemokines such as IL-8 and leukotriene B4 in the synovial fluid are the major chemoattractants that facilitate the translocation of neutrophils from the circulation into the joint. On entry into the synovial cavity, these cells are activated by immune complexes present in the synovial fluid and begin to secrete chemokines and cytokines. The most important proinflammatory cytokines produced by neutrophils are IL-1 and TNF-α. Activated neutrophils also secrete other

Table 3   Major Mediators of Inflammation and Tissue Destruction in Rheumatoid Arthritis

Name	Source	Target	Effect
Proinflammatory			
TNF-α	Activated T cells, macrophages, synoviocytes, granulocytes	Macrophages, synoviocytes, chondrocytes, endothelial cells, granulocytes	Target cell activation, enhancement of MHC class II expression and production of proteolytic enzymes, chemokines, and proinflammatory cytokines
IL-1	Activated macrophages, synoviocytes, various other cells	Macrophages, synoviocytes, chondrocytes, endothelial cells, granulocytes, T cells	Inhibition of matrix synthesis, enhancement of enzyme, chemokine, and cytokine production, stimulation of T cell and synoviocyte proliferation
IL-6	T cells and other cells activated by IL-1 or TNF-α	B and T cells, osteoclasts, hematopoietic precursors	Stimulation of T and B cell proliferation, osteoclast maturation, and synthesis of acute phase proteins
IL-17	Activated T cells	Endothelial cells, macrophages, synoviocytes	Stimulation of proinflammatory cytokine production and prostaglandin E2 secretion
Immunoregulatory			
IL-2	Activated Th1 cells	T and B cells	Stimulation of lymphocyte proliferation
IFN-γ	Activated Th1 cells	Macrophages, synoviocytes, chondrocytes	Induction of MHC class II expression
TGF-β	Macrophages, synoviocytes,	T and B cells, chondrocytes	
IL-15	Activated macrophages	T cells	Stimulation of T cell proliferation
Chemotactic			
MCP-1	Macrophages, synoviocytes	Mast cells, monocytes, T cells	Attraction of inflammatory leukocytes
IL-8	Macrophages, synoviocytes, other cells	Granulocytes, T cells	Attraction of inflammatory leukocytes, induction of neovascularization
RANTES	T cells, synoviocytes	Monocytes, T cells, dendritic cells, mast cells	Attraction and activation of target cells
Anti-inflammatory			
IL-1RAP (IRAP)	Monocytes, macrophages, granulocytes	IL-1RAP on several types of cells	Inhibition of IL-1 signaling via competition with the active cytokine for receptor binding
IL-4	Th2 cells	B cells, monocytes, macrophages	Inhibition of synthesis of proinflammatory cytokines, enhancement of B cell proliferation
IL-10	Th2 cells, macrophages	T cells, macrophages	Inhibition of synthesis of proinflammatory cytokines

TNF-α = ttumor necrosis factor-α, IL = interleukin, IFN-γ = interferon-γ, TGF-β = transforming growth factor-β, MCP-1 = monocyte chemotactic protein-1, RANTES = regulated on activation of normal T cell expressed and secreted, IL-1RAP = interleukin 1 receptor antagonist protein, MHC = major histocompatibility complex, Th1 = T helper 1

mediators capable of degrading extracellular matrix molecules, including proteolytic enzymes (collagenases, elastase, and cathepsin G) and reactive oxygen species (superoxide, hydroxyl radical, and peroxynitrite). HA, one of the macromolecular components of the cartilage matrix and the synovial fluid (Figure 3), is also a target of the degradative products of neutrophils. Depolymerization of HA by free radicals leads to reduced viscosity and partial loss of the lubricating and chondroprotective functions of synovial fluid in patients with RA.

Bone marrow–derived myelomonocytic precursors can differentiate into several types of cells such as granulocytes, mast cells, monocytes, macrophages, myeloid dendritic cells, and osteoclasts. Activated macrophages are present in high numbers in the inflamed joints. The direct role of macrophages in the pathogenesis of RA is suggested by the fact that, in addition to serving as antigen-presenting cells, macrophages produce metalloproteinases, proinflammatory and regulatory cytokines, chemotactic mediators (chemokines), and growth factors. Macrophage-derived mediators include IL-1, IL-6, IL-8, IL-15, TNF-α, macrophage inflammatory protein-1, macrophage chemotactic protein (MCP)-1, and granulocyte-macrophage colony stimulating factor (GM-CSF) (Table 3). The number of macrophages residing in the synovium of a patient with RA has been shown to correlate with the degree of cartilage damage and the radiographic progression of RA. Some macrophages and synoviocytes express toll-like receptors that recognize compounds produced by prokaryotes. These compounds include bacterial cell wall peptidoglycans, bacterial lipoproteins, lipopolysaccharide (endotoxin), and bacterial DNA. Although recognition of prokaryotic products by toll-like receptors can provide an explanation for the flare-up in RA activity that occurs with bacterial infections, aberrant expression or function of these receptors has been also considered a possible etiologic factor in RA.

Cells of the rheumatoid synovium and cartilage synthesize high amounts of COX-2, which, unlike the constitutively expressed COX-1, is associated with inflammation. COX-2 produces arachidonic acid metabolites, chiefly PGE2. In addition to mediating vasodilatation, edema, and joint pain, PGE2 can promote synoviocyte proliferation.

The Cytokine Network
The activity and function of the effector cells of the innate and adaptive immune system are under the control of an extensive network of proinflammatory and anti-inflammatory cytokines (**Table 3**). TNF-α, produced mainly by activated T cells, macrophages, neutrophils, and mast cells in the inflamed joint, represents a major convergence point in the regulation of inflammatory processes. TNF-α augments T cell and B cell proliferation and induces the production of other proinflammatory cytokines such as IL-1. TNF-α also stimulates MHC class II molecule expression on the surface of antigen-presenting cells, thus contributing to the perpetuation of the local immune response. TNF-α in the inflamed joint does not appear to mediate cartilage and bone damage. Rather, TNF-α synergizes with IL-1 in promoting the recruitment and activity of effector cells that are involved in tissue destruction.

IL-1 is produced primarily by synovial macrophages and activated T cells in the rheumatoid joint. The concentration of IL-1 in the synovial tissue and fluid of patients with RA positively correlates with disease activity. IL-1 is a major cytokine that mediates cartilage degradation by enhancing the production of MMPs and inhibiting the synthesis of extracellular matrix molecules necessary for tissue repair. The intrinsic control of IL-1 activity involves local production of a functionally inactive IL-1 analog, IL-1 receptor antagonist protein (IL-1RAP or IRAP). IL-1RAP can interfere with IL-1 signaling via competition with the active cytokine for binding to IL-1R on the cell surface.

Both IL-1 and TNF-α can induce synthesis of yet another proinflammatory cytokine, IL-6, in activated T cells, macrophages, and synovial fibroblasts. Because IL-6 promotes B cell differentiation, this cytokine likely plays a pathogenic role in the maintenance of RF production in RA. IL-6 also participates in the process of bone erosion through activation of osteoclasts.

Chemokines and Adhesion Molecules
Migration of specific leukocyte populations into the joint is governed by adhesion molecules and chemokines.

Proinflammatory chemokines include IL-8, which is abundantly produced in the rheumatoid synovium. In addition to attracting neutrophils, IL-8 promotes the formation of new blood vessels (neovascularization) in the hyperplastic synovium, thus supporting the expansion of rheumatoid pannus. Other chemokines produced in the inflamed joint, such as MCP-1 and regulated on activation of normal T cell expressed and secreted (RANTES), also have the ability to attract T lymphocytes, natural killer cells, and blood monocytes (**Table 3**).

By mediating cell-cell or cell-matrix interactions, adhesion molecules participate in a wide variety of pathologic processes in RA. Interactions between specific adhesion receptors and their ligands are required for the contact between T cells and antigen-presenting cells and for the recruitment of inflammatory cells to the joints. These interactions also play a role in neovascularization and attachment of the synovial pannus to cartilage. The major classes of adhesion molecules include selectins, integrins, and Ig superfamily members. In general, selectins mediate the rolling interactions of leukocytes with the vascular endothelium under blood flow. Integrins that mediate firm cell-cell and cell-matrix interactions can promote the arrest of inflammatory cells in the blood vessels, a committed step in leukocyte recruitment that is followed by migration of these cells across the vessel wall into the synovium. Certain integrins have preferential roles in the regulation of leukocyte traffic to the joints in RA. CD44, the primary cellular receptor for HA, is also a key adhesion molecule that directs the migration of activated leukocytes to inflamed tissues in chronic inflammation. CD44 mediates leukocyte rolling on HA, a matrix component whose expression is upregulated on the surface of endothelial cells under inflammatory conditions.

Mechanisms of Joint Destruction
Cartilage Destruction
Invasion of articular cartilage by synovial pannus (**Figure 1**) is a hallmark of RA. For as yet unknown reasons, the rheumatoid synovial tissue undergoes morphologic and functional transformation and exhibits tumor-like properties. Unlike synoviocytes isolated from normal human joints, fibroblast-type synovial cells derived from RA joints display anchorage-independent growth, loss of contact inhibition, invasiveness, and increased resistance to apoptosis. Rheumatoid synovial cells also show abnormal expression of signaling molecules that control cell proliferation and regulate the production of proinflammatory cytokines and matrix-degrading enzymes. In vivo, high concentrations of IL-1β, TNF-α, IL-6, IL-8, and GM-CSF are detected in the RA synovium. Rheumatoid synoviocytes represent the major cellular source of MMPs and cathepsins that are responsible for the degradation of type II collagen, proteoglycans, and fibronectin in cartilage. In addition to matrix degradation, serine and cysteine proteases (includ-

ing cathepsins) have the capacity to proteolytically activate MMP. Enhanced expression and activity of all of these enzymes contribute to the destructive behavior of synovium in RA. The activity of proteases is under the control of natural protease inhibitors such as TIMPs and serine protease inhibitors (serpins, α2-macroglobulin, and secretory leukoprotease inhibitor). However, the amount of proteolytic enzymes outbalances the amount of inhibitors, leading to a shift toward catabolic processes affecting the cartilage matrix in the rheumatoid joint. In addition to enzymatic degradation, cartilage macromolecules are subject to oxidative damage by reactive oxygen species released from activated granulocytes into the synovial fluid.

Bone Erosion

The pannus is actively involved in bone erosion, and cells in the pannus promote osteoclast recruitment and activation. Mature osteoclasts possess a lysosomal enzyme, tartrate-resistant acidic phosphatase, that enables these cells to resorb the inorganic compounds of the bone matrix and cathepsin K, which can digest the organic matrix, including collagen. Several proinflammatory mediators (IL-6, TNF-α, and GM-CSF) can promote osteoclast differentiation. The key mechanism of the regulation of osteoclastogenesis and osteoclast activity, however, involves a specific interaction between receptor activator of nuclear factor-kappa beta (NF-$\kappa\beta$) ligand [RANKL], a transmembrane protein expressed in osteoblasts, synovial fibroblasts, and activated T cells, and the soluble factor osteoprotegerin (OPG). OPG is a decoy receptor that blocks binding of RANKL to its cellular receptor, receptor activator of NF-$\kappa\beta$ (RANK), expressed in osteoclast progenitors and mature cells. Osteoclast differentiation requires RANK stimulation by RANKL. Binding of RANKL by OPG, therefore, inhibits osteoclastogenesis. In RA, RANKL expression is increased and OPG production is reduced resulting in increased osteoclastogenesis and focal resorption of cortical and subchondral bone in RA.

Principles of Drug-Based Medical Treatment

Nonsteroidal Anti-Inflammatory Drugs and Corticosteroids

Nonsteroidal anti-inflammatory drugs (NSAIDs) are potent inhibitors of COX-1 and COX-2, the enzymes responsible for the production of prostaglandins. NSAIDs effectively attenuate joint edema, vasodilation, and pain. Despite their clinical efficacy, there are considerable adverse effects of NSAIDs (gastrointestinal erosion, nephrotoxicity, and impaired blood coagulation) that do not permit long-term use of these drugs in certain patients. COX-2 inhibitors represent a new generation of NSAIDs that are distinguished from classic NSAIDs by their specificity for COX-2 and reduced toxicity. However, recent studies suggest an increased risk of thrombotic events in patients taking COX-2 inhibitors, so this must be balanced against the benefits.

The anti-inflammatory activity of the corticosteroids results, in part, from their inhibitory effect on the synthesis of prostaglandins and leukotrienes. Downregulation of genes encoding proinflammatory cytokines, inhibition of leukocyte migration, and blockade of neutrophil and mast cell degranulation also contribute to the robust anti-inflammatory effects of corticosteroids. Although they alleviate most inflammatory symptoms, long-term administration of steroids can lead to osteoporosis, hypertension, diabetes, and cataracts. Because these adverse effects are dose dependent, high-dose steroid monotherapy is no longer considered a treatment option in patients with RA. Low-dose corticosteroid therapy (10 mg of prednisone per day) is still used in 30% to 60% of patients with RA.

Disease-Modifying Antirheumatic Drugs

Disease-modifying antirheumatic drugs (DMARDs) comprise a broad category of small-molecule (synthetic) and large-molecule (biologic) agents that modify the clinical course of RA. Because of their clinical efficacy, DMARDs are more advanced therapeutics than NSAIDs. The most extensively applied small-molecule DMARDs in RA therapy are methotrexate and leflunomide, which have essentially eliminated the other types of these drugs (sulfasalazine, hydroxychloroquine, gold salts, and cyclosporine) from clinical use. Aggressive DMARD treatment in early RA results in a favorable clinical outcome, which is particularly obvious in patients with markers of poor prognosis such as expression of RA-associated HLA alleles. Clinical trials identified methotrexate as the DMARD that is most likely to induce a long-term response in most patients. In addition, the toxic effects of methotrexate (myelosuppression and hepatotoxicity) can be greatly reduced by the concomitant administration of folic acid without significant loss of efficacy. DMARDs can be used in monotherapy; however, in most patients, better results are achieved by the coadministration of these drugs with biologic agents.

Biologic DMARDs (also referred to as biologicals) are monoclonal antibodies, soluble receptors, or receptor antagonists that are capable of neutralizing the effects of proinflammatory cytokines. The prototype of anticytokine agents is infliximab, a chimeric (partially humanized) mouse monoclonal antibody against human TNF-α. Treatment with infliximab, alone or in combination with methotrexate, provides significant clinical benefit in most patients with RA. Soluble cytokine receptors can prevent cellular activation by competing with cell-surface receptors for the binding of cytokines. However, the half-life of soluble receptors in the circulation is short, and effective blockade of the cytokine receptor on the cell surface requires high concentrations of the soluble competitor. Etanercept, a fusion protein composed of a part of the human recombinant TNF receptor fused to the human IgG

Fc region to make a new protein, has an extended plasma half-life. Administration of etanercept has been reported to result in retardation of disease progression, even in refractory cases of RA. Anakinra, an IL-1RAP, has also proved to be effective in slowing disease progression; however, the short half-life of this agent requires frequent administration over an extended period. The superiority of DMARD therapy is reflected by the recent observation that aggressive treatment with small-molecule and/or biologic DMARDs at the early phase of the disease has improved the quality of life of patients with RA and reduced the need for joint arthroplasty surgery.

Drugs That Must Be Stopped Before Surgery

The major medications that must be stopped before surgery in patients with OA or RA are the same as those that must be discontinued in patients undergoing surgery with a high risk of bleeding. These medications are primarily those that affect blood clotting. The timing of when they should be stopped depends on their mechanism of action. Coumarin prevents gamma carboxylation of glutamic acid residues in key coagulation proteins such as factor X and prothrombin, which in turn prevents fibrin formation. Because new protein synthesis is required to replace the inactive factors, this takes 5 to 7 days. Heparin analogs act by forming complexes with antithrombin III and accelerate the inactivation of active thrombin and active factor Xa and thus prevent the conversion of fibrinogen to fibrin. Heparin is cleared rapidly. NSAIDs that inhibit COX-1 and prevent thromboxane A2 formation interfere with platelet aggregation. Aspirin is a suicide-inhibitor that acetylates the COX family of enzymes and irreversibly inactivates them. Because platelets do not synthesize proteins, new platelets must be synthesized before aggregation is improved. Other COX-1 inhibitors are competitive inhibitors; therefore, lowering their concentrations by stopping the drug for several half-lives (which varies from hours to days, depending on the drug) before surgery is enough to restore platelet aggregation.

Some drugs used to treat OA or RA can delay healing and/or increase the risk of infection. Glucocortoids at high concentrations, such as those that occur after interarticular injections, not only inhibit inflammation, but also inhibit repair; therefore, timing between such injections and surgery should be considered. Generally, oral steroids used for the treatment of RA are usually not stopped because of the complication of having to slowly withdraw them to prevent adrenal insufficiency. Although other drugs used to treat RA can interfere with healing (low-dose methotrexate) or increase the risk of infection (anti-TNF-α therapy), limited studies suggest that they do not need to be stopped before surgery. However, in all instances, the physician's decision must take into account the perceived risk of continuing or stopping the treatment of a specific patient.

Summary

Both OA and RA cause significant disability because of joint destruction but by very different mechanisms. OA initially involves the loss of cartilage, but changes in soft tissue and bone become dominant characteristics and contribute to pain and compromised function. Structural OA can become symptomatic and patients show different rates of disease progression. OA depends on systemic factors and extrinsic factors such as biomechanics and genetics. In OA cartilage, the balance of repair and breakdown is lost with increases in inflammatory cytokines and proteases and the mechanical properties of cartilage deteriorate. Medical therapies provide symptomatic relief with recent attempts to modify disease progression.

RA is a progressive disease of synovial joints with a strong genetic component and the involvement of autoantigens. In the synovium, regulatory and effector cells of the adaptive and immune system form a vicious cycle with an extensive cytokine network that perpetuates inflammation, generates large numbers of macrophages, homes specific lymphocytes to that joint, and modifies the synovial vascularity. Proteases are released that degrade cartilage, and cells at the bone interface recruit and activate osteoclasts, leading to chronic inflammation and bone cartilage destruction. The major drugs for managing RA slow inflammation and recently are aimed at the cytokines TNF-α and IL-1.

Selected Bibliography
Osteoarthritis
Aigner T, Kurz B, Fukui N, Sandell L: Roles of chondrocytes in the pathogenesis of OA. *Curr Opin Rheumatol* 2002;14:578-584.

Altman RD, Abramson S, Bruyere D, et al: Commentary: Osteoarthritis of the knee and glucosamine. *Osteoarth Cart* 2006;14:963-966.

Arokoski JPA, Jurvelin JS, Vaatainen U, Helminen HJ: Normal and pathological adaptations of articular cartilage to joint loading. *Scand J Med Sci Sports* 2000;10:186-198.

Bullough PG: The noninflammatory arthritides, in Bollough V (ed): *Orthopaedic Pathology*, ed 3. London, England, Mosby-Wolfe, 1997, pp 239-264.

Bullough PG: The pathophysiology of arthritis, in Bollough V (ed): *Orthopaedic Pathology*, ed 3. London, England, Mosby-Wolfe, 1997, pp 219-238.

Burr DB: The importance of subchondral bone in osteoarthrosis. *Curr Opin Rheumatol* 1998;10:256-262.

Cohen NP, Foster RJ, Mow VC: Composition and dynamics of articular cartilage: Structure, function, and maintaining healthy state. *J Orthop Sports Phys Ther* 1998;28:203-215.

Dieppe PA, Lohmander LS: Pathogenesis and management of pain in osteoarthritis. *Lancet* 2005;365:965-973.

Englund M, Roos EM, Roos HP, Lohmander LS: Impact of type of meniscal tear on radiographic and symptomatic knee osteoarthritis: A sixteen year follow-up of meniscectomy with the matched control. *Arthritis Rheum* 2003;48:2178-2187.

Felson DT: An update on the pathogenesis and epidemiology of osteoarthritis. *Radiol Clin North Am* 2004;42:1-9.

Felson DT, Lawrence RC, Dieppe PA, et al: Osteoarthritis: New insights. Part 1: The disease and its risk factors. *Ann Intern Med* 2000;133:635-646.

Felson DT, Lawrence RC, Hochberg MC, et al: Osteoarthritis: New insights. Part 2: Treatment approaches. *Ann Intern Med* 2000;133:726-737.

Ghosh P, Cheras PA: Vascular mechanisms in OA. *Best Pract Res Clin Rheumatol* 2001;15:693-709.

Glasson SS, Askew R, Sheppard B, et al: Deletion of ADAMTS-5 prevents cartilage degradation in a mouse model of osteoarthritis. *Nature* 2005;434:644-648.

Goldberg VM, Buckwalter JA: Hyaluronans in the treatment of osteoarthritis of the knee: Evidence for disease-modifying activity. *Osteoarthritis Cartilage* 2005;13:216-224.

Goldring MB: The role of the chondrocyte in OA. *Arthritis Rheum* 2000;43:1916-1926.

Klippel JH, Dequeker J, Dieppe PA: Disorders of bone, cartilage and connective tissue, in *Rheumatology*, ed 2. London, England, Mosby, 1998, p 8.

Knudson CB, Knudson W: Cartilage proteoglycans. *Semin Cell Dev Biol* 2001;12:69-78.

Lane NE, Nevitt MC: OA, bone mass, and fractures: How are they related? *Arthritis Rheum* 2002;46:1-4.

Loeser RF, Shakoor N: Aging or osteoarthritis: Which is the problem? *Rheum Dis Clin North Am* 2003;29:653-673.

Martin JA, Buckwalter JA: Aging, articular cartilage chondrocyte senescence and osteoarthritis. *Biogerontology* 2002;3:257-264.

McAlindon TE, LaValley MP, Gulin JP, Felson DT: Glucosamine and chondroitin for treatment of OA: A systematic quality assessment and meta-analysis. *JAMA* 2000;283:1469-1475.

Mengshol JA, Mix KS, Brinckerhoff CE: Matrix metalloproteinases as therapeutic targets in arthritic diseases: Bulls-eye and missing the mark? *Arthritis Rheum* 2002;46:13-20.

Mort JS, Billington CJ: Articular cartilage and changes in arthritis: Matrix degradation. *Arthritis Res* 2001;3:337-341.

Moskowitz RW, Howell DS, Altman RD, Buckwalter JA, Goldberg VM: *OA: Diagnosis and Medical/Surgical Management*, ed 3. Philadelphia, PA, Saunders, 2001.

Murphy G, Knauper V, Atkinson S, et al: Matrix metalloproteases in arthritic disease. *Arthritis Res* 2002;4(suppl 3):S39-549.

Peach CA, Carr AJ, Loughlin J: Recent advances in the genetic investigation of osteoarthritis. *Trends Mol Med* 2005;11:189-191.

Pelletier JP, Martel-Pelletier J, Abramson SB: OA, An inflammatory disease potential implication for the selection of new therapeutic targets. *Arthritis Rheum* 2001;44:1237-1247.

Poole AR: Can serum assays measure the progression of cartilage degeneration in OA. *Arthritis Rheum* 2002;46:2549-2552.

Poole RA: An introduction to the pathophysiology of OA. *Front Biosci* 1999;4:662-670.

Silver FH, Bradica G, Tria A: Do changes in the mechanical properties of articular cartilage promote catabolic destruction of cartilage and osteoarthritis. *Matrix Biol* 2004;23:467-476.

Valdes AM, Hart DJ, Jones KA, et al: Associate study of candidate genes for the prevalence and progression of knee osteoarthritis. *Arthritis Rheum* 2004;50:2497-2507.

Rheumatoid Arthritis

Aarvak T, Natvig JB: Cell-cell interactions in synovitis: Antigen presenting cells and T cell interaction in rheumatoid arthritis. *Arthritis Res* 2001;3:13-17.

Abramson SB, Amin A: Blocking the effects of IL-1 in rheumatoid arthritis protects bone and cartilage. *Rheumatology* 2002;41:972-980.

Choy EH, Panayi GS: Cytokine pathways and joint inflammation in rheumatoid arthritis. *N Engl J Med* 2001;344:907-916.

Firestein GS: Evolving concepts of rheumatoid arthritis. *Nature* 2003;423:356-361.

Fox DA: Etiology and pathogenesis of rheumatoid arthritis, in Koopman WJ (ed): *Arthritis and Allied Conditions: A Textbook of Rheumatology.* Philadelphia, PA, Lippincott Williams & Wilkins, 2001, pp 1085-1102.

Gabriel SE: The epidemiology of rheumatoid arthritis. *Rheum Dis Clin North Am* 2001;27:269-281.

Goldbach-Mansky R, Lipsky PE: New concepts in the treatment of rheumatoid arthritis. *Annu Rev Med* 2003;54:197-216.

Green MJ, Deodhar AA: Bone changes in early rheumatoid arthritis. *Best Pract Res Clin Rheumatol* 2001; 15:105-123.

Hale LP, Haynes BF: Pathology of rheumatoid arthritis and associated disorders, in Koopman WJ (ed): *Arthritis and Allied Conditions: A Textbook of Rheumatology.* Philadelphia, PA, Lippincott Williams & Wilkins, 2001, pp 1103-1127.

Harney S, Wordsworth BP: Genetic epidemiology of rheumatoid arthritis. *Tissue Antigens* 2002;60:465-473.

Harris ED Jr, Firestein GS, Sergent JS, Genovese MC, Budd RC (eds): *Kelley's Textbook of Rheumatology,* ed 7. Philadelphia, PA, WB Saunders, 2004.

Jasin HE: Mechanisms of tissue damage in rheumatoid arthritis, in Koopman WJ (ed): *Arthritis and Allied Conditions: A Textbook of Rheumatology.* Philadelphia, PA, Lippincott Williams & Wilkins, 2001, pp 1128-1152.

Kaplan C, Finnegan A: Osteoclasts, pro-inflammatory cytokines, RANK-L and bone remodeling in rheumatoid arthritis. *Front Biosci* 2003;8:D1018-D1029.

Klinman D: Does activation of the innate immune system contribute to the development of rheumatoid arthritis? *Arthritis Rheum* 2003;48:590-593.

Lee DM, Weinblatt ME: Rheumatoid arthritis. *Lancet* 2001;358:903-911.

O'Dell JR: Therapeutic strategies for rheumatoid arthritis. *N Engl J Med* 2004;350:2591-2602.

Panayi GS, Corrigall VM, Pitzalis C: Pathogenesis of rheumatoid arthritis: The role of T cells and other beasts. *Rheum Dis Clin North Am* 2001;27:317-334.

Sfikakis PP, Mavrikakis M: Adhesion and lymphocyte costimulatory molecules in systemic rheumatic diseases. *Clin Rheumatol* 1999;18:317-327.

Smith JB, Haynes MK: Rheumatoid arthritis: A molecular understanding. *Ann Intern Med* 2002;136:908-922.

Smolen JS, Steiner G: Therapeutic strategies for rheumatoid arthritis. *Nat Rev Drug Discov* 2003;2:473-488.

Williamson AA, McColl GJ: Early rheumatoid arthritis: Can we predict its outcome? *Intern Med J* 2001;31: 168-180.

Zhang Z, Bridges SL Jr: Pathogenesis of rheumatoid arthritis: Role of B lymphocytes. *Rheum Dis Clin North Am* 2001;27:335-353.

Chapter 23

Metabolic Bone Disease

Thomas A. Einhorn, MD

Introduction

Metabolic disorders of the skeleton result from imbalances between bone formation and bone resorption and from impairments in mineralization of bone. These disorders may be caused by cellular dysfunctions, genetic defects in the synthesis of type I collagen, overexpression of osteogenic morphogens, abnormalities in renal function, endocrinopathies, or the secretion of abnormal levels of bone-active substances from benign and malignant tumors. This chapter will provide an overview of the basic mechanisms that lead to the development of metabolic bone diseases, along with the basic foundation for understanding how specific cellular, biochemical, genetic, endocrinologic, and oncologic processes lead to clinical disorders.

Basic Principles of Bone Metabolism
Basic Cellular Biology of the Skeleton

The ability of bone to be formed and remodeled and to adapt to its environment depends on the regulation of cellular functions. Two stem cell populations contribute to the formation of cells that regulate skeletal metabolism, the mesenchymal and the hematopoietic stem cell pools. Mesenchymal stem cells give rise to osteoblasts and bone lining cells. The hematopoietic stem cell pool gives rise to osteoclasts. Osteoblasts secrete osteoid, a composite of proteins that includes structural proteins such as type I collagen, as well as smaller molecules such as cellular attachment factors, growth factors, and other signaling molecules. Bone lining cells primarily secrete neutral metalloproteinases. Osteoclasts resorb bone and are derived from osteoclast progenitors, which are mononuclear cells that undergo a genetic commitment to an osteoclastic lineage just before undergoing fusion to form multinucleated cells.

The bone remodeling cycle begins with the action of osteoclasts that attach to bone and begin their resorptive activities (**Figure 1**). Through a coupling mechanism that is as yet unknown, osteoblasts sense the need to form bone in response to osteoclastic bone resorption and initiate activities leading to the synthesis of osteoid. Osteoclasts are found in cavities on bone surfaces called resorptive pits or Howship's lacunae. They are characterized by a ruffled border and an extensively folded membrane. They attach to bone through the facility of α-v/β-3 integrin receptors on their membrane that recognize specific arginine-glycine-aspartate amino acid (RGD) sequences in the extracellular matrix of bone. This attachment results in a change in cellular conformation such that it takes on the configuration of an upside-down saucer sealing off a space under its membrane. The cell then releases protons by a carbonic anhydrase-dependent proton pump, lowering the pH and thereby facilitating the action of specific acid proteases, most notably cathepsin K, which degrade the extracellular matrix. In doing so, the osteoclast degrades both the mineral and the protein component of bone.

Osteoclasts respond to numerous regulatory agents known to induce bone resorption such as interleukin-1, interleukin-6, tumor necrosis factor-α, and prostaglandin E_2. Because osteoclasts lack receptors for parathyroid hormone (PTH) or 1,25-dihydroxyvitamin D, their response is believed to be mediated by cells of osteoblastic lineage. Osteoclasts do have receptors for, and respond directly to, calcitonin, colchicine, and gamma interferon.

Osteoblasts are bone-forming cells that synthesize and secrete unmineralized bone matrix (osteoid), regulate its mineralization, and control the flux of calcium and phosphate ions in and out of the skeleton. They are characterized by their expression of alkaline phosphatase, synthesis of type I collagen and osteocalcin, and the possession of specific receptors for proteins such as PTH, 1,25-dihydroxyvitamin D, and other bone-active substances. They appear to play a key role in regulating the activity of bone resorption by osteoclasts; thus, osteoblasts regulate bone remodeling through the control of both bone formation and resorption.

Once an osteoblast undergoes terminal cell division and is surrounded by a mineralized matrix, it becomes an osteocyte. Osteocytes are characterized by a higher

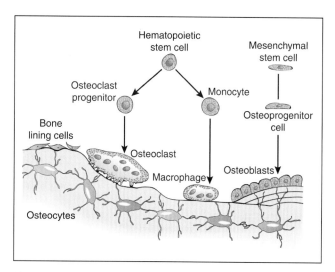

Figure 1   Schematic representation of the bone remodeling cycle. Beginning from the left, osteoclasts are responsible for the resorption of bone. Hematopoietic stem cells make a commitment to an osteoclastic lineage and the committed mononuclear osteoclast precursors fuse to form osteoclasts. Uncommitted mononuclear cells fuse to form tissue macrophages. In response to osteoclastic resorption, as well as environmental signals such as bone-specific hormones and growth factors, mesenchymal stem cells in the stromal stem cell pool differentiate to form osteoprogenitor cells and eventually osteoblasts. Osteoblasts secrete osteoid and then mediate its mineralization. Once this extracellular matrix is mineralized, the postdifferentiated osteoblasts become osteocytes. Although the role of osteocytes is not fully known, it is believed that they may transmit mechanical signals through bone matrix to regulate other cellular activities involved in bone remodeling.

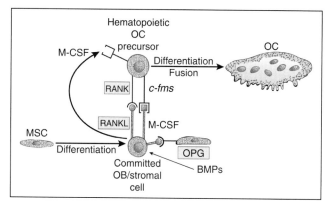

Figure 2   The regulation or coupling of bone formation to bone resorption involves a series of intracellular signaling mechanisms. Mesenchymal stem cells (MSCs) respond to a variety of hormones and growth factors in their microenvironment and differentiate into committed osteoblastic (OB) stromal cells. These cells are influenced by environmental signals such as bone morphogenetic proteins (BMPs), 1,25-dihydroxyvitamin D, and PTH. In response, they express an osteoclast differentiation factor known as receptor activator of NF-κβ ligand (RANKL) as well as M-CSF. When RANKL binds its receptor, RANK, on committed hematopoietic osteoclast (OC) precursors, in the presence of the binding of M-CSF to its protooncogene receptor, c-fms, osteoclast precursors differentiate and fuse to form osteoclasts. A decoy receptor, osteoprotegerin (OPG) can bind RANKL to downregulate osteoclastogenesis and osteoclast stimulation. OPG is produced by stromal cells.

nucleus-to-cytoplasm ratio, and are arranged concentrically around the central lumen of an osteon and between lamellae. They have extensive cell processes that project through canaliculi, establishing communications with other osteocytes and with osteoblasts that line the surface of bone. Although the function of osteocytes is not fully known, it has been suggested that osteocytes mediate the transmission of mechanical signals through bone and also participate in certain bone-resorptive activities.

Recent data have helped to advance knowledge of how osteoblasts regulate bone remodeling and resorption (**Figure 2**). Lacey and associates have shown that exposure of bone marrow cells and osteoblasts to substances such as PTH, prostaglandin E_2, and 1,25-dihdroxyvitamin D stimulates osteoclastic differentiation and ultimately osteoclastic activity through the expression of an osteoclast differentiation factor known as receptor activator of nuclear factor-kappaβ (NF-κβ) (RANK) ligand. Osteoblasts produce RANK ligand (RANKL), which binds to its receptor, RANK, on the surface of osteoclast precursors. When macrophage-colony stimulating factor (M-CSF), a cytokine also produced by bone marrow stromal cells and osteoblasts, binds to its receptor, c-fms, on the mononuclear osteoclast precursor cell, this cell matures and fuses with

other precursors leading to an increase in the number of osteoclasts and, consequently, increased bone resorption. In addition, RANKL can bind RANK on differentiated osteoclasts, further stimulating bone resorption. Osteoprotegerin inhibits differentiation of osteoclasts by binding RANKL as a decoy receptor and preventing its interaction with its receptor (RANK). Thus, remodeling of bone is accomplished through the action of osteoclastic bone resorption and osteoblastic bone formation; however, the regulation and governance of the process results from the way osteoblasts respond to the cellular, biochemical, and biomechanical influences of their microenvironment and transmit signals to osteoclasts and osteoclast progenitors.

The mechanical integrity of bone depends on the regulation of bone formation and resorption and the coupled and integrated activities of osteoblasts and osteoclasts. According to Wolff's Law, "form follows function" and thereby bone is formed in areas that undergo mechanical loading and is removed from areas in which loading does not occur. In osteoporosis, for example, this so-called coupling fails and bone is lost without being replaced. In osteopetrosis, bone is formed but insufficiently remolded, resulting in a mechanically brittle skeleton even though a substantial amount of mineralized bone is present. In states of high bone remodeling, such as in primary hyperparathyroidism, excessive osteoclastic activity can create stress risers in bone that weaken it mechanically. Thus, adequate coupling of bone formation and bone resorption in response to the locomotor and mechanical loading needs of the skeleton is required for normal function.

Mineral Homeostasis and Endocrine Function in Bone

The regulation of skeletal metabolism is a function of the action of three essential hormones—vitamin D, PTH, and calcitonin (**Figure 3**). In addition, the secondary influence of other factors such as thyroid hormones, estrogens, and hypothalamic control mechanisms in the central nervous system are also involved.

Calcium absorption from the gut results from the action of 1,25-dihydroxyvitamin D. This is the active metabolite in the vitamin D pathway and exists in two forms, 1,25-dihydroxyvitamin D_3, which is derived from cholecalciferol (vitamin D_3) found in the skin, and 1,25-dihydroxyvitamin D_2 which is derived from ergocalciferol (vitamin D_2) provided in the diet. Cholecalciferol is synthesized by the action of ultraviolet light on a skin sterol, 7-dehydrocholesterol. Only 10 minutes of exposure of ultraviolet light to the hands and face is sufficient to stimulate conversion to 10 mg of vitamin D_3, the minimum daily requirement. Cholecalciferol (or ergocalciferol) then circulates to the liver where, through the action of vitamin D-25 hydroxylase, the 25th carbon in the molecule becomes hydroxylated to form 25-hydroxyvitamin D. Under normal circumstances, approximately two thirds of the 25-hydroxyvitamin D synthesized is secreted into the serum and approximately one third is secreted into the bile. The bile-secreted 25-hydroxyvitamin D is then recaptured in the enterohepatic circulation and eventually nearly all the 25-hydroxyvitamin D produced circulates to the kidney. Hydroxylation of vitamin D in the liver can be inhibited by P450 mixed function oxidases if stimulated by drugs such as phenytoin.

When presented to the kidney, 25-hydroxyvitamin D undergoes additional hydroxylation of its 1α carbon to form 1,25-dihydroxyvitamin D. This active form of the metabolite then plays a role in stimulating biosynthesis of the intestinal and renal calcium-binding proteins. These proteins enhance active calcium transport in the gut and regulate calcium diuresis. The role of 1,25-dihydroxyvitamin D is involved in mineralization is not yet known. However, its role in enhancing absorption of intestinal calcium as well as phosphate is critical to bone and mineral homeostasis.

Serum levels of ionized calcium control the activation and secretion of PTH from chief cells in the parathyroid gland. As the activation of 1,25-hydroxyvitamin D by 25-hydroxyvitamin D-1α hydroxylase is under the control of PTH, serum levels of ionized calcium regulate PTH secretion; PTH secretion regulates 1,25-dihydroxyvitamin D synthesis; and 1,25-dihydroxyvitamin D synthesis controls intestinal calcium absorption, thereby establishing a regu-

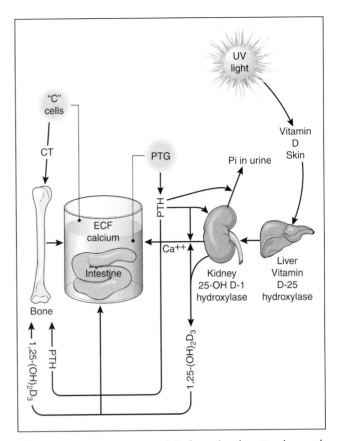

Figure 3   Mineral homeostasis in bone involves two ions, calcium (Ca) and phosphate (Pi), and three hormones, vitamin D and its metabolites, PTH and calcitonin (CT). Vitamin D is produced by the action of ultraviolet (UV) light on the skin. It then circulates to the liver where it is hydroxylated at its 25th carbon to form 25-hydroxyvitamin D. 25-hydroxyvitamin D then circulates to the kidney where it is hydroxylated at its 1-α carbon to form the active 1,25-dihydroxyvitamin D [1,25-$(OH)_2$ D_3]. This conversion step is under the control of PTH. 1,25-dihydroxyvitamin D increases intestinal calcium absorption and mediates mineralization of bone. As the extracellular fluid (ECF) concentration of Ca increases, the parathyroid gland (PTG) senses this and decreases the secretion of PTH. This reduces the amount of 1,25-dihydroxyvitamin D formed. Conversely, when serum and extracellular calcium levels are low, the parathyroid gland is stimulated, PTH is secreted, and more vitamin D activation occurs in the kidney. Under circumstances in which there is a rapid rise in serum calcium, the chief cells ("C cells") in the thyroid gland secrete calcitonin (CT), which downregulates osteoclastic bone resorption and thereby reduces the amount of calcium elaborated from the skeleton into the serum and ECF.

latory feedback group. Similarly, decreased levels of serum phosphate lead to increased 1,25-dihydroxyvitamin D synthesis, leading to phosphate homeostasis.

Under certain conditions in which there is a precipitous increase in serum calcium levels, calcitonin, a hormone secreted from the parafollicular cells of the thyroid gland, can cause an acute interruption of osteoclastic activity and thereby reduce the amount of calcium that is coming out of the skeleton and spilling into the serum.

Table 1   Risk Factors for Osteoporosis

Genetic	Behavioral
Caucasian race	Cigarette smoking
Fair skin and hair	Alcohol excess
Northern European heredity	Inactivity
Scoliosis	Malnutrition
Osteogenesis imperfecta	Caffeine use
Early menopause	Exercise-induced amenorrhea
Slender body build	High-fiber diet
	High-phosphate diet
	Medications (eg, glucocorticoids, thyroid hormone, diuretics, phenytoin)

Reproduced with permission from Gill SS, Einhorn TA: Metabolic bone disease of the adult and pediatric spine, in Frymoyer JW, Wiesel SW (eds): The Adult and Pediatric Spine, ed 3. Philadelphia, PA, Lippincott Williams & Wilkins, 2003, pp 121-140.

Calcitonin, a peptide hormone, interacts with receptors on the osteoclast, leading to direct inhibition of this cell. The general physiologic role of calcitonin is unknown, however, as it seems to play no role in steady-state calcium metabolism.

One of the more interesting developments in recent years has been new knowledge of how bone mass may be regulated through a hypothalamic control mechanism in the central nervous system. According to recent findings, leptin, a small polypeptide hormone secreted primarily by osteoblasts and acting mainly on the hypothalamus, appears to be essential in the control of body weight and, directly or indirectly, gonadal function. Studies have shown that leptin-deficient and leptin receptor-deficient mice are obese and hypogonadic and demonstrate an increase in bone formation leading to high bone mass. Hence, bone and body mass may be physiologically linked through the central nervous system and pharmacologic manipulation of the leptin pathway may prove to be a novel therapeutic approach for the treatment of metabolic bone diseases.

Estrogen deficiency is a recognized cause of postmenopausal loss of bone. How estrogens exert their protective effects on bone, however, is not fully understood. Like other steroid hormones, estrogens bind to specific intracellular receptors and regulate the transcription of defined sets of responsive genes. Recently, estrogen receptors were identified in both osteoblastic and osteoclastic bone cell populations. Estrogens increase DNA content, type I collagen synthesis, and alkaline phosphatase activity in osteoblasts while inhibiting the activation of adenylate cyclase by osteotropic agents such as PTH, prostaglandin E_2, and the β-adrenergic agonist isoproterenol. Thus, estrogen promotes the expression of traits associated with the formation of bone while reducing cellular responsiveness to hormones that may trigger the resorption of bone. As osteoblasts are involved in the regulation of osteoclas-

tic bone resorption as previously described, these mechanisms provide estrogen with the ability to control bone remodeling. The direct inhibition of osteoclastic activity by estrogen is less well understood.

Most recently, thyroid-stimulating hormone (TSH) has been shown to have a direct effect on skeletal remodeling. Although osteoporosis has traditionally been thought to be associated with hyperthyroidism as a secondary consequence of altered thyroid function, there is now evidence for direct effects of TSH on both components of skeletal remodeling, osteoblastic bone formation, and osteoclastic bone resorption, mediated via the TSH receptor found on osteoblast and osteoclast precursors. Even a 50% reduction in TSH receptor expression produces profound osteoporosis (bone loss) together with focal osteosclerosis (localized bone formation). These studies define a role for TSH as a single molecular switch in the independent control of both bone formation and resorption.

Disorders of Bone Metabolism
Osteoporosis

Osteoporosis is defined as a chronic, progressive disease characterized by low bone mass, microarchitectural deterioration and decreased bone strength, bone fragility, and a consequent increase in fracture risk. Recent studies have shown that the number of people age 50 years and older estimated to be at risk for osteoporosis and low bone mass is 44 million; this number represents 55% of the US population in this age group.

Although all men and women lose bone as they age, certain risk factors must exist and systemic or environmental conditions must occur for osteoporosis to develop. One major risk factor in women is a sensitivity of the skeleton to the cessation of estrogen production. Other risk factors include surgically-induced menopause, long-term calcium deficiency, secondary hyperparathyroidism, decreased physical activity, PTH excess, thyroid hormone excess, use of steroids, and alcohol abuse. Risk factors for this disease can be categorized into genetic (nonmodifiable) and behavioral (modifiable) factors (Table 1). The nonmodifiable poorly understood risk factors include the mechanisms underlying the genetic predisposition to osteoporosis among individuals who are fair skinned, slim, have hypermobile joints, are of northern European ancestry, or who have scoliosis. Cigarette smokers show a significantly increased incidence of bone loss and hip and vertebral fractures and this may be caused in part by the abnormal systemic handling of estrogen metabolites. Heavy alcohol users may develop osteoporosis as a result of calcium deficiencies or a direct depressive effect of alcohol on osteoblast function. In addition, environmental factors such as religious customs that require women to dress in ways that shield their bodies from sunlight may affect vitamin D synthesis. Moreover, diets that exclude dairy products may limit calcium absorption.

Table 2   Causes of Secondary Osteoporosis

Thyroid disease
Parathyroid disease
Hypothalamic hypogonadism
Diabetes mellitus
Human immunodeficiency virus infection
Steroid exposure (endogenous, iatrogenic)
Multiple myeloma (marrow packing tumors)
Leukemia
Prolonged bed rest or inactivity

Recent observations on clinical syndromes have further elucidated the role of genetics in the development of and protection from osteoporosis. These findings involve the low density lipoprotein receptor-related proteins (LRPs), which are a family of cell surface receptors involved in diverse biologic processes including lipid metabolism, retinoid uptake, and neuronal migration. A loss of function mutation in the LRP5 gene leads to the osteoporosis-pseudoglioma syndrome, an autosomal recessive disorder affecting bone mass and vision in children and making patients susceptible to fracture. However, if there is an autosomal dominant mutation in which valine is substituted for glycine at codon 171, a so-called gain-of-function mutation will occur. Indeed, recent recognition of a family with high bone mass and elevated levels of osteocalcin identified a kindred with this mutation. This finding suggests that genetic inheritance may play an extremely important role in skeletal health and disease.

Osteoporosis can be divided into primary and secondary forms. Primary osteoporosis, also known as idiopathic or involutional osteoporosis, occurs in many individuals as they age or after menopause. It is not related to any specific disease state or behavioral pattern. Secondary osteoporosis is caused by an abnormality in endocrine function, a neoplastic disease, a hematologic disorder, a mechanical disorder, a biochemical collagen disturbance, or a nutritional aberration. These conditions need to be treated or eliminated before therapy for osteoporosis is attempted (Table 2).

Most individuals attain their peak level of bone mass sometime between the ages of 16 and 25 years. Peak bone mass is the greatest amount of bone an individual will have in his or her lifetime and individuals with high peak bone mass are less susceptible to osteoporosis. The reason for this is that the ability of any specific rate of bone loss to lead to a critically low level or fracture threshold is dependent on the amount of bone present before the bone loss begins. Beginning at about age 30 years, both men

and women experience a gradual decline in bone mass, although the rate of bone loss is higher in women. When women reach menopause, there may be an accelerated rate of bone loss leading to osteoporosis. The turnover rate in trabecular bone is approximately eight times that of cortical bone because of the increase in surface area in comparison with cortical bone. Thus, imbalances in bone metabolism will generally affect trabecular bone more dramatically.

Treatment of osteoporosis is primarily aimed at preventing bone loss by maintaining adequate calcium intake and inhibiting osteoclastic activity. More recently, research has focused on developing drugs to increase bone formation. Agents with the capacity to inhibit bone loss include oral and intravenous bisphosphonates, estrogen, selective estrogen receptor modulators (SERMs), and calcitonin. See chapter 17 for more information on bisphosphonates. Estrogen is known to inhibit osteoclastic activity and may also stimulate osteoblastic bone formation. Although estrogen receptors have been identified on both of these cells, the mechanism by which bone resorption is inhibited, or bone formation stimulated by estrogen, is poorly understood. Present recommendations on the use of estrogen emphasize caution because of potential serious adverse side affects such as breast cancer, stroke, coronary heart disease, and pulmonary embolism. SERMs have been shown to improve bone mass by reducing bone resorption but their effects are not as profound as those of estrogen or bisphosphonates. The pharmacology of SERMs is sufficiently selective that the adverse effects of estrogens do not occur. Calcitonin inhibits osteoclastic activity by a direct cytotoxic action, the exact nature of which is as yet unclear. The most striking change is the destruction of clear zones and ruffled borders. In addition, calcitonin may disrupt cytoskeletal elements within the cell, further disabling its bone resorbing activity.

The only agent currently recommended for the enhancement of bone formation is the 1-34 amino acid fragment of PTH known as teriparatide. Although continuous exposure to PTH is known to induce bone resorption, pulsatile exposure enhances bone formation by direct stimulation of osteoblasts. Sodium fluoride, a drug that has been shown in the past to stimulate bone formation, does so by producing abnormal bone. Studies have shown that fracture incidence is not improved in patients exposed to this drug.

Osteomalacia and Rickets
Osteomalacia is a metabolic bone disorder caused by an accumulation of unmineralized osteoid on bone trabeculae as a result of impaired deposition of mineral. It may result from vitamin D deficiency, vitamin D resistance, impaired vitamin D synthesis or metabolism, metabolic acidosis, hypophosphatemia, intestinal malabsorption, acquired or hereditary renal disorders, intoxication with

Table 3	Causes of Osteomalacia

Vitamin D deficiency
  Dietary
  Malabsorption
    Intestinal disease
    Intestinal surgery
  Insufficient sunlight
Impaired vitamin D synthesis
  Liver disease
  Hepatic microsomal enzyme induction
  Phenytoin (eg, Dilantin)
  Renal failure
Metabolic acidosis
Fanconi's syndrome (renal tubular defect)
Hypophosphatemia
  Malabsorption
  X-linked hypophosphatemic rickets
  Oncogenic
  Oral phosphate-binding antacid excess
Mineralization inhibition
  Aluminum
  Iron
Hypophosphatasia

Reproduced with permission from Gill SS, Einhorn TA: Metabolic bone disease of the adult and pediatric spine, in Frymoyer JW, Wiesel SW (eds): The Adult and Pediatric Spine, ed 3. Philadelphia, PA, Lippincott Williams & Wilkins, 2003, pp 121-140.

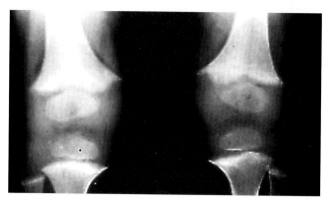

Figure 4 AP radiographs of the knees of a 4-year-old girl with hypophosphatemic rickets. Note widening of the growth plates.

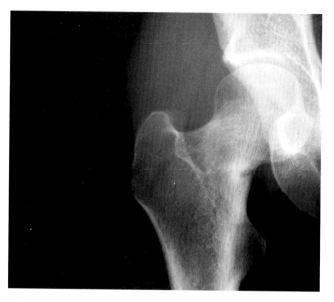

Figure 5 AP radiograph of the hip of a 35-year-old woman with osteomalacia. Note the radiolucent line at the inferior aspect of the femoral neck. This characteristic is consistent with a stress fracture in mechanically inferior bone, which is repaired with poorly mineralized osteoid.

heavy metals such as aluminum or iron, or other etiologies (Table 3). The childhood form of osteomalacia is termed rickets and it too has a multitude of causes. Rickets of the developing and growing skeleton may be caused by dietary deficiency of vitamin D; however, rickets has become rare since the widespread supplementation of dairy products with vitamin D. Other forms of rickets include vitamin D-dependent rickets, vitamin D malabsorption, X-linked hypophosphatemia, and renal osteodystrophy. Most children with rickets have characteristic growth disturbances.

Osteomalacia usually presents clinically with nonspecific complaints such as muscle weakness and diffuse aches and pains. Children with rickets often have enlargement of the costal cartilage (rachitic rosary), indentation of the lower ribs where the diaphragm inserts (Harrison's groove), and occasional pectus carinatum. These conditions result from impaired calcification of growth cartilage during endochondral ossification, leading to expansion of the zone of the hypertrophy and thus enlargement of the physis. The growth of children with rickets is often impaired while weight may be normal or higher for age-matched children. Long bone manifestations, particularly in the lower extremities, are also affected by enlargement of the zone of hypertrophy and leads to tibia vara (Figure 4). Spine manifestations of rickets include a long smooth dorsal kyphosis, known as the rachitic catback, and a slight to moderate scoliosis of limited progression.

Although the radiographic appearance of osteomalacia often mimics other disorders such as osteoporosis, certain specific findings often distinguish this disease. The presence of pseudofractures or Looser transformation zones is specific for osteomalacia. Looser zones are radiolucent areas of bone resulting from multiple microstress fractures that heal by the formation of osteomalacic bone, which is not mineralized (Figure 5). Looser lines are typically seen in the femoral neck, pelvic rami, and ribs. A high prevalence of cervical ossification of the posterior longitudinal ligament has been described in familial hypophosphatemic rickets, which may implicate abnormal calcium metabolism in ossification of these ligaments.

Different forms of osteomalacia result from distinct biochemical disturbances. However, the clinician can usually be alerted to the presence of this disease by an elevated serum alkaline phosphatase, low inorganic phosphate, or low serum bicarbonate level. Occasionally, serum calcium is also low but this is less common. Osteomalacia is almost always accompanied by low serum levels of 25-hydroxyvitamin D and 1-25-dihydroxyvitamin D.

In clinical practice, low bone mass, a propensity for fracture, the presence of Looser lines, and abnormalities in serum alkaline phosphatase, phosphate, and vitamin D metabolites is generally sufficient to establish a diagnosis of osteomalacia. However, in certain instances in which these findings are not always present, a transiliac bone biopsy may be necessary to confirm the diagnosis. The histologic hallmark of osteomalacia is an increase in the width and extent of osteoid seams with evidence of decreased rates of mineral apposition as determined by tetracycline labeling. Although tetracycline labels generally show discrete uptake in normal or even osteoporotic bone, the slow rate of mineralization prevents these labels from appearing separated in time, and results in a smudged appearance.

Vitamin D deficiency in osteomalacia is generally caused by insufficient vitamin D content in the diet as a result of restrictive dietary habits such as vegetarianism or diets low in fat (vitamin D is a fat-soluble vitamin). It is also common in elderly individuals and people with mild to severe malabsorption syndromes. These nutritional disorders are easily treated with vitamin D.

Other conditions that can cause osteomalacia include gastrointestinal abnormalities such as dumping syndrome, blind loops, or malabsorption resulting from intestinal bypass surgery. In addition, the use of anticonvulsant drugs such as phenytoin has been shown to cause osteomalacia by inducing the P450 mixed-function oxidases in hepatic cells that convert vitamin D to inactive polar metabolites. This reduces the production of 25-hydroxyvitamin D, resulting in insufficient amounts of this metabolite for conversion to the active 1,25-dihyroxyvitamin D form. Less common conditions such as metabolic acidosis leading to renal tubular leakage of phosphate, renal tubular dysfunction, inherited hypophosphatemia, or exposure to environmental inhibitors of phosphate (for example, phosphate-binding antacids) can lead to osteomalacia. A rare condition, known as oncogenic osteomalacia, is caused by different forms of mesenchymal tumors. These tumors are characteristically slow-growing, complex, polymorphous neoplasms that are subdivided into four groups: (1) phosphaturic mesenchymal tumor mixed connective tissue type (PMTMCT); (2) osteoblastoma-like tumors; (3) ossifying fibrous-like tumors; and (4) nonossifying fibrous-like tumors. PMTMCT is the most common type and is characterized by an admixture of spindle cells and osteoclast-like giant cells. Although typically benign, malignant forms have

been described. Fibroblast growth factor-23 message is abundantly expressed in these tumors and is used as a marker. Anatomically, the tumors are generally small, indolent, and located in remote regions such as the nasopharynx, sinuses, groin, and long bones. Aluminum-associated osteomalacia is common in hemodialysis–induced bone disease and will be discussed later in this chapter.

Treatment of osteomalacia and rickets depends on the specific metabolic defect and in most instances involves vitamin D therapy. For example, nutritional vitamin D deficiency is treated with high doses of cholecalciferol (vitamin D_3). Certain forms of osteomalacia in which hepatic, renal, or intestinal function is impaired require the addition of either calcifediol (25-hydroxyvitamin D_3), calcitriol (1,25-dihydroxyvitamin D_3), or both. These conditions may also require phosphate supplementation. When osteomalacia is caused by metabolic acidosis, a triturated dose of sodium bicarbonate is required. Tumor-induced osteomalacia requires removal of the tumor if possible but many times it is impossible to find. One form of tumor-induced osteomalacia involving a hemangiopericystoma has been treated successfully with subcutaneous administration of octreotide, a synthetic somatostatin analog. The treatment of rickets involves identifying the underlying pathology and directing therapy toward the specific category of rickets. Such therapy involves various combinations of calcium, vitamin D_3, phosphate, and 1,25-dihydroxyvitamin D_3, depending on the disorder.

Renal Osteodystrophy

Renal failure has profound effects on the skeleton. Moreover, hemodialysis treatment and the use of pharmacologic agents indicated in the management of patients on hemodialysis have additional effects on the skeleton. Renal osteodystrophy is initiated by two primary mechanisms induced by the loss of renal mass: an inability to hydroxylate 25-dihydroxyvitamin D to the active form (1,25-dihydroxyvitamin D), and phosphate retention caused by the lack of renal phosphate filtration. Failure to activate vitamin D metabolites results in osteomalacia for reasons noted in the prior section of this chapter. Loss of renal mass can also be associated with metabolic acidosis because one of the functions of the kidney is to regulate acid-base balance. The inability to filter phosphate results in phosphate retention. As serum phosphate increases, serum calcium is precipitated, leading to stimulation of PTH secretion and the deposition of calcific deposits in tendons, ligaments, and around joints. Continued stimulation of PTH secretion results in secondary hyperparathyroidism, leading to osteitis fibrosa cystica (Figure 6).

The treatment of patients with end-stage renal disease often involves hemodialysis as filtration of the circulation is a major function that is lacking in anephric patients. To manage the secondary hyperparathyroidism in these pa-

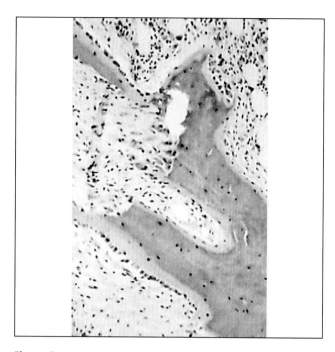

Figure 6   Bone biopsy from a patient with renal osteodystrophy and secondary hyperparathyroidism. This section shows typical findings of osteitis fibrosa cystica. Note extensive osteoclastic activity resulting in numerous osteoclasts found in Howship's lacunae. In response to this, there is abundant bone formation hallmarked by numerous osteoblasts lining the surfaces of bone. Because of this hyperactive bone remodeling state, there is also extensive marrow fibrosis present (hematoxylin and eosin, x25). *(Reproduced with permission from Jacobs SJ, Gilbert MS, Einhorn TA: The treatment of fractures in uremic bone diseases: Causes of failure and optimization of healing.* Contemp Orthop *1989;18:23-35.)*

tients, treatment often involves the use of phosphate-binding drugs. This may lead to a salting-out of serum ionized calcium and result in further stimulation of the parathyroid gland. In addition, the artificial filtration of blood by hemodialysis machines exposes the serum to aluminum; even small amounts of aluminum when deposited in the skeleton can cause adynamic bone disease and/or osteomalacia. The deposition of aluminum at mineralization fronts prevents the mineralization of newly formed osteoid.

Children with renal failure experience renal rickets, resulting in all of the classic findings of vitamin D-resistant rickets such as growth disturbance and varus deformities of the knees and ankles. As noted in the previous section, X-linked dominant hypophosphatemic rickets is a common cause of renal rickets. If the disorder is detected early in life, the skeleton may develop normally as treatment with phosphate and 1,25-dihydroxyvitamin D_3 usually maintains normal growth in these children. Hypophosphatemic rickets is usually caused by a renal tubular defect in phosphate reabsorption. Albright described a disorder termed "distant renal tubular acidosis" that has a dominant mode of inheritance with variable penetrance.

Patients usually show at least one of the following three features: kidney stones, hypophosphatemia, and osteomalacia. High doses of 1,25-dihydroxyvitamin D_3 and sodium bicarbonate are necessary to treat this condition.

Treatment of renal osteodystrophy is aimed at managing the aluminum or vitamin D-associated osteomalacia, or secondary hyperparathyroidism. Aluminum intoxication is typically managed with chelating agents such as deferoxamine. Treatment of secondary hyperparathyroidism is generally managed by optimization of the hemodialysis treatment and stabilization of serum calcium levels. Normocalcemia is maintained by a combination of phosphate-binding antacid treatment to counter the hyperphosphatemia produced by the lack of renal filtration and, in some patients, 1,25-dihydroxyvitamin D_3 therapy is used to increase intestinal absorption of calcium.

Paget's Disease of Bone

Paget's disease is the second most common metabolic bone disturbance after osteoporosis. It occurs in approximately 1 of 1,000 persons and affects an estimated 3% of individuals older than 55 years who are of northern European ancestry (United Kingdom, France, Germany, but also Australia and New Zealand). Although studies have failed to detect a genetic predisposition, there is a slight geographic clustering in the prevalence of this disease. People who have a family relative with Paget's disease are at increased risk of contracting it themselves. The male to female ratio is approximately equal.

The clinical characteristics of Paget's disease consist of pain, deformity, bony enlargement, and high-output cardiac failure. Although any bone may be affected by Paget's disease, the vertebrae, pelvic bones, and femora are the most common. Bone scans show that approximately 60% of patients have involvement of the lumbar spine, 47% have involvement of the thoracic spine and sacrum, and only 15% have involvement of the cervical spine. The pathologic lesion is characterized by excessive osteoclastic activity, with intense bone resorption and marrow replacement by hypervascular fibrous tissue. The altered bone remodeling caused by increased osteoclastic activity results in the formation of disorganized woven bone tissue with inferior mechanical properties (**Figure 7**).

The increased osteoclastic activity and compensatory osteoblastic bone formation leads to an increased urinary output of collagen breakdown by-products such as pyridinoline and N-telopeptides. The compensatory osteoblastic bone formation is accompanied by an increase in serum alkaline phosphatase and this is the serum marker most commonly used to follow the clinical course of this disease.

The increased cellular activity and turnover of bone matrix in Paget's disease may be phasic. Periods of excessive bone resorption may be followed by periods of increased bone formation resulting in characteristic histologic changes such as the presence of cement lines, and

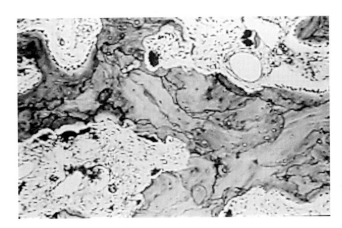

Figure 7 Photomicrograph of a histologic section of bone from a patient with Paget's disease. Note extensive osteoclastic activity and compensatory osteoblastic bone formation. The presence of so-called "cement lines" suggests periods of active and inactive metabolic states. The defect in bone remodeling homeostasis results in the development of disorganized woven bone leading to poor mechanical properties (hematoxylin and eosin, x25).

identifiable radiographic changes including patchy radiolucency and radiodensity. Clinically, Paget's disease is manifested by a wide array of presentations. Skeletal pain is most likely caused by the hypervascular state and hyperactive bone remodeling. Bony deformity results from the inferior mechanical properties of the disorganized osseous tissue. The high-output cardiac failure results from the hypervascular state and the development of arteriovenous fistulae. Involvement of the skull may result in cranial nerve compression leading to deafness; involvement of the spine can lead to localized back pain, radicular pain caused by encroachment of neural foramina, or spinal stenosis caused by bony overgrowth in the spinal canal.

The most common sites of involvement at the spine are at the level of the fourth and fifth lumbar vertebrae. When spinal stenosis occurs, it may be lateral or central or occur as a result of a compression of the nerve roots and/or spinal cord. Neural ischemia produced by the so-called arterial steal phenomenon, in which hypervascular pagetic bone "steals" blood from neural tissues, is also a possible etiology of spinal stenosis.

The etiology of Paget's disease remains unclear despite evidence suggesting a viral cause. Nuclear inclusion bodies have been demonstrated in the osteoclasts of patients with Paget's disease and shown to be morphologically similar to viruses in the paramyxovirus family such as measles, simian virus 5, respiratory syncytial virus, and human parainfluenza virus. However, a viral cause of Paget's disease has not been proven as no normal animal has been shown to develop Paget's disease as a result of experimental viral inoculation. Reports of a higher prevalence of Paget's disease in dog owners suggests an association with the canine distemper virus. Again, there is no direct proof of this hypothesis.

Malignant degeneration occurs in a minority of patients with Paget's disease and it is the most serious complication of this disorder. Incidences range from 1% to 10% and occurrence is more common in patients with polyostotic involvement. Pain is the most common presenting symptom. The most frequently occurring malignant tumor in pagetic bone is osteogenic sarcoma, followed by fibrosarcoma. Other less common tumors include chondrosarcoma, malignant fibrous histiocytoma, and reticulum cell sarcoma. The most common site of involvement is the femur, followed by the humerus, pelvis, and tibia. Malignant involvement of the spine is infrequent. Sarcomatous degeneration usually occurs after age 55 years and always develops in a bone that is already affected by Paget's disease. There have been several instances reported of a giant cell tumor or giant cell reparative granuloma in Paget's disease, which is a benign or low-grade malignant condition. Histologically, these tumors are filled with intracellular viral-like filamentous structures. They are partially sensitive to radiation and chemotherapy. Of particular interest is the fact that all patients in whom this particular giant cell tumor develops appear to be of Italian descent with ancestors originating from the province of Avellino. This finding lends credence to a viral or genetic etiology for this disease.

Treatment is targeted at reducing inflammation in mild cases and includes the use of nonsteroidal anti-inflammatory drugs and coxibs (cyclooxygenase-2 inhibitors). More active forms of Paget's disease require direct inhibition of osteoclastic activity with agents such as oral or intravenous bisphosphonates or calcitonin.

Osteopetrosis

Osteopetrosis (Albers-Schönberg disease or marble bone disease) is a rare metabolic bone disease characterized by brittle bones, an increased risk of fracture, and, in certain forms, impaired hearing and vision. It manifests as a diffuse increase in skeletal density and obliteration of marrow spaces (**Figure 8**). Histologically, the skeleton shows cores of calcified cartilage that are surrounded by areas of new bone; this new bone is normal but there is a deficiency of bone and cartilage resorption (**Figure 9**). Although the osteoclasts seem normal, they lack a functional ruffled border, rendering them incapable of conducting normal bone resorption. At least nine forms of osteopetrosis have been identified in humans. The three major forms of this condition are: (1) infantile or malignant osteopetrosis, which is inherited as an autosomal recessive condition; (2) adult or benign osteopetrosis, inherited as an autosomal dominant condition; and (3) carbonic anhydrase II deficiency, inherited as an autosomal recessive condition. The juvenile malignant form is characterized by severe anemia caused by obliteration of the marrow spaces, hepatosplenomegaly, thrombocytopenia, cranial and optic nerve palsy, and immune deficiency. Death usually occurs within

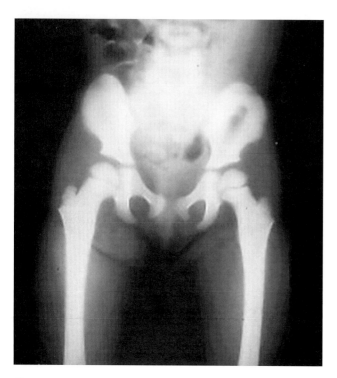

Figure 8   AP radiograph of the lower spine, pelvis, and femora from an 8-year-old child with osteopetrosis. Note increased skeletal density.

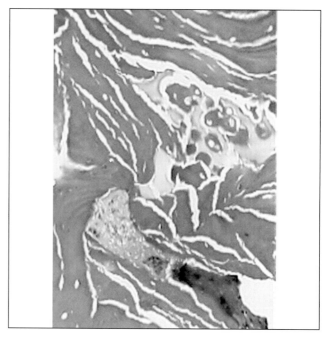

Figure 9   Photomicrograph of a histologic section from a patient with osteopetrosis. Note areas of calcified cartilage surrounded by areas of lamellar bone. The cracks in the bone occur in the process of histologic processing; the bone is so hard that normal histologic sectioning results in failure of the tissue (hematoxylin and eosin, x100).

the first 6 to 12 months of life as a result of anemia and sepsis. The adult tarda form, which is less severe than the infantile form, is attended by a lifelong risk of fractures that heal poorly. An even rarer adult form, carbonic anhydrase II deficiency, is associated with renal tubular acidosis. These patients can have cerebral calcifications that may result in mental retardation. As noted earlier in this chapter, the mechanism by which osteoclasts resorb bone involves a two-step process in which the cell first acidifies its microenvironment and then secretes acid hydrolases such as cathepsin K that operate in an acid milieu to resorb the mineralized bone matrix. The acidification process requires the intracellular conversion of water and CO_2 to carbonic acid, which then freely dissociates to bicarbonate and a free proton. Secretion of the free proton is how the cell acidifies its microenvironment. The conversion of water and CO_2 to carbonic acid requires carbonic anhydrase and if this enzyme is deficient, osteoclast function is significantly impaired.

Treatments of infantile osteopetrosis include bone marrow transplantation with an appropriate HLA-matched donor. The goal is restoration of patent marrow cavities with reversal of the hematologic abnormalities and defects in the immune system. A few isolated instances of high-dose 1,25-dihydroxyvitamin D_3 therapy accompanied by a low calcium diet have been shown to be successful. Although the mechanism is unclear, it is hypothesized that the 1,25-dihydroxyvitamin D_3 either stimulates the development of a ruffled border or, more likely,

increases the fusion of mononuclear osteoclast progenitor cells to form bone-resorbing osteoclasts. Long-term treatment of osteopetrosis with recombinant human interferon gamma has been shown to increase bone resorption by osteoclasts by increasing superoxide secretion. There is no known treatment of adult osteopetrosis.

Summary

Metabolic bone diseases occur as a result of genetic, endocrinologic, or behavioral causes that result in changes in osteoblast and osteoclast function. Because these cells are responsible for maintaining the structure and integrity of bone, alterations in bone matrix synthesis, mineral metabolism, or resorption of mineralized tissue will lead to diseases and conditions that affect normal skeletal development, mechanical integrity, and capacity to heal after injury. The most common metabolic bone disease encountered by orthopaedic surgeons is osteoporosis; patients with this condition have normal bone quality but, because of a variety of constitutive or behavioral causes, develop low bone mass. Osteomalacia and renal osteodystrophy result from the effects of environmental influences or systemic disease on mineral metabolism. Paget's disease and osteopetrosis are caused by specific defects in cell function. An understanding of these conditions will help orthopaedic surgeons to diagnose metabolic bone disease and plan appropriate surgical and nonsurgical treatments.

Selected Bibliography
Basic Principles of Bone Metabolism

Abe E, Marians RC, Yu W, et al: TSH is a negative regulator of skeletal remodeling. *Cell* 2003;115:151-162.

Baron R: General principles of bone biology, in Flavus MJ (ed): *Primer on the Metabolic Bone Diseases and Disorders of Mineral Metabolism*, ed 5. Philadelphia, PA, American Society for Bone and Mineral Research, 2003, pp 1-8.

Boyle WJ, Simonet WS, Lacey DL: Osteoclast differentiation and activation. *Nature* 2003;423:337-342.

Broadus AE: Mineral Balance and Homeostasis, in Flavus MJ (ed): *Primer on the Metabolic Bone Diseases and Disorders of Mineral Metabolism*, ed 5. Philadelphia, PA, American Society for Bone and Mineral Research, 2003, pp 105-111.

Ducy P, Schinke T, Karsenty G: The osteoblast: A sophisticated fibroblast under central surveillance. *Science* 2000;289:1501-1504.

Haberland M, Schilling AF, Rueger JM, Amling M: Brain and bone: Central regulation of bone mass: A new paradigm in skeletal biology. *J Bone Joint Surg Am* 2001;83:1871-1876.

Harada S-I, Rodan GA: Control of osteoblast function and regulation of bone mass. *Nature* 2000;423:349-355.

Holick MF: Vitamin D: Photobiology, metabolism, mechanism of action, and clinical applications, in Flavus MJ (ed): *Primer on the Metabolic Bone Diseases and Disorders of Mineral Metabolism*, ed 5. Philadelphia, PA, American Society for Bone and Mineral Research, 2003, pp 129-137.

Juppner H, Kronenberg HM: Parathyroid hormone, in Flavus MJ (ed): *Primer on the Metabolic Bone Diseases and Disorders of Mineral Metabolism*, ed 5. Philadelphia, PA, American Society for Bone and Mineral Research, 2003, pp 117-124.

Lacey DL, Timms E, Tan HL, et al: Osteoprotegerin ligand is a cytokine that regulates osteoclast differentiation and activation. *Cell* 1998;93:165-176.

Mundy GR, Chen D, Oyajobi BO: Bone remodeling, in Flavus MJ (ed): *Primer on the Metabolic Bone Diseases and Disorders of Mineral Metabolism*, ed 5. Philadelphia, PA, American Society for Bone and Mineral Research, 2003, pp 46-58.

Robey PG, Boskey AL: Extracellular matrix and biomineralization of bone, in Flavus MJ (ed): *Primer on the Metabolic Bone Diseases and Disorders of Mineral Metabolism*, ed 5. Philadelphia, PA, American Society for Bone and Mineral Research, 2003, pp 38-46.

Teitelbaum SL: Bone resorption by osteoclasts. *Science* 2000;289:1504-1508.

Disorders of Bone Metabolism

Basle MF, Rebel A, Fournier JG, Russell WC, Malkani K: On the trail of paramyxoviruses in Paget's disease of bone. *Clin Orthop Relat Res* 1987;217:9-15.

Bono CM, Einhorn TA: Orthopaedic complications of osteoporosis, in Flavus MJ (ed): *Primer on the Metabolic Bone Diseases and Disorders of Mineral Metabolism*, ed 5. Philadelphia, PA, American Society for Bone and Mineral Research, 2003, pp 388-398.

Boyden LM, Mao J, Belsky J, et al: High bone density due to a mutation in LDL-receptor-related protein 5. *N Engl J Med* 2002;346:1513-1521.

Case records of the Massachusetts General Hospital: Weekly clinicopathological exercises. Case 1-1986: A 67-year-old man with Paget's disease and progressive leg weakness. *N Engl J Med* 1986;314:105-113.

Delmas PD: Clinical use of selective estrogen receptor mudlators and other estrogen analogs, in Flavus MJ (ed): *Primer on the Metabolic Bone Diseases and Disorders of Mineral Metabolism*, ed 5. Philadelphia, PA, American Society for Bone and Mineral Research, 2003, pp 331-336.

Eastell R: Pathogenesis of postmenopausal osteoporosis, in Flavus MJ (ed): *Primer on the Metabolic Bone Diseases and Disorders of Mineral Metabolism*, ed 5. Philadelphia, PA, American Society for Bone and Mineral Research, 2003, pp 314-315.

Gallagher JC: Effect of estrogen on bone, in Flavus MJ (ed): *Primer on the Metabolic Bone Diseases and Disorders of Mineral Metabolism*, ed 5. Philadelphia, PA, American Society for Bone and Mineral Research, 2003, pp 327-330.

Glorieux FH: Hypophosphatemic vitamin D-resistant rickets, in Flavus MJ (ed): *Primer on the Metabolic Bone Diseases and Disorders of Mineral Metabolism*, ed 5. Philadelphia, PA, American Society for Bone and Mineral Research, 2003, pp 414-417.

Goodman WG, Coburn JW, Slatopolsky E, Salusky IB, Quarles LD: Renal osteodystrophy in adults and children, in Flavus MJ (ed): *Primer on the Metabolic Bone Diseases and Disorders of Mineral Metabolism*, ed 5. Philadelphia, PA, American Society for Bone and Mineral Research, 2003, pp 430-448.

Hadjipavlou A, Lander P: Paget disease of the spine. *J Bone Joint Surg Am* 1991;73:1376-1381.

Heaney RP: Nutrition and osteoporosis, in Flavus MJ (ed): *Primer on the Metabolic Bone Diseases and Disorders of Mineral Metabolism*, ed 5. Philadelphia, PA, American Society for Bone and Mineral Research, 2003, pp 352-355.

Herzberg L, Bayliss E: Spinal-cord syndrome due to non-compressive Paget's disease of bone: A spinal-artery steal phenomenon reversible with calcitonin. *Lancet* 1980;2:13-15.

Jan de Beur SM: Tumor-inducted osteomalacia, in Flavus MJ (ed): *Primer on the Metabolic Bone Diseases and Disorders of Mineral Metabolism*, ed 5. Philadelphia, PA, American Society for Bone and Mineral Research, 2003, pp 418-422.

Jensen J, Christiansen C, Rodbro P: Cigarette smoking, serum estrogens, and bone loss during hormone replacement therapy early after menopause. *N Engl J Med* 1985;313:973-975.

Kaplan FS, August CS, Fallon MD, et al: Successful treatment of infantile malignant osteopetrosis by bone marrow transplantation: A case report. *J Bone Joint Surg Am* 1988;70:617-623.

Key LL Jr, Rodriguez RM, Willi SM, et al: Long-term treatment of osteopetrosis with recombinant human interferon gamma. *N Engl J Med* 1995;332:1594-1599.

Liberman UA, Marx SJ: Vitamin D-dependent rickets, in Flavus MJ (ed): *Primer on the Metabolic Bone Diseases and Disorders of Mineral Metabolism*, ed 5. Philadelphia, PA, American Society for Bone and Mineral Research, 2003, pp 407-413.

Malluche HH, Smith AJ, Abrero K, Faugere M-C: The use of deferoxiamine in the management of aluminum accumulation in bone in patients with renal failure. *N Engl J Med* 1984;311:140-144.

Pettifor JM: Nutritional and drug-induced rickets and osteomalacia, in Flavus MJ (ed): *Primer on the Metabolic Bone Diseases and Disorders of Mineral Metabolism*, ed 5. Philadelphia, PA, American Society for Bone and Mineral Research, 2003, pp 399-407.

Rebel A, Basle A, Pouplard A, Malkani K, Filmon R, Lepatezour A: Bone tissue in Paget's disease of bone: Ultrastructure and immunocytology. *Arthritis Rheum* 1980;23:1104-1114.

Reeve J: Teriparatide (rhPTH(1-34) and future anabolic treatments for osteoporosis, in Flavus MJ (ed): *Primer on the Metabolic Bone Diseases and Disorders of Mineral Metabolism*, ed 5. Philadelphia, PA, American Society for Bone and Mineral Research, 2003, pp 344-349.

Riggs BL, Melton LJ III: Evidence for two distinct syndromes of involutional osteoporosis. *Am J Med* 1983;75:899-901.

Seufert J, Ebert K, Muller J, et al: Octreotide therapy for tumor-induced osteomalacia. *N Engl J Med* 2001;345:1883-1888.

Silverman SL, Chestnut CH III: Calcitonin therapy for osteoporosis, in Flavus MJ (ed): *Primer on the Metabolic Bone Diseases and Disorders of Mineral Metabolism*, ed 5. Philadelphia, PA, American Society for Bone and Mineral Research, 2003, pp 342-344.

Siris ES, Roodman GD: Paget's disease of bone, in Flavus MJ (ed): *Primer on the Metabolic Bone Diseases and Disorders of Mineral Metabolism*, ed 5. Philadelphia, PA, American Society for Bone and Mineral Research, 2003, pp 495-508.

Thomas J, Doherty SM: HIV infection: A risk factor for osteoporosis. *J Acquir Immune Defic Syndr* 2003;33:281-291.

Watts NB: Bisphosphonates for treatment of osteoporosis, in Flavus MJ (ed): *Primer on the Metabolic Bone Diseases and Disorders of Mineral Metabolism*, ed 5. Philadelphia, PA, American Society for Bone and Mineral Research, 2003, pp 336-341.

Whyte MP: Sclerosing bone disorders, in Flavus MJ (ed): *Primer on the Metabolic Bone Diseases and Disorders of Mineral Metabolism*, ed 5. Philadelphia, PA, American Society for Bone and Mineral Research, 2003, pp 449-466.

Chapter 24

Neuromuscular Diseases

Ranjan Gupta, MD
Tahseen Mozaffar, MD

Introduction

Orthopaedic surgeons often evaluate and treat patients with neuromuscular diseases, including both inherited and acquired disorders. Neurophysiology plays a role in diagnosing these conditions. Familiarity with the characteristics of common neuromuscular conditions is important to the orthopaedic surgeon, as is knowledge of factors influencing nerve regeneration.

Pathophysiology of Nerve Injury

After a nerve is injured, two main types of responses occur. The injury may affect the axon of the nerve cell (axotomy) or the injury may be limited to the myelin sheath (for example, demyelination). Both types of responses will result in the loss of neural function.

Axotomy

When a nerve is injured, the ensuing neural degeneration is not limited to the site of injury; an accompanying zone of injury occurs that is determined by the magnitude, duration, and severity of the noxious stimuli. Neurons and glial cells have a dynamic, reciprocal relationship that is significantly impacted by neural injury. The neural injury directly affects the axonal architecture and induces a process known as wallerian degeneration. After the axon is either transected or significantly injured, the distal stump undergoes wallerian degeneration to clear axonal and myelin debris and to create an environment that is hospitable to regeneration. The hallmark of the degenerative process is granular disintegration of the axonal cytoskeleton, which is triggered by increased axoplasmic calcium (**Figure 1**). Wallerian degeneration also produces numerous secondary responses. The nerve cell body responds with a significant alteration of metabolic activity with a decrease in production of neurotransmitters and an increase in production of proteins such as tubulin, actin, and growth-associated proteins. Normal adult Schwann cells do not divide and maintain a stable 1:1 relationship with axons.

Within 24 hours of injury, Schwann cells in the nerve segment distal to the site of injury begin to divide; a peak response occurs by 72 hours after injury. Schwann cells proliferate, forming the bands of Bunger within the distal segment of the nerve. These bands are cytoplasmic processes that interdigitate and line up in rows under the original basal lamina of the nerve fiber and guide the regenerating growth cone. To further facilitate regeneration, the myelin debris from the neural injury is removed. Macrophages, which accumulate by 72 hours after injury, are hematogenously recruited as the primary phagocytes of myelin. Early in the process, macrophages express major histocompatibility complex class II antigen; type 1a antigen is not initially phagocytic. Macrophages then penetrate the basal lamina, lose type 1a antigen expression, become phagocytic, produce interleukin-1, and stimulate Schwann cells to produce nerve growth factor. The segment of the nerve proximal to the site of neural injury will degenerate if the cell body dies, but will regenerate if the cell body survives.

Recovery From Axonal Neural Injury

Soon after neural injury, myelin thickness decreases relative to the axon diameter. Myelin thickness will later increase relative to axon diameter, but will still remain smaller than the preinjury thickness. The conduction velocity does not return to normal. Portions of the axonal cytoskeleton will sprout from the nodes of Ranvier, and a growth cone will develop from tips of the remaining axons. The regenerating unit will grow sprouts from a single axon. A sprout or growth cone will enter the distal segment with its surrounding Schwann cells and basal lamina. Axonal regeneration across the zone of injury is limited by the scar tissue between stumps; the scar tissue is obstructive to axonal advancement. This scar tissue also decreases the number of axons that reach the end organ, causes a delay in axon elongation, and increases the misdirection of axons. Within the segment distal to the injury

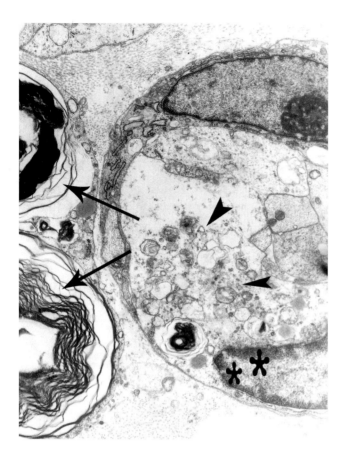

Figure 1   Electron microscopic image of a crush injury confirms wallerian degeneration with evidence of axonal injury (arrowheads point to granular disintegration of the cytoskeleton), myelin degradation (arrows), and condensed chromatin (stars).

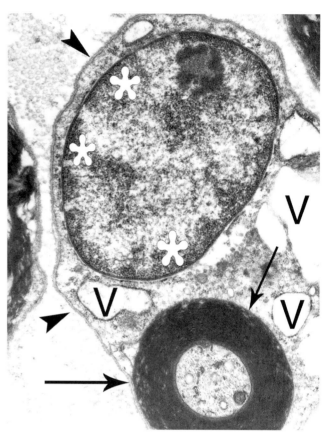

Figure 2   Electron microscopic image of a Schwann cell (identifiable by the surrounding basal lamina (arrowheads) and enclosed myelinated nerve (arrows)) undergoing apoptosis with large vacuolar cytoplasmic inclusions (V) and condensed chromatin (stars). In contrast to wallerian degeneration, the axon and the myelin remain intact (arrows) early after CNC injury.

site, a variable rate of axonal regeneration occurs based on the type and location of the nerve injury. On average, axonal growth occurs at 1 to 2 mm/day with a decreased rate of growth in distal regions. Axonal regeneration may be augmented by providing methods of guidance across the zone of injury. Guidance can be achieved with nerve tubes or axonal guidance channels, which can be made of arteries, veins, muscle, collagen, silicone, or polymer mixtures of various components of the extracellular matrix. Contact guidance is important in early axonal regeneration with extracellular matrix proteins (collagen, laminin, fibronectin) playing a role in cell-cell recognition. Neurotropic factors such as nerve growth factor are produced by Schwann cells and promote neurite survival. Other factors that promote growth of the axonal cone include surface-bound laminin and the basal lamina of Schwann and endothelial cells. Several studies in the literature detail the increased rate of axonal regeneration across a gap when a nerve guide tube is used to bridge the gap. Ongoing studies are underway to determine if these clinical results are reliably reproducible.

Demyelination

In contrast to an axonotomy or crush injury, a chronic nerve compression (CNC) injury, such as carpal tunnel syndrome, creates progressive demyelination and slowing of nerve conduction velocity. Recent studies have shown that CNC induces concurrent Schwann cell proliferation and apoptosis at the site of injury (**Figure 2**). Electron microscopic analysis confirms that dramatic changes occur in Schwann cells in the absence of axonal degeneration and axonal swelling, and before the ensuing alterations in nerve conduction velocity. In contrast to wallerian degeneration, which elicits a relatively immediate signal for macrophage recruitment, CNC provides a slow, sustained stimulus for macrophage recruitment. Early in the pathogenesis of disease, CNC injury induces significant Schwann cell turnover with minimal axonal injury.

Injury of Nerve Tissue

The prognosis for recovery from a nerve injury largely depends on the type and extent of the injury. In 1943, Seddon, a British orthopaedic surgeon, proposed a classifica-

Table 1   Comparison of Seddon and Sunderland Classification Systems of Nerve Injury

Sunderland	Details	Seddon	Prognosis	Recovery
Type I	No changes in axons, local conduction failure (block) Ischemia (short lived) Demyelinating (more persistent)	Neurapraxia	Good	Full
Type II	Axonal degeneration with wallerian degeneration Basil lamina, endoneurium, perineurium, and epineurium intact	Axonotmesis	Good	Full
Type III	Axonal degeneration with wallerian degeneration Basil lamina and endoneurium disrupted Perineurium and epineurium intact Scar tissue present	None	Fair	Incomplete
Type IV	Axonal degeneration with wallerian degeneration Scar tissue present Loss of endoneurium and perineurium Nerve in continuity because the epineurium is intact Severe loss of function	None	Poor	Poor (surgery needed)
Type V	Complete disruption of nerve and neural tube Elastic recoil of nerve ends	Neurotmesis	Poor	Poor (surgery needed)

tion system for traumatic nerve injuries based on his experience as the chief of the Medical Research Council Nerve Injury Unit at Oxford University during World War II. This system provided a means for classifying traumatic war-related nerve injuries.

Based on the Seddon system, localized nerve injuries can be classified into three categories: (1) neurapraxia, which is associated with a transient and temporary loss of nerve function caused by a conduction block (without disruption of axonal integrity); (2) axonotmesis, which is associated with axonal disruption but continuity of the nerve structure and Schwann cell basal lamina; and (3) neurotmesis, which is associated with axonal disruption with interruption of the Schwann cell basal lamina. Neurotmesis may be partial, with the continuity of the nerve maintained, or complete, in instances when the nerve is divided with complete disruption of the neural structures.

In 1951, Sunderland, an Australian anatomist and experimental neurologist, expanded on the Seddon classification system and proposed a new system. The Sunderland classification system, which was based on histopathologic studies, added two types of nerve injuries to the Seddon system. Details and a comparison of the two classification systems are shown in **Table 1**. The Sunderland system has five types of nerve injuries ranging from a mild type I injury to a very severe type V injury. Anatomic details of the Sunderland classification of nerve injury is graphically shown in **Figure 3**. Surgical treatment is usually not required in type I and II injuries because of the good potential for recovery of motor and sensory function. Recovery in type III injuries is often incomplete; nerve regeneration may fail because of the formation of excessive scar tissue, and surgery may be required to optimize nerve regeneration. Patients with type IV and V nerve injuries have a poor prognosis and recovery potential. Optimal surgical

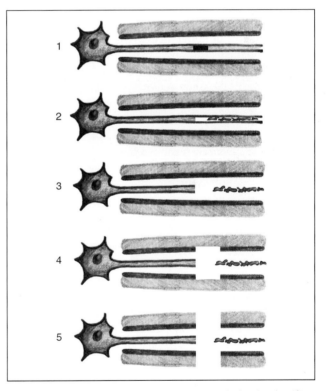

Figure 3   Schematic representation of Sunderland's classification of nerve injuries: (1) neurapraxia; (2) axonotmesis; (3) loss of nerve fiber continuity with intact perineurium; (4) loss of nerve fiber continuity with intact epineurium; and (5) complete nerve transaction (also known as neurotmesis).

repair often provides only minimal functional nerve recovery in adults. Early surgical intervention is needed for type IV and V injuries and should be planned based on an assessment of the extent of tissue damage. Type V injuries invariably result in neuroma formation.

Neurophysiologic Evaluation

Neurophysiologic or electrodiagnostic testing (EDX) is the natural extension of the neurologic examination and is used to confirm a tentative diagnosis of a peripheral nervous system disorder or to exclude other disorders with similar findings when a specific diagnosis is already suspected. EDX consists of nerve conduction velocity studies and needle electromyographic (EMG) examination. EDX is ideally suited to test the integrity of the peripheral sensory nerves and to assess the function of the motor unit (the lower motor neuron). EDX is useful in identifying and characterizing the disorders involving these two important units of the peripheral nervous system. It helps to quantify the extent of disease (in motor neuron disorders or in brachial plexopathies), to determine the severity of disease (in complete injuries of the peripheral nerves), and to evaluate the rate of disease progression (in motor neuron disease or peripheral neuropathies). EDX can also be used to follow treatment response and provide evidence of reinnervation (in compression or traumatic neuropathies). EDX is particularly useful for assessing uncooperative patients (such as children), patients with dementia or other neuropsychiatric disorders, and comatose patients; however, the information obtained in these situations will be limited because proper interpretation of the EMG study requires patient cooperation. In situations where preexisting conditions preclude a detailed examination (such as in patients on neuromuscular blockade), EDX may be used.

Because EDX can reliably differentiate between disorders of the nerve arising from either axonal dysfunction or myelin pathology, it provides important information for the initial determination of the etiology of the peripheral neuropathy. Mixed disorders affecting the motor and sensory nerves may be differentiated from disorders affecting only specific fiber types (motor nerves versus sensory nerves). With entrapment neuropathies, EDX may help determine the exact site of entrapment and dysfunction, such as within the cubital tunnel versus at the epicondyle in patients with ulnar nerve entrapment. **Table 2** details the various types of EDX that are used in the routine diagnosis of neuromuscular diseases.

Nerve Conduction Velocity Studies

Conventional nerve conduction velocity studies can only assess the integrity of the large myelinated nerve fibers ($A\alpha$ and $A\beta$ nerve fibers). Nerve conduction velocity studies are complementary to needle EMG studies; except in rare situations, it is difficult to make an accurate diagnosis without performing both examinations. Nerve conduction velocity studies are used to determine the physical integrity of the nerves, excitability thresholds, and dysfunction. These studies may be performed on any nerve; however, the median, ulnar, and radial nerves in the upper limbs, and peroneal, posterior tibial, plantar,

Table 2 Types of Electrodiagnostic Testing Used in the Diagnosis of Neuromuscular Diseases

Type of Test	Uses
Motor and sensory nerve conduction	Differentiation between axonal and demyelinating pathology Assessment of nerve integrity Assessment of nerve regeneration
Needle electromyography	Helps to differentiate radiculopathy from neuropathy Helps to differentiate myogenic conditions from neurogenic conditions Assessment of nerve regeneration
Late responses	Assessment of proximal segments of a nerve root
Repetitive nerve stimulation	Detects abnormalities in neuromuscular junction transmission
Motor unit number estimation	Estimates motor unit numbers: a useful measure of motor neuronal loss
Blink reflex	Neurophysiologic study of the blink response: assessment of afferent (trigeminal) and efferent (facial) pathways

femoral, and sural nerves in the lower extremities are most often studied. Some nerves are purely sensory, such as the sural, superficial peroneal, superficial radial, or saphenous nerves, whereas other nerves have a mixed sensory and motor function (such as the median, ulnar, and tibial nerves).

Measurement parameters common to these studies include the size of the evoked response, which is measured as amplitude in millivolts (mV) for motor nerve conductions and in microvolts (μV) for sensory nerve conductions; the latency of the response, which is measured in milliseconds (msec); and the rate of propagation of stimulus (conduction velocity), which is measured in meters per second (m/s).

Motor Nerve Conduction Velocity Studies

Motor nerve conduction velocity studies evaluate the evoked response elicited by supramaximal stimulation of a motor nerve. This response is the summation of activity from the muscle fibers (compound muscle action potential) and is recorded in an orthodromic (natural direction of the nerve's depolarizing current) manner distally from the muscle innervated by a nerve. This evoked response, also known as the M response, allows assessment of the motor axons distal to the stimulation, the neuromuscular junction, and the muscle fibers. Median, ulnar, peroneal, and tibial motor nerves are the most commonly tested because they provide consistent and reliable responses and are commonly involved in pathologic disorders.

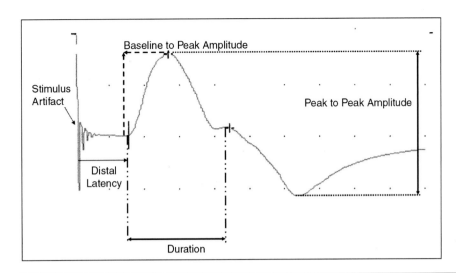

Figure 4   Characteristic responses of a compound motor action potential and parameters measured.

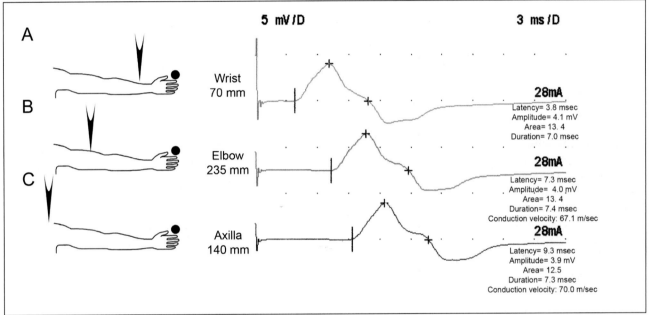

Figure 5   Typical motor nerve conductions from the median nerve taken across the wrist **(A)**, elbow **(B)**, and axilla **(C)**. The nerve is stimulated at locations indicated by arrows. All recordings are made in the muscles of the hand indicated by the dots. Latencies are observed at each stimulation site and the differential is used to determine conduction velocity across each joint. For this reason, there is no conduction velocity across the wrist in this example. Note that the excitability threshold, morphology of the waveform, its area, amplitude, and conduction velocity remain very consistent at different sites of stimulation.

Figure 4 shows a normal evoked motor nerve response and the parameters that are measured during such motor nerve conduction velocity studies including distal latency (the time taken from the stimulus until the response occurs), conduction velocity (distal latency divided by distance), and the compound motor action potential amplitude. The motor nerve evoked response is a summated compound response called compound motor action potential (CMAP) amplitude. Factors that influence motor unit integrity such as neuropathy or myopathy will influence CMAP. The CMAP amplitude is calculated by measuring the amplitude of the evoked motor response from baseline to the negative peak.

The duration of the CMAP is reflective of the range of conduction velocities in the various axons in the nerve supplying a motor unit and the synchrony of contraction of the muscle fibers. Duration of the CMAP is calculated from the onset of response through the end of the positive deflection. A loss of synchrony (resulting from increased variation in axonal conduction velocity) will result in longer duration CMAP, known as a dispersed potential.

During the performance of the motor nerve conduction velocity study, an inherent delay at the neuromuscular junction occurs; therefore, the measurement of distal conduction velocity is not reliable and an intermediate conduction velocity is calculated between a distal and a more proximal stimulation. The area of the response, in

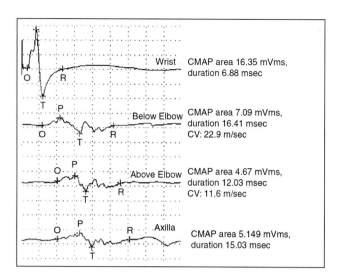

Figure 6   Conduction block. Motor nerve conductions in the ulnar nerve of a 53-year-old patient with chronic inflammatory demyelinating polyneuropathy. Note that the area of CMAP decreases by more than 50% between distal (wrist) and proximal (below elbow) stimulation without change in duration. O = onset; P = peak; T = trough; R = recovery; CV = conduction velocity.

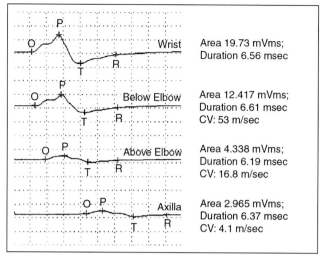

Figure 7   Contralateral ulnar nerve in the same patient as in Figure 6. CMAP shows change in both area and duration of more than 50% from baseline, suggestive of temporal dispersion. CV = conduction velocity.

Table 3   Factors Affecting Nerve Conduction

Temperature	Decrease in limb temperature prolongs distal latencies and slows conduction velocity Decrease in temperature increases amplitude of sensory nerve responses Warming up of extremities results in decrease neuromuscular junction transmission efficiency
Thickness of the myelin sheath	Decrease in myelin thickness results in prolonged distal latencies and slows conduction velocity
Age	At birth, conduction velocity in motor nerves is approximately one half of the adult value By age 1 year, conduction velocity is approximately two thirds of the adult value By age 3 to 4 years, conduction velocity is in the adult range Conduction velocity increases in children and parallels the increase in axonal size (maximal axonal size reached by age 5 years)
Length of the nerve	Latency is prolonged with increasing length; conduction velocity slows down with increasing length Latency is shorter and conduction velocity is faster in the proximal segment of the nerves, usually by 10% to 15%
Internodal distance	No clear relationship; changes in internodal distance may not have any effect on conduction velocity

Table 4   Normal Nerve Conduction Velocities in Different Age Groups

Age	Ulnar (range, in msec)	Median (range, in msec)	Peroneal (range, in msec)
0 to 1 week	32 (21-39)	29 (21-38)	29 (19-31)
1 week to 4 months	42 (27-53)	34 (22-42)	36 (23-53)
4 months to 1 year	49 (40-63)	40 (26-58)	48 (31-61)
1 to 3 years	59 (47-73)	50 (41-62)	54 (44-74)
3 to 8 years	66 (51-76)	58 (47-72)	57 (46-70)
8 to 16 years	68 (58-78)	64 (54-72)	57 (45-74)
Adults	63 (52-75)	63 (51-75)	56 (47-63)

to dispersion of the response. An example of normal motor nerve conduction is shown in **Figure 5**. The motor nerve conduction study of a patient with a chronic demyelinating neuropathy in which dispersion of the motor evoked response causes a drastic decrease in the area and increase in the duration of the response is shown in **Figure 6**. In the same patient a different motor nerve shows conduction block (a drop in the evoked motor response area without change in duration) but no dispersion (**Figure 7**). Both are signs of acquired demyelination. With inherited or uniform demyelination, conduction velocity is reduced in a symmetric manner. Even though latency will be prolonged and the conduction velocity slower, dispersion will not occur.

Each laboratory should define its own set of normative data for distal latency and conduction velocity because various factors influence these parameters (**Table 3**).

addition to the amplitude, helps to differentiate true loss of amplitude from apparent loss of amplitude secondary

Table 5   Pertinent Neurophysiologic Findings in Neuromuscular Disorders

Disease	Latency	Conduction Velocity	Amplitude of Response	F Waves	H Reflex
Axonal nerve	Normal*	Normal*	Decreased	Normal†	Decreased‡
Demyelinating nerve	Prolonged	Slow	Normal or decreased§	Prolonged or absent	Prolonged or absent
Muscle	Normal	Normal	Decreased	Normal	Normal or decreased‡
Neuromuscular junction	Normal	Normal	Normal or decreased‖	Normal	Normal

* In pure axonal disease, latency and conduction velocity should be normal. In severe axonal disease, some secondary demyelination invariably occurs, resulting in prolonged latency and slow conduction velocity.
† A few surviving axons are capable of generating an F-wave. In very severe axonal disease, F-waves may look normal.
‡ Because the efferent limb of the H-reflex is dependent on the integrity of the muscle from where the response is being recorded, H-reflex amplitude may be attenuated in severe axonal neurogenic or myogenic disorders. Latency of the reflex should remain normal.
§ Amplitude of motor or sensory response in demyelinating neuropathy may be decreased in the presence of (1) conduction block, (2) temporal dispersion of evoked response, and (3) secondary axonal damage.
‖ In neuromuscular junction disorders, routine nerve conduction may be normal and repetitive nerve stimulation at slow (3 Hz) or fast frequency (20 to 50 Hz) is usually required to demonstrate abnormalities. In botulism and in Lambert-Eaton myasthenic syndrome, both disorders of the presynaptic terminal at the neuromuscular junction, amplitude of the evoked motor nerve response may be decreased.

Table 4 shows the normal conduction velocity and distal latency in commonly tested nerves in adults.

Clinical Applications

Motor nerve conduction velocity studies provide objective measurements that characterize the severity of diffuse and focal disorders of peripheral nerves and can be used to identify and localize the sites of peripheral nerve damage from compression, ischemia, or other focal lesions. Focal nerve lesions can be characterized by conduction block with neurapraxia (weakness without atrophy), slowing of conduction velocity at a localized area, wallerian degeneration, and regeneration in the nerve.

Pertinent neurophysiologic findings in various neuromuscular disorders are shown in **Table 5**. The CMAP is reduced in lower motor neuron disorders, especially in lesions of the anterior horn cells and motor nerves, and in advanced stages of myopathy. In hysteria, malingering, or upper motor neuron disease, the CMAP is normal. CMAP assessment also is useful to measure neuromuscular junction transmission. In postsynaptic disorders of the neuromuscular junction, the CMAP deteriorates with repetitive nerve stimulation at slow or fast frequency because of failed or blocked transmission and loss of the safety threshold at the neuromuscular junction. In presynaptic diseases (such as botulism), repetitive nerve stimulation at fast frequency results in an incremental response in CMAP. This response is secondary to the activity-dependent release of the neurotransmitter, acetylcholine, which results in improvement of the CMAP.

Slowing of conduction velocity and prolongation of distal latency is characteristic of primary myelin disorders. Because secondary loss of myelin can occur in severe axonal disease, abnormal motor nerve conduction parameters should be carefully interpreted. In general, primary demyelination is characterized by normal CMAP, a conduction velocity less than 80% of the lower limit of normal, and a distal latency greater than 125% of the upper

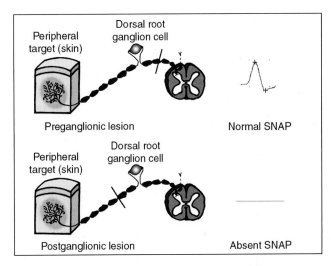

Figure 8   Sensory nerve action potential (SNAP) for preganglionic and postganglionic lesions.

limit of normal. In instances in which the CMAP amplitude is reduced (< 70% of the lower limit of normal), a more stringent criterion is recommended. A conduction velocity of less than 70% of the lower limit of normal and a distal latency greater than 150% of the upper limit of normal are required to support the diagnosis of a primary demyelinating disorder under conditions where CMAP amplitudes are reduced.

Sensory Nerve Conduction

One of the most important considerations in sensory nerve conduction studies is whether the defect is preganglionic or postganglionic. Ganglionic refers to the dorsal root ganglion, which is the primary sensory neuron. In postganglionic disorders, such as many brachial plexopathies, the continuity of the nerve with the dorsal root ganglion (the sensory neuron) is affected. The integrity of the nerve is challenged, resulting in abnormal sensory nerve

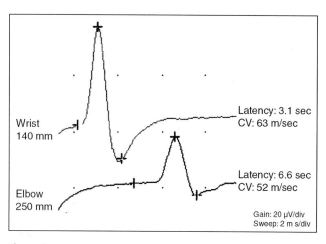

Figure 9 Examples of median nerve sensory potential recorded antidromically from the index finger with stimulation of the nerve at the wrist and elbow. CV = conduction velocity.

conduction velocity studies. In preganglionic lesions, such as a radiculopathy, prominent sensory symptoms occur without an alteration of sensory nerve conduction studies, secondary to the integrity of the sensory nerves and the connection with the dorsal root ganglia **(Figure 8)**. EDX is a useful tool to accurately localize the lesion.

Sensory nerve conduction velocity studies are performed by recording the sensory nerve action potential along the same nerve that is being stimulated **(Figure 9)**. As is the case with CMAP, sensory nerve action potential represents summated potentials of individual nerve fibers, and is usually more sensitive to both generalized and focal peripheral nerve disease than are motor nerve conduction studies. Sensory nerve conduction studies are technically more challenging because of the small size of the potentials and their susceptibility to extraneous artifacts. The variety of stimulating and recording techniques, especially digital averaging, have made it convenient to document reliable sensory potentials, even in the most challenging situations (such as intensive care units). Sensory nerve conduction also can be recorded antidromically (against the direction of the nerve impulses) or orthodromically (along the direction of the nerve impulses). It can be recorded with stimulation and recording from a purely cutaneous nerve, or may be recorded from a cutaneous nerve while stimulating a mixed nerve.

Latency, Amplitude, and Conduction Velocity
Secondary to the small magnitude of the response, it is often difficult to obtain a stable baseline measurement to determine onset latency. Even though the baseline measurement can be improved by using an averaging technique, most sensory nerve conduction velocity studies use peak-to-peak measurements (from initial negative to positive peaks) to estimate amplitude. It is advisable, especially in the absence of a stable baseline measurement, to

use an initial negative peak measurement for conduction velocity studies.

Most of the factors that influence motor nerve conductions may also influence sensory responses. Careful attention to these factors may improve the technical qualities of sensory studies. Deep tissue heating and warming is required to optimally correct temperature; most infrared lamps warm the skin and do not warm the deeper tissues, including nerves. Electrode placement and the type and quality of electrodes are equally important to obtain adequate sensory responses. Ring wire electrodes work well for the upper extremities, especially for digital nerves. Needle electrodes may be needed for deeper nerves.

Clinical Applications
Sensory nerve studies are generally more sensitive to nerve disorders than motor studies and can provide evidence for subclinical mononeuropathies and peripheral neuropathies. Sensory nerve conduction velocity studies are useful clinically to monitor toxicity from various medications, especially chemotherapy. Selective sensory fiber involvement may occur in paraneoplastic, toxic, and metabolic neuropathies. The major limitation of a conventional nerve conduction velocity study is its inability to adequately assess small fibers; these fibers are selectively involved in certain genetic, metabolic, and toxic neuropathies. In these instances, the study may show normal values despite the severity of sensory deficits.

Late Responses
Most of the information provided by motor and sensory nerve conduction velocity studies pertains to the distal nerve segments. It is difficult to directly evaluate nerve function in the proximal segments because of the difficulty with stimulation and recording. However, late responses provide useful information about these proximal nerve segments. Late responses are additional responses that occur with stimulation of motor nerves and follow the motor response (M-wave). F-waves, A-waves, and H-reflexes may be used to assess the peripheral nerves and spinal cord.

F-Waves
When motor nerves are supramaximally stimulated, in addition to orthodromic spread, action potentials also spread antidromically (centrally along motor axons toward the spinal cord) and generate motor units at the anterior horn cells. These motor units can be recorded at a defined latency after the M-wave (called F-waves) and can help to assess conduction in the proximal segments **(Figure 10)**. F-waves are most reliably recorded in median, ulnar, tibial, and sometimes peroneal motor nerves.

Latency, Amplitude, and Conduction Velocity
A minimum of 8 to 10 F-waves are recorded and minimum and maximum latency is measured. F-wave mini-

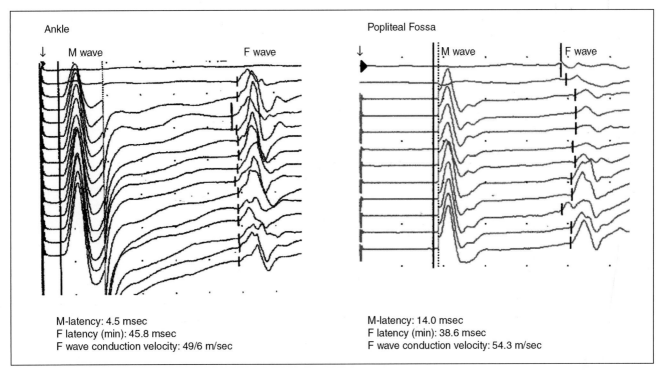

Ankle

↓   M wave   F wave

M-latency: 4.5 msec
F latency (min): 45.8 msec
F wave conduction velocity: 49/6 m/sec

Popliteal Fossa

↓   M wave   F wave

M-latency: 14.0 msec
F latency (min): 38.6 msec
F wave conduction velocity: 54.3 m/sec

Figure 10   Minimal F-wave latency recorded from the tibial nerve shortens with more proximal stimulation secondary to the decreased distance that the potential has to travel, whereas M-wave latency increases with more proximal stimulation.

mum latencies (and conduction velocities) are used to assess the function of the proximal nerves. For example, if F-wave latency is prolonged when distal conduction velocity is normal, slowing of conduction velocity along the proximal segment of the nerve compared with the distal segment is suggested. F-wave conduction velocity is a much more reliable measurement because it controls for the patient's height (distance covered by the stimulus) and peripheral conduction.

Clinical Applications

Peripheral nerve diseases usually produce F-waves with prolonged latency, and may produce normal peripheral conduction. If CMAPs are quite low, F-waves may be absent or may occur infrequently. If a few axons remain, F-wave variability is lost and a few large F-waves may repeatedly recur and will resemble A-waves. These repeated F-waves provide additional evidence of a severe, chronic neurogenic process.

F-waves are lost early in disorders that increase the excitatory threshold of peripheral nerves, such as demyelinating neuropathies. In Guillain-Barré syndrome, an acquired immune demyelinating neuropathy with predominantly proximal involvement, F-wave abnormalities are usually the earliest abnormality. Despite the severe loss of axons, F-waves may still be recorded in patients with Guillain-Barré syndrome in contrast to those with axonal neuropathies. The presence of F-waves helps to differentiate axonal neuropathies from demyelinating neuropathies.

A-Waves

A-waves (also known as axonal waves) are another late waveform occurring after the M-wave; latencies are generally between that of the M-wave and F-wave. A-waves also result from an antidromic action potential in the motor axon, but differ from F-waves in that they are mediated by peripheral or axonal backfiring by a collateral branch from the primary axon. Because A-waves are more constant than F-waves in occurrence and appearance, their presence often provides evidence of branched motor axons. A-waves can occur in normal individuals but are more common in patients with peripheral nerve disorders, especially demyelinating disorders.

H-Reflex

Unlike F-waves and A-waves, the H-reflex is a true reflex. It is a monosynaptic reflex response elicited by stimulation of Aα muscle spindle afferents that directly activate the neurons of anterior horn cells. Although similar to a tendon reflex, the H-reflex bypasses the muscle spindle. The difference between an H-reflex and an F-wave is shown in **Figure 11**.

Latency, Amplitude, and Conduction Velocity

In most adults, the H-reflex is recorded from the soleus muscle, using special stimulation requirements. Occasion-

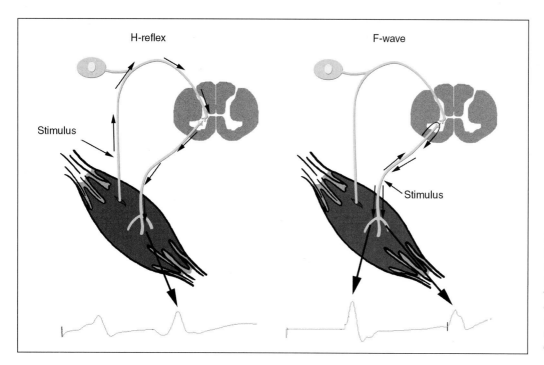

Figure 11 Unlike the H-reflex, which is a true reflex, the F-wave is propagated along only the motor fibers and occurs because of stimulation of one to three motor axons, which cause a late response.

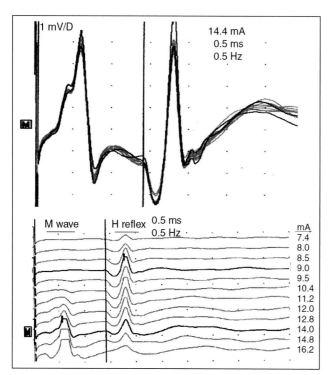

Figure 12 The H-reflex has both an afferent and an efferent limb. It behaves like sensory nerve conduction; with increasing intensity of the stimulus (shown in the right hand column of the lower figure), amplitude of the tibial nerve H-reflex becomes smaller, whereas the M-wave progressively becomes larger in amplitude.

ally in adults, the H-reflex also may be recorded from the flexor carpi radialis muscle. In infants and adults with hyperactive reflexes, the H-reflex may be recorded from most muscles. Because it is a late response, the H-reflex

follows the M-wave response. H-reflexes behave like sensory responses; with increasing stimuli, the H-reflex becomes smaller, whereas the M-wave progressively becomes larger (**Figure 12**). Unlike F-waves, H-reflexes are remarkably constant in latency and morphology; therefore, the onset latency of the H-reflex in an extremity can be reliably compared with that of the contralateral side. In tibial H-reflexes recorded from the soleus muscle, a difference of more than 1 msec between the right and left sides is considered abnormal.

Clinical Application

Because H-reflexes represent activation of a single root, these reflexes are helpful in more accurate localization of the proximal lesion. Loss of the tibial H-reflex represents dysfunction in the S1 root, whereas the loss of H-reflex from the flexor carpi radialis muscle represents dysfunction in the C7 root. The measurement of H-reflexes is less useful in patients with generalized large fiber sensory neuropathy. The primary application of H-reflex testing is to identify proximal slowing of sensory or motor axons in S1 and C7 radiculopathies in a select group of patients with normal sensory nerve conductions.

Electromyography

EMG records and analyzes the electrical activity generated in the motor units of the muscle when the muscle contracts or when muscle membranes are perturbed. Three forms of EMG are routinely used. Intramuscular needle EMG is the most commonly used clinical application. Single fiber EMG is used in highly specialized situations in clinical neurology, but has virtually no role in orthopaedic surgery. Surface EMG is mainly used for research.

Needle EMG examination is an essential component of EDX studies and is complementary to nerve conduction velocity studies. It is difficult to interpret nerve conduction velocity studies without the information from needle EMG examination and vice versa. EMG is needed to distinguish the various disorders of the lower motor neuron, such as anterior horn cell disorders from plexus disorders, or to distinguish peripheral neuropathy from radiculopathy. Based on specific information obtained from the needle EMG examination, an accurate distinction can be made between neurogenic and myogenic disorders. More importantly, needle EMG can be used to follow disease progression or to document reinnervation of a motor unit.

Needle EMG can be an uncomfortable test; therefore, it is important to be aware of the patient's medical history and to minimize patient discomfort. Needle EMG should be avoided in patients with coagulation disorders or extensive skin disease. If muscle biopsy is contemplated after the EMG examination, it should be done immediately after the needle EMG (within 6 hours) or should be done from a muscle not involved in the needle examination. The needle examination causes local inflammation and tissue damage that can be misinterpreted on histologic examinations.

The needle EMG examination involves multiple stages. The needle is first introduced into the muscle, which is used to evaluate insertional activity. The second phase involves assessment for abnormal spontaneous activity in the muscle. In the third phase, the needle remains in a resting position (supported but without movement) to detect fasciculations. The final stage requires assessment of volitional activity of the muscle, including motor unit potential (MUP) morphology, recruitment and interference frequencies, and firing rates.

The patient must be relaxed to adequately assess insertional activity and abnormal spontaneous activity. Evaluation of the volitional activity is dependent on the patient's cooperation and usually cannot be assessed in a comatose patient, children, and uncooperative adults.

Insertional Activity

As the needle is inserted into the muscle and passes through the muscle, it causes local depolarization of the muscle membrane and a local burst of activity that lasts for a finite period after cessation of needle movement (usually 300 to 500 msec, depending on the type of needle electrode used). Prolonged activity of more than 500 msec is considered abnormal and suggests either muscle membrane injury (denervation) or instability (myotonias). In contrast, reduced activity of less than 300 msec is suggestive of a qualitative change in muscle, such as replacement with adipose or fibrous tissue, and usually occurs in muscle with end-stage disease.

Spontaneous Activity

Spontaneous activity in the muscle is assessed by small but repeated movements in different planes of the muscle.

With each movement, the muscle membrane is depolarized; however, the electrical activity of the muscle does not continue beyond the movement of the needle. In resting healthy muscle, EMG activity usually cannot be measured at rest except at motor end-plate regions where two types of end-plate activity can be identified. End-plate noise represents nonpropagated end-plate depolarization (miniature end-plate potentials) caused by random release of transmitter from the major nerve terminals. End-plate spikes are nonpropagated single muscle fiber discharges caused by excitation in the intramuscular nerves.

Various abnormal spontaneous activities can be recorded in relaxed muscles; these activities are not related to end-plate activity and continue after insertional activity has ceased. These abnormal activities include fibrillation potentials (fibrillation and positive sharp waves), fasciculation potentials, myokymic discharges, myotonia, and complex repetitive discharges (**Table 6**). These potentials characterize various neuromuscular conditions (**Table 7**).

EMG Activity During Voluntary Movements

The MUP is the summated electrical activity of muscle fibers innervated by a single anterior horn cell in the region of the needle electrode (**Figure 13**). Only a small portion of the fibers in a motor unit are near the electrode; those at a distance contribute much less to the MUP. The firing pattern and appearance define MUPs. Those under voluntary control exhibit a characteristic semirhythmic firing pattern in which the firing rate is continuously changing by small amounts. The firing pattern of the MUP is described by the rate of discharge and recruitment. Recruitment can be characterized by the recruitment frequency (the frequency of firing of a unit when the next unit is recruited [begins to discharge]). This recruitment frequency is a function of the number of units capable of firing and is 7 to 12 Hz for motor units in a normal muscle during mild contraction. Recruitment also may be described by the ratio of the rate of firing of the individual motor units to the number of units that are active. Recruitment frequency decreases in neurogenic diseases, whereas firing rate is increased to compensate for reduced recruitment.

MUPs are described by specific measurements including duration, amplitude, number of phases (the number of times the response crosses the baseline), and rise time (the rate of rise of the fast component). These specific measurements vary with several physiologic, histologic, and technical factors including location of the muscle (small distal muscles tend to have larger amplitudes compared with more intermediate or proximal muscles), fiber density, the state of muscle innervation, and type of recording electrodes (concentric needle electrodes record smaller, fewer polyphasic potentials compared with monopolar needle electrodes, which record larger, more polyphasic potentials).

Table 6   Types of Abnormal Spontaneous Activity That Occurs on EMG Examination

Fibrillation potentials	Action potential of single muscle fibers twitching spontaneously in the absence of innervation Typically biphasic or triphasic brief spike (1 to 5 msec in duration and 20 to 200 μV) Can also present as positive sharp waves (biphasic, long duration) Occurs predominantly in neurogenic conditions; develops 1 to 3 weeks following denervation May occur in myopathic conditions; related to destruction of intramuscular nerves
Myotonia	Action potential of muscle fibers firing spontaneously in a prolonged manner after external excitation Characteristically waxing and waning in amplitude and in frequency Caused by prolonged muscle membrane depolarization Occurs only in myopathic disorders
Fasciculation potentials	Random discharge of a motor unit Typically random, often single (doublets and triplets may occur) Vary tremendously in amplitude, morphology, and rate of discharge Can occur in normal individuals When pathologic, signifies acute denervation Occurs in motor neuron disease and acute root disorders
Myokymic discharges	Fine, undulation movement related to spontaneous muscle potentials Appearance of normal motor unit potential, fired with a fixed pattern and rhythm Occur in bursts of 2 to 10 potentials firing at 40 to 60 Hz with a burst frequency of 0.1 to 10 Hz Occur in neurogenic conditions
Complex repetitive discharges	Bizarre high frequency discharges that start abruptly and end abruptly Occur through ephaptic activation of adjacent muscle fibers or split fibers Can abruptly change morphology but have uniform frequency (2 to 40 Hz) Can occur in both myogenic and neurogenic disorders

Table 7   Diseases Characterized by Fibrillation Potentials

Neurogenic Disorders
Anterior horn cell disorders
Polyradiculopathies
Radiculopathies
Plexopathies
Peripheral neuropathies, especially axonal
Mononeuropathies

Myogenic Disorders
Myositis (including polymyositis and dermatomyositis)
Duchenne and Becker's muscular dystrophy
Myotonic myopathies
Critical care myopathy
Rhabdomyolysis
Metabolic myopathies, especially acid-maltase disease
Periodic paralyses
Muscle trauma

Muscle Diseases Associated With Myotonic Discharges
Myotonic dystrophy
Myotonia congenita
Schwartz-Jampel syndrome
Periodic paralyses
Polymyositis
Acid maltase disease

Disorders Associated With Fasciculation Potentials
Normal
Benign (fatigue)
Benign with cramps
Metabolic Disorders
Tetany
Thyrotoxicosis
Anticholinesterase medication
Lower Motor Neuron Diseases
Amyotrophic lateral sclerosis
Root compression
Peripheral neuropathy

Abnormal Voluntary Motor Unit Potentials

Abnormalities in voluntary MUPs may manifest as abnormalities in morphology (short-duration MUPs or long-duration MUPs) or in recruitment patterns. Polyphasic MUPs may occur. Single potentials that have a mean duration less than the normal range are called short-duration potentials and are commonly low in amplitude (small amplitude). Short-duration potentials often manifest rapid (early) recruitment with minimal effort but may have reduced recruitment, normal amplitude, or both. Although short-duration MUPs commonly occur in primary muscle disorders, they may occur as nascent potentials (often accompanied by satellite potentials) in early reinnervation after nerve damage. Individual MUPs that have a mean duration greater than the normal range are called long-duration MUPs. Long-duration MUPs occur in neurogenic diseases that involve increased fiber density in a motor unit or loss of firing synchrony. Conditions associated with MUP abnormalities and changes that occur are shown in **Table 8** and **Figure 14**.

Abnormal recruitment patterns may also differentiate neurogenic disease from myopathic disease. Reduced recruitment occurs with any disease process that destroys axons or blocks their conduction, or that destroys a sufficient proportion of the muscle resulting in the loss of whole motor units. This pattern occurs in all neurogenic disorders, and may be the only abnormal finding in conduction block. In myopathy, early recruitment occurs with more

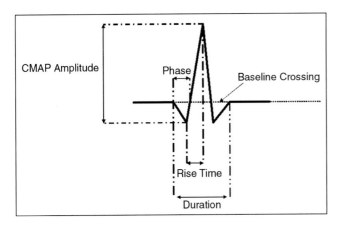

Figure 13   Characteristics of a MUP. The rise time is an important determinant of the quality of the MUP. Potentials with rise times greater than 500 msec are reflective of distant potentials and should not be used for qualitative and quantitative assessment of EMG potentials.

Table 8   Motor Unit Potential Morphologic Abnormalities

Disorders Associated With Short-Duration Motor Unit Potentials
Myasthenia gravis
Myasthenic syndrome
Early reinnervation after nerve damage
Late-stage neurogenic atrophy
Muscular dystrophies (all forms)
Myositis
Myopathies (most forms)

Disorders Associated With Long-Duration Motor Unit Potentials
Motor neuron diseases
Axonal neuropathies with reinnervation
Chronic radiculopathies
Chronic mononeuropathies
Reinnervation following a neuropathy
Chronic myositis

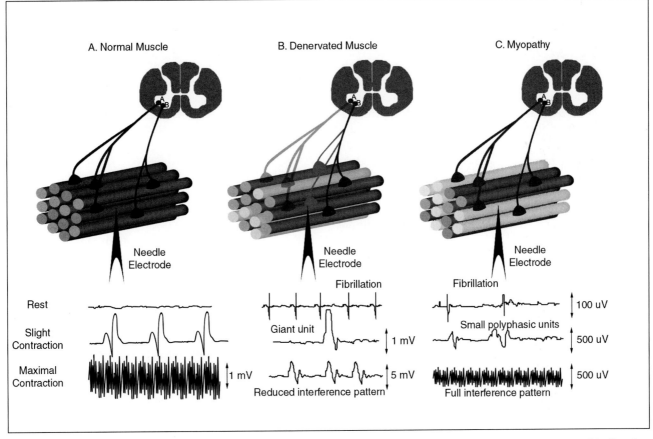

Figure 14   Characteristic EMG abnormalities in neuropathies compared with myopathies. Both neurogenic and myopathic disorders can result in abnormal spontaneous potentials such as fibrillation potentials. Neurogenic potentials show reduced recruitment, whereas myopathic potentials show early recruitment. MUP morphology in neuropathy depends on whether reinnervation has occurred; chronic neuropathies show large amplitude broad duration polyphasic potentials. Myopathies in general show short duration polyphasic potentials, often with small amplitudes. The Interference pattern is full myopathy, whereas it is invariably reduced in neuropathy.

motor units activated than would be expected for the force exerted. The rate of firing and recruitment frequency relative to the number of motor units is normal in myopathy.

Evaluation of Neuromuscular Disorders

Anterior Horn Cell Disorder

Poliomyelitis, although the archetypal anterior horn cell disorder, is now a rare disease. Currently, orthopaedic surgeons usually treat patients with continuing disabilities from past poliomyelitis infection or, in rare instances, those with postpolio syndrome. More recently, epidemics of West Nile virus-related poliomyelitis have occurred; this form of poliomyelitis is clinically indistinguishable from the traditional polio-related poliomyelitis virus and tends to affect elderly patients and those with chronic medical conditions.

The most common anterior horn cell disease in the United States is amyotrophic lateral sclerosis (ALS), also known as Lou Gehrig's disease. ALS is an uncommon but often fatal neurodegenerative disorder that is characterized by the presence of upper motor neuron signs (spasticity and exaggerated deep tendon reflexes) and lower motor neuron signs (flaccid weakness with muscle atrophy, fasciculations, and decreased deep tendon reflexes). Morbidity and mortality are caused by bulbar and respiratory muscle weakness along with the resultant dysphagia and respiratory failure. The diagnosis of ALS is clinically established and confirmed by neurophysiologic testing. EMG shows widespread acute and chronic denervation in the affected myotomes. In motor neuron disease, axial paraspinal muscles are often affected, especially thoracic paraspinal muscles (normally not affected by neurogenic changes related to degenerative changes in the spine). It is important to sample the thoracic paraspinal muscles. The differential diagnosis includes syringomyelia and severe cervical myelopathy; both of these conditions can manifest with upper and lower motor neuron signs.

Radiculopathy

In radiculopathy, root involvement is common, either from degenerative joint disease of the cervical and lumbar spines or from inflammatory lesions (such as Guillain-Barré syndrome or neoplastic meningitis). Radiculopathies can cause profound sensory or motor disturbances. Even though pain is prominent in root disorders related to disk disease, it is uncommon in Guillain-Barré syndrome, which is characterized by sensory symptoms and severe progressive muscle weakness. Sensory nerve conduction velocity studies are often normal in root disorders because these are preganglionic lesions. Radiculopathies are preganglionic lesions, whereas plexopathies are postganglionic and thus affect sensory nerve conduction velocity studies. Nerve conduction studies may be completely normal in radiculopathies unless severe motor

axon loss occurs. EMG abnormalities follow myotomal patterns.

Brachial Plexopathy

Involvement of the plexus can occur in traumatic lesions, from inflammatory causes (usually postviral), from neoplastic infiltration, or from radiation injury. Plexopathies produce very severe sensory and motor deficits; the nerve conduction studies are equally abnormal. Because the plexus represents a postganglionic segment of the sensory axon, sensory nerve conductions are abnormal in plexopathies. Needle EMG examination shows widespread denervation in multiple muscles spanning multiple nerves with no myotomal pattern. Axial paraspinal muscles are not involved, differentiating brachial plexopathy from severe radiculopathy. In radiation-induced plexopathy, myokymia (a rhythmic EMG discharge) is common.

Peripheral Neuropathy

Neuropathies may involve single nerves (mononeuropathy), multiple single nerves (multiple mononeuropathies), or multiple nerves in a confluent manner (polyneuropathy). Entrapment of a single nerve affects the motor and sensory fibers of that particular nerve. Carpal tunnel syndrome is the most common example of such a neuropathy. Often, the sensory fibers are initially affected with late motor involvement. Axonal loss occurs only with severe forms of nerve compression. In contrast, ulnar entrapments tend to have more motor manifestations, with sensory potentials often normal or unaffected.

Multiple mononeuropathies usually occur in peripheral nerve vasculitis. This pattern is important to recognize because nerve biopsy is often needed before treatment for immunosuppression is initiated. Polyneuropathies are common and may have multiple causes. Finding a treatable or readily reversible condition is often emphasized. Pathologic processes causing polyneuropathies include axonal or demyelinating conditions. Demyelinating neuropathies, if acquired, are usually immune in origin and have a better potential for treatment. Deficiency states (such as vitamin B_{12} deficiency or hypothyroidism), toxicity, or immune conditions should be evaluated in the workup for these neuropathies. Neurophysiologic studies play an important role in determining the underlying pathology and in providing a focus for the diagnostic workup.

Myopathy

Myopathies, like polyneuropathies, can have many causes. Patients are usually evaluated for evidence of inflammatory muscle disease or inherited muscular dystrophy because these conditions have high treatment potential or genetic implications. Patients with myopathies may also require orthopaedic or rehabilitative surgery. Needle EMG examination will differentiate myopathy from a pure motor axonal neuropathy and will show specific myopathic changes including short duration and small amplitude polyphasic potentials, which manifest the characteristic signs of early recruitment. Fibrillation potentials may be found in certain forms of myopathy, especially those associated with muscle fiber necrosis or membrane defects. Muscle creatine phosphokinase is often elevated in these conditions.

Axonal Regeneration

Multiple factors are involved with axonal regeneration. The axonal growth cone receives significant guidance from contact-mediated cues. Growth cones are oriented by diffusible chemotrophic molecules secreted by intermediate or final targets. Extracts of denervated muscle have increased neuron survival and promoted neurite extension in vitro. The distal stump of transected nerve releases substances that promote and direct regenerating axons. Selective adhesion also occurs between developing neurons and the glycoproteins L1, G4, neurofascin, and contactin. Inhibitory interactions occur between the growth cone and surrounding inhibitory molecules that restrict growth across a particular surface.

Without specificity of reinnervation, there is lack of functional recovery secondary to axonal misdirection. Mechanical alignment with surgery improves both contact recognition and neurotropic cues. Neurotropism describes the diffusion of factors released from distal targets that guide axons to their appropriate targets. Neurotrophism describes the random growth of axon growth cones; only the axons entering the correct pathway or target will receive trophic factors and continue to regenerate and subsequently myelinate. Although axonal regeneration occurs, the ensuing muscle alteration contributes to the lack of recovery because of a loss of motor fibers/units and the loss of the ability of muscle fiber to increase in size and reverse atrophy after reinnervation. Long-term denervation results in loss of muscle fibers and increased formation of connective tissue and scarring. Many surgeons consider performing early tendon transfers while the nerve is attempting to regenerate.

Nerve Repair

The objectives of surgical nerve repair are to maximize the number of axons regenerating across the injury site and to maximize the accuracy of reinnervation. Primary nerve repair, either immediate repair or repair within several hours of injury, is the treatment of choice if appropriate conditions are present. These conditions include a clean wound, a healthy tissue bed, the availability of a surgeon and appropriate surgical equipment and staff, and a physically and emotionally stable patient. Primary nerve repair is appropriate for patients with sharp nerve transection because crushed segments must be excised. In an open fracture, the nerve may be explored (for example,

radial nerve exploration with an open humeral fracture). A delayed primary repair is performed within 5 to 7 days and is most appropriate with avulsion or crush injuries in which the zone of injury is not clear at time of injury. These procedures may require nerve grafting. Secondary nerve repairs are performed more than 7 days after injury.

Commonly accepted principles of nerve repair include quantitative preoperative and postoperative clinical assessment of both motor and sensory systems. This assessment may be accomplished with evaluation of pinch/grip strength, static and moving two-point discrimination (innervation density), and measures of threshold vibration and pressure stimulus. Standard microsurgical techniques include the use of a microscope and loupes, microsurgical instruments, and appropriate sutures. An epineurial repair is usually performed for mixed sensory and motor fascicles when it is not possible to define the individual groups of fascicles. This repair is performed by identifying proximal and distal nerve ends in a bloodless field. Fascicular or vascular landmarks are identified with the epineurial sleeves joined to oppose the neural contents. After nerve ends are trimmed, an attempt is made to align the axons. The repair is performed with the first suture placed farthest from the surgeon and a second suture placed 180° from the first suture. Uniform tension is created with additional sutures placed sparingly. For most nerve repairs, 8-0, 9-0, or 10-0 sutures are recommended. When a particular fascicle is recognized as mediating a specific function, a surgeon may attempt a grouped fascicular repair. Higher magnification is needed for grouped fascicular repair because the nerve ends are inspected to determine the alignment of fascicles to allow matching, trimming, and repair of fascicular groups. It is rare to perform individual fascicular repair secondary to the extensive subsequent scarring that occurs. Direct muscular neurotization has been shown to produce limited recovery. The superiority of epineurial repair compared with group fascicular repair techniques has not been proved. The potential benefits of fascicular repair may be lost because of increased surgical manipulation and the repair of inappropriate fascicles; poor outcomes may result.

Fascicle matching techniques include intraoperative nerve stimulation whereby the proximal sensory and distal motor fascicles are identified. This technique requires patient cooperation and has achieved limited success. Histochemical identification is an alternative technique for fascicle matching. Acetylcholinesterase is present in the axoplasm of myelinated motor axons and many unmyelinated axons, but not in sensory axons. Carbonic anhydrase is present in myelin and the axoplasm of sensory axons. By performing immunohistochemical staining for these proteins, it may be possible to differentiate sensory and motor axons up to 9 days after injury. A limitation of this technique is the sacrifice of nerve tissue from the proximal and distal stumps. Histochemical identification also requires 1 to 2 hours of intraoperative processing;

however, patient cooperation is not needed. This technique has been most often used for late nerve reconstruction. Most of these techniques of fascicle identification are not routinely performed. Critical evaluation of surgical results has shown that the most important factor affecting recovery after nerve injury is the age of the patient. It is not known why younger patients will usually have a better functional outcome than adults with similar injuries. Other variables such as postoperative motor and sensory reeducation have achieved mixed results. The functional recovery of nerves injured by a gunshot wound is about 70%.

Nerve repair must be tension free. The current belief is that the ends of the peripheral nerve should be approximated with the use of two 8-0 sutures. If these sutures do not provide adequate immediate strength to retain nerve approximation, an interposition nerve graft is warranted if tension-free repair is not possible. Although changes in joint position are commonly used to reduce tension at the repair site, the extremity should be kept in neutral position when judging if an interpositional nerve graft is required. It is important to recognize the difference between a nerve gap and a nerve defect. A nerve gap is the distance between proximal and distal nerve ends, whereas a nerve defect reflects the actual amount of lost tissue and must be recognized before surgical repair. A nerve graft is performed when an end-to-end repair cannot be performed without undue tension across the nerve defect. The ideal graft should have large fascicles, little connective tissue, separate parallel fascicles, and a large diameter. It should include large-caliber axons, have an accessible location, little variability, and little branching. The functional outcome after a nerve graft will decrease as the length of the graft increases. Potential donor nerves include the sural, anterior branch of the medial antebrachial cutaneous, lateral antebrachial, and the terminal branch of the posterior interosseous nerves. The role of vascularized nerve grafts has not been established; however, potential indications for use of these grafts include large nerve gaps, very proximal injuries, compromised tissue beds (radiated tissue), and large caliber donor nerve grafts.

Because current surgical repair techniques achieve mixed outcomes and variable improvements in function, peripheral nerve tissue engineering may produce superior results compared with current standard techniques. Current alternatives include cadaveric nerve allografts, acellular allografts, and a variety of synthetic axonal/nerve guidance channels. The use of allografts are often limited by host immunogenic complications and currently do not appear to have significant potential for improved results compared with autografts. Although nerve guidance channels were initially made of nonbiodegradable materials such as silicone, the more recent versions are made of components of the nerve extracellular matrix and basal lamina such as laminin and fibronectin. To enhance neurotropic and neurotrophic support for regenerating axons,

the nerve growth channels have been coated with Schwann cells to provide nerve growth factor, brain-derived growth factor, and insulin-like growth factor-1. Further studies are needed to evaluate Schwann cell interaction with the components of the nerve growth channels within the dynamic mechanical nature of the host environment. Attempts to create the natural environment for growth cones with the implementation of innovative biodegradable scaffolding techniques may lead to superior results and offer better functional outcomes for patients. Although there are reports of increased rates of axonal regeneration across a gap when a nerve guide tube is used to bridge the gap, these axonal guidance channels are primarily used for gaps with digital nerve repairs, and further investigation is required prior to widespread use.

Summary

Nerve injuries continue to be difficult to treat, as functional recovery after neural injury has mixed results. It is important to recognize the different mechanisms of nerve injury that occur after acute and chronic insults as this shall influence treatment and expected outcomes. Just as radiographs provide objective data about bony pathology, electrophysiologic testing provides analogous data about nerve pathology. A combination of nerve conduction studies and electromyography is critical to fully appreciate the nature of a neural injury and the potential for recovery. A better appreciation of the mechanisms and biology of neural injury will help to improve the ability to treat these injuries in the future.

Selected Bibliography
Pathophysiology of Nerve Injury

Bodine S, Lieber R: Peripheral nerve physiology, anatomy, and pathology, in Buckwalter J, Einhorn T, Simon S (eds): *Orthopaedic Basic Science: Biology and Biomechanics of the Musculoskeletal System*, ed 2. Rosemont, IL, American Academy of Orthopaedic Surgeons, 2000, pp 617-682.

Chafik D, Bear D, Bui P, et al: Optimization of Schwann cell adhesion in response to shear stress in an in vitro model for peripheral nerve tissue engineering. *Tissue Eng* 2003;9:233-241.

Griffin JW, Drucker N, Gold BG, et al: Schwann cell proliferation and migration during paranodal demyelination. *J Neurosci* 1987;7:682-699.

Gupta R, Gray M, Chao T, Bear D, Modafferi E, Mozaffar T: Schwann cells upregulate vascular endothelial growth factor secondary to chronic nerve compression injury. *Muscle Nerve* 2005;31:452-460.

Gupta R, Lin YM, Bui P, Chao T, Preston C, Mozaffar T: Macrophage recruitment follows the pattern of inducible nitric oxide synthase expression in a model for carpal tunnel syndrome. *J Neurotrauma* 2003;20:671-680.

Gupta R, Rowshan K, Chao T, Mozaffar T, Steward O: Chronic nerve compression induces local demyelination and remyelination in a rat model of carpal tunnel syndrome. *Exp Neurol* 2004;187:500-508.

Gupta R, Steward O: Chronic nerve compression induces concurrent apoptosis and proliferation of Schwann cells. *J Comp Neurol* 2003;461:174-186.

Kandell E, Schwartz J, Jessell T: *Principles of Neural Science*. New York, NY, McGraw-Hill, 2000, p 1414.

Injury of Nerve Tissue
Sunderland S: *Nerve Injuries and Their Repair: A Critical Appraisal*. New York, NY, Churchill Livingstone, 1991.

Neurophysiologic Evaluation
Daube J: *Clinical Neurophysiology*. Philadelphia, PA, Lippincott Williams, 1998.

Kimura J: *Electrodiagnosis in Diseases of Nerve and Muscle: Principles and Practice*. New York, NY, Oxford University Press, 2001, p 991.

Sethi R, Thompson L: *Electromyographer's Handbook*. Boston, MA, Little Brown, 1989, p 199.

Evaluation of Neuromuscular Disorders
Dyck PJ, Thomas PK, Griffin JW, Low PA, Poduslo JF: *Peripheral Neuropathy*. Philadelphia, PA, WB Saunders, 1993, p 1721.

Axonal Regeneration
Stoll G, Muller HW: Nerve injury, axonal degeneration and neural regeneration: Basic insights. *Brain Pathol* 1999;9:313-325.

Nerve Repair
Kline D, Hudson A (eds): *Nerve Injuries: Operative Results for Major Nerve Injuries, Entrapments, and Tumors*. Philadelphia, PA, WB Saunders, 1995.

Lee SK, Wolfe SW: Peripheral nerve injury and repair. *J Am Acad Orthop Surg* 2000;8:243-252.

Index

Index

Fluoroquinolones, 316
fnb gene, 301
Focal adhesion kinase, 11, 16
Fondaparinux, 322
Foot, ligaments of, 289*f*
Force-velocity relationships, 234–235, 235*f*
Forces
    definition, 50–51
    moments, 51–52, 51*f*
Forearm, 54*f*, 118, 230*t*
Forging
    cobalt alloys, 74
    of metal alloys, 71
    solid metal, 72*f*
    titanium alloys, 75
Fracture hematomas, 334
Fractures
    fixation
        biomechanics of, 339–341
        external, 340–341
        plates, 65–66, 339–340
    healing, 333–337, 344–346
    inflammatory response, 334
    long bone, 111–112
    patterns of, 154
FRADA (frataxin) gene, 42
Fragile X syndrome, 41
Free-body diagrams, 52
    deltoid forces, 56–57
    glenohumeral joint, 53*f*
    hip abductor forces, 55–56, 56*f*
    spine forces, 57–58, 58*f*
Free radicals, 78, 78*f*, 302
Fretting corrosion, 66
Friedreich's ataxia, 41–42
Frizzled protein, 139
Frizzled receptor, 9
Frizzled-related proteins, 9, 403

G

G proteins, 7, 11
Gage lengths, 60
Gain-of-function mutations, 28, 419
Gait analysis, 52
Galvanic corrosion, 65–66, 73
Gamma radiation sterilization, 77–78
Gap junctions, 15, 142, 195
Gas plasma sterilization, 78
Gatifloxacin, 316
Gaucher's disease, 170*t*
GC boxes, 4
Gender
    ligament injuries and, 211
    osteoarthritis and, 398
    spinal motion and, 279
Gene Tests website, 26*t*
Gene therapy, 10
Genes. *See also* specific diseases; specific genes
    alternative splicing pathways, 4
    causing musculoskeletal abnormalities, 26*t*–27*t*
    expression, 3–5
    levels of regulation, 3
    organization of, 3–4
    osteoarthritis and, 398, 403
    promoters, 4
    repressible, 3

Geneticists, 43–44
Gentamicin, 316
Germline mutations, 18–19
Glasses, bioactive, 82
Glenohumeral joint, 53*f*
    biomechanics, 267–269
        humeral contact position, 268*f*
        rotation, 267*t*
        surface motion, 268
Glenoid, 268, 268*f*
GLI 3 gene disorders, 33–34
Gli receptor, 7
Glial cells, 247
Glial fibrillary protein, 247
Glucocorticoids, 326–327, 411
Glucosamine sulfate, 329, 352, 405
α-Glycerophosphate dehydrogenase (αGP) assay, 236, 238
Glycosaminoglycans (GAGs), 138, 164–165, 178, 181
GNAS1 gene, 34
Goldman-Hodgkin-Katz equation, 246
Golgi organs, 196–197
Golgi tendon organs, 256
Good Manufacturing Practices regulations, 69
Gracilis muscles, 228
Graded potentials, 246
Grafting. *See also* Allografts; Autografts
    bone substitutes, 341–344, 341*f*
    ligaments, 214–216
    nerves, 442
    tendons, 214–216
    whole tissue in, 354
Granulocytes, 407
Gray matter, spinal, 251
Greig cephalopolysyndactyly syndrome, 33
Growth arrest, 125
Growth factors. *See also* specific growth factors
    bone grafts and, 341–344
    calcium release and, 145
    in extracellular matrices, 138
    in fracture healing, 344
    musculoskeletal system, 5–9
    osteoblast differentiation and, 149*f*
    phosphoproteins in, 138
Growth hormone, 7
Growth hormone receptor, 119
Growth plates
    anatomy, 129–130
    biochemistry of, 117–118
    blood supply, 121
    cell proliferation in, 118
    chondrocytes, 15
    function, 117–118
    growth arrest, 125
    infections, 300
    injury classification of, 124, 124*f*
    mechanical loading and, 123–125
    physeal closure, 122
    premature closure, 124*f*
    structure, 117–118, 117*f*
    zones, 117–118, 117*f*
Guillain-Barré syndrome, 435
Guttmacher syndrome, 33

H

H-reflex, 436*f*
H-zone (sarcomere), 225

Haemophilus influenzae type B, 300, 302
Hamate, 272
Hampton's hump, 109
Hamstring muscles, 228
Hand
    anatomy, 275–279
    function, 275–279
    sphere of influence, 272*f*
Hand-foot genital syndrome, 33
Hands, mechanoreceptors, 253*f*
Haversian canals, 131, 131*f*, 133, 133*f*, 146
Healos, 343
Heat shock proteins, 39
Heberden's nodes, 397
HECT (homologous to E6AP carboxyl terminus) family, 6
Height, diurnal changes, 283
Helfet test, 286–287
Helix-turn-helix transcription factors, 5
Hematopoietic stem cells, 415
Hemiosteons, 133*f*, 146
Hemochromatosis, 170*t*
Hemodialysis, 421
Hemoglobinopathies, 333
Hemophilia, osteoarthritis in, 170*t*
Heparin, 109, 320–321, 321*t*, 411
Heparin-antithrombin III, 106*f*
Hepatitis B virus, 310–311, 341
Hepatitis C virus, 310–311, 341
Hereditary arthro-ophthalmopathy, 31
Hereditary motor sensory neuropathies, 39–40
Hereditary multiple exostoses, 19, 42
Hereditary spastic paraplegias, 38–39
Heuter-Volkman Law, 123–124
Hip, abductor forces, 55–56
Hip arthroplasty, 169
Hip dysplasia, 399
Hip fractures, 105
Hip joint
    anatomy, 283–284
    function, 283–284
    neck-shaft angle, 284*f*
    planes of motion, 284, 284*t*
Hirudin, 322
HLA-DR haplotypes, 10, 20, 406
Homan's sign, 107
Homeobox *(HOX)* genes, 33–34, 41, 116
Homeodomain transcription factors, 5
Homeostasis, definition, 350
Hormonal status, 398. *See also* Gender
Hot isostatic pressing, 71, 74
Howship's lacuna, 142, 145, 148, 415
HSP60 gene, 39
Human genome, size of, 3, 25
Human Genome Database (GDB) website, 26*t*
Human immunodeficiency virus (HIV), 309–311, 312*t*, 341
Human T cell lymphoma/lymphotrophic virus type-1 (HTLV-1), 309
Humeral head, forces on, 55*f*, 57*f*
Humeroulnar joint, 269–270
Humerus, rotations of, 55, 266, 267*f*, 268*f*
Humoral immunity, 302
Huntington's disease, 41
Hyalgan, 329
Hyaluronan, 164*f*, 183
Hyaluronan receptor family, 12
Hyaluronic acid
    for arthritis, 329–330
    in cartilage injuries, 352

chondrocyte content, 401
    in ligament scar formation, 212
    in meniscal healing, 183
    in osteoarthritis therapy, 405
Hyaluronidase, 302
Hydrocortisone, 326
Hydrogels, biodegradable, 79
Hydroxyapatite (HA)
    in bone, 136
    CD44 and, 409
    cements, 82
    depolymerization of, 408
    implant coating with, 82, 367
Hydroxyproline, 147
Hypercoagulability, 106–107, 332
Hyperparathyroidism, 421–422
Hypertrophic arthritis. *See* Osteoarthritis
Hypertrophic cartilage, 337
Hypochondroplasia, 28, 29*f*
Hypophosphatemia, 123, 420, 422
Hypophosphatemic rickets, 34–35, 123
Hypothesis testing
    description, 92–93
    errors in, 93–94, 94*t*, 98
    statistical issues, 92–97
Hypoxemia, 108
Hysteresis, 68, 196

I

I-band (sarcomere), 225, 226*f*
I-κB kinases (IKKs), 371
Idraparinux, 322
imatinib, 387
IMMIX extenders, 343
Immobilization, tendon, 202*f*, 203
Immune responses
    adaptive, 302
    to metal ions, 372–373
    to osteomyelitis, 302
    process of, 21*f*
    rheumatoid arthritis and, 406–407
Immune system, innate, 407–408
Immunobiology, 20–22
Impedance plethysmography, 108
Implants
    biologic responses to, 365–377
    cell-coated, 367
    coatings, 82
    corrosion modes, 65–66
    corundum-blasted, 367
    fatigue in, 67
    fixation, 365–366
    as foreign bodies, 368
    metal ion release, 372–373
    osteointegration, 365–367
Indian hedgehog *(Ihh)* gene, 334
    cartilage development and, 8*f*
    expression of, 338
    in extracellular matrices, 338
    musculoskeletal system, 7
    suppression, 7
Indian hedgehog (Ihh) protein, 7, 118–119
Inductive coupling (IC), 345
Infections
    in orthopaedics, 299–314
    pathogenesis, 299–300

Multidrug resistance (*MDR*) genes, 19, 386–387
Multipennate muscles, 227
Multiple epiphyseal dysplasia, 30, 32
Muscle spindles, 200, 256, 256*f*
Muscles. *See also* Skeletal muscle
    fiber length, 231*f*
    fiber types, 254*t*
Musculoskeletal system
    abnormalities in, 26*t*–27*t*
    anisotropic behaviors, 68
    cell-matrix interactions, 11–12
    cytokines, 9–11
    fibroblast growth factors in, 8
    growth factors, 5–9
    immunobiology of, 20–22
    Indian hedgehog protein, 7
    insulin-like growth factors in, 7–8
    transcription factors, 3–5
    tumors of, 382–386, 383*f*
    VEGF in, 8–9
    Wnt family proteins, 9
Mycobacterium sp., 302
    M. africanum, 307–309
    M. avium complex, 301*t*
    M. bovis, 301, 307–309
    M. tuberculosis, 301*t*, 307–309
Myelin
    debris, 427
    formation of, 248
    function, 248
    function of, 430
    membrane resistance and, 246
    structure of, 247
Myelin-associated glycoprotein, 247, 249
Myelin basic protein, 249
Myelin protein 0 gene, 39
Myo D, 5
Myofibrillar ATPase (MATPase) assay, 236–238, 237*f*
Myofibrils, 223–224
Myofilaments, 224–225
Myopathies, 439*f*, 440–441
Myosin, 233, 237*f*, 238
Myotome formation, 115
Myotonic dystrophy, 41–42
myotonin gene, 42
Myxoid chondrosarcomas, 19, 385
Myxoid liposarcomas, 19, 384

N

N-myc gene, 385
Nail-patella syndrome, 37*t*
National Health and Nutrition Examination Surveys (NHANESII and NHANESIII), 123
National Library of Medicine, 88
Navicular bone, 291
Necking phenomenon, 60
Neisseria gonorrhoeae, 300, 302
Neoadjuvant chemotherapy, 386
Neomycin, 316
Neonates, osteomyelitis in, 300, 303
Neoplasia, 18–19
Nernst equation, 246
Nerve conduction velocity studies, 430, 432*t*
Nerve fiber classification, 247–248, 248*f*
Nerve growth factor, 427

Nerves
    action potentials, 232
    conduction blocks, 432*f*
    crush injuries, 428*f*
    description, 245
    grafting, 442
    histology, 249*f*
    injury to, 428–429
        classification of, 428–429, 429*t*
        pathophysiology of, 427–428
    regeneration, 433, 441
    repair, 441–442
Neural cell adhesion molecules, 248
Neurapraxia, 429, 429*f*
β-Neuregulins, 248
Neurofibromatosis (NF), 42
Neurofibromin, 42
Neurofilament-light (*NF-L*) gene, 39
Neuroma formation, 429
Neuromuscular diseases. *See also* specific diseases
    fibrillation potentials and, 438*t*
    neurophysiologic evaluation, 430–440
    neurophysiologic findings, 433*t*
Neuronal apoptosis inhibitory protein, 41
Neurons. *See* Nerves
Neuropathic arthropathies, 170*t*
Neuropathies, 432, 439*f*
Neurotmesis, 429, 429*f*
Neurotransmitters, 247
Neutrophils, 407
Newton's laws, 52
Newtons (N), 50
NF genes, 18
Nickel
    in cobalt alloys, 74
    in steel alloys, 73
    toxicity of, 372
Niobium, 75
Nitric oxide, 169, 183
Nocardia sp., 302
Nociceptors, 253*t*
Nodes of Ranvier, 39, 247, 427
Noggin protein, 140
Noggin receptor, 338
Non-Hodgkin's lymphoma, 386
Nonparametric tests, 95–96
Nonsteroidal anti-inflammatory drugs (NSAIDs)
    adverse side effects, 351–352
    articular cartilage repair and, 351
    characterization, 327–328
    dosages, 328*t*
    in rheumatoid arthritis, 410
    side effects, 328
    before surgery, 411
Noradrenalin, 144
Norian Skeletal Repair System, 343
Normal distribution, 95, 95*f*
Normal stress, definition, 58
NTX, bone resorption and, 147
Nuclear factor kappa B (NFκB)
    control of, 5
    in inflammatory bone loss, 371
    osteoclast differentiation and, 148
    in osteolysis, 370
Nuclear factor kappa B (NFκB) gene, 248
Nucleus proprius, 252
Nucleus pulposus, 259

Index

Index